1/5
6/10

NEWCASTLE COLLEGE LIBRARY

02188988

WITHDRAWN

KU-479-873

NEWCASTLE COLLEGE LIBRARY

02188988

Dance Anatomy and Kinesiology

Karen Clippinger, MSPE

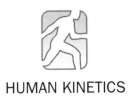

HUMAN KINETICS

Library of Congress Cataloging-in-Publication Data

Clippinger, Karen S.
   Dance anatomy and kinesiology / Karen Clippinger.
      p.   cm.
   Includes bibliographical references and index.
   ISBN-13: 978-0-88011-531-5 (hard cover)
   ISBN-10: 0-88011-531-9 (hard cover)
   1. Dance--Physiological aspects.   2. Dancing injuries--Prevention.   I. Title.
   RC1220.D35C55 2007
   617.1'02--dc22

                              2006012441

ISBN-10: 0-88011-531-9
ISBN-13: 978-0-88011-531-5

Copyright © 2007 by Karen Sue Clippinger

All rights reserved. Except for use in a review, the reproduction or utilization of this work in any form or by any electronic, mechanical, or other means, now known or hereafter invented, including xerography, photocopying, and recording, and in any information storage and retrieval system, is forbidden without the written permission of the publisher.

The Web addresses cited in this text were current as of July 2006, unless otherwise noted.

Acquisitions Editor: Judy Patterson Wright, PhD; **Developmental Editor:** Ray Vallese; **Assistant Editor:** Derek Campbell; **Copyeditor:** Joyce Sexton; **Proofreader**: Joanna Hatzopoulos Portman; **Indexer:** Marie Rizzo; **Permission Manager:** Carly Breeding; **Graphic Designer:** Bob Reuther; **Graphic Artist:** Kathleen Boudreau-Fuoss; **Cover Designer:** Robert Reuther; **Photographer (cover):** © Angela Sterling Photography; **Photographer (interior):** Karen Clippinger, unless otherwise noted; **Photo Editor:** Shawn Robertson; **Art Manager:** Kelly Hendren; **Illustrators:** Mario Zemann and D. Skip Clippinger, unless otherwise noted; figures 2.3 and 2.6 by Jason M. McAlexander, MFA; **Printer:** Sheridan Books

Title/chapter-opening page montage photos courtesy of Keith Ian Polakoff (top and bottom) and Patrick Van Osta (middle). Dancers, from top to bottom: Holly Clark, Jennifer Fitzgerald, and Dwayne Worthington.

Printed in the United States of America   10   9   8   7   6   5

The paper in this book is certified under a sustainable forestry program.

LIBRARY
NEWCASTLE COLLEGE
NEWCASTLE UPON TYNE

Class   617 · 102

BARCODE   02188988

Human Kinetics
Web site: www.HumanKinetics.com

United States: Human Kinetics, P.O. Box 5076, Champaign, IL 61825-5076
800-747-4457
email: humank@hkusa.com

Canada: Human Kinetics, 475 Devonshire Road Unit 100, Windsor, ON N8Y 2L5
800-465-7301 (in Canada only)
email: info@hkcanada.com

Europe: Human Kinetics, 107 Bradford Road, Stanningley, Leeds LS28 6AT, United Kingdom
+44 (0) 113 255 5665
email: hk@hkeurope.com

Australia: Human Kinetics, 57A Price Avenue, Lower Mitcham, South Australia 5062
08 8372 0999
e-mail: info@hkaustralia.com

New Zealand: Human Kinetics, Division of Sports Distributors NZ Ltd., P.O. Box 300 226 Albany,
North Shore City, Auckland
0064 9 448 1207
e-mail: info@humankinetics.co.nz

Dedicated to my parents, Delphine and Everett,
for instilling in me the love of learning;

my son, Shawn,
for keeping learning fresh and alive;

my many teachers and colleagues
for their generous sharing of their knowledge; and

dancers everywhere
for adding inspiration to my life.

Contents

Preface

Dance is physically demanding and involves many styles of movement. The vocabulary of dance requires tremendous versatility, strength, range of motion, balance, neuromuscular coordination, and kinesthetic awareness. To measure a successful performance is difficult. It is not simply a matter of how high a dancer jumps or how fast a dancer runs, but rather includes elusive qualities such as expressiveness, movement connectivity and phrasing, aesthetic demands for specific body segment positioning, dynamic versatility, and stage presence. This is to say that the dancer is an artist as well as a technician. However, the human body is still the instrument of expression, and some basic anatomical and biomechanical principles apply to optimal performance. Hence, this text has been written to provide scientific information that dancers can use to better understand their bodies and consequently reduce injury risk while they enhance longevity and performance.

This book emerged from the difficulty that I and many colleagues had in finding a single text that could be used to teach anatomy and kinesiology classes for dancers. Many dancers are visual learners and so often request texts that are rich in graphic materials. However, there was also the desire for the written material to be adequate in depth, as scientifically accurate as possible, and specific for dancers. This text has been developed to meet these criteria and to provide many practical exercises to allow dancers to apply the material on their own bodies.

Scope, Structure, and Organization

The focus of this book is dance movement, so selected aspects of the broader disciplines of anatomy and kinesiology that are most vital for developing an understanding of dance movement are included. For example, human anatomy is the science of the structure of the human body and traditionally covers all of the systems of the body. However, the scope of this text is narrowed to cover just the skeletal and muscular systems. Similarly, kinesiology can be considered the science of human motion and traditionally involves the study of the principles of anatomy and mechanics in relation to human movement. Even though the broader use of kinesiology includes anatomical principles, anatomy is listed separately in the title of this text because of the greater focus given to anatomy than seen in some kinesiology texts. Kinesiology is included in the title of this text because of the more applied focus and inclusion of aspects of mechanics that generally exceed the scope of traditional anatomy texts. Mechanics is a branch of physics concerned with energy and forces and their effect on bodies and motion. When mechanics is applied to the study of the anatomical structure and function of living organisms, such as human beings, it is called biomechanics. This text selectively includes aspects of biomechanics that relate to movements of joints, dance technique, and injury prevention.

Chapter Content

This book contains eight chapters. The first two chapters provide a foundation for the rest of the text by presenting anatomical and kinesiological concepts and terminology that are particularly relevant for dance and that are utilized in the remaining text. Chapter 1 covers bones, joints, body orientation terminology, and joint movement terminology. Chapter 2 focuses on muscle structure, levers, types of muscle contractions and their function in human movement, and an approach to learning muscle names and actions.

Chapters 3 through 7 deal with the various regions of the body. The first of these chapters (chapter 3) focuses on the spine because of its central structural and functional role in movement. The next three chapters (chapters 4 through 6) cover the lower extremity, moving proximally to distally from the hip to the knee and then to the ankle and foot. A single chapter (chapter 7) covers the upper extremity. The lower extremity is discussed first and in more detail because of the preponderance of injury in this area, the important use of the lower extremity for weight bearing and force generation in many dance forms, and the tendency to emphasize the spine and the lower extremity in dance anatomy and kinesiology courses due to time constraints.

Each of these five chapters addresses the primary bones, joints, muscles, alignment deviations, and mechanics for the given region, with special considerations for dance. Sample strength and flexibility exercises are also presented. These exercises are included to help the reader better understand the function and location of muscles as well as the purpose of classic strength or flexibility exercises for improving dance technique and helping prevent common injuries. In the final section of each of these chapters, common dance injuries for the given region are described. The purpose of these injury sections is not for self-diagnosis and self-treatment. Rather, they provide a better understanding of the anatomical basis of selected injuries so that teachers and dancers have a sound basis for evaluating risk, deciding on temporary modification, or designing sequential class progressions that will allow execution of dance repertoire with the desired aesthetic and lower injury risk. Through the material in the injury sections the dancer can be better informed when seeking treatment from a qualified medical professional should an injury occur.

The concluding chapter of this book provides a schema that will help readers analyze full-body dance movements. The purpose of this chapter is to present a tool that can be used to increase understanding of strength, flexibility, and technique issues that will influence optimal execution of a dance movement. This understanding will allow the dancer and dance instructor to be more specific in cueing and in the use of supplemental exercises so that dance performance is enhanced.

Special Elements

Various special elements appear throughout most chapters to provide practical applications of selected key concepts covered in the given chapter. Some of these special elements can easily be utilized in a lab format in academic settings. The special elements include the following:

- **Concept Demonstrations** select key concepts that are often difficult to grasp and provide movement experiences that the reader can perform to aid learning.
- **Tests and Measurements** provide examples of tests that are used for evaluation of areas such as ligamental injury, muscular strength, or flexibility. Although many of these tests require specialized training to perform and are not meant to be performed by the reader without such training, they have been included because they clearly illustrate the function or constraint provided by a given structure.
- **Dance Cues** reflect on the potential anatomical basis of some cues that are commonly used when teaching dance technique.

- **Attachments tables** provide the pronunciation, proximal attachment(s), distal attachment(s), and key action(s) of the primary muscles covered in this text. This special element is included in chapters 3 through 7, positioned closely to the picture and verbal description of the given muscle to aid the reader with deducing the line of pull and potential action(s) of the given muscle.
- **Study Questions and Applications** are designed to aid with learning the material presented in the chapter and with checking that key concepts are understood.

Dance Terminology

Throughout the text, dance movements are often described using terminology from ballet. This was done because of the greater standardization of this terminology. However, simplified versions of this terminology (e.g., front développé vs. développé devant) without reference to the facing of the body are used to make the information more accessible to dance medicine professionals and dancers from other dance forms, who often use ballet terminology less formally. But this common use of ballet terminology is not meant to limit the application of the information to ballet technique; dancers can make parallel applications to similar movements in the dance form of their choice.

How to Use This Book for Different Goals

Although the original impetus for this book was to provide a text for university courses, it is also intended for other dancers, for dance teachers, and for those who provide health care for dancers. Potential benefits for the teacher include a clearer picture of anatomical and kinesiological factors that will help the teacher better communicate technique challenges, a better understanding of what to look for in students to identify potential technique problems, and exercises that can be given to students to help them better achieve technical success. Potential benefits for the dancer include a better understanding of technique challenges such as proper turnout and alignment and a clearer understanding of individual strengths and weaknesses, as well as of ways to improve the areas of weakness. Potential benefits for health care providers include a better understanding of how injury prevention and treatment relate to dance technique.

In an attempt to meet the disparate needs of the potential readers just described, this book is designed to allow for different levels and emphasis as the book is used. For example, the student new to anatomy may focus on the illustrations and the summary charts of primary muscles and their functions while using the sections on strength exercises, flexibility exercises, and injuries only for reference. In contrast, the more knowledgeable reader may focus on details such as the secondary actions of muscles, implications of joint mechanics for technique and injury, and the many references provided for more in-depth study.

Similarly, in surveying colleagues teaching dance anatomy and kinesiology courses in academic settings, I found that courses were taught in many different ways. For example, some teachers gave little or no coverage to the upper extremity while others included a basic survey of the area. Some teachers included primarily anatomy, while others provided greater emphasis on injuries and mechanics and still others on corrective exercises and cueing. So, again, the book is designed with consistent headings within chapters in order to allow teachers to select the sections of the chapters they want to emphasize in their courses while leaving other sections as optional supplemental reading.

In summary, it is hoped that this book will become a valuable resource that can be used on different levels as knowledge and circumstances change. In the past, much of dance was taught by imitation of proficient dancers and teachers, with cueing often based on intuition and personally derived experiential assumptions. This text is designed to bring greater scientific knowledge and understanding to dance so that assumptions can be evaluated and honed to reflect an ideal blend of science and art. It is also designed to show the value of the scientific perspective so that as new research and knowledge evolve in dance, readers can have a framework within which to apply this information. Such a blend of science and art can allow teaching to become more effective and empower dancers to realize their unique individual potentials so that technical proficiency will less limit their artistic vision.

Acknowledgments

I would like to thank the many colleagues who have provided valuable input to this book, and especially Katherine Daniels (Cornish College of the Arts), Scott E. Brown (Sinai Hospital of Baltimore and Johns Hopkins University), Terese Freedman (Mount Holyoke College), and Ralph Rozenek (California State University, Long Beach), for their review of all or portions of this text. Deepest gratitude is expressed to D. Skip Clippinger and Mario Zemann for the countless hours they spent rendering illustrations for this book, essential for enriching and clarifying the theoretical concepts presented in this text. Sincere thanks are also expressed to Francia Russell (Director of Pacific Northwest Ballet School) for her long support of my work, particularly in the early years, and the pivotal role she and Pacific Northwest Ballet played in the evolution of my work with dancers.

I also greatly appreciate all the talented photographers who provided inspiring images of dancers in motion, as well as other individuals who contributed photographs or helped me acquire the photographs used in this text. Particular appreciation is expressed to Francia Russell and Lia Chiarelli for their assistance with photo acquisition of Pacific Northwest Ballet dancers and Angela Sterling (photographer for Pacific Northwest Ballet) for providing the photographs of Pacific Northwest Ballet dancers used on the cover, each chapter opening, and some chapter interiors. Gratitude is also expressed to photographers Keith Ian Polokoff and Patrick Van Osta for use of their photos in the montage at the opening of the book and each chapter, as well as their contribution of other photos used within chapter interiors. Appreciation is also expressed to Alonzo King's Lines Ballet and Robert Rosenwasser for their assistance with acquisition of photos.

I would also like to thank the dancers who are depicted in the photos and especially (1) the dancers of Pacific Northwest Ballet; (2) Maurya Kerr (currently dancing with Alonzo King's Lines Ballet) and Jennifer Owen (currently dancing with BalletMet Columbus) for use of photos demonstrating exercises and correct technique taken by me when they were students at Pacific Northwest Ballet School; and (3) Jennifer Fitzgerald (CSULB dancer), Merett Miller (Sacramento Ballet dancer), and Dwayne Worthington (CSULB MFA dancer) for modeling for strength, flexibility, and technique exercises. Appreciation is also expressed to Shawn Robertson for his assistance with editing and cataloging my photos.

Lastly, I would like to thank California State University, Long Beach and particularly Judy Allen (Dance Department Chair) and Donald Para (Dean, College of the Arts) for their support of this work, as well as the many individuals at Human Kinetics that helped to make this text become a reality.

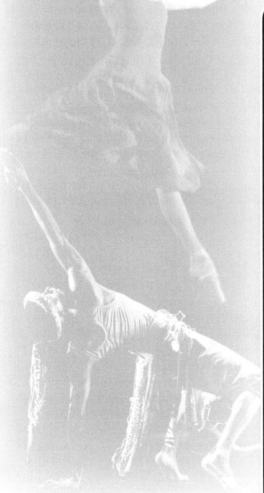

CHAPTER ONE

The Skeletal System and Its Movements

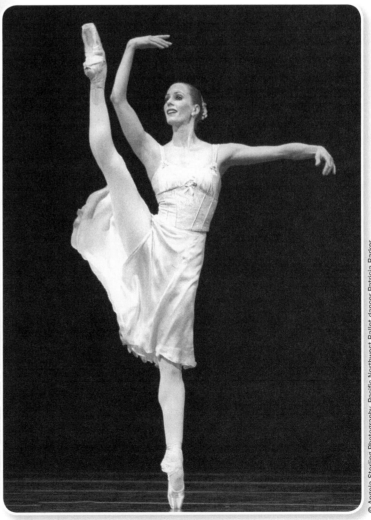

© Angela Sterling Photography. Pacific Northwest Ballet dancer Patricia Barker.

We start our discussion of dance anatomy and kinesiology in this book by looking at the skeletal system. The skeletal system provides the structural framework of the human body, and its joints permit the varied movements we explore in dance vocabulary. In movements such as the high kick shown in the photo on page 1, bones function in both their support and movement functions. The bones and associated joints of the gesture leg allow for the large movement occurring at the right hip, while those of the support leg are key for providing stability so that the dancer can remain upright despite a very small base of support. The support function of bones requires that they be strong, and understanding of bone remodeling is key for preventing loss in bone strength commonly seen in female dancers. The role of bones in joints is key for understanding and describing human movement. Topics covered in this chapter will include the following:

- Primary tissues of the body
- Bone composition and structure
- Bone development and growth
- The human skeleton
- Joint architecture
- Body orientation terminology
- Joint movement terminology
- Skeletal considerations in whole body movement

The concepts and terminology provided in this chapter will be utilized and applied in more depth in later chapters. Hence, this chapter can serve both as an introduction and as a reference for when this information is readdressed.

Primary Tissues of the Body

The body is composed of four different primary tissues, each with its own particular structure to help it carry out its required functions. These four primary tissues include muscle, nervous, epithelial, and connective tissues. **Muscle tissue** is characterized by its ability to contract and is found in the heart, in various organs (e.g., in the smooth muscle in the gastrointestinal tract), and in the many skeletal muscles of the body. **Nervous tissue** is composed of cells (neurons) that are able to generate and conduct electrical messages, as well as other cells (neuroglia) that help support these neurons. **Epithelial tissue** is composed of cells that fit closely together to form continuous sheets, or membranes, that cover and line surfaces of the body or form glands. **Connective tissues** generally function to bind, support, insulate, and protect structures and can be further divided into **connective tissue proper, cartilage, bone,** and **blood.**

While the first three types of tissues are composed mainly of cells, connective tissue is characterized by the presence of large quantities of nonliving material in the space between connective tissue cells (**extracellular matrix;** L. *extra,* outside of), which contains different fibers and other constituents that dictate its form and function. For example, bone has calcium salts within its extracellular matrix that provide it with the type of strength needed to support body weight. Some types of connective tissue proper have closely packed bundles of protein fibers (collagen), giving them the type of strength necessary for their function of binding bone to bone (ligaments) or muscles to bones (tendons). Blood, the atypical connective tissue, has plasma as its extracellular matrix; its fibers become apparent only during the process of blood clotting.

These primary tissues of the body can be grouped together into anatomical or functional units called **organs.** An organ is a structure that performs a specific function for the body and is composed of two to four of the primary tissues. Examples of organs are the heart and brain. Furthermore, organs that work closely together for a common purpose can be grouped according to a common function into **systems,** including the skeletal system, muscular system, and nervous system. The skeletal system will be addressed in this chapter, and the muscular system will be addressed in chapter 2. The **skeletal system** is composed of all of the bones of the body, related cartilages and ligaments, and the joints that connect these bones together.

Bone Composition and Structure

In the average individual, bone makes up about 15% to 20% of total body weight (Huwyler, 1999). Bone is characterized by its strength and rigidity, and it is one of the strongest connective tissues in the body. Unlike that of other tissues, the extracellular matrix of bone contains **calcium salts.** These minerals compose about 60% to 70% of bone weight (Hall, 1999; Rasch, 1989) and impart to bone its great **compressive** (L. *pressus,* to press together) strength, the ability to resist a force that would tend to push together or crush a bone. This extracellular matrix also contains **collagen fibers** (G. *koila,* glue + *gen,* producing).

Collagen imbues bone with its great **tensile** strength (the ability to resist a pulling force that would tend to pull a bone apart; L. *tensio,* to stretch) and flexibility. The composition of bone can be compared to that of reinforced concrete, with the collagen playing the role of the steel and the calcium crystals serving the role of the sand and rock. The compression strength of bone is actually greater than that of reinforced concrete (Guyton, 1976), and the tensile strength of very dense bone is estimated to be 230 times greater than that of muscle of a similar cross section (Rasch and Burke, 1978).

Functions of Bone

The composition of bone allows it to serve in the following key functions.

- Support: Bones provide an internal framework for the body that is essential for stability and form.
- Protection: Some bones protect fragile structures within. For example, the skull helps protect the brain; the rib cage, the heart and lungs; and the pelvic girdle, vital internal organs.
- Movement: Many bones serve as levers to enhance movement capabilities (see Muscles, Levers, and Rotary Motion in chapter 2 [p. 44] for more information). Having long levers in our body allows our limbs to move through a large distance, at a fast speed, or both.
- Blood cell production: Some bones contain tissue (red bone marrow) that is responsible for the production of red blood cells. Red blood cells are vital for the transport of oxygen and carbon dioxide.
- Mineral storage: Various important minerals such as calcium, phosphorus, and magnesium are stored within the bones. When necessary, hormones can stimulate release of some of these minerals into the blood for the body to use. These minerals are vital for important processes such as blood clotting, nerve transmission, muscle contraction, and energy metabolism.

Types of Bone

Bones come in a large variety of shapes and sizes. They can be classified according to their shape into the five types described next and illustrated in figure 1.1.

- **Long bones** are tubular in shape and much longer than they are wide. They are found in the limbs, where they serve as levers to enhance movement. For example, the "thigh" bone, or femur, is a long bone (figure 1.1). Other examples include the clavicles, humerus, radius, ulna, and metacarpals and phalanges of the upper limb or extremity and the tibia, fibula, and metatarsals and phalanges of the lower limb or extremity (figure 1.4). The long bones in the lower extremity are generally larger and stronger to meet their weight-bearing needs, while those in the upper extremity are generally smaller and lighter to meet their role in reaching and in manipulation of objects.

- **Short bones** are cubical in shape and are found in the upper portion of the hand (carpals; see figure 1.4) and feet (tarsals; see figures 1.1 and 1.4). These bones aid with shock absorption, transmission of forces, and small complex movements.

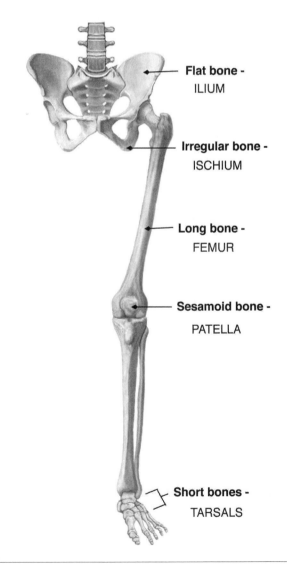

Flat bone -
ILIUM

Irregular bone -
ISCHIUM

Long bone -
FEMUR

Sesamoid bone -
PATELLA

Short bones -
TARSALS

FIGURE 1.1 Types of bones in the skeleton (anterior view).

• **Flat bones** are relatively thin and flat, but often slightly curved in shape. These bones commonly protect important soft underlying structures (such as the brain), and their shape also allows for extensive attachment of muscles. Examples include the upper portion of the pelvis (ilium) seen in figure 1.1 and the ribs, sternum, scapulae, and some of the bones of the skull shown in figure 1.4.

• **Irregular bones** do not fall into the preceding three classifications and exhibit complex and varied shapes. Their shape is adapted to special purposes; and they serve a variety of functions including protecting the spinal cord, supporting body weight, transmitting loads, providing sites for muscle attachment, and facilitating movement. Examples include the vertebrae and lower portions of the pelvis (ischium and pubis) shown in figures 1.1 and 1.4.

• **Sesamoid bones** (G. *sesamoeides,* like sesame) are bones that form within a tendon. They help protect the tendon from excessive wear due to rubbing against the underlying bone, and they change the angle of the tendon so that the muscle can produce more effective force. Examples include the "kneecap," or patella (figure 1.1), which is encased in the tendon of the quadriceps femoris, and two small bones within the tendon of the flexor hallucis brevis, located under the base of the big toe and discussed in chapter 6. Because these sesamoid bones are relatively flat, many texts include them in the class of "flat bones" just described, while other texts put them in a class of their own.

Structure of Bone

Bone does not have uniform composition. For example, the relative percentage of mineralization varies between bones, as well as within a given bone to help it better serve its functions. In general, bones have an outer layer of very dense bone called **compact bone** and an inner layer of less dense bone called spongy, trabecular, or **cancellous bone.** The compact bone provides strength and stiffness. Cancellous bone (L. a grating, lattice) contains many open spaces between thin processes of bone (trabeculae). These **trabeculae** (L. *trabs,* a beam) form a type of latticework that corresponds to the lines of stress occurring within the bone. This architecture provides bones with additional strength and shock-absorbing capacity, while allowing the bones to be much lighter than if they were composed solely of compact bone.

Structure of a Typical Long Bone

The compact bone, cancellous bone, and other structures present in a typical long bone are shown in figure 1.2. Learning these structures is key for understanding bone growth and health. The shaftlike part, called the **diaphysis** (G. a growing between), has thick walls of compact bone and a hollow cavity called the **medullary cavity** (L. marrow). The layer of compact bone thins toward the extremities of the long bone. The enlarged ends of the bones are called the **epiphyses** (G. *epi,* upon + *physis,* growth). These broadened epiphyses provide extensive area for muscle attachment. They also offer larger surface areas for articulation with adjacent bones, enhancing joint stability. The surfaces of the epiphyses that actually come in contact with opposing bones are covered with a thin layer of specialized connective tissue called **articular cartilage.** Articular cartilage helps lessen forces and allows joints to move more smoothly (see Synovial Joints on pp. 12 and 13 for more information). Rather than housing a hollow cavity, the epiphyses are filled with cancellous bone. The spaces of both the cancellous bone and the medullary cavity are filled with a soft, fatty substance called **bone marrow.** Some of this marrow (red marrow) is the type that is vital for making red blood cells.

In bone that is still growing, there is a plate of cartilage separating each epiphysis from the diaphysis.

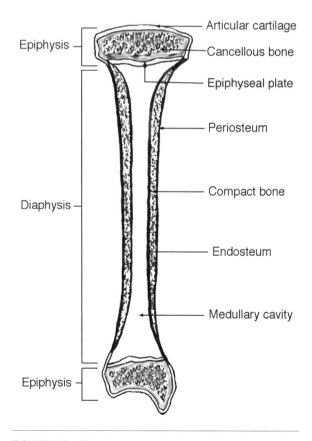

FIGURE 1.2   Structure of a typical long bone (longitudinal section).

This is termed the **epiphyseal plate** (G. *epi*, upon + *physis*, growth) or **"growth plate"** (see Bone Development and Growth for more information). In the adult these epiphyseal plates have been replaced with bone, and the diaphysis has fused with the epiphysis. The bone used in this fusion is very dense and is visible as an epiphyseal line on X rays.

With the exception of the portion of the epiphyses covered with articular cartilage, the whole outside of the bone is covered by a fibrous membrane called the **periosteum** (G. *peri*, around + *osteon*, bone). The inner layer of the periosteum contains cells that are capable of laying down new bone (osteoblasts). The periosteum is richly supplied with blood vessels, which are essential for bone nutrition. It also provides a site for attachment of muscles and ligaments to the bone. Muscles generally do not attach right into the bone; rather their connective tissue extensions, such as the tendon, attach to the periosteum, which in turn has small fibers that penetrate into the bone (Sharpey's fibers). The periosteum can be readily injured, and due to its abundant nerve supply may be responsible for much of the pain associated with shin splints, bone bruises, and fractures.

The **endosteum** (G. *endon*, within + *osteon*, bone) is a membrane lining the internal bone surfaces including the medullary cavity and the canals passing through the compact bone. Like the periosteum, it contains cells that can help with bone growth and repair. These cells, located in the endosteum and periosteum of growing bones, are particularly important for growth of bones in terms of girth versus length (see Bone Development and Growth for more information).

Structure of Other Types of Bones

Similar to long bones, the short bones, irregular bones, and flat bones have an outer layer of compact bone covered by periosteum. Underneath this layer of compact bone lies cancellous bone that is covered by endosteum. These types of bones are not cylindrical in shape and so have no epiphyses, diaphysis, or medullary cavity. However, they do contain bone marrow between their trabeculae. Some of the flat bones contain red marrow, the type of marrow capable of generating red blood cells.

Bone Development and Growth

During fetal development, specialized connective tissue (mesenchyme) can be directly turned into bone, termed **intramembranous ossification** (L. within a membrane; *os*, bone + *facia*, to make), but more commonly is turned into cartilage models of bones that are then mostly replaced with bone as the child develops. This latter type of ossification is termed **endochondral ossification** (G. *endon*, within + *chondros*, cartilage), and it is this type of ossification that is responsible for the increase in length of long bones. Endochondral ossification originates at a site near the center of the shaft of the cartilage model that is called the **primary ossification site.** This ossification begins at the end of the second month of intrauterine life (Hall-Craggs, 1985) and proceeds in both directions away from the center to form the diaphysis. Shortly before or after birth, one or more **secondary ossification centers** appear toward the extremities of the long bone, which ossify the epiphysis.

As growth proceeds, a plate of cartilage remains between the diaphysis and epiphyses: the epiphyseal plate or "growth plate" previously described. This epiphyseal plate maintains its thickness by balancing the growth of cartilage on its epiphyseal side with the replacement by bony tissue on its diaphyseal side. This process prevents fusion and allows growth in length of the bone to continue until the adult size of that particular bone is achieved. At this time, the production of new cartilage declines; the cartilaginous epiphyseal plates are replaced by bone; and the diaphysis fuses with the epiphyses. The "growth plates" are now considered "closed." This **closure of the epiphyseal plates** generally occurs progressively from puberty to maturity. Although there is much individual variability, most of the long bones of the limbs achieve closure between approximately age 15 and 25 (Goss, 1980); it occurs as much as four years earlier in a female than a male (Kreighbaum and Barthels, 1996).

In addition to growth in length, long bones also undergo remodeling and growth in circumference, termed **appositional growth.** The osteoblasts in the deep layer of the periosteum lay down new bone (intramembranous ossification), while cells in the endosteum (osteoclasts) resorb bone. This process allows the bone to grow "outward," increasing its girth while slightly expanding the medullary cavity to make a thicker and stronger bone while preventing the bone from becoming too heavy. Although this expansion in girth occurs at the greatest rate before maturity, it continues throughout adulthood. A summary of this growth of long bones in circumference and length appears in figure 1.3.

Bone Remodeling

In addition to growing in length and width, bone is also continually remodeling. Approximately 5% to

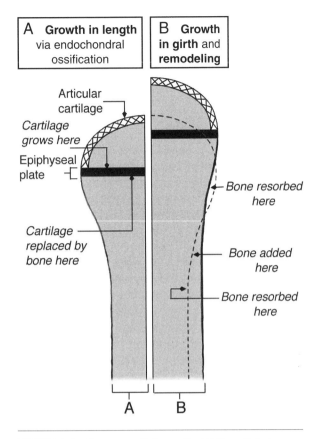

A Growth in length via endochondral ossification	B Growth in girth and remodeling

FIGURE 1.3   Bone growth in youth. (A) Growth in bone length via endochondral ossification; (B) growth in bone girth via appositional growth and maintenance of proportions via remodeling.

7% of our bone mass is recycled in a week, and as much as a half a gram of calcium can enter or leave the adult skeleton in a single day (Marieb, 1995). So, although bone is very hard, it is very alive and is continually changing in response to many factors including the mechanical stresses to which it is exposed. This relationship of stress to bone development was actually expressed a long time ago (in 1892) by Julius Wolff. **Wolff's law** holds that changes in the internal architecture of bone and the external conformation of bone will occur in accordance with mathematical laws and in response to the forces acting on bones. The primary forces acting on bones are believed to relate to the contraction of muscles and the loading of bones in weight-bearing activities.

It appears that the longitudinal stresses (compression) related to weight bearing are particularly potent for instigating bone deposition and may be due to the **piezoelectric effect** (G. *piez* , to press + electricity). In the 1950s it was shown that when bone is placed under stress, an electrical gradient is generated. The side of the bone under compression becomes electronegative while the side under ten-

sion becomes electropositive, creating an electrical potential that appears to stimulate bone deposition (Enoka, 2002; Mercier, 1995). Although Wolff's law has gone through some modifications in more recent years to include additional factors, the concept is still germane. Healthy bones remodel in response to mechanical demands; they lay down new bone where needed and resorb bone where it is not needed.

With Wolff's law in mind, it is not surprising that bone density is very much influenced by activity. The mechanical stresses associated with walking, running, and dancing provide an important stimulus to encourage maintenance of healthy bone density, and bone density has been shown to be differentially increased in relation to the associated stresses of those activities. For example, some runners may show increased bone density in the lower leg bones; tennis players may show increased bone density of the arm bones on their dominant side; and ballet dancers may show thickening of the shaft of the second metatarsal bone of the foot.

Although the most potent effect on bone density appears to relate to high-impact weight-bearing physical activity, forceful muscle contractions without weight bearing can also positively influence bone density; and greater bone density has also been shown to be associated with stronger muscles and greater muscle mass (Andreoli et al., 2001; Frost, 2000; Stewart and Hannan, 2000). Conversely, even young children who are hospitalized, individuals of any age whose limbs are immobilized in casts, and healthy young individuals involved in space flight (Hall, 1999; Roy, Baldwin, and Edgerton, 1996; Zernicke, Vailas, and Salem, 1990) experience loss of bone density (osteopenia) that can lead to gross structural weakening of bones (increased porosity in bone termed **osteoporosis**), probably due to inadequate forces borne by bone. For example, bed rest of four to six weeks can result in significant bone density losses that are not fully reversed with six months of normal weight-bearing activity; and astronauts may lose up to 19% of their weight-bearing bone on extended missions.

Bone remodeling and density are also influenced by race, age, calcium availability, hormones, and gender. For example, in terms of ethnicity, African Americans tend to have greater bone density than Caucasians, which is conjectured to be linked to greater muscle mass in African Americans (Burr, 1997; Hall, 1999). In terms of age, bone deposition outweighs bone resorption in healthy children, resulting in net growth in bones. In younger adults, bone resorption and bone deposition proceed at similar rates. In older adults, bone resorption predominates, resulting in loss in bone density and osteoporosis. However, for normal bone growth to proceed in children, and for normal peak mineral mass to develop in young adulthood, adequate dietary intake of calcium and other nutrients is essential. Furthermore, even if there is adequate calcium available and normal peak bone density is achieved, osteoporosis develops earlier, tends to be more severe, and is four times more common in women than men (Dudek, 1997). In terms of gender, adult females generally begin with about 30% less bone mass than men (Rasch, 1989), start decreasing bone density at an earlier age, and lose bone at a greater rate than males. Osteoporosis affects approximately 40% of women after the age of 50 (Hall, 1999); and in elderly females, spinal bone density is often 40% of that at 20 years of age (Abernethy et al., 2005). At age 80, women have one chance in five (Kenney, 1982) of sustaining a fracture of the hip (neck of the femur), and osteoporosis-related fractures and associated complications are among the leading causes of death in the elderly population (Hall, 1999).

Unfortunately, this vulnerability of women to osteoporosis is of particular concern to dancers, and not just in later life. Although moderate activity has been shown to increase bone density, strenuous physical training combined with other factors still under investigation, such as low energy availability, extremely low percentage body fat, or failing to menstruate normally, can result in loss of bone density rather than a gain in bone density (Myszkewycz and Koutedakis, 1998; Williams, 1998). Estrogen appears to be protective for bone density, and so dancers who are low in estrogen production or not menstruating (athletic amenorrhea) would be at risk for lower bone density. This risk for early bone loss is heightened by the common tendency for dancers to smoke cigarettes and ingest large quantities of caffeinated beverages, including soft drinks (Clippinger, 1999). This loss of bone density, part of the female athlete triad (American College of Sports Medicine, 1997), can occur with dancers as young as in their teens, resulting in losses in bone density normally not seen until after the fifth decade and markedly increasing susceptibility to stress fractures (Khan et al., 1999). Some of this loss in bone density may be irreversible, and loss of bone density in young dancers is particularly concerning when one realizes that approximately 50% of bone mineralization and 15% of adult height are normally established during the teenage years (Hall, 1999).

Hence, dancers should be particularly conscientious about eating a nutrient-dense diet with adequate caloric and calcium content. Recommended daily calcium intakes vary, according to source, gender, and age, between 800 and 1,500 milligrams; and a 1994 National Institutes of Health consensus panel recommends 1,200 to 1,500 milligrams daily for young adults between the ages of 11 and 24 years (Beck and Shoemaker, 2000; Clark, 1997). One of the easiest ways to obtain adequate levels of calcium is to regularly ingest three or four servings of milk products per day. Any of the following foods provides about 300 milligrams of calcium: 8 ounces

TESTS AND MEASUREMENTS 1.1

Measurement of Bone Density

Various tests can be used for detecting osteoporosis through the measurement of bone density. In the 1940s, plain X rays were used (Kaufman, 2000). However, since demineralization of bone is not apparent until about 40% of the bone has been lost, other methods have been developed that are more sensitive and can detect changes at a much earlier stage. One of the more precise tests currently used is termed dual-energy X-ray absorptiometry (DXA). This method uses X-ray beams that have two distinct energy peaks—one that will be absorbed more by soft tissue and the other by bone. This allows for the soft tissue component to be subtracted and the bone mineral density to be determined. However, many other tests are also available, some of which are less expensive and more accessible. In dancers, testing of multiple sites is often recommended, as results from various sites may differ (Khan et al., 1996). For example, due to the frequent loading of the lower extremity associated with dancing, the bone density in the femur might appear normal while a site in the upper extremity may be low. Dancers who have amenorrhea or have other reason for concern should discuss with their attending physicians what their concerns are, whether testing is indicated, and what test would be best for them.

(0.2 liters) of milk, 1 cup of yogurt, or 1 ounce (28 grams) of Swiss cheese. So one can easily achieve 1,200 milligrams of calcium by having four of such dairy options or three dairy options plus other selections that add up to the needed additional 300 milligrams (see table 1.1). To foster goals of staying lean, low or nonfat varieties of these dairy products can be selected (for more specific recommendations, see Nancy Clark's *Sports Nutrition Guidebook* [1997]). For dancers who cannot tolerate or do not like dairy products, one can see from looking at table 1.1 that it is difficult to meet recommended values. In such cases, consultation with a nutritionist and discussion of supplementation with the dancer's physician are recommended.

Stress Fractures

While exercise usually serves as a stimulus for increasing bone density, there are times when the breakdown of bone exceeds the repair and remodeling of bone and a stress fracture occurs. A **stress fracture** is a microscopic fracturing of the bone resulting in a thin crack that is so small, it is not even initially apparent on an X ray. When a bone undergoes excessive repetitive submaximal stress, it responds with increased osteoclast activity. These osteoclasts resorb bone as the first step before laying down a stronger new matrix. In the process, they temporarily leave the bone weaker. If stress is too great, the outer portion of the bone (cortex) may crack, creating a stress fracture.

Theoretically, stress fracture risk can be increased by factors that negatively impact bone health, and so all of the factors just discussed relating to bone density, including being female, a history of menstrual disturbance, less lean mass in the lower limb, inadequate calcium intake, a low-fat diet, and smoking, can heighten stress fracture risk (Bennell et al., 1996; Clarkson, 1998; Hershman and Mailly, 1990; Taube and Wadsworth, 1993). Female athletes have been reported to have a 1.5 to 3.5 times

TABLE 1.1   Calcium Content of Selected Foods (Approximate)

	Serving size	Calcium content (mg)	Calories
Dairy products			
Low-fat yogurt			
Plain	1 cup	415	145
Fruit-flavored	1 cup	340	230
Ricotta cheese (part skim)	1/2 cup	335	170
Low-fat milk	1 cup	300	120
Swiss cheese	1 oz	270	105
Cheddar cheese	1 oz	205	110
American cheese	1 oz	175	105
Low-fat cottage cheese	1/2 cup	70	100
Cream cheese	2 tbsp	20	100
Protein foods			
Processed tofu with calcium sulfate	4 oz	145	70
Eggs	2 large	56	160
Cooked lentils	1 cup	50	210
Almonds	12-15	40	90
Peanut butter	2 tbsp	20	190
Hamburger patty	3 oz	10	200
Chicken	3 oz	10	140
Vegetables and fruits			
Collard greens	1/2 cup	180	30
Bok choy, cooked	1/2 cup	125	15
Broccoli	1/2 cup	70	20
Orange	1 medium	55	70
Green beans	1/2 cup	30	15
Orange juice	1 cup	27	110
Calcium fortified orange juice	1 cup	300	110
Mashed potatoes	1/2 cup	25	100
Carrots	1/2 cup	24	24
Lettuce	1/4 head	20	27
Apple	1 medium	10	80
Grains			
Whole-wheat bread	2 slices	40	130
Cooked rice	1/2 cup	10	80
Bagel (water)	1 3 in.	8	165

Sources: Clark (1997) and U.S. Department of Agriculture (1981).

greater risk of stress fractures than male athletes (Browning, 2001), and a study of ballet students found that young females had about twice the risk of developing stress fractures as young males and that this risk is further heightened during adolescence; 70% of the stress fractures in female dancers occurred during the late adolescent period of 15 to 19 years of age (Lundon, Melcher, and Bray, 1999). Furthermore, a study of female dancers found an older age of onset of menstruation (menarche), and the incidence of menstruation stopping (secondary amenorrhea) was twice as high among dancers with stress fractures as compared to dancers without stress fractures (Warren et al., 1986). Even more dramatic, another study of professional ballet dancers found a female dancer who had amenorrhea longer than 6 months had an estimated risk for stress fracture 93 times that of a dancer who did not have amenorrhea (Kadel, Teitz, and Kronmal, 1992).

Training errors, such as an increase in exercise intensity or duration that is too great, can also be important (Brukner, Bradshaw, and Bennell, 1998), and one study of runners with stress fractures found 27% of cases developed after rapid commencement of training (Taunton, Clement, and Webber, 1981). Another study of runners found training errors in 22.4% of 320 stress fractures (Matheson et al., 1987). Although not substantiated, in dance, a sudden increase in workload (especially pointe work or jumps); rapid changes in dance style, technique, or floor surfaces; and excessive fatigue may contribute to stress fracture risk. One study of professional ballet dancers showed a 16 times greater risk for those dancing more than 5 hours per day when compared with those dancing less than 5 hours (Kadel, Teitz, and Kronmal, 1992).

Stress fracture prevalence has been reported to be as high as 61% in professional ballet dancers (Warren et al., 1986), and further research will be necessary to understand the relative significance of the various causative factors in dancers. In the interim, current study results suggest that application of sound training principles, swift medical referral when amenorrhea is present, healthy nutritional practices including adequate calcium intake, and smoking cessation can aid in the prevention and treatment of stress fractures.

The Human Skeleton

There are 206 bones in the adult human skeleton, 177 that can engage in voluntary movement (Hamilton and Luttgens, 2002). The major bones of the skeleton are shown in figure 1.4.

The Axial and Appendicular Skeleton

The skeleton has two major divisions—the **axial skeleton** (L. relating to an axis) and the appendicular skeleton. As its name implies, the axial portion forms the central upright "axis" of the skeleton, and includes the skull, vertebral column, sternum, and ribs (figure 1.4A). The **skull** contains 28 bones, which form the face (facial bones) and remainder of the skull (cranial bones). This book will simplify this area and simply refer to the bones of the skull as a unit. The skull provides an essential protective function for the vulnerable brain and plays an important part in housing the senses of sight, smell, taste, and hearing. The **sternum** (commonly referred to as the breastbone; G. *sternon,* the chest) and the 12 ribs with their adjoining cartilages help form the **thorax,** which provides important protection for the lungs and heart. Thirty-three **vertebrae** form the **vertebral column** (commonly referred to as the spine). The segmented property of the spine allows it to be flexible and capable of a wide variety of movements. Consecutive vertebrae form a canal that houses and protects the very important and fragile spinal cord.

The **appendicular skeleton** is composed of the bones of the limbs (appendages), which are hung upon or attached to the axial skeleton as seen in figure 1.4B. The appendicular skeleton contains two additional subdivisions, the paired upper extremity and the paired lower extremity. The **upper extremity** is composed of the bones of the **shoulder girdle,** upper arm, lower arm, wrist, and hand. The shoulder girdle consists of the paired **clavicles** (commonly called collarbones) and **scapulae** (L. the shoulder blades). The upper arm bone is called the **humerus** (L. shoulder), while bones of the lower arm are the **radius** (on the thumb side; L. rod, ray) and **ulna** (L. arm). The upper part of the hand contains two rows of small bones called the **carpals** (eight bones); followed by five rays of bone found in the "palm" of the hand, called the **metacarpals;** and the 14 digits of the fingers called the **phalanges.**

The **lower extremity** is composed of the bones of the pelvic girdle, thigh, lower leg, and the ankle-foot. The **pelvic girdle** is composed of two paired hip bones called os innominatum or **os coxae** that connect to each other in the front and to the sacrum behind. In the young child, each os coxae is made up of three separate bones: the **ilium** (upper wing-like portion of the pelvis), **ischium** (lower portion), and **pubis** (front portion). These bones later fuse together. The thigh bone is called the **femur,** and the lower leg bones are the **tibia** and **fibula.** The tibia is

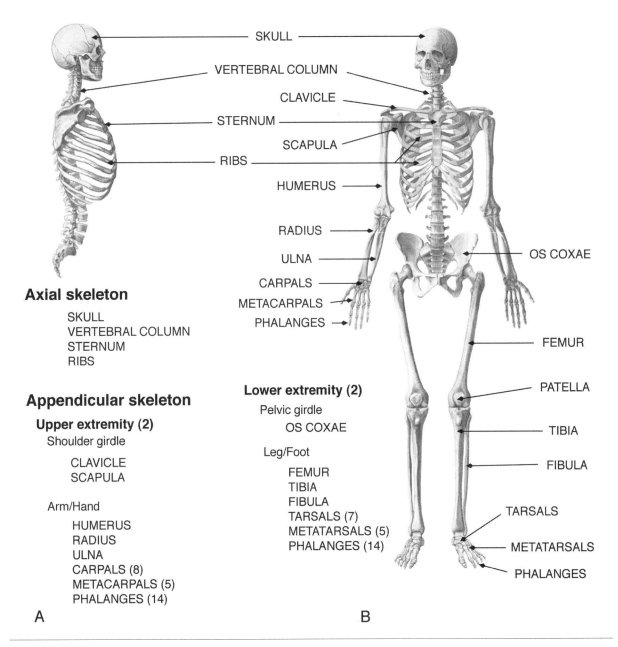

SKULL

VERTEBRAL COLUMN

CLAVICLE

STERNUM

SCAPULA

RIBS

HUMERUS

RADIUS

ULNA

CARPALS

METACARPALS

PHALANGES

OS COXAE

FEMUR

PATELLA

TIBIA

FIBULA

TARSALS

METATARSALS

PHALANGES

Axial skeleton

SKULL
VERTEBRAL COLUMN
STERNUM
RIBS

Appendicular skeleton

Upper extremity (2)

Shoulder girdle

CLAVICLE
SCAPULA

Arm/Hand

HUMERUS
RADIUS
ULNA
CARPALS (8)
METACARPALS (5)
PHALANGES (14)

Lower extremity (2)

Pelvic girdle

OS COXAE

Leg/Foot

FEMUR
TIBIA
FIBULA
TARSALS (7)
METATARSALS (5)
PHALANGES (14)

A   B

FIGURE 1.4   Major bones of the human skeleton. (A) Lateral view of axial skeleton and (B) anterior view of complete skeleton.

the larger of the bones, and is the primary weight-bearing bone of the lower leg. The fibula acts like a strut, placed to the outside of the tibia. The **patella,** or kneecap, is located in front of the lower part of the femur. The ankle-foot region has seven bones located in the ankle and upper foot area called the **tarsals;** five rays of bone located in the main body of the foot, called the **metatarsals;** and 14 digits located in the toes, called the phalanges. Note the similarity of the arrangement of the foot and hand; the difference is that the hand has one more carpal than the foot has tarsals.

Bony Markings

In addition to the names just mentioned for the bones of the skeleton, names are often used for specific sites on a given bone. This labeling is helpful for describing the specific location of blood vessels and nerves, or attachments of tendons, ligaments, or fascia. Such sites are commonly depressions, openings, projections, or processes as described in table 1.2. This terminology will be applied as individual joints are described more fully in following chapters of this book.

TABLE 1.2 Bony Markings

Name	Definition	Example
Depressions and openings		
Fossa	A hollow or depression	Iliac fossa
Foramen	A hole or passage through a bone	Obturator foramen of pelvis
Sinus	A cavity or spongelike space in a bone	Sinus tarsi in foot
Projections and processes that help form joints		
Condyle	Rounded projection at the end of a bone that enters into formation of a joint	Condyles of tibia
Facet	Smooth, flat area where a bone comes in contact with another bone	Facets of vertebrae
Head	Spherical projection beyond a narrow necklike portion located at the end of a bone that enters into formation of a joint	Head of femur
Projections and processes to which muscles attach		
Crest	A large ridge	Crest of ilium
Epicondyle	Eminence located above a condyle	Epicondyles of femur
Line	A less prominent ridge	Linea aspera of femur
Malleolus	A rounded process	Lateral malleolus of fibula
Spinous process or spine	A sharp spine-like projection	Spine of scapula
Trochanter	Very large projection	Greater trochanter of femur
Tubercle	A small rounded projection	Lesser tubercle of humerus
Tuberosity	A rounded projection	Ischial tuberosity

Joint Architecture

The human skeleton is composed of various bones joined together to form segments or links. The connection between adjacent bones or cartilage is termed a joint or, more technically, an **articulation.** These articulations have two primary but divergent functions: to bind the skeleton together and to provide mobility. There are many different kinds of articulations, with varied types of connections and motions present.

Classification of Joints

Joints can be classified according to the type of connective tissue that binds them and the presence or absence of a joint cavity (Marieb, 1995). In this structure-based classification system there are three classes of joints—fibrous, cartilaginous, and synovial (see table 1.3).

Fibrous Joints

Fibrous joints are held tightly together by either very short fibers (sutures), cords (ligaments), or sheets (interosseous membranes) of fibrous connective tissue. In each case, the fibrous connective tissue directly connects the adjacent bones and there is no space between the bones. Sutures allow no true movement, but only "give," while the other two types of fibrous joints allow a variable amount of movement depending on the length of their fibers. The type of connective tissue involved (dense regular connective tissue) can withstand great tensile stress. Examples of fibrous joints include the sutures of the skull, the middle joint between the bones of the forearm (middle radioulnar), and two of the joints between the bones of the lower leg (middle tibiofibular and distal tibiofibular joints).

Cartilaginous Joints

Cartilaginous joints are united directly by cartilage (fibrocartilage or hyaline cartilage); and, similarly

TABLE 1.3   Types of Joints

Examples	Description
Fibrous joints	
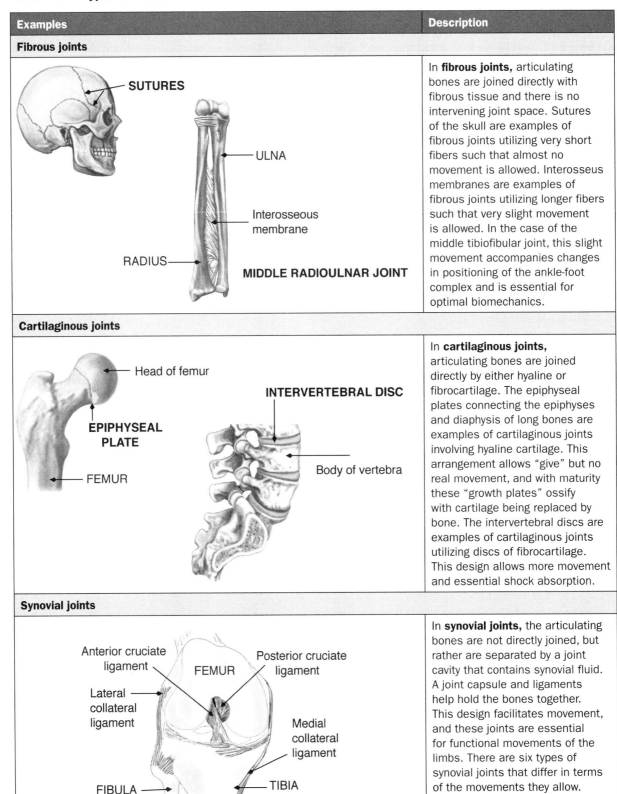 SUTURES · ULNA · Interosseous membrane · RADIUS · **MIDDLE RADIOULNAR JOINT**	In **fibrous joints,** articulating bones are joined directly with fibrous tissue and there is no intervening joint space. Sutures of the skull are examples of fibrous joints utilizing very short fibers such that almost no movement is allowed. Interosseus membranes are examples of fibrous joints utilizing longer fibers such that very slight movement is allowed. In the case of the middle tibiofibular joint, this slight movement accompanies changes in positioning of the ankle-foot complex and is essential for optimal biomechanics.
Cartilaginous joints	
Head of femur · INTERVERTEBRAL DISC · **EPIPHYSEAL PLATE** · FEMUR · Body of vertebra	In **cartilaginous joints,** articulating bones are joined directly by either hyaline or fibrocartilage. The epiphyseal plates connecting the epiphyses and diaphysis of long bones are examples of cartilaginous joints involving hyaline cartilage. This arrangement allows "give" but no real movement, and with maturity these "growth plates" ossify with cartilage being replaced by bone. The intervertebral discs are examples of cartilaginous joints utilizing discs of fibrocartilage. This design allows more movement and essential shock absorption.
Synovial joints	
Anterior cruciate ligament · Posterior cruciate ligament · FEMUR · Lateral collateral ligament · Medial collateral ligament · FIBULA · TIBIA · **THE KNEE JOINT**	In **synovial joints,** the articulating bones are not directly joined, but rather are separated by a joint cavity that contains synovial fluid. A joint capsule and ligaments help hold the bones together. This design facilitates movement, and these joints are essential for functional movements of the limbs. There are six types of synovial joints that differ in terms of the movements they allow. The knee joint is an example of a synovial joint that is considered a modified hinge joint and primarily allows motion in one plane and around one axis.

12

to the situation with fibrous joints, there is no space between the adjacent bones. Like bone, cartilage cells are surrounded by an extracellular matrix containing collagen fibers. However, unlike bone, this matrix is not calcified and is more like a firm gel in consistency. This gives cartilage less rigidity and more shock-absorbing capacity. Examples of cartilaginous joints (fibrocartilage type) include the joints between the bodies of the vertebrae (the intervertebral discs) and the pubes (pubic symphysis). This fibrocartilage type of joint involves a pad or disc of fibrocartilage, a design that allows slight movement as well as shock absorption. The epiphyseal plate, previously discussed with long bones, is also a cartilaginous joint, only of the hyaline cartilage type. The latter joint allows no true movement but adds a "give" to the associated bones.

Synovial Joints

Synovial joints differ from fibrous and cartilaginous joints in that adjacent bones are not directly connected to each other and there is actually a space between the articulating bones. This space is called the **joint cavity.** Although this space is very small, it generally allows a large degree of motion. Synovial joints are the most common type of joint in the human body, and almost all of the joints found in the limbs are synovial in nature. Synovial joints are particularly important for the study of human movement, and thus are the focus of this book. Examples of synovial joints include the shoulder, elbow, wrist, hip, knee, and ankle. The typical structure of a synovial joint is described next and is depicted in figure 1.5.

A characteristic of synovial joints is that the ends of the bones that come together to form the joint are covered with articular cartilage. Articular cartilage is a thin layer of hyaline cartilage covering the joint surfaces that helps decrease friction and aids in shock absorbency. The extracellular matrix of hyaline cartilage has characteristics between those of a solid and a liquid and has the ability to adapt to stress—actually exuding some of its fluid in response to loading (Whiting and Zernicke, 1998), spreading the load and reducing the stress at any contact point by 50% or more (Hall, 1999). According to one estimate, it also reduces friction at joints to only approximately 17% to 33% of the friction of a skate on ice under the same load. Articular cartilage does not contain its own blood supply and is dependent on nourishment from the synovial fluid and underlying vascular bone. In some areas where this cartilage is thick (such as the backside of the patella), nourishment may not be adequate and degeneration can occur. In general, once growth has ceased, cartilage

cell division is infrequent, and damage is generally repaired by fibrous tissue.

Synovial joints are surrounded by a sleevelike structure made of fibrous tissue called the **articular** or **joint capsule.** This capsule varies markedly in thickness and composition between joints to favor either mobility or stability. The fibrous tissue composing the capsule contains irregularly arranged collagen fibers and some elastic fibers in its matrix (dense irregular connective tissue), which give it strength and allow it to withstand tension applied in many directions. The capsule generally attaches to the bones, via the periosteum, at the margins of the articular cartilage.

The capsule is lined on the inside with **synovial membrane.** This membrane is a vascular, fragile, smooth tissue (loose connective tissue) that produces **synovial fluid.** This synovial fluid (G. *syn,* together + L. *ovum,* egg) has a consistency similar to egg white and helps to lubricate the joint and decrease wear and tear. Studies indicate that synovial fluid will change its characteristics (viscosity) such that when either the temperature or the velocity of joint movement is low, it will offer more resistance to movement (Levangie and Norkin, 2001). Conversely, when the temperature is higher (such as after warm-up) or the velocity of movement is higher, less resistance to movement is provided. Synovial fluid also is important for nourishment of articular cartilage, and it contains cells that respond to the presence of a foreign object or infection. When injury or irritation occurs, an abundant secretion of synovial fluid follows, which can produce noticeable swelling. It is the presence of the

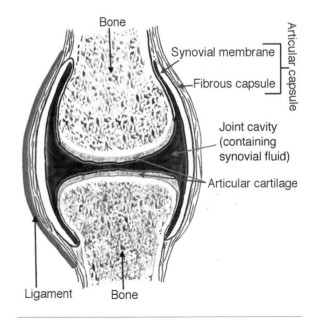

FIGURE 1.5   Structure of a typical synovial joint (longitudinal section).

synovial membrane and synovial fluid that gives rise to the name of this type of joint, "synovial" joint.

Synovial joints are generally reinforced by **ligaments.** Ligaments (L. *ligamentum,* a band) are strong bands of fibrous tissue that bind the articulating bones together. They contain abundant collagen fibers arranged in a lengthwise manner (dense regular connective tissue), which provide them with good tensile strength. Ligaments serve as passive constraints to prevent dislocations and add greater stability to joints. They also tend to limit the direction and extent of motion allowed at a given joint. These ligaments can be deep to (intracapsular), part of (capsular), or outside of (extracapsular) the joint capsule. The cruciate ligaments of the knee are examples of intracapsular ligaments; and the collateral ligaments of the knee (figure 5.3 on p. 240) are examples of extracapsular ligaments. The glenohumeral ligaments of the shoulder (figure 7.7 on p. 380) are examples of capsular ligaments.

Some synovial joints contain another specialized structure called a **fibrocartilage disc** (alternately termed **articular disc**). As the name suggests, this structure is composed of fibrous cartilage. Fibrous cartilage has more collagen fibers in its extracellular matrix and hence is stronger than hyaline cartilage. In some joints this fibrocartilage structure is shaped more like a circumferential ring than a disc and is called a **labrum.** These fibrocartilage structures are located within the joint and function to enhance joint congruency, joint stability, and joint shock absorbency. They are present only in select synovial joints such as the knee (meniscus), shoulder (glenoid labrum), and hip (acetabular labrum). Two examples are shown in figure 1.6.

Many synovial joints have other associated structures that aid in their function, such as fat pads, bursae, tendon sheaths, and retinacula. As their name suggests, **fat pads** are an accumulation of somewhat encapsulated fatty tissue (adipose tissue). They aid with cushioning and shock absorption and can be found at various places such as the hip, knee, and under the heel. A **bursa** (L. a purse) is a connective tissue sac lined with synovial membrane and containing a thin film of synovial fluid that functions to help reduce friction. Bursae often protect soft tissue such as tendons or skin from underlying hard bone, and there are approximately 150 present in the human body (McCarthy, 1989). For example, there is a bursa between the back of your heel bone and the overlying tendon, and one between the patella and the overlying skin. Synovial tissue can also be used to protect tendons via a double-layered sac-like covering called a **tendon sheath.** These tendon sheaths are

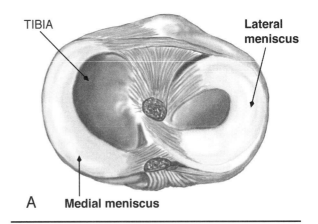

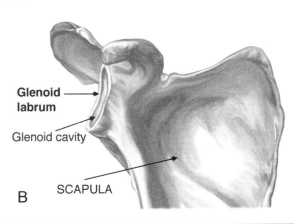

FIGURE 1.6   Fibrocartilage structures associated with synovial joints. (A) Menisci of the knee (right knee, superior view) and (B) glenoid labrum of shoulder (right scapula, anterior view).

often found surrounding tendons that come into close association with bones such as the long tendons of the hand and foot. A **retinaculum** (L. a band, a halter) is a thickened band of connective tissue that helps hold tendons in place. Retinacula are also prevalent around the ankle and foot. Examples of these structures associated with the foot are shown in figure 1.7.

Subclassification of Synovial Joints

Despite sharing the common structure just described, synovial joints vary considerably in their shape and the movements they allow. Table 1.4 illustrates one commonly used classification system for basic types of synovial joints and their associated movements. Here, the six types of synovial joints are described only in terms of their shape. However, their shape has important implications for movement capacity (noted in parentheses in table 1.4) and will be discussed after the necessary terminology is covered in the next two sections of this chapter.

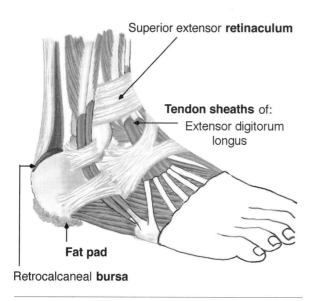

Superior extensor **retinaculum**

Tendon sheaths of:
Extensor digitorum
longus

Fat pad

Retrocalcaneal **bursa**

FIGURE 1.7   Associated structures of the foot.

- **Gliding** or **plane joints** contain joint surfaces that are generally flat or slightly curved in shape. Examples of gliding joints occur between some of the carpal bones (intercarpal joints), tarsal bones (intertarsal joints), and the articular processes of the vertebrae (facet joints).

- **Hinge joints** are composed of a spool-shaped surface that fits into a concave surface. Examples of hinge joints are the ankle, elbow, and knee (the latter is a modified hinge).

- **Pivot joints** are composed of an arch- or ring-shaped surface that rotates about a rounded or peg-like pivot. Examples of pivot joints occur in the upper forearm (upper radioulnar joint) and between the first and second vertebrae of the spine (atlantoaxial joint).

- **Condyloid** or **ellipsoid joints** consist of an oval-shaped condyle that fits into an elliptical cavity. An example of a condyloid joint occurs at the wrist (radiocarpal joint) and knuckles of the hands (#2–#5 metacarpophalangeal joints) and feet (metatarsophalangeal joints).

- **Saddle joints** are composed of a saddle-shaped bone that fits into a socket, which is concave-convex in the opposite direction. An example of a saddle joint occurs at the thumb (first carpo-metacarpal joint).

- **Ball-and-socket joints** consist of a ball-shaped head that fits into a socket. Ball-and-socket joints are the most freely movable type of joint in the body. Examples of ball-and-socket joints occur at the shoulder joint and hip joint.

Body Orientation Terminology

Before we consider the specific movements allowed by the synovial joints just described, it is helpful to learn some basic anatomical terminology. This terminology can be used to describe the location of anatomical structures, body segments, or the body as a whole. Key terminology includes the center of mass, line of gravity, anatomical position, anatomical directions, anatomical planes, and anatomical axes.

The Center of Mass and Line of Gravity

The **center of mass** of the body is the single point of a body about which every particle of its mass is equally distributed. This can be thought of as the point at which the body could be suspended or supported where the body would be totally balanced in all directions. When studying bodies subject to gravity (such as human movement on Earth), the center of mass may also be termed the **center of gravity** (CG). During upright standing with the arms down by the sides, the center of mass or center of gravity of the body is approximately located just in front of the second sacral vertebra and at about 55% of a person's height (Smith, Weiss, and Lehmkuhl, 1996).

The **line of gravity** is an imaginary line running vertically from the center of mass of the body toward the ground. Gravity is the attraction of the mass of the earth for the mass of other objects, and due to the effect of gravity, every particle of the body has a vertical force vector. However, these individual force vectors can be simplified into one force vector for the entire body. This single force vector acting on the whole body is termed the line of gravity of the body. Since the line of gravity of the body must run through the center of mass of the body, its position in space constantly changes as the body changes its position and configuration during movement.

These concepts of the center of mass and line of gravity can be applied to body segments, as well as the body as a whole. For example, the center of mass of the trunk, thigh, leg, and foot segments can be derived. One can then establish the line of gravity of each of these segments by dropping a vertical line from the center of mass of the given segment. These concepts of the center of mass and line of gravity are key for the analysis of alignment, forces, and movement. They will be used in later chapters, including the calculation of resistance torque when lifting a dumbbell or another dancer (see figure 2.12 on p. 48).

TABLE 1.4   Types of Synovial Joints

Examples	Description
Uniaxial joints	
Hinge	In hinge joints, a spool-shaped surface fits into a concave surface allowing motion in one plane (flexion-extension in the sagittal plane). Example: elbow joint.
Pivot	In pivot joints, an arch- or ring-shaped surface rotates about a rounded pivot allowing motion in one plane (rotation in the horizontal plane). Example: upper radioulnar joint.
Biaxial joints	
Condyloid	In condyloid joints, an oval-shaped condyle fits into an elliptical cavity allowing motion in two planes (flexion-extension in the sagittal plane and abduction-adduction in the frontal plane). Example: knuckles (metacarpophalangeal joints) in hands.
Saddle	In saddle joints, a saddle-shaped bone fits into a socket that is concave-convex in the opposite direction allowing motion in two planes (generally involving specialized movement terminology). Example: thumb (first carpometacarpal joint).
Triaxial joints	
Ball-and-socket	In ball-and-socket joints, a ball-shaped head fits into a socket allowing motion in three planes (flexion-extension in the sagittal plane, abduction-adduction in the frontal plane, and external rotation-internal rotation in the horizontal plane). Example: shoulder joint.

Examples	Description
Triaxial joints *(continued)*	
Gliding 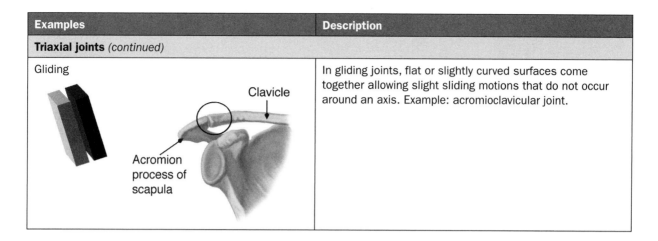 Clavicle Acromion process of scapula	In gliding joints, flat or slightly curved surfaces come together allowing slight sliding motions that do not occur around an axis. Example: acromioclavicular joint.

Anatomical Position

Anatomical position is a reference position or starting position that is used for movement terminology. **Anatomical position** is an erect standing position; the feet face front (either together or slightly separated), and the arms are down by the sides with the palms facing forward so that the thumbs face outward and the fingers are extended. Anatomical position is illustrated in figure 1.8. This position of the arms allows movements such as bending and straightening (technically termed flexion-extension) of the elbow, wrist, and fingers to occur in the same spatial direction (plane) as other major joints of the body such as the shoulder and hip. This makes learning movements easier and more logical.

Two other terms are commonly used to describe positions of the body—prone and supine. As seen in table 1.5, **prone** refers to lying face downward on the stomach, while **supine** refers to lying face upward on the back. These two terms are particularly useful when one is describing exercises.

Directional Terminology

The other key terms defined in table 1.5 and selectively illustrated in figure 1.8 are used to describe the relationship between parts of the body in anatomical position, or the location of the given structure in reference to other structures. Note that these terms occur in pairs with opposite meanings. So, **superior** means closer to the head or "above" while **inferior** means farther from the head or "below." **Anterior** or ventral means toward the front of the body while **posterior** or dorsal means toward the back of the body. For example, the bony projection used for evaluation of pelvic alignment, found on the front and top portion of the pelvis, is termed the anterior superior iliac spine (ASIS); that found on the back of the pelvis is termed

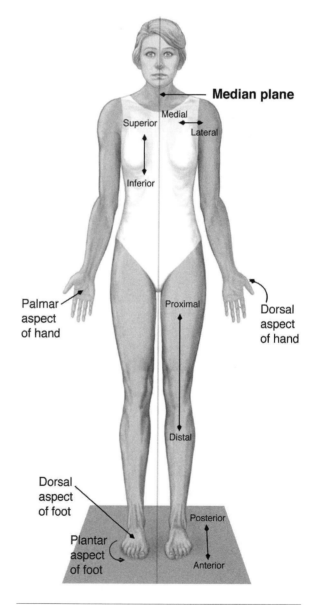

FIGURE 1.8 Anatomical position and directional terminology.

TABLE 1.5   Anatomical Position and Directional Terminology

Term	Definition
Positional terminology	
Anatomical position	Standing with feet and palms facing front
Supine	Lying on the back
Prone	Lying face downward
Directional terminology	
Superior (cranial)	Above/toward head
Inferior (caudal)	Below/toward feet
Anterior (ventral)	Front side/in front of
Posterior (dorsal)	Back side/in back of
Medial	Closer to the median plane/toward midline
Lateral	Farther from the median plane/toward side
Proximal	Closer to root of limb, trunk, or center of body
Distal	Farther from root of limb, trunk, or center of body
Superficial	Closer to or on the surface of body
Deep	Farther from the surface of body
Palmar	Anterior aspect of hand in anatomical position
Dorsal (for hands/feet)	Posterior aspect of hand in anatomical position; top aspect of foot when standing in anatomical position
Plantar	Bottom aspect of foot when standing in anatomical position

the posterior superior iliac spine (PSIS). **Medial** refers to closer to the midline while **lateral** refers to farther from the midline. For example, the rounded bony projection of the inferior femur, located on the inside of the knee, is termed the medial condyle; the projection located on the outside of the knee is termed the lateral condyle. **Proximal** means closer to the root of the limb or trunk, while **distal** means farther from the root of the limb or trunk. For example, the joint between the radius and the ulna that is located close to the elbow is termed the proximal or superior radioulnar joint, while the joint located close to the wrist is termed the distal or inferior radioulnar joint. **Superficial** refers to closer to the surface of the body, while **deep** refers to farther from the surface of the body. For example, the abdominal muscle called the rectus abdominis is superficial relative to the deep abdominal muscle called the transverse abdominis.

Some additional specialized terminology is used for clarification in some parts of the body such as the hands and feet. For example, during standing in anatomical position, the posterior side of the hand is referred to as the **dorsal** aspect or surface while the anterior side is termed the **palmar** aspect. For the lower extremity, during standing in anatomical position the top side of the foot is termed the dorsal aspect while the bottom aspect is termed the **plantar** aspect.

Anatomical Planes

The concept of planes is used to help describe basic movements of the body and its segments. In this context, a plane can be thought of as an imaginary flat surface such as a sheet of cardboard that passes through the body in a given direction. In anatomical position there are three imaginary reference planes that are perpendicular to each other and divide the body in half by mass. These **cardinal planes** or principal planes each pass through the center of mass of the body. These cardinal planes correspond to the three dimensions in space and are termed the sagittal, frontal, and horizontal planes as illustrated in figure 1.9. The cardinal **sagittal plane** is also termed the **median** or midsagittal plane, and it is a vertical plane that divides the body into equal right and left portions. The cardinal **frontal,** or coronal, plane is a vertical plane that runs perpendicular to the sagittal plane and divides the body into anterior and posterior portions of equal mass. The cardinal **horizontal** or transverse plane runs transversely through the body such that it is perpendicular to the sagittal and frontal planes. During upright standing the horizontal plane is parallel to the floor. It divides the body into superior and inferior portions of equal mass.

In addition to these cardinal planes, there can be other sagittal, frontal, or horizontal planes that run parallel to their cardinal counterpart but differ in that they do not pass through the center of mass of the body and do not divide the body in half by mass. These other planes are helpful for describing many functional movements in which different segments of the body are moving in planes parallel to a given cardinal plane. While some texts term these noncardinal planes **secondary planes** (Smith, Weiss, and Lehmkuhl, 1996) or segmental planes (Kreighbaum and Barthels, 1996), for purposes of simplicity this text includes cardinal and noncardinal planes within the terms sagittal, frontal, and horizontal planes as described in table 1.6.

Anatomical Axes and Associated Movements

When movement occurs in a plane, it is always occurring around an axis that is perpendicular to this plane. Hence, there are three imaginary anatomical **reference axes,** each associated with one of the three basic planes—sagittal, frontal, and horizontal—previously described. When one is describing motion about these axes in their respective planes, movement can be of the whole body or of a body segment. Examples of such movements in the sagittal plane are shown in figure 1.10. With whole body movement the axis generally runs through the center of mass of the body, as with a forward somersault (figure 1.10A), or through a point of external support. Examples of a point of external support are the hands on a parallel bar during a swinging motion, the hands on the floor in a walkover (figure 1.10B), and the feet on the floor in the preparation phase of a jump. With movement of body segments, the axis runs through the joint, again in a direction perpendicular to the

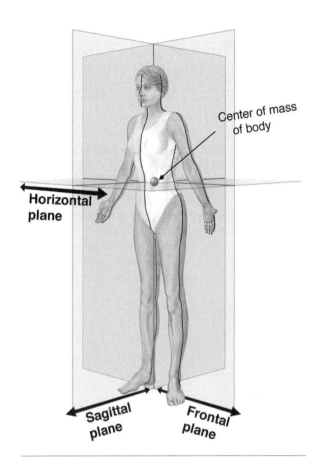

FIGURE 1.9   The three cardinal planes of the body and their axes.

plane in which the movement occurs. To picture the relationship between an axis and the motion it allows, imagine a pencil running through your joint in the direction associated with that given axis. Then try to imagine what type of movement it would allow and in what plane this movement would occur (table 1.7). Mediolateral axes for the wrist, elbow, shoulder, hip, knee, and ankle joints are shown in figure 1.10C that would allow movements at these joints in a sagittal plane.

• Mediolateral axis (frontal axis). A **mediolateral** (ML) axis runs in a side-to-side direction in a frontal plane, perpendicular to a sagittal plane and allowing motion in a sagittal plane. An ML axis through the

TABLE 1.6   Basic Anatomical Planes

Name	Definition
Sagittal plane(s)	A vertical plane dividing body into right and left portions
Median plane	The midsagittal plane dividing the body into equal right and left portions
Frontal plane(s)	A vertical plane dividing the body into front and back portions
Horizontal plane(s)	A transverse plane dividing the body into upper and lower portions

"Bend the Knees to the Side"

During work in turnout, some teachers use directional cues to help students try to maximize their turnout. During standing in parallel position with the feet, the knees will bend or flex "forward" in a sagittal plane. However, with ideal turnout, the hips would be externally rotated sufficiently to allow the knees to bend "sideward" so that this movement would occur in a plane closer to the frontal. Sometimes using this spatial cue of "reaching the knees to the side" or "bending the knees to the side" can help dancers use more turnout and find muscles that can help with maximizing turnout. However, as discussed later (chapters 4 and 5), it is important that the positioning of the knee be appropriate for the individual dancer's turnout and be achieved through emphasis on external rotation of the femur at the hip joint versus excessive rotation of the tibia at the knee joint.

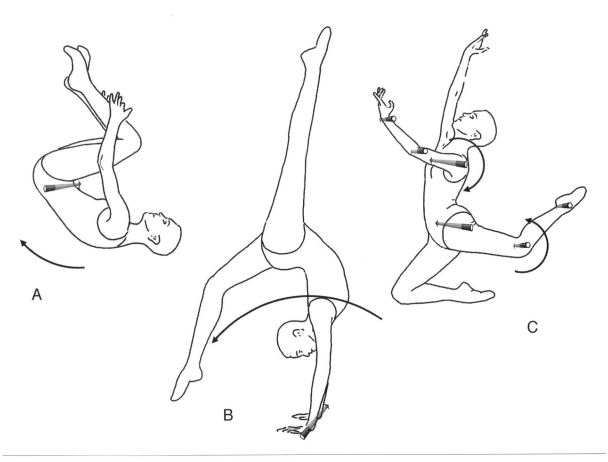

FIGURE 1.10 Movement of the body in a sagittal plane about a mediolateral axis through (A) the center of mass of the whole body, (B) an external point of support, and (C) a joint.

TABLE 1.7   **Basic Anatomical Axes**

Name	Definition	Plane of motion	Movement example (axis running through hip joint)
Mediolateral (ML)	Passes through body from side to side	Sagittal	Parallel dégagé (front)
Anteroposterior (AP)	Passes through body from front to back	Frontal	Parallel dégagé (side)
Vertical	Passes through body from top to bottom	Horizontal	Turning out while standing in first position

knee would allow the motion of bending the knee (knee flexion) in a sagittal plane such as used in a first-position parallel plié. Examples of dance movements occurring primarily in sagittal (L. *sagitta,* an arrow, in the line of an arrow shot from a bow; e.g., in an anteroposterior direction) planes are a parallel brush (dégagé) to the front; torso "contractions"; raising the arm from a position down by the side, forward, to an overhead position (shoulder flexion); a forward roll; a forward leap; and performing a triplet moving forward. These can be thought of as movements of body segments (an example for the torso is provided in figure 1.11A) or the whole body in primarily a forward and backward direction.

• Anteroposterior axis (sagittal axis). An **anteroposterior** (AP) axis runs in a front-to-back direction in a sagittal plane, perpendicular to a frontal plane and allowing motion in a frontal plane. For example, the AP axis running through the shoulder allows the movement of raising the arm to the side (shoulder abduction) in a frontal plane. Examples of dance movements occurring primarily in a frontal plane

are a parallel brush (dégagé) to the side, a lateral bend of the torso (figure 1.11B), a jumping jack, a cartwheel, and a Russian split. These can be thought of as movements of body segments or the whole body in a side-to-side or lateral direction.

• Vertical axis (longitudinal axis). A **vertical axis** runs in a superior-inferior direction, perpendicular to a horizontal plane and allowing motion in a horizontal plane. For example, the vertical axis running through the spine (from top to bottom) allows the movement of trunk rotation in the horizontal plane. Examples of dance movements occurring primarily in horizontal planes are a torso twist (figure 1.11C), turnout (hip external rotation), a turn (pirouette), and a turning jump. These can be thought of as movements of body segments or the whole body in a twisting or turning manner.

Students new to anatomical terminology often do well at picturing these planes relative to anatomical position as shown in figure 1.9, but have difficulty understanding how these planes correlate with functional

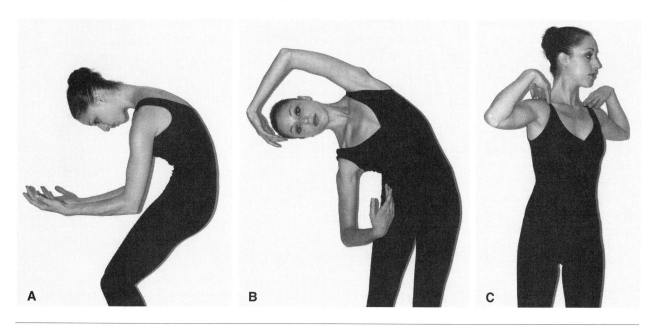

A   B   C

FIGURE 1.11   Dance vocabulary showing movement of the trunk in the (A) sagittal, (B) frontal, and (C) horizontal plane.

movement. To aid with this understanding, it is first important to remember that these planes are in reference to the body. So, if you turn the entire body, these planes shift without any consideration for the space in which you are standing. Hence, a parallel back attitude would be in the sagittal plane whether you were facing the front of the room, the side of the room, or the front diagonal of the room. Second, it is important to realize that with most joints key to the study of human movement, motion involves rotation of one bone relative to another bone (angular motion). Because bones are secured relative to other bones at joints, the bones rotate about this joint when they receive force (see Muscles, Levers, and Rotary Motion on p. 44 for more information). So, to establish the plane of motion, picture the imaginary surface that the entire rotating bone segment is sweeping along. It sometimes helps to imagine that you had chalk on that segment and then imagine what plane the segment would "draw." For example, when you are standing in anatomical position and lifting the thigh to the front and then back down, the thigh segment "draws" a sagittal plane as seen in figure 1.13. In contrast, when you are lifting the leg to the side and then back down, the thigh segment "draws" a frontal plane as seen in figure 1.14. Lastly, when you are rotating the leg along the long axis of the femur, the end of the leg (e.g., the foot) "draws" a horizontal plane as seen in figure 1.16.

Planes and Axes in Complex Movement

Understanding these three reference planes and associated axes is very helpful for analyzing movement. However, it is important to realize that joint axes are often complex and involve subtle shifts in different ranges of motions. Therefore, the concept of reference axes is not exact but rather provides a useful approximation helpful for picturing movement. Furthermore, many complex dance movements utilize several planes with different body segments and often involve planes between the sagittal, frontal, and horizontal planes. For example, aesthetics are often enhanced through addition of rotation to the trunk when it is arched or tilted rather than vertically positioned (figure 1.12). Planes other than the basic sagittal, frontal, and horizontal planes are termed **diagonal,** or oblique, planes. In such cases the axis is perpendicular to the particular diagonal plane and different from the three reference axes previously described.

Joint Movement Terminology

The movements at joints about the axes and in the planes just described have specific names. With

the exception of gliding joints, all synovial joints can permit two or more of the following six basic joint movements: flexion, extension, abduction, adduction, external rotation, and internal rotation. The logic of these terms is best seen relative to anatomical position. As with position terminology, these terms occur in pairs that have opposite meanings. The pairings for movement terminology are flexion-extension, abduction-adduction, and external rotation-internal rotation. Each of these pairs reflects movement that occurs in the same plane and about the same axis, but in the opposite direction. For example, flexion-extension could be reflected by bringing the arm to the front (shoulder flexion) or bringing the arm back (shoulder extension), with both movements occurring in the sagittal plane about an ML axis. A description of these fundamental movements follows, and a summary is provided in table 1.8.

- **Flexion** (L. *flecto,* to bend) involves bringing anterior surfaces toward adjacent anterior surfaces, or posterior surfaces toward adjacent posterior sur-

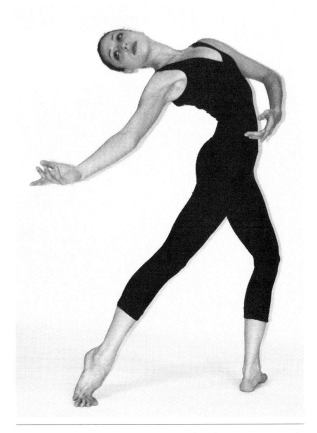

FIGURE 1.12 Dance vocabulary showing movement of the trunk that does not occur in the basic planes, but rather in diagonal planes.

CSULB dancer Jennifer Fitzgerald.

TABLE 1.8   Joint Movement Terminology

Name	Definition
Basic movements	
Flexion	Bringing the anterior or posterior surface of a body segment toward the anterior or posterior surface of an adjacent body segment (bending)
Extension	Moving from a flexed position toward the anatomical position (straightening)
(Hyperextension)	Moving in extension past the anatomical position
Abduction	Moving away from the midline of the body
Adduction	Moving toward the midline of the body
(Circumduction)	Describing a cone with the apex at the joint; combines flexion, abduction, extension, and adduction
External rotation	Turning anterior surface outward
Internal rotation	Turning anterior surface inward
Specialized movements	
Right lateral flexion (spine)	Side-bending of the trunk to the right or moving from a position of left lateral flexion toward anatomical position
Left lateral flexion (spine)	Side-bending of the trunk to the left or moving from a position of right lateral flexion toward anatomical position
Right rotation (spine)	Turning the anterior surface of the head or trunk to the right
Left rotation (spine)	Turning the anterior surface of the head or trunk to the left
Pronation (forearm)	Turning the palm backward
Supination (forearm)	Turning the palm forward
Horizontal abduction (shoulder and hip)	Movement of the limb away from the midline in a horizontal plane when the limb is flexed to a 90° position
Horizontal adduction (shoulder and hip)	Movement of the limb toward the midline in a horizontal plane when the limb is flexed to a 90° position
Dorsiflexion (ankle-foot)	Bringing the toes and top of the foot up toward the shin (flexing the foot)
Plantar flexion (ankle-foot)	Bringing the toes and bottom of the foot downward (pointing the foot)
Inversion (foot)	Lifting the medial portion of the foot upward
Eversion (foot)	Lifting the lateral portion of the foot upward

faces. In most joints, such as the spine, hip, elbow, wrist, or joints between the digits of the fingers (interphalangeal joints), it is the anterior surfaces of the segments that are brought closer together or "approximated" with flexion. For example, bringing the front of the forearm toward the front of the upper arm is elbow flexion. However, with selected joints, such as the knee, it is the posterior surfaces of the segments that are approximated with flexion. Flexion is also sometimes described as decreasing the angle between two bones or, colloquially, as "bending" the joint. Flexion occurs in the sagittal plane around an ML axis as seen in figure 1.13.

• **Extension** (L. *extensio,* to stretch out) is the opposite motion to flexion, although occurring in the same sagittal plane and around an ML axis as seen in figure 1.13. Extension can be described as bringing anterior surfaces away from adjacent anterior surfaces, or posterior surfaces away from adjacent posterior surfaces, back toward anatomical position. It can also be thought of as increasing the angle between adjacent bones or, colloquially, as "straightening" the joint from a bent position. Straightening the knee from a bent position during rising from a plié or executing a développé is an example of knee extension. Straightening a joint beyond anatomical position is

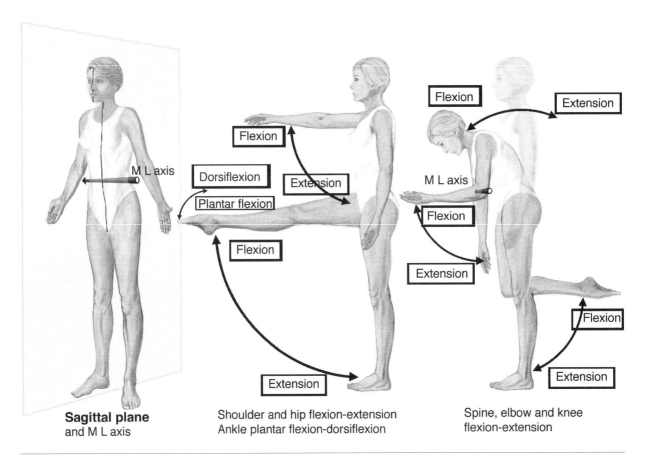

Sagittal plane
and M L axis

Shoulder and hip flexion-extension
Ankle plantar flexion-dorsiflexion

Spine, elbow and knee
flexion-extension

FIGURE 1.13 Joint movements in the sagittal plane about a mediolateral (ML) axis: flexion-extension and plantar flexion-dorsiflexion.

termed hyperextension. For some joints (such as the knee, elbow, or fingers), extension from anatomical position (hyperextension) is not possible except in very flexible individuals. Hyperextension is not a new movement but rather just a continuation of extension beyond anatomical position, and in movement analysis the term *extension* encompasses hyperextension. Flexion-extension occurs in some uniaxial (hinge) joints, all biaxial (condyloid and saddle) joints, and all triaxial (ball-and-socket) joints.

• **Abduction** (L. *abducens,* drawing away) involves moving a segment of the body away from the median plane or midline of the body. This movement is still considered abduction throughout its full range, even if it seems to be coming back toward the midline in its excursion beyond 90° (e.g., raising the arm to the side and continuing to an overhead position when bringing the arms to a high fifth position). Abduction occurs in the frontal plane around an AP axis as seen in figure 1.14.

• **Adduction** (L. *ductus,* to bring toward) is the opposite motion to abduction, although it still occurs in the same frontal plane around an AP axis

as seen in figure 1.14. Adduction can be described as returning the body segment back toward anatomical position and the midline of the body. For example, adduction would involve bringing the arm down to the side from an overhead position. To remember this terminology it is helpful to associate adduction with "add"ing that body part into the midline, while to abduct someone means to unlawfully carry the person "away." So, to abduct a body segment is to take it "away" from the midline. Abduction-adduction occurs in all biaxial (condyloid and saddle) and triaxial (ball-and-socket) joints but is not possible in any uniaxial joint. Abduction-adduction occurs at such joints as the shoulder and hip.

• **Circumduction** (L. *circium,* around + *ductus,* to draw) is not a new movement per se, but rather a compound movement that simply combines the four basic movements just described while utilizing multiple planes. Circumduction is a sequential combination of flexion, abduction, extension, and adduction (in that order or in the reverse order). In circumduction, the body segment describes a cone, with one end of the segment making a circle (base

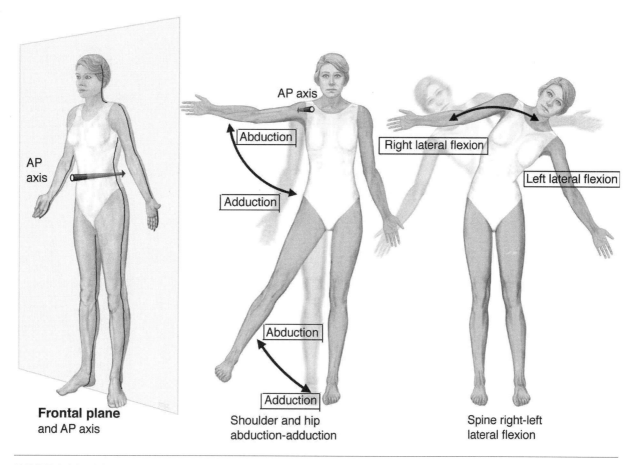

FIGURE 1.14 Joint movements in the frontal plane about an anteroposterior (AP) axis: abduction-adduction and right lateral flexion-left lateral flexion.

of the cone) while the other end stays stationary (apex of the cone). For example, circumduction of the shoulder occurs when you trace a circle with your middle finger as seen in figure 1.15B.

- **External rotation** involves moving the anterior surface of a limb outward or away from the midline of the body. It is also termed lateral rotation or outward rotation and is the primary motion used at the hip to establish turnout. External rotation occurs in a horizontal plane around a vertical (longitudinal) axis through the body segment as seen in figure 1.16. The fact that a longitudinal axis is involved is important for understanding rotation, as well as the difference between rotation and circumduction. For rotation, both ends of the segment stay at the same point in space and the segment just twists along the long axis. For example, rotation of the shoulder occurs when the entire arm is twisted while the middle finger stays at the same place rather than making a circle (circumduction), as shown in figure 1.15A. In dance, external rotation of the hip occurs during turning out from a parallel first position. In contrast, circumduction of the hip is utilized when

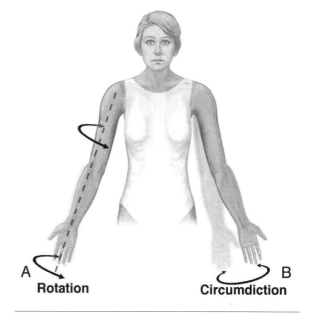

FIGURE 1.15 Distinguishing between shoulder rotation and circumduction. (A) Rotation involves twisting along the longitudinal axis of the limb with the middle finger rotating in place, while (B) circumduction involves a cone-shaped movement path with the middle finger tracing a circle.

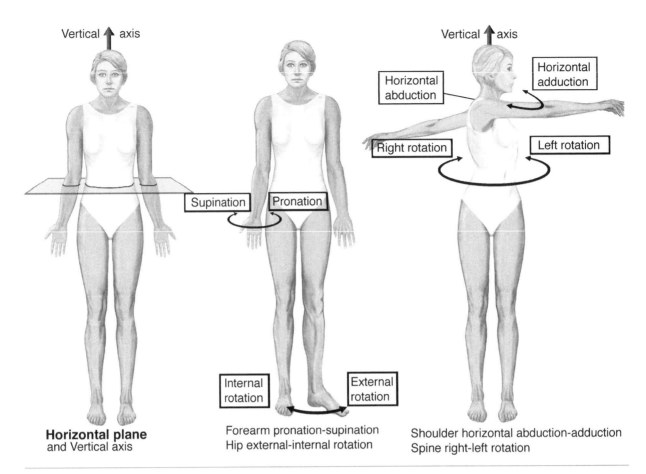

Vertical axis

Horizontal
abduction

Horizontal
adduction

Right rotation

Left rotation

Supination   Pronation

Vertical axis

Internal
rotation

External
rotation

Horizontal plane
and Vertical axis

Forearm pronation-supination
Hip external-internal rotation

Shoulder horizontal abduction-adduction
Spine right-left rotation

FIGURE 1.16   Joint movements in the horizontal plane about a vertical axis: internal rotation-external rotation, pronation-supination, right rotation-left rotation, and horizontal abduction-adduction.

the dancer performs a circling motion with the foot on the floor (circular portion of rond de jambe à terre).

• **Internal rotation** is the opposite motion to external rotation, although still in the horizontal plane and about a longitudinal axis through the body segment as seen in figure 1.16. Internal rotation involves bringing the anterior surface of the limb inward, toward the midline of the body, such as is used in jazz dance when the thigh is rotated inward so that the knee faces medially. It is also termed medial or inward rotation. Unlike what occurs with some of the other movement pairs discussed, the limb can readily be either internally or externally rotated from anatomical position, and anatomical position is often regarded as the neutral position. External-internal rotation occurs in some uniaxial (pivot) joints and all triaxial (ball-and-socket) joints. External rotation-internal rotation occurs at such joints as the shoulder and hip.

Specialized Joint Movement Terminology

At some joints, additional terminology is used to describe motions. This specialized terminology is usually used for certain joints in an effort to clarify the direction of movement or to describe movement that is slightly different from the six basic movements just discussed. For example, since the midline runs through the head and trunk segments, much of the basic terminology does not work well for describing movements of the spine. Hence, during bending the torso to the side in the frontal plane, abduction-adduction does not clearly describe what is occurring, and right or left lateral flexion is alternatively used. So, **right lateral flexion** is the movement of bending the torso to the right, while returning from this position to anatomical position or bending to the left is termed **left lateral flexion** as seen in figure 1.14. Similarly, external and internal rotation in the transverse plane are not adequate characterizations for the spine or head, and rotation is described as right or left rotation from the perspective of the dancer who is moving. So, **right rotation** is movement of the anterior surface of the head or trunk so that it faces right, while **left rotation** is movement of the anterior surface of the head or trunk so that it faces left as seen in figure 1.16.

CONCEPT DEMONSTRATION 1.1

Fundamental Joint Movements

While standing in anatomical position, perform the following movements.

· **Movements in the sagittal plane.** Perform flexion of the fingers, wrist, elbow, shoulder, and hip joints in which the distal segment is the moving segment. Note that this involves forward movement of the distal segment of the joint from anatomical position in a sagittal plane such that anterior surfaces of the joint segments are approximating. Then, extend these joints, returning to anatomical position. Note that this occurs in a backward direction in a sagittal plane. Can these joints be extended from anatomical position? Now flex the knee joint. Note that although movement occurs in a sagittal plane, flexion of the knee involves a backward movement of the distal segment with posterior surfaces of the segments approximating, while extension involves a forward motion. In some cases, such as when the hand or foot is weight bearing and fixed, the proximal segment moves alone or simultaneously with the distal segment. Perform flexion of the hip in which the proximal segment moves and the distal segment remains stationary.

· **Movements in the frontal plane.** Perform abduction of the shoulder and hip joints in which the distal segment of the limb (hand and foot) is allowed to move. Note that these movements involve movement from anatomical position away from the midline of the body in a frontal plane. Then, adduct these joints, returning to anatomical position. Note that adduction of these joints involves a movement toward the midline of the body in the frontal plane. Can these joints be adducted from anatomical position? Now perform abduction and adduction of the hip joint in which the foot is fixed and the pelvis is the moving segment. How do these movements relate to the dance terminology "sitting in your hip"?

· **Movements in the horizontal plane.** Perform internal rotation of the shoulder and hip joint in which the distal segment (hand and foot) is free to move. Note that this involves movement of the anterior surface of the limb toward the midline in a horizontal plane. Then, perform external rotation of the shoulder and hip, returning back to anatomical position. Can external rotation be performed from anatomical position? Note how similar amounts of internal and external rotation can occur from anatomical position, in contrast to the other movement pairs. How do these movements relate to the dance terminology "turnout"? Now perform rotation at the hip joint in which the pelvis moves while the foot remains fixed.

In the upper extremity, two specialized movement pairs are used to describe movements in the horizontal plane about a vertical axis: pronation-supination and horizontal abduction-adduction (see figure 1.16). **Pronation** refers to internal rotation of the forearm so that the palm faces backward while **supination** refers to external rotation of the forearm so that the palm faces forward. Anatomical position utilizes a position of forearm supination. Horizontal abduction-adduction is terminology that has been developed because of the common use of the arms at shoulder height during functional movement. If the arm is flexed to a 90° position at the shoulder joint, movement of the arm laterally in the horizontal plane is termed **horizontal abduction** or horizontal extension. Movement in the opposite direction from a lateral position anteriorly (toward the midline of the body) is termed **horizontal adduction** or horizontal flexion.

In the lower extremity, this same terminology of horizontal abduction-adduction can be used for movements of the thigh in the horizontal plane from a position of 90° of hip flexion. With the foot, terminology of plantar flexion and dorsiflexion is used in place of flexion-extension due to the controversy regarding which side of the foot should be considered "anterior." **Plantar flexion** of the foot at the ankle joint corresponds to what dancers term "pointing" the foot, while **dorsiflexion** corresponds to what dancers term "flexing" the foot. So, remember that "P" in pointing goes with "P" in plantar flexion. These movements occur in the sagittal plane around an ML axis as seen in figure 1.13. Additional specialized terminology for both the upper and lower extremity is addressed in chapters covering the respective joints.

Joint Movements Associated With Specific Types of Synovial Joints

Now that planes, axes, and joint movement terminology have been covered, the movement capacity of synovial joints can be added to their shape-based description. Synovial joints can be subclassified according to whether they have one, two, three, or no axes—uniaxial, biaxial, triaxial, and nonaxial, respectively. The number of axes a joint has also parallels the number of planes in which that joint allows motion, which is termed **degrees of freedom** (df) and determines the types of movement allowed from anatomical position.

Gliding joints are considered nonaxial joints as they allow only slight gliding or sliding motion that does not occur about an axis. Hinge and pivot joints are uniaxial joints allowing movement in one plane (1df). Hinge joints allow the movements of flexion-extension in the sagittal plane, while pivot joints allow rotation in the horizontal plane. Condyloid and saddle joints are biaxial joints allowing movement in two planes (2df). Condyloid joints generally allow flexion-extension in the sagittal plane and abduction-adduction in the frontal plane (although specialized terminology is used for some of these movements). For the saddle joint (first carpometacarpal joint), specialized movement terminology is used that will be addressed in chapter 7. The ball-and-socket joint is the only type of triaxial joint, allowing movement in three planes (3df). Movements allowed are flexion-extension in the sagittal plane, abduction-adduction in the frontal plane, and external rotation-internal rotation in the horizontal plane. Notice that triaxial joints differ from biaxial joints through the addition of rotation. The association of movement capacity and joint type is summarized in table 1.4 (p. 16).

Skeletal Considerations in Whole Body Movement

Additional concepts come into play when one examines the contribution of bones and joints to functional movements such as those used in dancing. Three particularly key considerations are joint stability and mobility, close-packed and loose-packed positions of joints, and closed and open kinematic chain movements.

CONCEPT DEMONSTRATION 1.2

Types of Synovial Joints and Their Movements

While standing in anatomical position, identify the following joints and perform their movements. Refer to figure 1.9 as needed.

- **Uniaxial joints.** Perform the movements of the forearm that are allowed by the elbow joint. What type of synovial joint is it? In what plane and about what axis does movement of this joint occur? Now, perform movements of the forearm that are allowed by the upper radioulnar joint. In what plane and about what axis does movement of this joint occur?

- **Biaxial joints.** Perform the movements of the hand that are allowed by the wrist joint. What type of synovial joint is it? In what two planes and about what two axes does movement of this joint occur? Now, perform movements of the thumb and note similarities and differences from the wrist joint. Can either of these joints be actively rotated?

- **Triaxial joints.** Perform the movements of the upper arm that are allowed by the shoulder joint. What type of synovial joint is it? In what three planes and about what three axes does movement of this joint occur? How does rotation differ from circumduction? What plane is utilized with triaxial joints that is missing with biaxial joints? How does this combination of uniaxial, biaxial, and triaxial joints further the stability and mobility demands of the upper extremity in gestural movements and weight-bearing movements in dance?

Close- and Loose-Packed Joint Positions

· **Loose-packed position of the fingers.** While sitting, bend your elbows to 90° with your palms facing upward and the fingers in line with the metacarpals. Spread the fingers and then bring them back in. Note the degree of abduction and adduction of the fingers that can occur in this loose-packed position of the metacarpophalangeal joint.

· **Close-packed position of the fingers.** Bring the fingers up to face the ceiling while keeping the rest of the hand in place (90° of metacarpophalangeal joint flexion). Now, try to spread the fingers and notice how limited abduction and adduction of the fingers are in this close-packed position of the metacarpophalangeal joints. What advantages could the change in mobility present in different positions offer functions performed by the hand?

Joint Stability and Mobility

Joint stability can be defined as the ability of a joint to withstand forces and avoid being separated (disarticulated) without injury. This is a very important property of joints, from a perspective of both defining movement capacity and promoting safety. When forces exceed the stability of a joint, injury to the various tissues can occur. Two common types of injury are injury to the ligament, termed a **sprain,** and injury to the muscle, termed a **strain.**

In contrast to joint stability, **joint mobility** can be defined as the range of motion allowed prior to tissue restraints. The functional capacity of joints to move through a full range of motion, also termed **flexibility,** is an important aspect of physical fitness and essential for allowing the achievement of dance aesthetics. Key factors that influence relative joint stability versus mobility include the joint architecture (type of joint, shape and depth of articulation); arrangement of the ligaments and capsule; vacuum created in the joint due to the negative atmospheric pressure; extensibility of the muscles, tendons, and fascia crossing the joint; neural factors that influence the resistance to movement; effects of gravity; and, in some cases, occlusion of adjacent soft body parts or impingement of bone against bone. These factors are discussed in more detail and as they relate to specific key joints in subsequent chapters. However, it is important to note that although dancers often imagine that continuing to increase joint mobility should be their goal, excessive mobility can be associated with decreased stability and increased injury risk. Instead, the goal should be a balance of joint stability and mobility, which will allow for protection of joints while still meeting desired dance aesthetics.

Close-Packed and Loose-Packed Positions of Joints

Joint stability is also influenced by the specific position of a given joint, and articulating surfaces of synovial joints have a position that offers the greatest mechanical stability. This position is termed the **close-packed position** and often occurs at the extreme in the range of motion, such as full extension of the elbow, knee, wrist, or fingers (interphalangeal joints); flexion of the metacarpophalangeal joints; and dorsiflexion of the ankle. In this close-packed position the following conditions generally occur: (1) The joint surfaces have the greatest contact area and fit (congruency); (2) a majority of key ligaments are under tension; (3) the capsule is taut; and (4) the joint is under compression and difficult to separate (Smith, Weiss, and Lehmkuhl, 1996). In close-packed positions stability is facilitated, and often little or no muscular contraction is required to maintain the position during weight bearing. This offers advantages in terms of energy expenditure that can be very valuable in positions such as upright standing. In all other positions, the joint surfaces have less contact and are termed **loose-packed.** In loose-packed positions key capsular and ligamental structures are slack, and motion, rather than joint stability, is facilitated.

Closed and Open Kinematic Chain Movements

In the human body many joints occur in series and often their movements occur together, rather than in isolation. This has led to the use of the engineering term "closed kinematic chain," in which a series

DANCE CUES 1.2

"Stand So That Your Bones Support Your Weight"

Some forms of modern dance encourage students to achieve standing alignment emphasizing support by bones and minimizing muscle contraction to maintain an upright position. Although standing involves many joints, for simplicity we focus on the knee at this point. During standing with the knees straight, a close-packed position of the knee is present, allowing the bones and passive constraints to primarily create stability. However, if the knees are bent either in a standing position or to begin a movement, muscle contraction is immediately required to prevent the knees from buckling. While some schools of dance that emphasize efficiency favor this cue and a more passive approach with standing, other schools prefer a more active stance ("pulling up on the knees") utilizing slight levels of muscle contraction as discussed in chapter 5.

of rigid links are interconnected by a series of pin-center joints such that motion of one link will produce predictable motion in the other joints of the system (Levangie and Norkin, 2001). In the human body, a **kinematic chain** (G. *kinēmatica,* things that move) is represented by a series of joints that link successive body segments or bones. The concept of a **closed kinematic chain,** or closed kinetic chain, is operative when the distal segment is fixed while the proximal segments move, such as when one is in an erect weight-bearing position. In this case, when the knee bends, simultaneous motion in the ankle and hip also occurs. In contrast, when the distal segment moves in space, such as in performing brushes (dégagés), motion at the hip can occur in isolation, without necessarily involving motion of the knee. This is termed an **open kinematic chain,** or open kinetic chain, movement. With this type of movement, the motion of adjacent joints is not predictable, as they may move either independently or together.

In dance, the upper extremity is more commonly used in an open kinematic chain manner such as when the dancer is making gestural movements. However, when used in an open manner, there is often a required linking of segments to achieve the desired aesthetic for use of the arms. This aesthetic often varies markedly between different dance forms and even different choreography within the same dance form. Less frequently the arms are used in a closed kinematic manner, such as when one is

performing weight-supported positions like a handstand. In dance, the lower extremity is commonly used both as a closed and as an open kinematic system, often changing in different phases of the movement or between sides of the body. An example of the former is in a stag leap: Prior to the takeoff the lower extremity is working in a closed manner, while in the air the legs are acting as an open kinematic chain. An example of the latter occurs at the barre; the support leg is working in a closed manner, while the gesture leg is often working as an open kinematic chain as seen in figure 1.17.

The concept of kinematic chains has important implications for understanding movement, injury, and rehabilitation. In terms of movement, one important implication has to do with the potential movement allowed by the whole limb. The total degrees of freedom available for the performance of a multijoint movement is considered the summation of the degrees of freedom derived from all adjacent joints in the chain. So, for example, kicking a ball could be considered to involve an 11-degree-of-freedom system relative to the trunk, with 3df derived from the hip, 2df from the knee, 1df from the ankle, 3df from the tarsals, and 2df from the toes (Hamill and Knutzen, 1995). This summation concept is essential to allow for the complex movements and adjustments required by dance. Implications for injury and injury rehabilitation is addressed in following chapters.

CONCEPT DEMONSTRATION 1.4

Closed and Open Kinematic Chain Movements

Begin standing in fifth position with the arms in low fifth, and perform the following movements, distinguishing between open and closed kinematic chains.

- **Lower extremity movement.** Plié and then bring the left foot up to touch the right knee (retiré). The right leg is working as a closed kinematic chain. How is the left leg working? How does the concept of open and closed kinematic chains relate to the terminology of the support and gesture leg used in dance?

- **Upper extremity movement.** Bring the arms overhead, from low to high fifth position. What type of kinematic chain does the arm movement represent? How could arm movement be changed in dance to create a condition in which the distal segment is fixed?

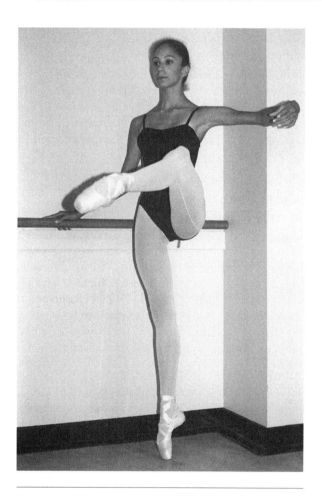

FIGURE 1.17 Open and closed kinematic chain movements. The foot of the support leg is fixed on the ground, and the right leg is functioning as a closed kinematic chain. In contrast, the left foot and the left hand are free to move, and hence these limbs are functioning as open kinematic chains.

Maurya Kerr as a student at Pacific Northwest Ballet School.

Summary

The skeletal system is composed of the bones of the body, the related cartilages and ligaments, and the joints that connect these bones together. Bones can be classified according to their shape as long, short, flat, and irregular bones. Their shape is in accordance with their functions of providing support, protection, sites for muscle attachments, and levers for movement. Although bones have great compressive and tensile strength, they are constantly being remodeled in accordance with applied stresses and the availability of calcium and other key nutrients.

A total of 206 bones come together to form the skeleton. The skeleton can be divided into the axial skeleton and the appendicular skeleton (upper extremity and lower extremity), and adjacent bones within these divisions are connected by fibrous, cartilaginous, or synovial joints. Synovial joints contain a joint cavity and primarily give rise to the movements we associate with the limbs. These synovial joints can be further classified according to their shape and the number of axes and planes of movements they allow. Standardized terminology has been developed to clearly describe the planes, axes, and associated movements of joints. In functional movement, joints serve dual functions of stability and mobility. The demands of these opposite functions can in part be met by the change in stability offered by close- and loose-packed positions. In functional movement, joints often work in conjunction with other joints, rather than in isolation. The concepts of open and closed kinematic chains help describe the potential linkings of adjacent joints.

Study Questions and Applications

1. Describe how long bones grow in width and in length.

2. List and locate, on your own body, the bones that constitute the (a) axial skeleton, (b) upper extremity, and (c) lower extremity.

3. Classify each of the bones that constitute the lower extremity as long, short, flat, or irregular.

4. Standing in anatomical position, demonstrate three dance movements that occur in each of the following planes: sagittal, frontal, and horizontal.

5. Review the joint movements described in table 1.8 and select two movements from dance that exemplify each of these joint movements.

6. Draw a typical synovial joint and label its components. Then, describe the function of each of these components.

7. Contrast and compare the types of joints found in the upper extremity and lower extremity.

8. Describe how the presence of loose- and close-packed positions of the joints could be helpful to meet differing movement demands of joints required by dance.

9. Design a movement sequence that incorporates both open and closed kinematic chain movements for the hip, knee, and ankle. Identify when these joints are working in an open and a closed kinematic chain.

10. A dancer has been having a difficult time performing a pushing movement of the arm with the desired aesthetic. Her teacher has noted that her movement looks "jerky" and lacks the desired smooth coordination.

    a. Describe what joint motions should be occurring at the shoulder, elbow, and wrist.

    b. Describe how the idea of a kinematic chain relates to this movement.

    c. Describe how the movement aesthetic would be different under the following conditions:

       1. Sequential movement starting from the distal and proceeding to the proximal joint

       2. Sequential movement starting from the proximal joint and proceeding to the distal joint

       3. Movement beginning at the elbow, followed by movement at the other two joints

       4. Simultaneous movement at all three joints so that the end position of each joint is reached at the same moment

    d. Identify appropriate cues that could be utilized to try to implement the desired technique adjustments.

CHAPTER TWO

The Muscular System

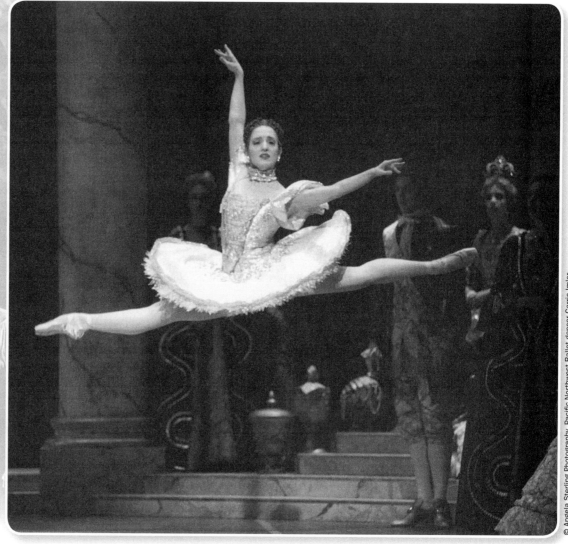

© Angela Sterling Photography. Pacific Northwest Ballet dancer Carrie Imler.

In this chapter we examine the muscular system. It is the muscular system that produces movements of the skeletal system. We could not walk or dance without the motive force provided by our muscles. Muscles have a unique ability to produce tension that is translated to bones to produce joint movement. In addition, muscles can offer constraints to motion when the limits of their extensibility are approached. Hence, adequate flexibility, as well as strength, is essential for the expansive movements encompassed in dance. The large leap (grand jeté en avant) shown in the photo on page 33 exemplifies these demands for both muscular strength and flexibility to project the body through space and achieve the desired lines of the body segments. Learning about how muscles work is key for understanding and describing human movement. Topics covered in this chapter include the following:

- Skeletal muscle structure and function
- Microstructure of skeletal muscle and muscle contraction
- Muscle architecture
- Muscle attachments to bone
- Muscles, levers, and rotary motion
- Types of muscle contraction (tension)
- Muscular considerations in whole body movement
- Learning muscle names and actions

Skeletal Muscle Structure and Function

Muscle cells are the only cells capable of producing active tension and contracting. **Contractility** is the unique ability of muscle tissue to shorten. Some recent texts substitute "the ability to produce tension" for "contractility," since tension produced by muscles does not always result in a shortening of muscles (see Types of Muscle Contraction [Tension] on p. 50 for more information). It is this property of contractility that generates movement of the human body, as well as allows for movements in the heart and other internal organs. There are three types of muscle tissue—smooth muscle, cardiac muscle, and skeletal muscle—shown in table 2.1. **Smooth muscle** forms part of the walls of hollow organs (e.g., bladder, uterus, stomach) and various systems of tubes (e.g., within the circulatory, digestive, respiratory, and reproductive systems). Contraction of smooth muscles helps move substances through organs (such as food through the stomach) and through tubes (such as blood through arteries). Under a light microscope, smooth muscle cells appear long, narrow, and spindle shaped, with a single central nucleus. The cells are very closely aligned to form sheets, and as their name suggests, lacking in cross-striations. Smooth muscle contraction is not under voluntary control; hence this type of muscle is termed involuntary muscle. It also has the ability to maintain tone and contract automatically, without stimulation from the nervous system.

Cardiac muscle is the type of muscle found in the walls of the heart. The contraction of cardiac muscle helps pump blood via blood vessels to the lungs and other parts of the body. Under the light microscope, cardiac muscle fibers have bands, termed striations, that run across the width of the cell. Cardiac muscle fibers are also short and branched with unique junctions, termed intercalated discs, at the abutment of the ends of adjacent cells. Cardiac muscle cells generally contain a single nucleus (uninucleate) but sometimes two (binucleate). Similar to smooth muscle, cardiac muscle is not under voluntary control (involuntary), and due to specialized cells (pacemaker cells) is able to contract automatically, without stimulation from the nervous system.

Skeletal muscle is the type of muscle that attaches to the bones of the skeleton and gives rise to movements at joints. Although influenced by gender, body type, and activity, these muscles make up approximately 40% to 45% of an average adult's body weight (Hall, 1999). Under the light microscope, a skeletal muscle cell is very long, narrow, and cylindrical, with many cross-striations and many nuclei (multinucleate). Unlike smooth and cardiac muscles, which generally work with little conscious control, skeletal muscles are called voluntary because many can be controlled at will. Unlike smooth and cardiac muscles, they cannot contract automatically and instead rely on stimulation from a nerve. Skeletal muscles are also important for the maintenance of posture and positions, stability of joints, shock absorption, support and protection of internal tissues, control of pressures within cavities, and production of body heat. Greater than 75% of the energy utilized with muscle contraction is released as heat (McGinnis, 2005). Because of its importance for human movement, this book focuses on skeletal muscle, and any further reference to muscle will be to skeletal muscle only.

Properties of Skeletal Muscle Tissue

In addition to contractility, skeletal muscle is characterized by the following properties: irritability, extensibility, and elasticity. **Irritability** is the ability to receive and respond to a stimulus, commonly from

TABLE 2.1   Three Types of Muscle Tissue

	A. Smooth muscle	B. Cardiac muscle	C. Skeletal muscle
Appearance	Closely aligned, long, spindle-shaped cells with central nuclei Nonstriated Smooth muscle cell Nuclei	Short, branching, generally uninucleate cells that interdigitate at intercalated discs Striated Myocardial cell Intercalated disc Nucleus	Very long, cylindrical, multinucleate cells Striated Skeletal muscle cell Nuclei
Location	Walls of hollow organs and tubes Smooth muscle of stomach (Longitudinal layer) (Circular layer) (Oblique layer)	Walls of heart Cardiac muscle of heart	Primarily attaches to bones and occasionally to skin Skeletal muscle of gastrocnemius
Function	Propels substances or objects through organs or tubes	Propels blood through blood vessels	Movement, posture, joint stability, shock absorption, facial expressions
Control	Involuntary Automatic contractions	Involuntary Automatic contractions	Voluntary Requires nerve stimulation to contract

35

an associated nerve. The classic response of muscle to this stimulus is to produce tension or contract. The properties of extensibility and elasticity can be better understood if we look at a mechanical model of muscle.

The Mechanical Model of Muscle

A three-component mechanical model has been developed to explain the behavior of muscle (figure 2.1). The ability of muscle to contract resides within very small protein structures found within the muscle cell that are further discussed in the next section of this chapter. These structures are termed the **contractile component** (CC) or **active component** of muscle. However, muscle also contains two **elastic components**—the parallel elastic component and the series elastic component. The contribution of these elastic components does not require active contraction, and hence they are also termed **passive components.** As its name suggests, the parallel elastic component (PEC) lies parallel to the contractile component and is composed of many structures including the connective tissue in muscle, the muscle cell membrane (sarcolemma), and an elastic protein closely associated with the contractile proteins of muscle (titin). Conversely, the series elastic component (SEC) lies in series with the contractile component and consists primarily of the tendon (about 85%), with a much smaller contribution from some of the structures of the contractile component (Alter, 2004; Enoka, 2002; Kreighbaum and Barthels, 1996; Levangie and Norkin, 2001).

These elastic components can be modeled as a spring (figure 2.2), and mechanical energy that is stored in the elastic component of muscle when a stretch is applied can be recovered when the stretch is released (recoverable deformation), just as a spring will quickly recoil to its unextended position when the tension is removed. These elastic components give rise to muscle's property of elasticity. **Elasticity** is the ability of a muscle to return to its resting length after being stretched. In addition, the connective tissue associated with muscle has another property, termed viscosity. **Viscous** or plastic properties are usually modeled by a hydraulic cylinder (dash pot) as shown in figure 2.2 and reflect puttylike behavior, in which the elongation produced by a force remains after the force is removed (permanent deformation). Together, the elastic and viscous properties of connective tissue are termed **viscoelastic,** and it is this viscoelastic response that gives rise to muscle's property of extensibility as seen in figure 2.3. **Extensibility** or distensibility is the ability of muscle to be stretched or to increase in length beyond resting length. The average muscle fiber can be stretched 1.5 times its resting length (Hamilton and Luttgens, 2002). The

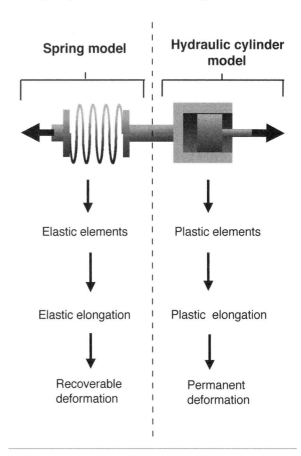

FIGURE 2.2 Viscoelastic properties of connective tissue.

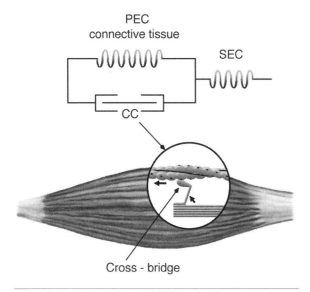

FIGURE 2.1 Three-component mechanical model of muscle.

muscle cannot lengthen on its own; rather a force such as gravity or the contraction of another muscle is required to create this elongation. This characteristic of extensibility is key for allowing the dancer to improve the range of motion permitted at a given joint—that is, flexibility.

The study of this viscoelastic characteristic of muscle has been instrumental in developing current theories of muscle behavior and recommendations for effective muscle conditioning programs such as those for improving flexibility. When a muscle and its related connective tissue are stretched, elongation of both the elastic and viscous elements occurs. However, when the stretch is discontinued the elastic elongation recovers, and only the plastic elongation remains (Taylor et al., 1990). While the elastic elements are influenced only by the magnitude of the applied force, the viscous elements are influenced by temperature, as well as the rate and duration of the applied forces. The behavior of this component can be compared to that of Silly Putty or stiff taffy. A force (i.e., pulling the taffy apart) that is applied slowly and for a long duration, with the taffy warm, produces greater elongation and less tendency for breaking. Thus, to emphasize increases in flexibility that persist over time, the goal is to maximize plastic elongation. This can be achieved by the use of a slow, lower-force, longer-duration stretch applied to warmed muscles. In terms of duration, three repetitions of a 30-second stretch appear to provide most of the potential length changes associated with a given stretch (Garrett, 1991). Conversely, to emphasize greater force production of a muscle, the goal is to maximize elastic elongation. This can be achieved through application of a rapid, higher-force stretch, immediately preceding a shortening (concentric) contraction of the same muscle (see Stretch-Shortening Cycle on p. 54 for more information).

Microstructure of Skeletal Muscle and Muscle Contraction

The structural unit of a muscle is the muscle cell. It has been estimated that the human body contains approximately 270 million muscle cells (Wells and Luttgens, 1976). Because these muscle cells are long and very thin, they are often called muscle fibers. An individual muscle cell generally has a diameter ranging from approximately 0.0004 to 0.004 inches (0.01 to 0.1 millimeters). In contrast, many muscle cells range between 1 and 3 inches (approximately 2.5-7.6 centimeters) in length, and select muscles may be up to even 24 or 28 inches (60 or 70 centimeters) in length (Hamilton and Luttgens, 2002; Rasch and Burke, 1978; Smith, Weiss, and Lehmkuhl, 1996). Skeletal muscle fibers grow in both length and diameter from birth to adulthood, with a five times increase in diameter possible during this period (Hall, 1999). Strength training using heavy resistance and low repetitions can also result in substantial increases in muscle cell diameter, termed **hypertrophy** (G. *hyper*, over + *trophy*, nourishment).

To understand how muscle cells are capable of causing a contraction, it is necessary to look at a single muscle cell on a microscopic level. Each muscle fiber contains specialized protoplasm termed the sarcoplasm, within which is embedded very thin fibers called **myofibrils** (G. *mys*, muscle) that run the length of the muscle cell but are only about four-millionths of an inch (1-2 micrometers) wide (Hamill and Knutzen, 1995). These myofibrils are arranged in a parallel formation within the muscle cell and consist of still finer threads called **myofilaments** (G. *mys*, muscle + L. *filamentum*, thread) that can be either **thick** (primarily containing the protein **myosin**) or **thin** (primarily containing the protein **actin**). These myosin and actin filaments exhibit different light properties under the view of a polarizing microscope and interdigitate in a manner that gives rise to alternating dark and light bands, imparting to skeletal muscle fibers their characteristic striated appearance. As can be seen in figure 2.3, the lighter I band contains only thin filaments (actin), while the darker A band contains thick filaments throughout, with thin filaments extending as far as the H zone. The H zone of the A band contains only thick filaments (myosin) and is lighter than the other portion of the A band. Each I band is bisected transversely by a Z line, and one end of each actin filament within this I band is attached to this Z line. These actin and myosin filaments are organized in repeating segments longitudinally that are termed sarcomeres. The **sarcomere** (G. *sarco*, muscular substance + *meros*, part) is a compartment between consecutive Z lines and is the functional unit of muscle contraction.

The Sliding Filament Theory

The most widely held theory of muscle contraction is called the **sliding filament theory** (Huxley, 1969). As its name implies, this theory holds that the filaments just discussed are the mechanism by which muscles contract. Each myosin filament is surrounded by six actin filaments. Myosin filaments contain crossbridges, and actin filaments contain active sites as shown in figure 2.3. When the muscle is not activated,

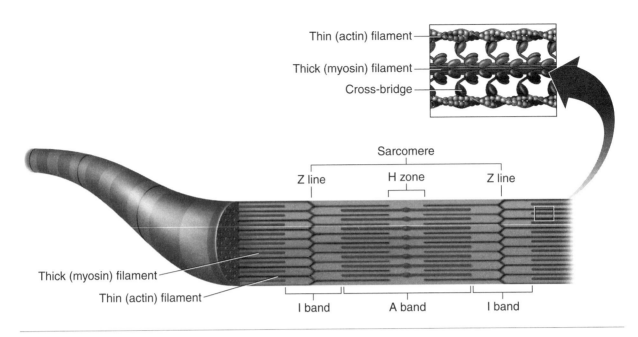

Thin (actin) filament
Thick (myosin) filament
Cross-bridge

Sarcomere

Z line   H zone   Z line

Thick (myosin) filament
Thin (actin) filament

I band   A band   I band

FIGURE 2.3   Microstructure of a skeletal muscle fiber.

Reprinted, by permission, from R.S. Behnke, 2006, *Kinetic anatomy,* 2nd ed. (Champaign, IL: Human Kinetics), p. 14.

the active sites on the actin are blocked. The sliding filament theory holds that activation of a muscle causes a release of calcium from within the muscle fiber. This calcium release changes the configuration of protein molecules (troponin and tropomyosin) so that the active sites on actin are exposed and become available for the myosin cross-bridges to attach to. This attachment, termed coupling, triggers a splitting of the energy molecule adenosine triphosphate (ATP), producing rapid "flexion" of the myosin cross-bridge, which pulls the actin filaments a short distance toward the center of the sarcomere. The cross-bridge then uncouples, and retracts, and the myosin is recharged with another molecule of ATP. It is now ready to react with another active actin site. In this process of cross-bridge coupling, flexion, and uncoupling, the Z lines are drawn in toward the A bands, and the H zone narrows or even disappears as seen in figure 2.4.

Although the amount of shortening of each sarcomere unit is small, the cumulative effect of shortening of the many sarcomere units in series can be marked. For example, a muscle fiber similar in length to that of the biceps brachii has been estimated to have about 40,000 sarcomere units in series; and the sum effect of their shortening would be approximately 1.6 inches (4 centimeters), equivalent to about 40% of the length of the muscle from its position at rest (Smith, Weiss, and Lehmkuhl, 1996). These coupling, flexion, uncoupling, retraction, and recharging processes, known as **cross-bridge cycling,** are

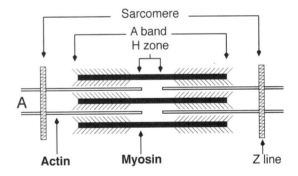

Sarcomere
A band
H zone

A

Actin   Myosin   Z line

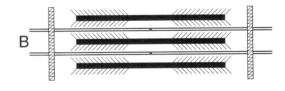

B

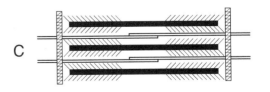

C

FIGURE 2.4   Schema of muscle contraction. (A) Resting state, (B) slight contraction, (C) greater contraction.

repeated hundreds of times in a second to produce the shortening of the sarcomere associated with muscle contraction. And the amount of tension generated by a muscle depends on the average number of links between actin and myosin at a given moment.

As soon as activation of the muscle fiber ends, calcium is rapidly pumped from the vicinity of the myofilaments. This drop in calcium concentration restores the blocking of the sites on actin, returning the filaments to their relaxed, "resting" state.

Muscle Fiber Type

Although all muscle fibers are capable of contracting as just described, there are some important differences in their contractile properties and energy use that are reflected by their classification into two basic types—slow-twitch (Type I) and fast-twitch (Type II) (American College of Sports Medicine [ACSM], 2001). Type II fibers can be further divided into two major subtypes: Type IIa and Type IIb. A third subtype has been identified but appears to occur infrequently, and its characteristics are still under investigation (Wilmore and Costill, 2004). Hence, it will not be further addressed in this text. Type I fibers emphasize energy systems that utilize oxygen (aerobic metabolism), allowing them to remain active for prolonged periods. Type I fibers have a slower contraction time and smaller cross-sectional area, and produce less tension, but have a higher resistance to fatigue than Type II fibers. These fibers are particularly important for carrying out sustained contractions or repetitive low-intensity muscle contractions such as those used with posture, walking, or endurance events (e.g., running a marathon).

In contrast, **Type IIb** fibers favor energy systems that do not depend on oxygen (anaerobic pathways) and are characterized by having the fastest contraction time, the largest diameter, and the greatest force production, but the greatest fatigability of all fiber types. These fibers are particularly important for carrying out short-duration, high-intensity muscle contractions such as used with weight training or with sprint or power events such as the 100 m dash. Lastly, **Type IIa** fiber properties lie between those of Type I and Type IIb fibers, with generally a slightly slower contraction time, smaller diameter, and less force production, but a higher resistance to fatigue than Type IIb fibers. Type IIb fibers become key when a limited endurance element is added to activities, such as with running a mile. Because the characteristics of Type IIa fibers are in between those of Type I and Type IIb fibers, some texts list their characteristics as intermediate. However, because many of these characteristics are still closer to those of Type IIb than Type I fibers, other texts list many of their characteristics as the same as those of Type II. This text combines these approaches to reflect characteristics more closely aligned to Type IIb (hence their name) but different in the direction of Type I fibers as seen in table 2.2.

Although most human muscles contain both slow-twitch and fast-twitch fibers, different proportions exist in line with functional demands. For example, the gastrocnemius is used predominantly for powerful activity such as jumping and has about 50% fast-twitch and 50% slow-twitch fibers in the average individual. In contrast, in the soleus muscle, which is used in more sustained activity and serves key postural functions, the proportion of slow-twitch fibers may be as great as 85% (Smith, Weiss, and Lehmkuhl, 1996). The difference in the role of

TABLE 2.2 Skeletal Muscle Fiber Characteristics

Characteristics	Muscle fiber type		
	Type I	Type IIa	Type IIb
Muscle fiber diameter	Small	Intermediate/large	Large
Color	Red (dark)	Red	White (pale)
Contractile speed	Slow	Fast	Fast
Force production	Low	Intermediate/high	High
Fatigue resistance	High	Moderate	Low
Energy efficiency	High	Intermediate/low	Low
Aerobic capacity	High	Moderate	Low
Anaerobic capacity	Low	High	Highest

such muscles has led to the use of the terms **tonic** or **postural** to describe muscles that have a greater presence of slow-twitch fibers and **phasic** or **nonpostural** to describe muscles that have a greater presence of fast-twitch fibers.

In addition to varying between muscles, percentages of slow-twitch fibers and fast-twitch fibers differ between individuals. Most sedentary individuals have a similar proportion of fast-twitch and slow-twitch fibers in many muscles. However, since fast-twitch fibers are important for generating fast, powerful muscle contractions, athletes like sprinters generally have high proportions of fast-twitch fibers (55-75%). In contrast, since slow-twitch fibers are important for producing repetitive contractions without fatigue, endurance athletes such as distance runners have high proportions (60-90%) of slow-twitch fibers (Powers and Howley, 1990; Takashi, Kumagai, and Brechue, 2000). For example, the gastrocnemius muscle in some elite sprint runners has been shown to be composed of 73% fast-twitch fibers while the gastrocnemius in elite female distance runners contained 69% slow-twitch fibers (Wilmore and Costill, 2004). Ethnicity may also be a factor. For example, individuals of African American descent have been shown to have a higher percentage of fast-twitch fibers than individuals of Caucasian descent (ACSM, 2001).

How much of this composition of fibers is genetically determined and how much of it can be changed by training is still an area of controversy. At this point it appears that genetics is the most fundamental determinant of quantity and distribution of fibers, but heavy training may alter some of the properties of given fibers to allow them to better meet the demands produced by the specific training regime (Gordon and Pattullo, 1993; Nieman, 1999; Wilmore and Costill, 2004). So, for example, dancers who genetically have a higher percentage of fast-twitch fibers may be able to naturally generate more force and potentially jump higher, while dancers with higher percentages of slow-twitch fibers may have advantages in adagio or repetitive movements such as relevés. However, with appropriate training, all dancers can improve their ability to some degree to meet specific dance demands.

Muscle Architecture

In addition to fiber type, the architecture of a given muscle is important for meeting specific demands. Two architectural characteristics that are particularly important are muscle cross-sectional area and fiber arrangement.

Muscle Cross-Sectional Area

Basically, a muscle with more muscle fibers will be capable of producing more force than one with fewer fibers. Muscle fibers usually lie parallel to each other, and so the cross-sectional area reflects to some degree the number of fibers and relates to force production. Although this idea of a direct relationship between cross-sectional area and the number of muscle fibers is complicated by different fiber arrangements and the fact that different fibers have different diameters due to fiber types and hypertrophy, the concept still holds that a larger muscle with a greater cross-sectional area can produce more force than a smaller muscle with a smaller cross-sectional area. So, for example, the gluteus maximus can produce more force than one of the hamstring muscles, in part due to a greater cross-sectional area. Furthermore, strength training will generally cause an increase in the cross-sectional area within the same muscle (hypertrophy) and will allow for greater force production.

Fiber Arrangement

Muscle fibers in a whole muscle occur in two primary arrangements—fusiform and penniform—with many variations within each of these types. With **fusiform** (L. *fusus*, spindle + *forma*, form), also termed longitudinal arrangements, muscle fibers run close to parallel with the muscle's long axis as seen in figure 2.5A. This structure allows for relatively few fibers per unit area, and so offers a disadvantage in terms of force production capacity. However, in this arrangement muscle fibers are generally longer, and so there is an advantage in terms of how much shortening of the muscle can occur. When sarcomeres are fully contracted, they can reduce the length of a muscle fiber by 30% to 70% of its original resting length, with the average muscle fiber shortening about 50% (Hamill and Knutzen, 1995; Levangie and Norkin, 2001; Pitt-Brooke, 1998). So, for example, a 50% shortening of a muscle fiber of the sartorius, which is about 17.6 inches (448 millimeters) long (Enoka, 2002), would represent about 8.8 inches (224 millimeters) of shortening; 50% shortening of the vasti muscle fibers (penniform muscles), which are about 2.8 inches (72 millimeters) long, would only represent a decrease in length of about 1.4 inches (36 millimeters). Furthermore, due to the lengthwise arrangement of fibers, shortening of fibers translates into almost equivalent shortening of fusiform muscles as a whole. Hence, muscles with such an arrangement favor moving the limbs through space with greater range or speed. Examples of fusiform muscles are

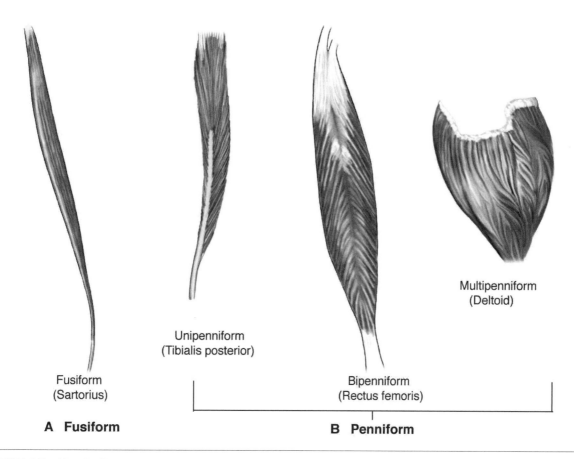

A Fusiform

Fusiform
(Sartorius)

Unipenniform
(Tibialis posterior)

B Penniform

Bipenniform
(Rectus femoris)

Multipenniform
(Deltoid)

FIGURE 2.5 Muscle fiber arrangement. (A) Fusiform, (B) penniform.

the biceps brachii, pectineus, adductor brevis, and the very long and thin sartorius muscle.

In contrast, with **penniform** (L. *penna*, feather + *forma*, form) or pennate muscles, fibers run at an angle relative to the muscle's longitudinal axis as seen in figure 2.5B. This diagonal arrangement, similar to the design of a feather, allows more fibers in a given volume of muscle (greater physiological cross-sectional area) and hence the ability to produce greater force. However, since these fibers tend to be shorter and are also at an angle to the long axis of the muscle, a 50% shortening of a fiber in these muscles results in less shortening of the muscle as a whole. So greater force production is gained at the cost of reduced speed and range of motion. Approximately three-fourths of the muscles in the human body follow this penniform arrangement, including many muscles of the limbs such as the gluteus maximus, quadriceps femoris, deltoid, tibialis posterior, and gastrocnemius.

Muscle Attachments to Bone

Connective tissue, including the endomysium, perimysium, and epimysium, is intimately related to muscle tissue and is key for providing form and for attaching muscles to their respective bones. As shown in figure 2.6, individual muscle cells are covered by a very fine sheath termed the **endomysium** (G. *endon*, within + *mys*, muscle), while bundles of about 100 to 200 muscle fibers (fascicles) are covered by a dense connective sheath termed the **perimysium** (G. *peri*, around + *mys*, muscle) and the whole muscle itself is covered by another membrane called the **epimysium** (G. *epi*, upon + *mys*, muscle). The central part of a muscle, which tends to be thicker and in which the contractile cells predominate, is called the **muscle belly.** Toward the ends of the muscle belly, the muscle cells end; but the connective tissue coverings continue to attach the muscle to one or more bones: directly (e.g., trapezius, figure 2.7A), via a cordlike or flat band called a **tendon** (e.g., biceps brachii, figure 2.7B), or via a sheetlike structure of fibrous tissue called an **aponeurosis** (e.g., latissimus dorsi, figure 2.7C). Tendons (L. *tendo*, to stretch out, extend) are the most common form of attachment and serve to concentrate the pull of the muscle to a small area on the bone. Tendons are very strong. Their tensile strength has been estimated to be 4,169 pounds (1,891 kilograms) per square inch in an adult

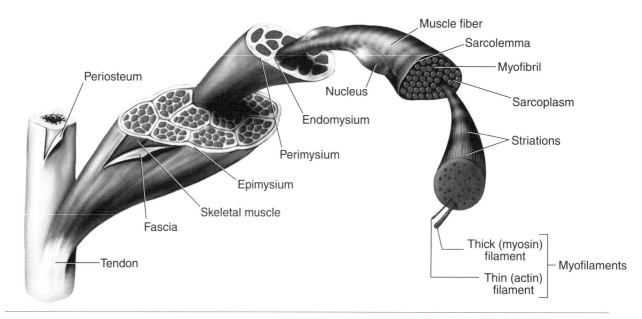

FIGURE 2.6   Structure of skeletal muscle and related connective tissue.

Reprinted, by permission, from R.S. Behnke, 2006, *Kinetic anatomy,* 2nd ed. (Champaign, IL: Human Kinetics), p. 14.

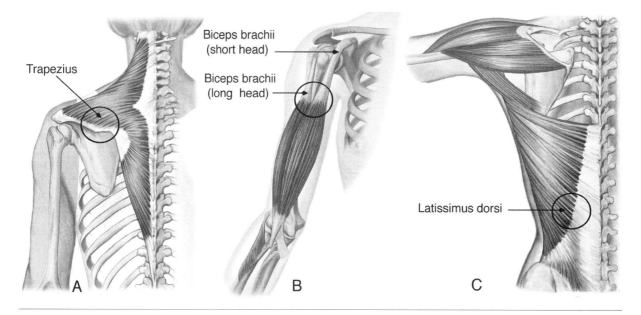

FIGURE 2.7   Attachments of muscles onto bones (A) directly, or indirectly through a (B) tendon or (C) aponeurosis.

(Rasch and Burke, 1978), and the Achilles tendon can resist tensile loads equal to or greater than steel of similar dimensions (Hamill and Knutzen, 1995). Due to the large forces transmitted by tendons and aponeuroses (G. *apon,* from + *neuron,* sinew), the attachment of a tendon often gives rise to a raised tubercle, and an aponeurosis to a line or ridge on the bone to which it attaches.

Origin and Insertion

These connective tissue attachments of muscles to bones have historically been termed the **origin** and **insertion** of a muscle; the origin generally stays stationary as the segment containing the insertion moves. However, more recent texts, including this text, have elected to substitute the terms **proximal** attachment and **distal attachment.** While this termi-nology works well for the extremities, it is sometimes necessary to use additional terminology for the head, neck, and trunk, such as superior attach-ment/inferior attachment or medial attachment/lateral attachment. The use of these alternative terms to origin and insertion better reflect the con-cept that when a muscle contracts, it exerts equal force on each attachment and tends to pull both attachments toward each other. Which end actually moves depends on the other forces that come into play, such as the relative mass of the adjacent seg-ments or the stabilizing action of adjacent muscles, and whether the distal segment of the limb is fixed or moving. For example, when flexing the elbow as you lift a weight (biceps curl), the proximal attachment stays stationary, and it is the forearm and distal attach-ment of the biceps brachii that move. In many everyday movements of the limbs (espe-cially of the upper extremity), this pattern occurs where the distal segment moves while proximal segments are readily stabilized due to greater mass. It is also generally the easiest way to think about learning the actions of a given muscle and can be termed the **customary action** of a muscle. However, there are cases in functional movement where the distal segment is stationary and the proximal segment moves, or where both segments simul-taneously move. When the proximal segment moves, it can be termed a **reversal of customary action** of a muscle. A pull-up offers an example of a reversal of customary action for the biceps brachii, where the proximal segments and attachments (humerus and trunk) move, while the distal segment (forearm) stays sta-tionary with the hands fixed on the pull-up bar. Similarly, lifting the thigh to the front while the trunk stays station-ary (figure 2.8A) would reflect customary action, whereas lift-ing the trunk while the thigh stays stationary would reflect

reversal of customary action of the iliopsoas muscle (figure 2.8B).

Line of Pull of a Muscle

The location of the proximal and distal attachments of a muscle relative to the axis of the joint is funda-mental in determining the type of joint movement that will occur. Although technically the line of action or **line of pull** of a muscle is the net effect (resultant) of applied forces on a common point of attach-ment of every fiber contained within a given muscle (Levangie and Norkin, 2001), one can roughly approximate this resultant force, or "pull," by draw-ing an imaginary double-headed arrow with its base at each attachment and pointing toward the center of the muscle as seen in figure 2.9A. In instances in

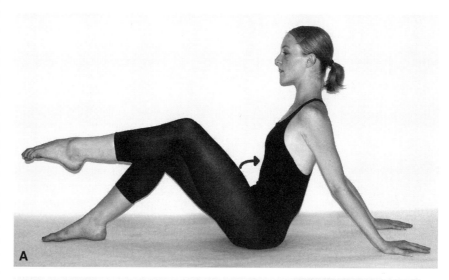

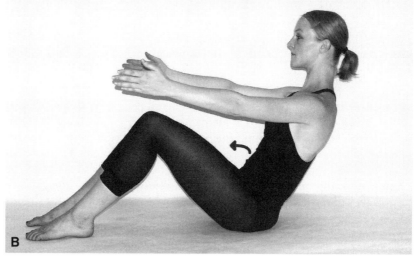

FIGURE 2.8   Customary and reverse muscle actions of the iliopsoas. (A) Raising the thigh and (B) raising the trunk.

Sacramento Ballet dancer Merett Miller.

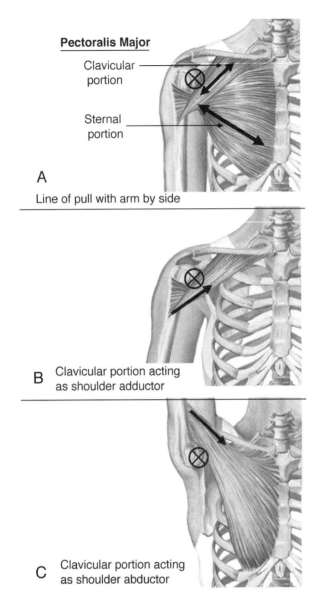

Pectoralis Major

Clavicular portion

Sternal portion

A

Line of pull with arm by side

B Clavicular portion acting as shoulder adductor

C Clavicular portion acting as shoulder abductor

FIGURE 2.9   Change in line of pull and action of the pectoralis major with different angles of shoulder abduction.

which muscles have broad attachments, the arrow would be drawn to bisect the broad attachment. In some cases with very broad or multiple proximal or distal attachments, multiple arrows may need to be used, and different portions of the muscle may have different actions due to different lines of pull relative to the axes of movement. In such instances, the usual way of reflecting this difference in action is to divide the muscle into portions such as the upper (clavicular) and lower (sternal) portions of the pectoralis major (figure 2.9A). Although simplistic, and not inclusive of all of the factors involved in an accurate mathematical analysis of a muscle's line of

pull, this is an effective tool for deducing the actions of a given muscle in the tradition of Platzer (1978) and Kreighbaum and Barthels (1996). Readers are encouraged to approach learning muscle actions in this manner rather than by rote memorization to make the learning process easier, to provide a self-check procedure, and to promote retention. If just the location and line of pull of a muscle are learned, the actions can be figured out logically, or conjectured actions can be evaluated. To facilitate this process, summary figures showing the approximate line of pull of primary muscles of their respective joints are provided in chapters 3 through 7.

When applying this line of pull analysis to a specific movement, rather than a specific muscle, the double-headed arrow is replaced by an arrow with one head. The direction of this arrow reflects the pull of the muscle on the body segment that is moving in the given movement.

It is also important to realize that the line of pull of a muscle may change its relation to the axis of rotation of a given joint in different ranges of motion, causing the muscle to change its action. For example, the upper (clavicular) portion of the pectoralis major acts as an adductor of the shoulder when the arm is low as seen in figure 2.9B; but when the arm is brought above shoulder height (90° shoulder abduction), the line of pull shifts to above the axis of rotation of the shoulder and the clavicular portion of the pectoralis major becomes an abductor of the shoulder as seen in figure 2.9C. In dance, the same change in the line of pull occurs when raising the arms to the side from low to high fifth, and the dancer can palpate contraction of the pectoralis major in the upper ranges of the movement.

Muscles, Levers, and Rotary Motion

When force is applied to a system that is not restricted at some point, motion occurs along a straight line; that is, **linear motion** occurs. However, as previously described, in the human body, bones are restricted at joints; therefore when a muscle contracts, its attachments produce rotation of the associated bone or body segments about its joint axis or axes. This form of motion is called **rotary** or **angular motion,** and it occurs in all types of synovial joints except gliding joints. Learning about angular motion and levers is important for appreciating how changing the body configuration, such as having the knee bent versus straight, profoundly influences the forces required to execute a movement.

Different Actions of Pectoralis Major

The differing functions of the clavicular and sternal portions of the pectoralis major can be demonstrated with the following exercise.

- **Shoulder flexion and extension.** Sit with your hands clasped at shoulder height with both elbows extended. Pull down with the right arm (shoulder extension) and up with the left arm (shoulder flexion) simultaneously such that no net movement of the shoulders occurs. Note the lower sternal portion of the pectoralis major contracting on the right side of your chest and the upper clavicular portion of the pectoralis major contracting on the left side of your chest.

- **Shoulder horizontal adduction.** Press both your hands and arms toward each other so that no net movement of the shoulder occurs (isometric horizontal adduction). Note the clavicular and sternal portions of the pectoralis major contracting on both the right and left sides of your chest.

It is easier to understand rotary motion if we look at how a lever works. Put simply, a **lever** is a rigid bar revolving about a fixed point called the **axis,** pivot, or fulcrum. In the human body, bones serve as levers, and the interposed joint serves as the axis (A). Muscles attach to the levers or bones, and when they contract they generally produce rotary motion about the fixed or relatively fixed axis of the joint (in reality, the axis of joints tends to shift slightly with different ranges of motion). This tendency of muscles to produce rotation in one direction, termed **effort** (E), is countered by the tendency of the **resistance** to produce rotation in the opposite direction (R). Which of these three components—effort, axis, or resistance—is between the other two determines which of the three classes a lever belongs to as shown in figure 2.10. It is easier to remember the difference between levers if you remember that the middle components spell "ARE" when you proceed from first- to third-class levers. So, with a **first-class lever** the axis is in the middle, and effort and resistance are on opposite sides of this axis. This arrangement can be used for balance or to gain either effective force or range of motion, depending on the relative distances of effort and resistance from the axis. Seesaws, scissors, and crowbars can function as first-class levers. In the body, the atlanto-occipital joint (A) functions in a first-class lever system, where the weight of the head (R) is balanced by the extensor muscles of the head/neck (E).

With a **second-class lever,** the resistance is between the axis and effort, making the distance of the effort from the axis always greater than the distance of the resistance. This arrangement magnifies the effective-ness of the effort, allowing for less force to be used to overcome a given resistance. The wheelbarrow, nutcracker, and lug nut wrench can all function as second-class levers. This type of lever probably does not exist in its pure form in the human body. However, there are cases in closed kinematic chain movements in which the muscle acts on the proximal segment while the distal segment (e.g., foot or hand) is fixed, so that the distal portion of the body acts like a third-class lever. For example, in a relevé, the dancer rises on the toes (metatarsophalangeal joints—A) when the weight of the body (R) is overcome by contraction of the calf muscles (E).

In the **third-class lever,** the effort lies between the resistance and the axis, making the distance of the resistance from the axis always greater than the distance of the effort. This arrangement favors range of motion and speed, at the expense of the effective-ness of the force. Tweezers and many sport implements (bats, rackets, paddles) are used as third-class levers. Most muscles of the human body when they act in open kinematic chain movements function as third-class levers. An example is the deltoid muscle (E) acting to produce abduction of the arm (R) at the glenohumeral joint (A).

Torque (Moment of Force)

Adding a little more detail to this concept, the capacity or effectiveness of a force to produce rotation is termed **torque** (L. *torqueo,* to twist) or **moment of force.** The amount of torque acting to rotate a given system can be calculated by multiplying the amount of force times the perpendicular distance

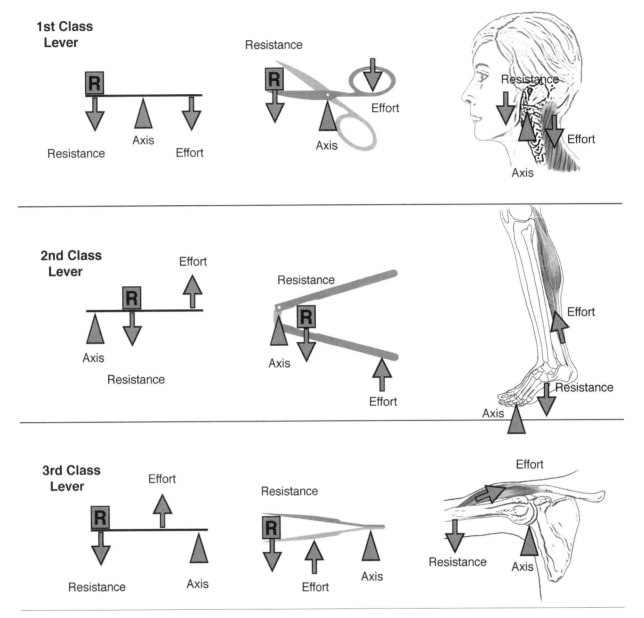

FIGURE 2.10   Three classes of lever systems used in human movement.

from the line of action of the force to the axis of rotation or potential rotation. This latter quantity (perpendicular distance from the line of force to the axis of rotation) is termed the force arm or **moment arm.** The key point here is that it is not just the magnitude of the force but also how far away from the axis (e.g., the joint) that this force is acting that is vital in determining its effect. So, when analyzing joint movement, the force resulting from muscle contraction can be termed the effort (E); the line of this force would be the line of pull of the muscle, and the point of application of this force would be the muscle attachment to the bone. So, as can be seen in figure 2.11, torque of the muscle (T) =

effort (E) × effort arm (EA). However, this torque related to contraction of the muscles trying to effect a given motion is countered by the torque related to the resistance to this motion. When the torque of the resistance is due to external forces such as the effect of gravity on a dumbbell or a body segment, then the torque of the resistance = resistance (R) × resistance arm (RA).

Mechanical Advantage

The relation of the moment arm of the effort to the moment arm of the resistance has important consequences for the potential to overcome resistance and

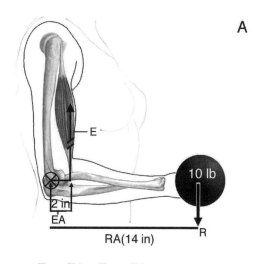

A

$$E \times EA = R \times RA$$

$$E = \frac{R \times RA}{EA} = \frac{10 \text{ lb} \times 14 \text{ in}}{2 \text{ in}} = 70 \text{ lb}$$

$$\text{Mechanical advantage} = \frac{EA}{RA} = \frac{2 \text{ in}}{14 \text{ in}} = \frac{1}{7} \quad B$$

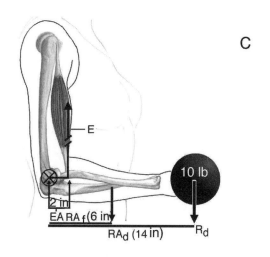

C

$$E \times EA = R_1 \times RA_1 + R_2 \times RA_2$$

$$E = \frac{R_f \times RA_f + R_d \times RA_d}{EA}$$

$$E = \frac{(3 \text{ lb} \times 6 \text{ in}) + (10 \text{ lb} \times 14 \text{ in})}{2 \text{ in}} = 79 \text{ lb}$$

FIGURE 2.11   Levers and torque. (A) Biceps force required to counter dumbbell torque; (B) mechanical advantage; (C) biceps force required to counter forearm and dumbbell torque.

is called the **mechanical advantage** (EA/RA). If the effort arm and resistance arm were of equal length, then this would yield a mechanical advantage of 1 and would mean that if you wanted to hold a 15-pound (6.8-kilogram) weight, it would take about 15 pounds of muscle force to counterbalance this weight. However, throughout most human limbs, third-class levers predominate, where EA is much smaller than RA as shown in figure 2.11A. Since in third-class levers the effort is located between the axis and resistance, RA always must be greater than EA and the mechanical advantage must always be less than 1 (figure 2.11B). Furthermore, muscle attachments are usually very close to the joint (axis), making EA very small relative to RA with mechanical advantages often 0.1 or even lower (Smith, Weiss, and Lehmkuhl, 1996).

This gives the limbs very low mechanical advantage where very large forces have to be generated to overcome relatively small resistances. For example, as shown in figure 2.11C, about 79 pounds (351 N) of force must be exerted by the biceps brachii to counterbalance holding a 10-pound (4.5-kilogram) weight in the hand. This calculation, in contrast to the calculation shown in figure 2.11A, takes into account the contribution of the weight of the forearm, as well as the weight of the dumbbell. When doing a calculation where the external weight is large (e.g., lifting another dancer), the weight of the arm may be excluded for purposes of simplicity and because its contribution to the torque produced by the resistance is relatively small. However, in other instances, such as when lifting a lower limb in dance class (e.g., side extension), consideration of the weight of this limb is vital, and it is primarily the torque produced by the weight of the leg that must be overcome by the muscles of the hip in order to effect the desired movement.

However, whether the weight of the limb is key or not, the point remains that large forces have to be generated by muscles to overcome much smaller resistances, and the triceps brachii must exert about 222 pounds (987 N) of force in order for the hand to press down with 20 pounds (89 N) of force on a scale. In cases in which the elbow is extended and the resistance arm is greater, the torque produced by a 10-pound weight would be approximately 20 foot-pounds at shoulder height as shown in figure 2.12A, and about 300 pounds (1,335 N) of tension in the deltoid may be necessary to raise the arm to this height (Rasch and Burke, 1978). So, in human limbs this prevalence of third-class levers represents a grave disadvantage in terms of mechanical advantage and has important implications for injury predisposition. However, this arrangement does foster a large range

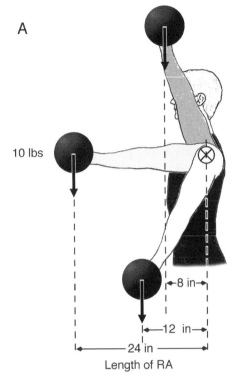

A

10 lbs

←8 in→

←12 in→

←————24 in————→

Length of RA

T 20° = 10 lb × 24 in = 240 in.lbs = 20 ft.lbs

T 90° = 10 lb × 12 in = 120 in.lbs = 10 ft.lbs

T 155° = 10 lb × 8 in = 80 in.lbs = 6.7 ft.lbs

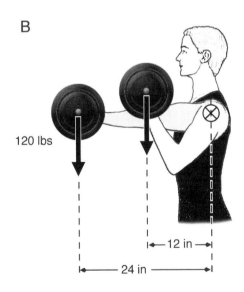

B

120 lbs

←12 in→

←————24 in————→

T elbows straight = 120 lb × 24 in = 2,880 in.lbs
= 240 ft.lbs

T elbows bent = 120 lb × 12 in = 1,440 in.lbs
= 120 ft.lbs

FIGURE 2.12 Change in resistance torque with (A) change in shoulder joint angle and (B) change in shoulder and elbow joint angle.

of motion of the end of the lever and a potential advantage in terms of speed of movement of this distal segment. So, although a large amount of force of the deltoid would be required to overcome the 10-pound dumbbell, a small amount of shortening of the deltoid would result in a much greater excursion of the hand. This ability to move the hand or foot through a very large range of motion, and if desired, at a very high velocity, is commonly utilized in dance and many other human movements.

Equilibrium Versus Movement

Lastly, the relationship of the net torque of the muscle relative to the resistance has important implications for joint movement. In essence, if the torque of the muscle is exactly equal to the torque of the resistance, the system is in **equilibrium** (Fr. *aequus*, equal + *libra*, a balance) and no net movement will occur. If the torque of the muscle (effort) is greater than the torque of the resistance, joint rotation will occur in the direction of the muscle's pull. And, if torque of the resistance is greater than that of the muscle, joint rotation will occur in the direction of the resistance (table 2.3).

Applying these concepts to dance, when you hold another dancer at shoulder height, the torque of the muscles must be equal to the torque of the dancer (e.g., weight of dancer × perpendicular distance to shoulder joint axis). When you lift the dancer, muscle torque is greater than resistance (dancer) torque; and when you lower the dancer, muscle torque is less than the torque produced by the dancer. Furthermore, as illustrated in figure 2.12B, if you imagine the 120-pound weight is a dancer, moving the dancer closer to you when you lift would dramatically reduce the torque produced by the dancer and the amount of muscle force needed to lift the dancer. Conversely, moving the dancer farther away when you lift would dramatically increase the muscle force required to carry out the movement. Taking this concept into consideration, it is easy to understand how functional human movement often incorporates bending the limbs (elbows, knees) to shorten the lever arms when reducing resistance torque would be advantageous. It also explains why a very long-limbed person would have to exert significantly greater muscular effort than one with shorter limbs to lift a dance partner of a given weight.

Angle of Muscle Attachment

While the moment arm of the resistance is key in determining resistance torque, the effectiveness of

The Influence of Moment Arms on Torque

Perform the following movements while sitting or standing.

· **Use of a long moment arm.** Hold your dance bag or another heavy object at shoulder height with your elbows extended. Think about the distance your bag is from your shoulder, that is, the moment arm of the resistance, and the large torque that this bag would exert. Note the amount of muscular effort that is required to hold the bag in place.

· **Shortening the moment arm.** Bend your elbows, bringing your bag close to your chest at shoulder height. Notice the change in the moment arm of the resistance. Why does your bag feel lighter, and why is less muscular effort required to hold it at shoulder height?

· **Application to other dance movements.** Now consider the weight of your leg as the resistance. How would bending your knee for a développé versus lifting the leg with your knee straight make it easier to lift the leg higher?

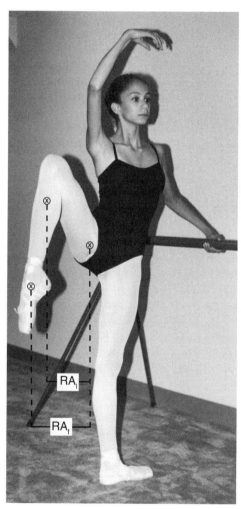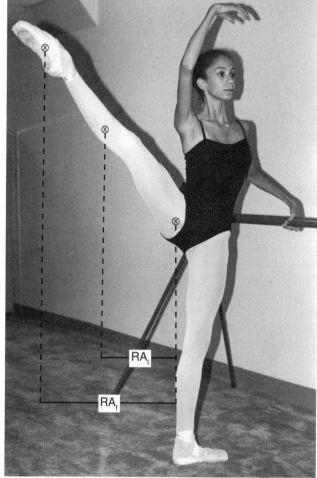

RA_l = moment arm of leg
RA_f = moment arm of foot

TABLE 2.3   Relationship of Net Torque, Joint Movement, and Type of Muscle Contraction

Type of Muscle Contraction	Concentric	Isometric	Eccentric
	Elbow flexion E R ⊗ A	No elbow movement E R ⊗ B	Elbow extension E ⊗ R C
Torque Relationship	E x EA > R x RA	E x EA = R x RA	R x RA > E x EA
Net Movement	Counterclockwise rotary movement in direction of muscle pull	No movement	Clockwise rotary movement in direction of resistance

the muscle force in producing desired rotation is greatly influenced by the angle of the muscle's attachment relative to the bone. The muscle force or effort has a direction determined by its angle of attachment and a magnitude determined by how hard the muscle is contracting, and hence is a **vector.** A basic property of vectors is that they can be resolved into vertical or perpendicular and horizontal or parallel components. In the human body, the perpendicular component of the muscle effort will tend to produce rotation of the joint and hence is termed the **rotary component,** as shown in figure 2.13. At all angles of pull other than 90°, the **parallel component** (running parallel to the distal bone and through the axis of the joint) of the muscle effort will tend to pull the distal bone toward the joint (stabilizing) or away from the joint (dislocating), depending on the joint angle. So, at angles less than 90°, only part of the muscle effort will produce rotation (rotary component), while part contributes to joint stability (parallel component), as seen in figure 2.13A. This offers a disadvantage for movement but an advantage for joint stability that can be particularly useful when the limbs are weightbearing. When a muscle's angle of pull is perpendicular (90°) to the bone on which it is pulling, virtually all of the muscle's effort will contribute to joint rotation (figure 2.13B), an optimal situation in favor of movement. Lastly, when the muscle's angle of pull is greater than 90°, again only part of the muscle effort will produce joint rotation (rotary component), while part acts to dislocate the joint (parallel component), as seen in figure 2.13C. For

this reason, a joint that is loaded in extreme flexion, such as during dance floorwork, is at heightened risk for injury. However, careful simultaneous use of muscles that tend to dislocate the joint in the opposite direction can be used to help protect and stabilize the joint.

Types of Muscle Contraction (Tension)

The relationship of net torque of the muscle relative to the net resistance previously discussed can also be associated with types of muscle contraction or tension. Before looking at possible types of muscle contraction, it is important to remember the sliding-filament theory and to recall that this muscle tension can only pull the ends of the muscles toward each other (termed the law of approximation) and not push them away. This gives rise to the commonly used statement that "muscles can only pull and not push." However, although the same internal process of cross-bridge formation is occurring within a muscle cell, the muscle as a whole may shorten, lengthen, or stay the same length, depending on whether the torque resulting from the contraction of the muscle is more than, less than, or the same as the resistance torque. These differences have traditionally been described as types of muscle contractions. However, because contraction implies "shortening," some authors prefer the terminology "types of muscle tension."

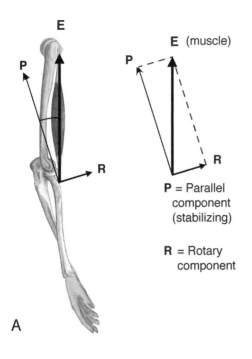

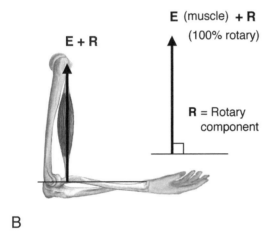

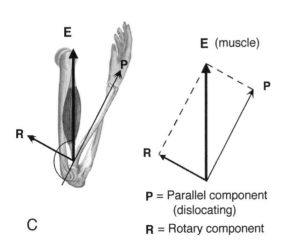

FIGURE 2.13   Influence of angle of muscle attachment on rotary and parallel components of muscle force.

Dynamic Muscle Contraction

Dynamic muscle contraction or tension occurs when there is a change in length of the involved muscle and accompanying observable joint movement. There are two types of dynamic (historically termed **isotonic**) contractions—concentric and eccentric.

Concentric Contraction

A **concentric muscle contraction** or tension involves a shortening of the muscle and resultant visible joint movement (e.g., flexion, abduction) in the direction of the action of the primary muscle. Concentric (G. *con*, with + *kentron*, center) loosely means "toward the center"; and with this type of contraction, both attachments of the muscle will tend to be pulled toward each other as the muscle shortens. On the sarcomere level, actin is being pulled toward the center of the sarcomere with each successive cross-bridge formation. This is the classic way we think of muscle contraction, and the concentric contraction is the basis for charts that list the action or actions of a given muscle. With concentric contractions the torque from the muscle or muscle group is greater than that of the resistance, and joint movement is in the same direction as the torque generated by the muscle or muscle group. For example, a concentric contraction occurs in a biceps curl exercise on the up-phase of the movement (table 2.3A) because the torque of the elbow flexors (including the biceps brachii) is greater than the resistance torque produced by the weight of the dumbbell and forearm.

Concentric contractions are commonly used on the up-phase of movements in dance such as rising from a plié, the takeoff phase of a jump, or raising the arms overhead.

Eccentric Contraction

An **eccentric contraction** or tension involves a "lengthening" of the muscle (i.e., the distance between origin and insertion gets greater) as visible joint motion is occurring. Eccentric (G. *ek*, out + *kentron*, center) loosely means "away from the center," and with eccentric contractions the resistance is "lengthening" the muscle while the muscle is contracting to control the effect of the resistance. On the sarcomere level, the actin go away from the center of the sarcomere, and cross-bridges are broken and then reformed as the muscle lengthens (Levangie and Norkin, 2001). In most cases, the muscle is not actually "lengthening" beyond resting length, but rather gradually decreasing the degree of contraction from its shortened (contracted position) toward its resting length. With eccentric contractions,

"Pull Up Your Knees"

While some schools prefer a more relaxed stance, other schools of dance encourage students to "pull up the knees" on the support leg when working at the barre or center floor. This cue is often further elaborated by encouraging students to not let the thigh muscles be "relaxed," the kneecaps be "loose," or the support knee bend or "wobble." From an anatomical perspective, tightening the quadriceps femoris muscle can pull the patella upward, add the desired tension to the thigh, offer joint stability (large parallel stabilizing component), and prevent the knee from bending. Although a maximum contraction of the quadriceps is not recommended due to the aesthetic in many dance forms to avoid overdevelopment of the thighs and from a perspective of desired movement efficiency, a slight contraction of the quadriceps can help stabilize the support knee and prepare the muscles for necessary rapid slight adjustments as the gesture leg is moving. Tensing muscles around a joint can enhance some of the muscle receptors' sensitivity to stretch and markedly enhance proprioception at that joint (Irrgang and Neri, 2000). It can also help counter the tendency that some dancers have of relying too much on passive constraints such as the ligaments for stability.

Some dancers, however, tend to create a hyperextended position of the knee when they contract the quadriceps. In these cases, cueing to "lightly pull the kneecap up versus back," or cueing to "gently pull up both the front and back of your knees" may be helpful. In the latter case the desire is to generate a slight co-contraction of the quadriceps and hamstrings that can create a balanced stability and readiness with the hamstrings (knee flexors) acting to prevent potential knee hyperextension that is sometimes associated with excessive contraction of the quadriceps femoris. Some examples of electromyography recordings from the quadriceps femoris, hamstrings, and adductors from selected dancers are shown later in the chapter to demonstrate the individual differences in muscle activation associated with standing "in preparation" in turned-out first position (see Tests and Measurements 2.1 on p. 64).

---

the torque produced by the resistance is greater than the torque produced by the muscle, and the direction of movement is opposite to that of the muscle torque and in the same direction as that of the resistance.

In human movement, this type of contraction is commonly used to control the effects of gravity, to decelerate body segments, and to help absorb shock loads (Dye and Vaupel, 2000). For example, in the down-phase of the biceps curl (table 2.3C), gravity is the external force that is producing the movement, and the elbow flexors are working eccentrically to help control the movement. If the elbow flexors were not used, gravity would make the weight drop very rapidly, potentially causing joint injury. In this case the resistance torque is greater than that of the muscles. It is important to notice that even though elbow extension is occurring (due to the effects of gravity), it is the elbow flexors and not the elbow extensors that are being used to control this extension. So, the same muscle group is working on the up-phase as on the down-phase, only with a concentric and eccentric contraction, respectively. Eccentric contractions are

commonly used on the down-phase of movements in dance, such as the descent of a plié, landing from a jump, or lowering the arms from overhead to the sides of the body.

Static (Isometric) Muscle Contraction

A **static** or **isometric contraction** (G. *iso*, same + *metron*, measure) loosely means "equal length" and involves a partial or complete contraction of a muscle where no visible joint movement occurs. On a sarcomere level, there is a small initial pulling of the actin toward the center of the sarcomere until the slack is taken out of the muscle-tendon complex as a whole, and then cross-bridge formation cyclically occurs at the same sites. So, although there is active tension being generated by the involved muscle, the torque generated by the muscle is being exactly counterbalanced by that of the resistance such that no net movement occurs. The resistance can be from internal forces generated from contracting muscles with oppposite actions or the result of an external force such as another person, a weight, or gravity.

Concentric, Eccentric, and Isometric Muscle Contractions

Perform a very slow développé to the front.

- **Analysis of contraction type.** Analyze whether an isometric, concentric, or eccentric contraction of the hip flexors would be used on the following phases of the movement:
  - Up-phase
  - Hold-phase
  - Down-phase
- **Influence of tempo.** Perform this same movement more quickly and speculate on any changes in muscle action that might occur, particularly on the down-phase.

DANCE CUES 2.2

"Release and Recover"

Some styles of choreography encourage dancers to "drop" or "release" their body weight and then "catch" or "recover" the weight to create a pause or change in the direction of the movement. When the center of mass of a body segment such as the head, arm, or upper torso is moved out of equilibrium, such as by bringing the segment forward, gravity will tend to make it fall toward the floor. In dance, this dilemma can be dealt with in many ways. One approach is to use the muscles that oppose the influence of gravity eccentrically in a constant, controlled manner so that the movement can be stopped at any instant. Another approach is to momentarily let the body segments "fall" under the influence of gravity, and then rapidly use the muscles that oppose gravity eccentrically to decelerate the segments in accordance with the desired movement path. Although the look and feel of the movements are quite different, it is important to realize that muscles are still required to shape the movement and oppose gravity. So, care should be taken to avoid cues suggesting that muscles are not used, or that you can move from your bones alone. If we did not use our muscles we would collapse to the floor and would be unable to get up.

For example, an isometric contraction of the elbow flexors would be operative when one is holding the dumbbell at a given angle and not letting that joint angle change (table 2.3B). Isometric contractions are also used posturally to maintain a position of parts of the body or the whole body. For example, in upright standing, the soleus muscle generally contracts isometrically to prevent the body from falling forward. In dance, isometric contractions play a vital role in preventing undesired compensations of the body, as well as maintaining desired positions of the body and its segments. For example, when the dancer is working at the barre, isometric contractions are commonly used to maintain desired positions of the support leg, torso, and the arm on the barre.

Muscular Considerations in Whole Body Movement

Much of this chapter has focused on principles related to a single muscle. However, in most functional movement there is well-orchestrated contribution of many muscles at many joints. When trying to understand such whole body movements, some additional important considerations include use of the stretch-shortening cycle, the different roles muscles can play when they are acting simultaneously, how muscles can work as force couples, and the unique challenges that arise with muscles that cross multiple joints.

Stretch-Shortening Cycle

In some movements, a muscle is used eccentrically immediately preceding use of the same muscle concentrically. This is termed the **stretch-shortening cycle** (SSC), or prestretch. When an active muscle is stretched, mechanical energy is stored in the elastic component of the muscle, which is then released during the immediately following shortening contraction, resulting in greater force production (Asmussen and Bonde-Petersen, 1974; Bosco and Komi, 1979; Komi, 1979). Recall that the elastic components of muscle can be modeled as a spring. So, you can envision this phenomenon by imagining stretching a spring. When you let go, the spring will recoil and pull back together. Additional factors, including neural considerations and chemical energy from preloading the muscle, also probably contribute to enhanced force output; and the relative potential contribution of these and other factors is still under investigation (Cronin, McNair, and Marshall, 2000; Enoka, 2002; Smith, Weiss, and Lehmkuhl, 1996). Whatever the mechanism, this enhanced force can be marked; and in very rapid, small jumps from both feet, it was calculated that only 40% of the force was due to the concentric contraction of the muscle while approximately 60% of the force was due to these elastic and other factors (Thys, Cavagna, and Margaria, 1975). In addition, release velocity and jump height have been shown to improve 12% to 18%, and mean power output in a strength training exercise improved 8% to 16% with the use of SSC (Cronin, McNair, and Marshall, 2000). Furthermore, use of SSC has been shown to allow for lower energy requirements (e.g., greater efficiency) in a given movement.

An example of use of the SSC in dance is the use of a quick demi-plié prior to a jump. The gluteus maximus, hamstrings, quadriceps femoris, and calf muscles would work eccentrically on the down-phase of the plié and then concentrically on the up-phase. This principle is used frequently in dance, allowing for greater movement efficiency and potentially contributing to the "effortless" aesthetic desired in some dance forms, as well as greater force production for explosive movements. To optimize use of this property, the prestretch should be of a relatively small magnitude (e.g., lowering the body 8-12 inches [20-30 centimeters] in the plié), rapidly applied, with minimal delay (less than 0.4-1.0 second), and without a pause or relaxation of the muscle at the end of the stretch (e.g., at the bottom of the plié) between the eccentric and concentric contraction. While some dancers appear to naturally utilize a timing that facilitates enhanced force from the SSC, other dancers could benefit by small changes in their preparatory movements. Common errors include hesitating rather than utilizing a quick reversal of directions at the bottom of the plié and suboptimal depth of the preparatory plié. Training regimes that focus on this response of muscle (e.g., plyometrics) have been shown to enhance performance and may reduce injury incidence in muscles such as the hamstrings that are required to perform rapid stretch-shortening phases in movements like jumping and sprinting (Smith, Weiss, and Lehmkuhl, 1996).

Muscle Roles

When muscles work together at the same time, there are four primary potential roles they can play—mover (agonist), antagonist, synergist, or stabilizer. These roles are specific to a given movement and not a given muscle. Hence, the same muscle can serve in a different role with different movements.

Mover (Agonist)

A **mover,** or **agonist** (G. *agon,* contest), is a muscle or muscles whose contraction actually produces the desired joint movement. There may be many muscles that are capable of producing this desired movement. Traditionally the term **prime mover(s)** or **primary muscle(s)** is reserved for those muscles that are most important or effective in producing the movement, and the terms **assistant mover(s)** or **secondary muscle(s)** are used for those muscles that are less effective or that are called into play in specialized circumstances such as when more force is needed. However, these distinctions often are controversial and complex, and so which agonists are considered primary or secondary may differ between different sources. In raising the leg to the back (e.g., parallel attitude), the agonists are the hip extensors including the hamstrings as seen in figure 2.14.

Antagonist

An **antagonist** (G. *anti,* against + *agon,* contest) is a muscle or muscles with an action opposite to the action of the prime mover. Antagonists are often positioned on the side of the joint opposite to the

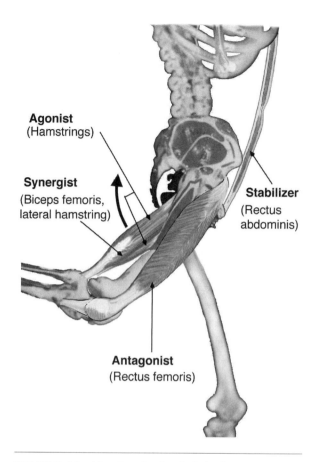

Agonist
(Hamstrings)

Synergist
(Biceps femoris,
lateral hamstring)

Stabilizer
(Rectus
abdominis)

Antagonist
(Rectus femoris)

FIGURE 2.14   Muscle roles in whole body movement (lateral view).

agonists. In raising the leg to the back, the antagonists are the hip flexors including the rectus femoris as seen in figure 2.14. Generally, antagonists relax while the prime movers contract. However, antagonists sometimes work together with agonists—termed **co-contraction**—when a part must be held rigid, when very precise movement is required, and during deceleration of body parts. An example of the latter occurs during running, where the antagonist (hip extensors) would initially relax to allow the prime movers (hip flexors) to bring the thigh forward in the swing phase but then would contract eccentrically to decelerate the thigh before it reaches its full height to the front.

Synergist (Neutralizer)

A **synergist** (G. *syn*, together + *ergon*, work) is a muscle that works together with the agonist(s) to help achieve the movement goal. The role of the synergist is described differently in different texts. This text will confine the meaning of synergist to a muscle whose action serves to neutralize an undesired secondary action of the prime mover(s). When raising the leg to the back in a parallel attitude, the medial

hamstrings (semimembranosus and semitendinosus) have actions of hip internal rotation as well as hip extension. To achieve the desired parallel position of the leg, the lateral hamstring (biceps femoris) can act as a synergist, with its secondary action of hip external rotation neutralizing the undesired internal rotation of the other hamstrings as shown in figure 2.14.

A further useful distinction is between a true and a helping synergist. If the synergist only neutralizes the undesired action and does not help with the desired action, it is called a **true synergist.** However, if it helps with the desired action and neutralizes the undesired action, it is called a **helping synergist.** The back attitude synergy just described is an example involving a helping synergist, since the lateral hamstring aids with the desired action of hip extension while it neutralizes the undesired hip internal rotation.

Stabilizer (Fixator)

A **stabilizer,** or fixator, is a muscle that contracts isometrically to support or steady a body part against forces related to muscle contraction, gravity, soft tissue constraints, momentum, or recoil from the movement. The first of these potential functions, stabilization against the forces related to muscle contraction, occurs with most movements. Remember that when a muscle contracts, it tends to pull both of its ends toward its center. However, often the desire is to have movement occur only at one end of the muscle, and stabilizers can work to anchor the necessary bone or body part to allow that to happen. For example, in a kick to the front (grand battement), stabilizers (abdominal muscles) work to prevent the proximal attachment of the iliopsoas muscle (a hip flexor that attaches to the lower spine proximally) from arching the low back, as the iliopsoas' distal attachment on the femur effects the desired action of lifting the thigh (hip flexion).

An example in which gravity is the primary factor occurs with push-ups. Abdominal muscles must be contracted to stabilize the pelvis and spine and prevent the tendency for the low back to arch and the body to sag due to the effect of gravity. An example in which soft tissue constraints are instrumental occurs during raising of the leg to the back in a parallel attitude. As the leg is raised backward, the hip flexors offer passive resistance as they are being stretched and tend to pull the pelvis into an anterior tilt and produce an arching of the low back unless the abdominal muscles are used to stabilize the pelvis as seen in figure 2.14. Appropriate timing and magnitude of stabilization are an important element of skilled dance performance, and very specific positioning and movement of many joints are often desired.

Muscles as Force Couples

The technical definition of a **force couple** is two forces that are equal in magnitude and opposite in direction and are located at a distance from the axis such that they produce rotation. An example of a force couple is the use of the hands on the steering wheel of an automobile to produce rotation of the wheel as seen in figure 2.15A. In dance, a force couple is formed by the feet to produce rotation of the body for turns such as a pirouette. When referring to muscles in the body, "force couples" can be more loosely used to describe muscles located at different positions relative to a joint axis but that act together to produce rotation in the same direction. In such anatomical force couples, the lines of pull of muscles are not necessarily directly opposite in direction and equal in magnitude. Examples of force

couples used whenever the arms are raised overhead are shown in figure 2.15B. The upper trapezius and serratus anterior muscles as well as the upper trapezius and lower trapezius can work as force couples to produce upward rotation of the scapula necessary for raising the arms overhead (see Scapulohumeral Rhythm on p. 397 for a more detailed discussion on the function of these particular muscles).

Special Considerations With Multijoint Muscles

Muscles can cross one or multiple joints, and the number of joints crossed dramatically influences the muscle's contribution to movement. As their names

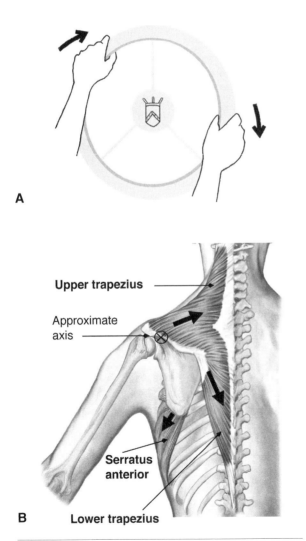

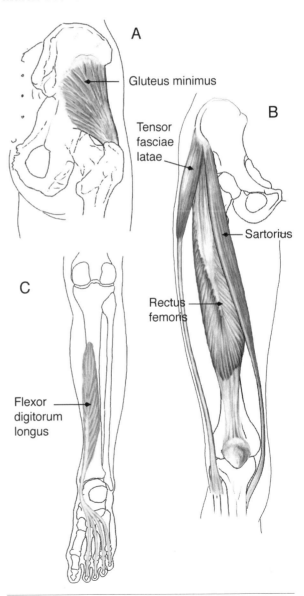

FIGURE 2.15   Force couples. (A) Hands on steering wheel and (B) muscles of scapula (posterior view).

FIGURE 2.16   Number of joints crossed by muscles. (A) Single-joint (posterolateral view), (B) two-joint (anterior view), and (C) multijoint muscles (posterior view).

suggest and as illustrated in figure 2.16, a **single-joint (uniarticulate) muscle** crosses only one joint, while a **two-joint (biarticulate) muscle** crosses two joints and a **multijoint (multiarticulate) muscle** crosses two or more joints. A single-joint muscle can produce motion only at the one joint it crosses. For example, the gluteus minimus shown in figure 2.16A crosses only the hip joint and so can produce movement only at the hip joint. In contrast, a multijoint muscle can produce motion at all the joints that it crosses. With a two-joint muscle, both of its tendons are pulled nonselectively toward the belly of the muscle, resulting in the tendency to cause movement at both of its joints. This can be advantageous from a perspective of efficiency when both actions are simultaneously desired, such as when both functions (hip flexion and knee extension) of the two-joint rectus femoris (figure 2.16B) are used when kicking.

Using one function of the muscle concentrically and the other eccentrically at the same time can also offer an advantage for two-joint muscles. For example, in locomotion, when the leg is initially swung forward (concentric hip flexion), the knee is often in a flexed position (knee extensors working eccentrically). This combination stretches the rectus femoris over the knee while shortening is occurring across the hip. In essence, this enhances the efficiency of the rectus femoris by keeping the whole muscle at a length where it can generate more muscle tension, as well as allowing for greater force due to the use of the stretch-shortening cycle. Other examples of muscles that cross two or more joints—that is, multijoint muscles—are the sartorius, tensor fascia latae (figure 2.16B), hamstrings, gastrocnemius, biceps brachii, the long head of the triceps brachii, and many muscles of the hands and feet, such as the flexor digitorum longus shown in figure 2.16C.

Active and Passive Insufficiency

However, despite this advantage in terms of efficiency, multijoint muscles hold a disadvantage in terms of allowing either fully active or fully passive range of motion at two or more joints simultaneously. Regarding the former, **active insufficiency** occurs when active contraction of the muscle is unable to produce as much range of motion as could be produced if an external force (e.g., gravity, momentum, another body part, or another person) was responsible for the movement. This limitation is due to the fact that the average muscle fiber can shorten only about half

---

Active Insufficiency

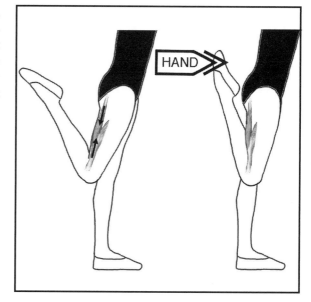

· **Establishing active insufficiency.** Create active insufficiency with the hamstring muscles by performing both of its joint actions (knee flexion and hip extension) together. Stand on your left foot and lift the right foot off the ground and flex the right knee as fully as possible. Then, with the knee fully flexed, try to lift the leg as high as possible to the back (hip hyperextension) as if doing a parallel back attitude.

· **Angle of knee flexion.**

– You will find that either the hamstring starts to cramp or the knee starts to decrease its degree of flexion as the thigh is raised higher toward the ceiling. Why?

– Holding the end position, use your hand to bring your right heel toward your buttocks. Why can you bend the knee further when you use your hand?

CONCEPT DEMONSTRATION 2.5

Passive Insufficiency

- **Establishing passive insufficiency.** Create passive insufficiency with the hamstring muscles by establishing a position opposite to the actions the hamstrings produce (e.g., hip flexion and knee extension) by lying on your back and using your arms to bring one leg up toward your shoulder while your knee is maintained in an extended position until a mild stretch is felt at the back of the leg (see figure 2.23B on p. 67). Note this endpoint.

- **Adding knee flexion.** Then bend your knee slightly and note that the leg can be brought higher.
  - Why can you bring the leg higher with your knee bent?
- **Application to other dance movements.**
  - Noting the degree of passive range that your body exhibits with your knee straight, how could this affect your ability to perform high kicks to the front or split leaps?
  - If a dancer has less than 90° of hip flexion possible due to passive insufficiency, how would this influence the dancer's ability to stretch the hamstrings while sitting with the legs straight to the front or in second position?

of its resting length, and this limit of shortening can readily be reached when a muscle is shortening across two or more joints simultaneously. In addition, muscle has difficulty producing high contractile force when in a very shortened position (length–tension relationship), and so strength of that muscle will influence how much range of movement can be achieved. Active insufficiency can be demonstrated by simultaneous performance of both actions of a two-joint muscle, such as hip flexion and knee extension for the rectus femoris as seen in figure 2.17A.

Lombard's Paradox

Another special consideration with a two-joint muscle comes into play when the required motion at one joint is in the opposite direction to that produced by that muscle. This condition is termed **Lombard's paradox** (Rasch, 1989). The classic example used with Lombard's paradox is co-contraction of the hamstrings and the quadriceps femoris, such as during rising from a plié or standing up from sitting in a chair. The hamstrings can produce the desired action of hip extension but the undesired action of knee flexion. On the other hand, the rectus femoris produces the desired action of knee extension but the undesired action of hip flexion. So how can the desired action of hip extension and knee extension occur from their co-contraction? One would think that if they were used together they would just neutralize each other's action and

no resultant movement would occur. However, this is not the case. The explanation for this apparent paradox is that multijoint muscles often have a more pronounced effect, due to having better leverage and producing greater torque, at one of the joints that they cross as shown in figure 2.18. In the case of the hamstrings, this muscle has a longer moment arm and so creates a greater torque at the hip than the knee, with its action of hip extension predominating. Conversely, the rectus femoris has a longer moment arm and so creates a greater torque at the knee than the hip, with its action of knee extension predominating. Hence, their co-contraction can result in the desired motion rather than either no motion or undesired motions. So, a two-joint muscle can be utilized that has its primary action coincident with the desired action at one joint, while another muscle works synergistically to overcome the undesired motion and create the desired action at the second joint.

Learning Muscle Names and Actions

Now that some key principles of how muscles function have been covered, the next step in understanding movement is to learn the names, locations, and actions of specific muscles. There are approximately 434 muscles in the human body, with about 75 pairs

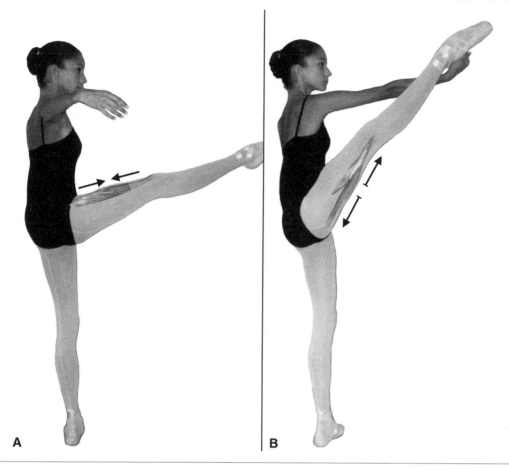

FIGURE 2.17   Active and passive insufficiency of two-joint muscles. (A) Active insufficiency of the rectus femoris; (B) passive insufficiency of the hamstrings.

responsible for movements of the body and posture (Hall, 1999). An overview of selected primary muscles and the one or two most important actions for some

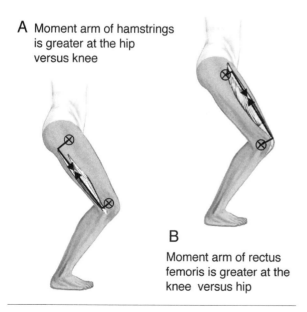

A Moment arm of hamstrings is greater at the hip versus knee

B Moment arm of rectus femoris is greater at the knee versus hip

FIGURE 2.18   Lombard's paradox.

of these muscles that are more commonly known is provided in figures 2.19 and 2.20. These and other muscles are then presented in more detail by region with a drawing, description of their attachments, and a more detailed description of their actions in chapters 3 through 7. Chapter 8 provides more in-depth figures and summary charts of major muscles, useful for movement analysis. Although the process of learning muscles can seem overwhelming for someone new to anatomy, it is made easier if logic rather than just pure rote memorization is used. A recommended approach to learning individual muscles follows.

1. **Use Latin and Greek roots to provide information.** Note that many of the words used in anatomy, including the names of muscles, have their roots in Latin or Greek. When learning about specific muscles it is often helpful to understand the meaning of these roots. The meaning of selected word roots is provided in table 2.4 and included for key muscles in chapters 3 through 7. If one understands the meaning of these roots, the name of a muscle often provides useful information about that muscle's characteristics.

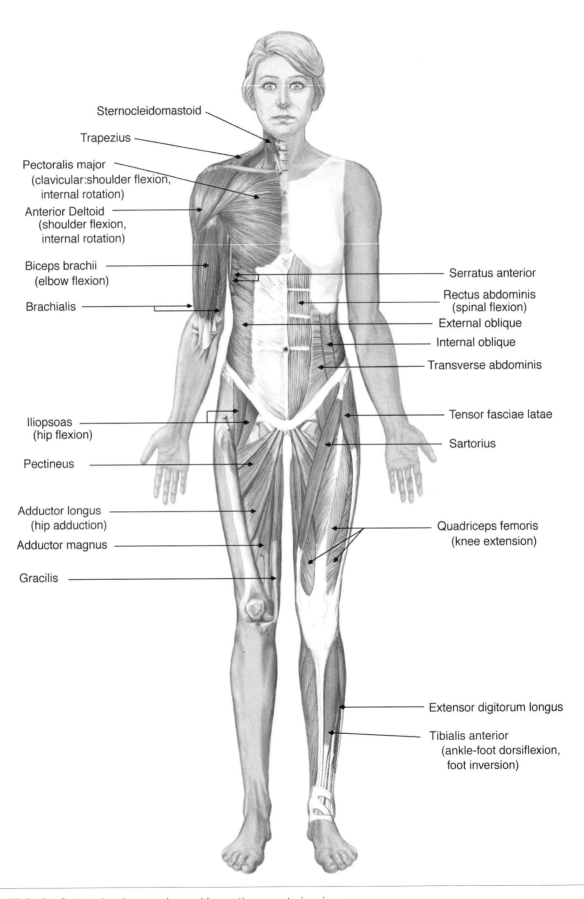

FIGURE 2.19   Selected major muscles and key actions—anterior view.

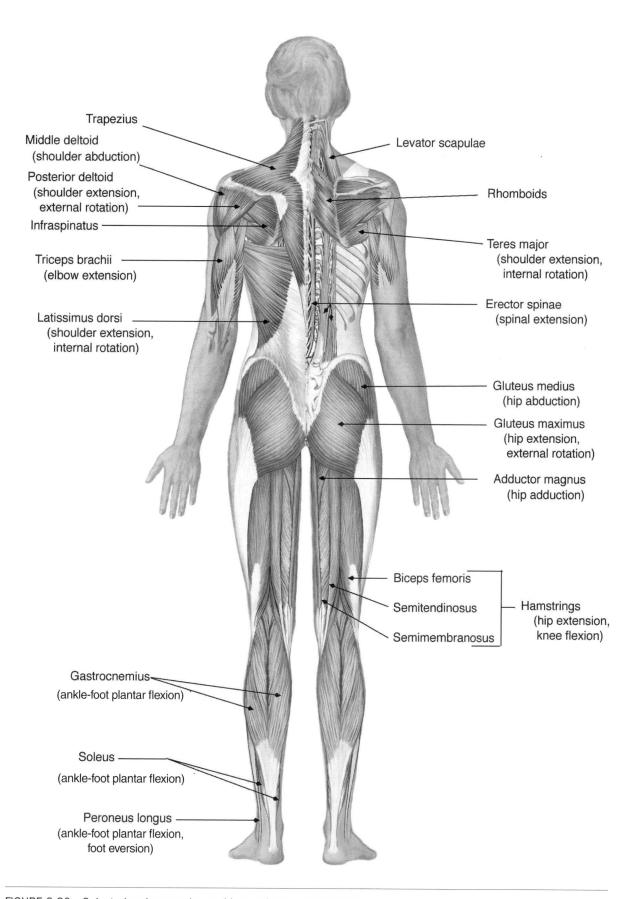

FIGURE 2.20 Selected major muscles and key actions—posterior view.

Latin and Greek roots provide the following clues about a muscle:

- Action: adductor longus (adductor = to adduct or bring toward the midline), levator scapulae (levator = to lift)

- Direction of fibers: rectus abdominis (rectus = straight), obliquus internus abdominis (obliquus = slanting or oblique)

- Location: triceps brachii (brachium = arm), pectoralis major (pectoris = chest)

- Number of divisions/proximal attachments (heads): quadriceps femoris (quadriceps = having four heads), triceps brachii (triceps = having three heads), biceps brachii (biceps = having two heads)

- Shape: deltoid (delta = shaped like the letter delta, triangular)

- Size/relative size: gluteus maximus (maximus = largest), adductor brevis (brevis = short)

2. **Learn the muscle name and location.** While keeping the meaning of useful word roots in mind, learn the name and location of the specific muscle.

3. **Estimate the muscle's line of pull, and deduce its action(s).** From knowing the muscle's location and approximate attachments, estimate its line of pull. Then, note where this line of pull is relative to the axis of the joint to deduce what type of movement would be produced at that joint when the muscle shortens (e.g., concentric contraction). Try to understand the logic, rather than just memorize the actions. For example, in many cases, muscles located anterior to the joint produce flexion; muscles located posterior to the joint produce extension; muscles lateral to biaxial or triaxial joints produce abduction; and muscles medial to these types of joints produce adduction (exceptions include muscles at the knee joint and scapulae). Muscles producing external rotation are often located posteriorly, and those producing internal rotation are often located anteriorly; but this relationship is less consistent.

Initially it is helpful to try to deduce just the primary one or two actions some of the more commonly known muscles would have and cross-check these

TABLE 2.4   Word Roots and Muscle Names

Word root	Meaning	Sample muscle
abducens	leading away from	abductor hallucis
biceps	two-headed	biceps femoris
brachium	upper arm	brachialis
brevis	short	adductor brevis
delta	triangle	deltoid
gracilio	slender	gracilis
latissimus	the broadest	latissimus dorsi
levator	lifter	levator scapulae
longissimus	the longest	longissimus of erector spinae
longus	long	adductor longus
magnus	larger	adductor magnus
major	the larger	teres major
maximus	the largest	gluteus maximus
minimus	the smallest	gluteus minimus
minor	the smaller	pectoralis minor
obliquus	oblique, slanting	obliquus internus abdominis
pectoris	chest	pectoralis major
peroneus	belonging to fibula	peroneus longus
piriformis	pear-shaped	piriformis
quadriceps	having four heads	quadriceps femoris
rectus	straight	rectus abdominis
rhomboids	rhomboid	rhomboideus major
serratus	serrated	serratus anterior
sterno	sternum	sternocleidomastoid
tensor	stretcher	tensor fasciae latae
teres	round	teres minor
triceps	three-headed	triceps brachii
vastus	large	vastus medialis

deductions with the actions listed in figures 2.19 and 2.20. However, a more in-depth understanding of muscles requires an appreciation of their secondary actions and use in functional movements. Knowledge regarding many of these more complex actions of muscles has been derived from various methods of research including electromyography (EMG). **Electromyography** (G. *electron*, amber [electricity] + *mys*, muscle + *grapho*, to write) utilizes electrodes inserted into the muscle (e.g., needle electrodes) or applied to the skin over a given muscle (e.g., surface

Deducing Muscle Actions From Their Attachments

Use figures 2.19 and 2.20 for reference.

· **Action of the middle deltoid muscle.** Find the middle deltoid in figure 2.20, and use this to locate the muscle on your body or a skeleton. Place your thumb on the estimated midpoint of the proximal attachment and your little finger of the same hand on the estimated midpoint of the distal attachment to establish the line of pull of the muscle. Now bring the distal attachment toward the proximal attachment and see what shoulder joint movement occurs. Check this action with that listed on figure 2.20.

· **Action of the anterior deltoid and posterior deltoid.** Repeat this procedure with the anterior deltoid (figure 2.19) and posterior deltoid (figure 2.20).

· **Reversal of customary action.** This procedure demonstrates the customary actions of muscles (with concentric contractions) in which the distal segment is the moving end. This is the easiest way to learn muscle actions. However, keep in mind that in instances such as when the hand is fixed (closed kinematic chain), these muscles can produce movement of the proximal segment (reversal of customary action) or both segments simultaneously (e.g., push-up, pull-up, dips).

Attachments and Primary Actions of the Deltoid Muscle

Muscle	Proximal attachment(s)	Distal attachment(s)	Primary action(s)	
Deltoid (DEL-toid)	Anterior: clavicle (lateral aspect) Middle: scapula (acromion process) Posterior: scapula (spine)	Humerus (deltoid tuberosity)	Anterior:	Shoulder flexion Shoulder horizontal adduction Shoulder internal rotation
			Middle:	Shoulder abduction Shoulder horizontal abduction
			Posterior:	Shoulder extension Shoulder horizontal abduction Shoulder external rotation

electrodes) to help record the electrical activity of muscles during various movements or conditions (see Basmajian and DeLuca, 1985). The greater the contraction of the muscle, the greater the frequency and amplitude of the recorded potentials. Results of some of these studies will be referred to in ensuing chapters, and additional research methods helpful for movement analysis will be addressed in chapter 8.

4. **Determine the muscles that could produce a given joint movement.** In addition to learning the action(s) of a given muscle, it is important to reverse that process and learn which muscles could produce a given joint movement. This is important for movement analysis. A summary table for each region is provided in chapters 3 through 7 to help with this process. A cumulative summary is also provided in chapter 8. When performing this process, for now focus on just the prime movers. A more detailed analysis can take into account secondary muscles, synergists, and stabilizers; this more detailed approach will be reserved for chapter 8. Furthermore, simplify this process of analysis by first identifying the functional group of muscles that would perform the movement (e.g., hip flexors, hip extensors, hip abductors) as seen in table 2.5, and then selecting one to three specific primary muscles that perform this desired joint movement.

5. **Take into account the influence of gravity and the type of muscle contraction.** When one is practicing this process of analyzing a movement, it is important to remember that the influence of gravity must be taken into account. In many phases of dance movements, gravity is fundamental in producing the movement, and muscles are used to control this

Electromyography

Examples of EMG records of three muscle groups for dancers directed to stand in first position, "prepared," as if they were in class, is shown. Records from two professional ballet dancers and two advanced modern dancers were selected to show the range in response with the same position. With this version of testing, the magnitude of the tracing of a muscle during a given movement is compared to that of a maximum voluntary contraction of the same muscle with the same electrode application.

Key:

A = hip adductor (adductor longus)

Q = quadriceps femoris (vastus medialis)

H = hamstrings (biceps femoris)

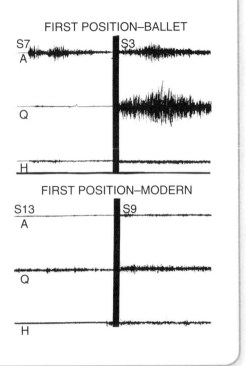

TABLE 2.5   Simplified Movement Analysis of Demi-Plié in Parallel First Position

Phase	Hip joint motion	Hip muscle group	Type of contraction (sample muscles)	Knee joint motion	Knee muscle group	Type of contraction (sample muscles)
Up-phase	Hip extension	Hip extensors	Concentric (gluteus maximus, hamstrings)	Knee extension	Knee extensors	Concentric (quadriceps femoris)
Down-phase	Hip flexion	Hip extensors	Eccentric (gluteus maximus, hamstrings)	Knee flexion	Knee extensors	Eccentric (quadriceps femoris)

Selected key joints: Hip, knee

movement set into play by gravity. For students new to anatomy, this is a difficult concept to grasp. It is helpful to consider whether the movement of the body or its segments is primarily (1) opposite to the direction of gravity (upward) or (2) in the same direction as gravitational forces (downward). For slow, controlled movements, movements opposite to the direction of gravity are generally produced by concentric muscle contraction of muscles whose action is the same as

the direction of movement, while movements in the same direction as gravity will be produced by gravity and controlled by eccentric contraction of muscles whose action is in the opposite direction to the joint movement occurring.

For example, in a plié in first position (figure 2.21), the up-phase would be going against gravity, and the knee extensors (quadriceps femoris) would be working concentrically to produce knee exten-

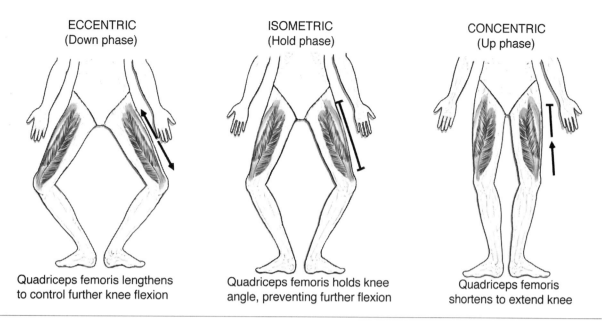

ECCENTRIC
(Down phase)

Quadriceps femoris lengthens
to control further knee flexion

ISOMETRIC
(Hold phase)

Quadriceps femoris holds knee
angle, preventing further flexion

CONCENTRIC
(Up phase)

Quadriceps femoris
shortens to extend knee

FIGURE 2.21   Types of muscle contraction in which gravity plays a primary role.

sion. In contrast, the down-phase would be produced by gravity, and the knee extensors would be working eccentrically to control knee flexion and prevent the dancer from collapsing to the floor. So, even though opposite motion is occurring at the joint (knee extension on the up-phase and knee flexion on the down-phase), the same muscle group is being used for both phases (concentrically on the up-phase to produce the movement and eccentrically on the down-phase to control and resist the flexion tendency produced by gravity). So, one approach to movement analysis is to determine what muscle group is working on the concentric phase of the movement; this will tell you the muscle group responsible for the movement both on the up-phase (concentrically) and on the down-phase (eccentrically). A basic schema for this approach is provided in table 2.5 with the plié performed in a parallel position and analysis limited to the hip and knee joints for purposes of simplicity. Another way of thinking of this is to note that when eccentric contractions are involved, muscles are working that have the opposite action to the direction of movement that is actually occurring. Also remember that when gravity would tend to produce a given movement and no movement is occurring, isometric muscle contractions are generally in play.

In slow movements of body segments that are perpendicular to gravity (horizontal or parallel to the floor), gravity does not have the same effect, and muscles are often used concentrically to produce movements and to maintain the limb in the horizon-

tal plane in both directions of the movement (e.g., horizontal abduction and adduction). In fast movements, the interplay of muscles and gravity becomes more complex; and concentric use of muscles to accelerate segments, co-contraction of antagonists to control movement, and eccentric contractions to decelerate body segments combined with gravitational forces often come into play. Understanding the importance of gravity on muscle function is essential for accurate movement analysis and will be further discussed in chapter 8.

6. **Application to exercise design.** Another way to reinforce the understanding of a muscle's action(s) and location is to design exercises for strengthening a given muscle, stretching a given muscle, or preventing injury to that muscle or a related structure. Chapters 3 to 7 contain samples of such exercises. When one is designing a strength exercise, at least one of the primary actions of the muscle must be opposed by the resistance. In order for the exercise to be effective, this muscle must be challenged (overloaded) sufficiently such that muscle failure is approached within relatively few repetitions but muscle injury is avoided. The American College of Sports Medicine recommendations (1998) are to perform 8 to 12 repetitions of a variety of exercises. Some of the more difficult examples of strength exercises provided in the following chapters may initially require that fewer repetitions be performed (four to six repetitions) so that excessive muscle stress is avoided.

The resistance utilized in strength exercises can take many forms, such as body weight, ankle weights, dumbbells, springs, elastic bands, or guided weight apparatus. In the case of the first three forms of resistance, an effective exercise also depends on appropriate positioning of the body so that the action of the muscle is opposed by gravity. For example, when one is performing shoulder external rotation with the elbows by the sides, an upright position of the torso will allow effective opposition if a band is being used for resistance, but not if a dumbbell is the resistance. Instead, using a side-lying position of the body would allow gravity to better resist the action of shoulder external rotation. Similarly if one is trying to strengthen the hip extensors, lowering the leg from 90° would be hip extension but not effective for strengthening the hip extensors. As seen in figure 2.22A, this movement is going in the same direction as gravity and would actually require eccentric contraction of the opposite muscle group, the hip flexors, to control the lowering of the legs. To make the hip extensors the prime movers, the leg would have to be lifted to the back in order to be working against gravity as seen in figure 2.22B. However, in the standing position the range of motion is quite limited without necessitating a marked anterior tilt of the pelvis and hyperextension of the lumbar spine, which could be of concern if a heavy resistance was being used. Furthermore, greater challenge to the hip extensors will be provided when the leg lifts higher such that the moment arm for the resistance is longer. To allow more range of motion with a long

moment arm working against gravity, but less back stress, hip extensor strengthening can be performed with the torso leaning forward (such as with forearms resting on a barre) or kneeling with the hands on the floor as seen in figure 2.22C.

In the design of strength exercises for two-joint muscles, the exercise may incorporate movement at just one of the joints or may combine the movements at both joints. In the latter case, the positioning used at one joint can influence which muscle of a functional group is being emphasized. For example, the hamstrings can be strengthened by an exercise using only knee flexion such as knee curls, an exercise using only hip extension such as back leg lifts, or an exercise that combines both actions such as seen in figure 2.22C. In this latter exercise, the knee is just bent slightly to try to help the dancer "find" the hamstring muscle. Then, the leg is lifted higher (hip extension), focusing on using this same muscle group to lift the leg. This approach can be used to help the dancer emphasize use of the hamstrings versus the gluteus maximus. In contrast, if the knee is bent to an extreme range as seen in figure 2.22D, the hamstring will be so shortened across the knee joint that it will be difficult for it to be effective in generating force for hip extension. This intentional production of active insufficiency for the hamstrings can be used to perform hip extension with a greater use of the gluteus maximus.

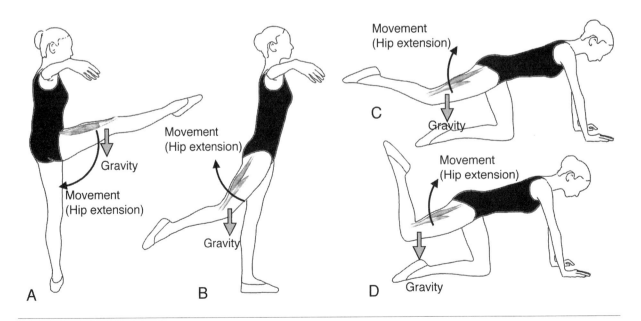

FIGURE 2.22   Influence of body position on hip extensor strengthening. (A) Ineffective relationship to gravity, (B) effective relationship to gravity but small range of motion, (C) effective positioning with hamstring emphasis, and (D) effective positioning with gluteus maximus emphasis.

When one is designing a stretching exercise for a given muscle, the approach is different. Here a position is utilized that is opposite to, versus the same as, at least one of the primary actions of the muscle such that the given muscle is put in a position of elongation. As previously described, three repetitions of a 30-second slowly applied stretch of low to moderate intensity appear to be an effective approach for improving flexibility. This method of stretching, where a position is maintained, is termed **static stretching.** Another effective approach, termed PNF contract-relax (proprioceptive neuromuscular facilitation), utilizes a 5- to 10-second contraction of the target muscle immediately followed by a 10- to 20-second stretch, with this sequence repeated three times (Shrier and Gossal, 2000; Tanigawa, 1972; Wallin et al., 1985). While this is frequently used for stretching outside of class, fewer repetitions and shorter-duration stretches are commonly employed within the dance class for a majority of muscle groups due to other programming considerations such as class flow, maintenance of the elevated temperature of the body, and time constraints because of the many other essential class objectives.

With two-joint muscles, the desired position of stretch is often achieved by incorporating elongation of the muscle across both joints, at least to some degree. For example, when stretching the hamstring muscle, a more flexible dancer would likely use a position of hip flexion and knee extension to produce an effective intensity of stretch on the hamstrings such as seen in figure 2.23A. However, this combined use might create too great an intensity of a stretch or not allow appropriate positioning of the body for a less flexible individual. In such a case, the knee can be slightly bent to allow correct positioning and an appropriate intensity of stretch either in a sitting position or in a supine position as shown in figure 2.23B. Gravity can be utilized in many ways during stretching of muscles. However, positions will often be used in which gravity tends to approximate either the proximal or the distal body segment such that stretch intensity is increased. In the sitting hamstring stretch shown in figure 2.23A, gravity will tend to bring the trunk (proximal segment) closer to the thigh to increase hip flexion and stretch intensity. In the supine hamstring stretch shown in figure 2.23B, gravity will tend to bring the thigh (distal segment)

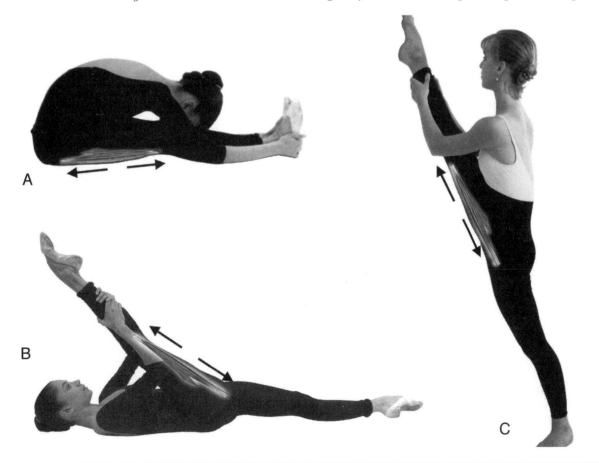

FIGURE 2.23   Influence of body position on hamstring stretching. (A) Sitting, (B) supine, and (C) standing.

toward the trunk to increase hip flexion and stretch intensity. In the advanced standing hamstring stretch shown in figure 2.23C (performed with the foot of the upper leg resting on a wall), gravity will intensify the stretch (hip flexion) when the trunk is leaned forward. However, as flexibility progresses and the dancer gets closer to the wall, gravity plays less of a role and the arms are classically used to pull the torso further forward.

When one is considering appropriate exercises for injury prevention and treatment, it is essential to understand the underlying mechanics or principles that are associated with a given injury. For example, as will be discussed in chapter 5, improper movement (tracking) of the patella is believed to underscore some injuries involving the kneecap. The quadriceps femoris muscle, and specifically the vastus medialis, is vital for correct movement of the patella, and hence specific strengthening of the quadriceps femoris is one recommendation for prevention of such problems. The addition of the sections on injuries to chapters 3 through 7 is not to suggest that readers who are not medical professionals diagnose and treat their own injuries or those of their students/associates. Diagnosis and treatment of injuries should be performed only by qualified medical professionals. Rather, the intent of these sections is to elucidate some of the theorized relationships between injuries and the anatomy and mechanics discussed in the given chapter so that dancers can be more effective in preventing injuries and have a better understanding of why certain exercises might be recommended in medically prescribed rehabilitation programs.

Summary

Skeletal muscle gives rise to movements at joints. Skeletal muscle contains both elastic and contractile components. The elastic components play an important role in stretching muscle and in the passive contribution to muscle force. The contractile components are the active elements of muscle. According to the sliding-filament theory, a coupling of small filaments within the muscle produces muscle tension or contraction. The skeletal muscles are attached to bones via tendons or aponeurosis, and so muscle contraction can be translated into rotary motions at joints. Depending on the balance of torque related to muscle effort and torque related to resistance at a given joint, muscle contractions can be dynamic (concentric or eccentric) or static (isometric). These different types of muscle contractions help muscles serve their varied roles as prime movers, antagonists, synergists, and stabilizers.

Individual muscles vary in their relative percentage of slow-twitch and fast-twitch fibers, cross-sectional area, and fusiform or penniform fiber arrangement in accordance with functional demands for greater force production, greater speed/range of motion, or greater postural control. When learning individual muscles it is helpful to take into account the meaning of Latin or Greek word roots utilized in their names and locations. The location of the proximal and distal attachments of a muscle creates a "line of pull," and from the relationship of this line to the axis of the joint one can deduce the possible actions of a muscle. Knowledge of the actions of muscles can also be used to analyze movements and predict the muscles that would function as prime movers in a given movement. To be accurate, such an analysis must take into account the role of gravity and the types of muscle contractions occurring in different phases of the movement. Knowledge of muscle actions can also be used to design effective strength exercises and flexibility exercises, and to better understand why certain exercises would be valuable for prevention and treatment of common dance injuries.

Study Questions and Applications

1. List the four properties of skeletal muscle and explain their practical significance for dance.

2. Make a diagram of the contractile mechanism of a muscle cell and label and define the following structures: A band, I band, H zone, Z line, actin, myosin, and sarcomere.

3. Describe the sliding-filament theory and how it relates to concentric, eccentric, and isometric muscle contractions.

4. Examine a pirouette, and describe when the calf muscles (gastrocnemius and soleus) would be working concentrically, isometrically, and eccentrically.

5. What difference in muscle fiber types would you expect to see in a world-class marathon runner versus a high jumper?

6. If the EA for a given muscle is 1.5 inches (3.8 centimeters) and the RA is 15 inches (38 centimeters), what would the mechanical advantage be? What is the significance of this mechanical advantage in terms of the muscle force needed to effect movement against the resistance?

7. Describe how the relationship of the torque associated with muscle effort and the torque associated with the resistance changes with concentric, eccentric, and isometric contractions.

8. Distinguish between a synergist and stabilizer, and provide two examples from dance.

9. Using figures 2.19 and 2.20 for reference, identify a muscle that can serve as an antagonist to the following muscles: pectoralis major, gluteus maximus, erector spinae, biceps brachii, and quadriceps femoris.

10. Describe how the serratus anterior and trapezius work as a force couple.

11. Using figure 2.14 for reference, locate the proximal and distal attachments of the rectus femoris on the skeleton. Use these attachments to mentally construct the line of pull of the rectus femoris, and deduce the actions the rectus femoris could have at the hip joint and knee joint. Use figure 2.19 to check your deductions.

12. Apply the concept of active and passive insufficiency to the rectus femoris. Provide two examples of movements in dance in which these phenomena would be operative and what you could do to lessen the constraints.

13. Using the schema provided in table 2.5, perform a simplified movement analysis for raising the arms to the front from low fifth to high fifth.

14. A dancer wants to improve her form in a grand jeté. Her teacher notes that her back knee tends to bend and both legs do not reach adequate height to give the desired line in the jump.

    a. Describe what joint motions are occurring at the hip and knee of the front leg and the back leg.

    b. Describe how raising the front leg straight versus with a developing movement would affect the moment arm of the leg and potential height of the front leg.

    c. Taking into account the concept of active insufficiency, identify muscles that should be strengthened to help increase the height the front leg can be raised. Taking into account the desired hip joint motion of the back leg, identify muscles that should be strengthened to help increase the height to which the back leg can be raised. Which of these muscles would also tend to bend the knee of the back leg, and what muscle group could serve as a synergist to neutralize this undesired knee flexion? Looking at the desired position at the height of the leap, identify the muscles that would need very high levels of flexibility. Provide a cue to help the dancer achieve the desired line of the back leg.

CHAPTER THREE

The Spine

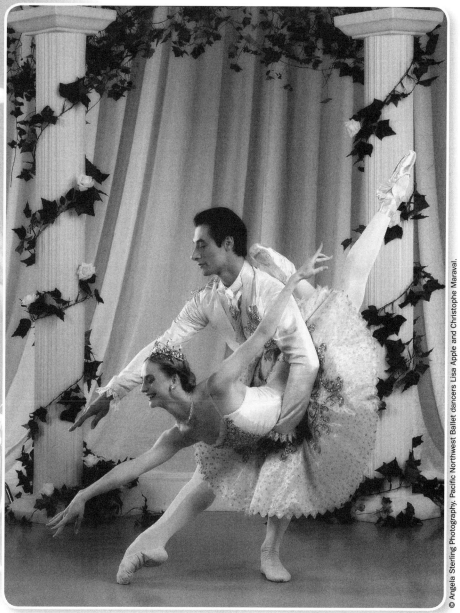

© Angela Sterling Photography. Pacific Northwest Ballet dancers Lisa Apple and Christophe Maraval.

The spine, or vertebral column, is the central organizing structure of the skeleton and the most fundamental element of the axial skeleton. For this reason it is the first anatomical region discussed in this text. The vertebral column as a whole articulates with the head, ribs, and pelvis, whereas individual vertebrae articulate with each other. These various articulations allow for movements of the head, trunk, and pelvis. Due to its central location, the spine also functions to provide vital support for upright posture, and to transmit forces to and from the upper and lower extremities. In dance, great demands are placed on the spine to maintain the desired positioning of the torso and help support another dancer during partnering as shown in the photo on page 71. In addition to strength, dance movements such as arabesques or jazz layouts require exceptional spinal flexibility and complex neuromuscular coordination to achieve the desired aesthetics of the movement. With dance, in contrast to many sports, great attention is also paid to positioning or alignment of the spine whenever the limbs are in movement. Hence, better understanding of both how to move and how to stabilize the spine can enhance dance skill.

This chapter will present basic anatomy and mechanics of the spine that influence optimal performance and injury vulnerability. Topics covered will include the following:

- Bones and bony landmarks of the spine
- Joint structure and movements of the vertebral column
- Description and functions of individual muscles of the spine
- Ideal spinal alignment and common deviations
- Spinal mechanics
- Muscular analysis of fundamental spinal movements
- Key considerations for the spine in whole body movement
- Special considerations for the spine in dance
- Conditioning exercises for the spine
- Back injuries in dancers

Bones and Bony Landmarks of the Spine

The spine extends from the skull to the tip of the tailbone (coccyx). It is composed of 33 consecutive small bones called **vertebrae** (L. joint) and hence is commonly called the **spinal column** or **vertebral column.** These vertebrae are arranged in five contiguous regions and are numbered consecutively by region as seen in figure 3.1. Seven vertebrae are located in the neck region and are called **cervical vertebrae** (C1-C7) (L. *cervix,* neck); 12 are in the region of the chest or thorax and are called **thoracic vertebrae** (T1-T12) (G. *thorax,* chest); five are in the low back region and are called **lumbar vertebrae** (L1-L5) (L. *lumbus,* loin); five form the **sacrum** (L. sacred bone) at the back of the pelvis; and the lowest four (three to five) are only partially formed and make up the **coccyx,** or tailbone. Since in the adult the five sacral vertebrae are fused to form the sacrum and the four coccygeal vertebrae fused to form the coccyx, only the upper 24 (7 cervical, 12 thoracic, and 5 lumbar) are movable. Although the number of cervical vertebrae tends to be constant, numerical variations of thoracic, lumbar, and sacral vertebrae occur in approximately 5% of otherwise normal people (Moore and Agur, 1995).

The vertebrae found in each of these regions differ in both shape and size in accordance with function. For example, the vertebral column as a whole is shaped like an extended pyramid such that the vertebrae get progressively larger from cervical to lumbar regions. This arrangement has functional significance since each vertebra must bear the weight of all the body parts above it, until the spine rests on the sacrum, where the weight of the body is transferred. Since the weight of the body is transferred to the pelvic girdle via the sacrum, the bones of the coccyx do not have to support the weight of the upper body and are much smaller.

Although there is variance in structure by region, a typical vertebra consists of a vertebral body, vertebral arch, and seven processes as shown in figure 3.2A. The **vertebral body** is the large, cylindrical anterior portion of the vertebra, through which most of the weight of the body is transmitted. Extending posteriorly from the body is a hollow partial ring termed the **neural arch** or **vertebral arch,** formed by two pedicles and two laminae. The **pedicles** (L. *pes,* foot) are short, broad processes that extend back from the body of the vertebra to attach to the broad, flat plates of bone called **laminae** (L. a thin plate). This vertebral arch and the posterior surface of the body of the vertebra form the walls of the very important opening, the **vertebral foramen** (L. an aperture). The vertebral foramen from successive vertebrae of the vertebral column form the **vertebral canal** or **spinal canal,** which houses and provides protection for the spinal cord and its related membranes, vessels, and nerve roots. Small indentations located on the upper (supe-

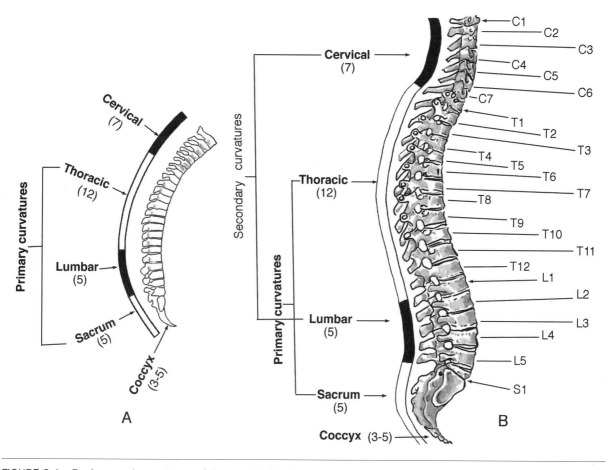

FIGURE 3.1   Regions and curvatures of the vertebral column (lateral view) (A) at birth and (B) during adulthood.

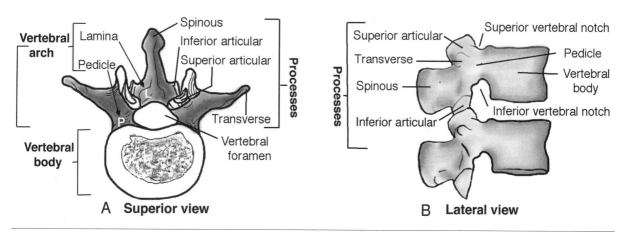

FIGURE 3.2   Typical lumbar vertebra. (A) Superior view, (B) lateral view.

rior vertebral notch) and lower (inferior vertebral notch) portions of the pedicles of adjacent vertebrae form smaller openings called **intervertebral foramina** as seen in figure 3.2B, which provide passageways for the nerves to leave the spinal cord.

The vertebral arch also gives rise to seven processes—one spinous, two transverse, two superior articular, and two inferior articular. The **spinous process** projects backward and downward from the junction of the paired laminae. The spinous processes are the projections you can feel, or **palpate,** when you run your finger down the back of your neck and trunk. The spinous process that is particularly large at the base of the neck belongs to C7, and due to its distinctive shape is termed the **vertebra prominens** (L. prominent). The paired **transverse processes** project posterolaterally from the junction of the pedicles and the laminae. The spinous and transverse processes form important sites for the attachment of ligaments and muscles of the vertebral column, and they function to increase the mechanical advantage of these structures by allowing for an attachment farther away from the axis of rotation. The paired **superior and inferior articular processes** are located at the junctions of the pedicles and laminae. As their name suggests, these processes form joints with the vertebrae immediately above and below.

Joint Structure and Movements of the Vertebral Column

The vertebrae are generally joined to adjacent vertebrae both at the vertebral bodies and at the vertebral arches. These joints are collectively termed the intervertebral joints. There are also some additional specialized joints that occur in specific regions of the vertebral column and serve to help connect the skull, ribs, and pelvis to the spine.

Joints Between the Vertebral Bodies

The bodies of adjacent vertebrae from the second cervical vertebra to the first sacral vertebra are connected by cartilaginous joints, and the interposed cartilage is termed the **intervertebral disc.** Each intervertebral disc consists of an outer ring, termed the **annulus fibrosus,** and an inner gelatinous mass, termed the **nucleus pulposus** as shown in figure 3.3. The annulus (L. *annulus,* ring) fibrosus is composed of concentric sheets or lamellae of fibrocartilage. The fibers run in approximately the same direction in a given band but in the opposite direction in any two adjacent bands as shown in figure 3.3A. This structural arrangement provides strength to the disc to help it withstand forces and limit excessive motion in many directions. The nucleus pulposus (L. the inside of a thing + fleshy) is a deformable gel-like core that is about 80% water in a healthy disc (Deckey and Weidenbaum, 1997) and allows for rocking and rotating motion between adjacent vertebrae, as well as essential absorption of compression forces for the vertebrae.

During weight bearing, the nucleus pulposus is compressed and exerts a large centrifugal force on the fibers of the annulus as seen in figure 3.3B. The nucleus pulposus contains charged molecules (proteoglycans) that tend to pull water into the disc—important to counter the tendency for water to

be pushed out of the disc by the compression associated with weight bearing. However, with repetitive loading, a small amount of water is lost from the disc such that the spine undergoes up to an 0.8-inch (2-centimeter) loss in height during the day (Hall, 1999), which is restored when pressures are relieved such as during sleep and recumbency. Conversely, when compression is decreased due to the loss of gravity during space flight, astronauts can undergo a temporary increase in the height of the spine of approximately 2 inches (5 centimeters).

Each end of the disc is centrally closed by a thin cartilaginous plate (vertebral **endplate**) that is firmly adhered to the body of the adjacent vertebrae (figure 3.3). The inner zone of the annulus fibers is attached to this endplate, while the outer peripheral zone attaches directly into the bony tissue of the vertebral body (**epiphyseal ring**). When the spine is subjected to very large compression forces, these vertebral endplates can sometimes fracture (Panjabi, Tech, and White III, 1980).

The intervertebral disc constitutes 20% to 33% of the total height of the vertebral column (White III and Panjabi, 1978), with disc thickness varying in dif-

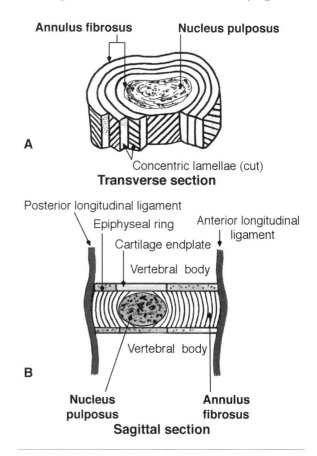

Annulus fibrosus   **Nucleus pulposus**

A

Concentric lamellae (cut)
Transverse section

Posterior longitudinal ligament
Epiphyseal ring   Anterior longitudinal
Cartilage endplate   ligament
Vertebral body

Vertebral body

B

Nucleus   **Annulus**
pulposus   **fibrosus**
Sagittal section

FIGURE 3.3   The intervertebral disc. (A) Transverse section, (B) sagittal section.

ferent regions from about 0.1 inch (3 millimeters) in the cervical region to about 0.3 inches (9 millimeters) in the lumbar region (Levangie and Norkin, 2001). In the cervical and lumbar regions the discs are thicker anteriorly and help form the anteriorly convex curvatures found in these regions. In the thoracic region the discs are more even in thickness, and the posteriorly convex curvature in this region is more due to the wedge shape of the vertebral bodies.

The bodies of the vertebrae and intervertebral discs are further connected by ligaments—the anterior longitudinal ligament and the posterior longitudinal ligament as seen in figure 3.4. The **anterior longitudinal ligament** is a strong, broad fibrous band that extends from the inner (pelvic) surface of the sacrum up to the skull. This ligament covers and connects the anterior aspects of the vertebral bodies and the intervertebral discs. It functions to help limit the extent of spinal hyperextension, maintain stability, and prevent forward bulging of the annulus of the intervertebral disc as seen in figure 3.5A. The **posterior longitudinal ligament** is a narrower fibrous band, having about half the strength of the anterior longitudinal ligament (Levangie and Norkin, 2001). This ligament runs along the posterior aspect of the vertebral bodies, within the vertebral canal. It is attached to the intervertebral discs and the posterior edges of the vertebral bodies from C2 to the sacrum. The posterior longitudinal ligament helps limit extreme spinal flexion and posterior protrusion of the intervertebral discs as seen in figure 3.5B. However, the posterolateral corner of the annulus

is poorly covered and represents a weak area where disc protrusion frequently occurs.

Joints Between the Vertebral Arches

The superior articular process of one vertebra articulates with the inferior articular process of the vertebra above to form the facet joints, more technically termed zygoapophyseal or apophyseal joints (figures 3.2 and 3.5A). These **facet joints** are synovial joints of the gliding variety. Hence, they allow small gliding movements in various directions. The shape and facing of the given articular processes are key in determining the extent and direction of movement

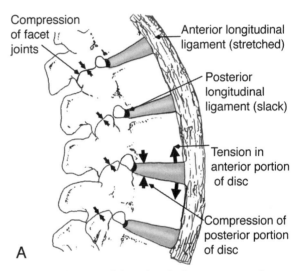

A
Lateral view with spine in hyperextension

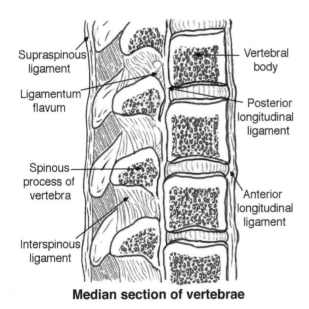

Median section of vertebrae

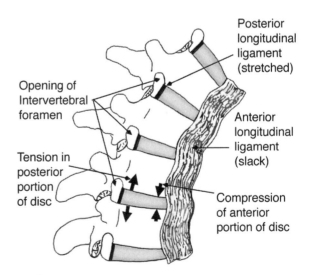

B   **Lateral view with spine in flexion**

FIGURE 3.4   Primary ligaments of the spine (intertransverse ligament not visible in this section).

FIGURE 3.5   Influence of (A) hyperextension and (B) flexion on key spinal structures.

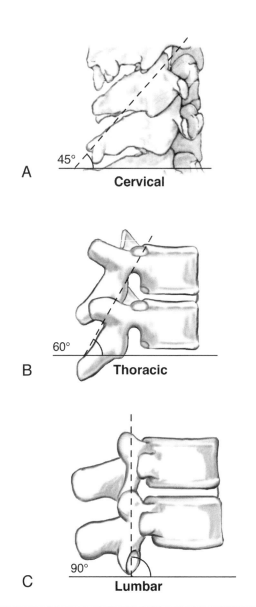

A 45° **Cervical**

B 60° **Thoracic**

C 90° **Lumbar**

FIGURE 3.6   The role of the facet joints in spinal movement (lateral view). Orientation of facets in (A) cervical and (B) thoracic regions allows for more free rotation, while (C) orientation in the lumbar region limits rotation.

possible between adjacent vertebrae and tend to vary significantly in different regions of the spine as seen in figure 3.6. For example, in the lumbar region, the more vertical alignment of the facet joints limits the degree of possible rotation (figure 3.6C), while in the thoracic (figure 3.6B) and cervical regions (figure 3.6A) the facet orientation allows more free rotation. While the forces on the facet joints are relatively small in standing and sitting, during bending and lifting the lumbar facets take on a greater role in spinal stability by helping prevent one vertebra from sliding forward on another (Fiorini and McCammond, 1976). These facet joints can also undergo

greater forces with hyperextension, lateral flexion, and rotation; they have been shown to provide about 40% of the spine's ability to resist rotational torsion and must withstand 30% of the compression forces accompanying hyperextension (Hall, 1999).

The facet joints are given further support by a thin articular capsule and by more distant ligaments of varying width and strength as seen in figure 3.4. These ligaments span between adjacent transverse processes (**intertransverse ligaments** [L. *inter,* between]), laminae (**ligamentum flavum**), deeper portions of the spinous processes (**interspinous ligaments**), and tips of the spinous processes (**supraspinous ligament** [L. *supra,* above]). In the neck region, the supraspinous ligament merges with the **ligamentum nuchae** (L. *nucha,* back of the neck) and actually provides a site for muscle attachment (Moore and Agur, 1995). The ligamentum flavum (L. *flavus,* yellow) also is unique in that its relatively high elastic content (giving rise to its yellowish color) allows it to aid with straightening the spine after it has been flexed.

The various ligaments of the spine, including those between the bodies and vertebral arches, have been shown to be under tension during erect positions and are very important for helping provide stability to the vertebral column as a whole. The pre-tension of these ligaments, in conjunction with the presence of the intervertebral discs, helps resist the tendency for the vertebral column to collapse. In addition, the muscles, discussed shortly, are fundamental for integrity as well as movements of the spine.

Specialized Vertebral Joints

There are some specialized joints associated with the vertebral column. These joints help link the head, ribs, and pelvis to the spine.

Craniovertebral Joints

The **craniovertebral joints** (G. *kranion,* skull)—the atlanto-occipital and atlantoaxial joints—involve the skull and the two most superior cervical vertebrae (C1 and C2). These two uppermost vertebrae lack an interposed intervertebral disc, are not typical in shape, and are specialized to meet their function of helping support and move the head. The first cervical vertebra is ringlike, without a body or spinous process, as seen in figure 3.7A. Because it receives the weight of the head, C1 is called the **atlas** (after the mythical giant who is said to have supported the pillars of heaven). Its superior concave, oval articular facets join with two rockerlike projections located on the lower skull (occipital condyles) to form the

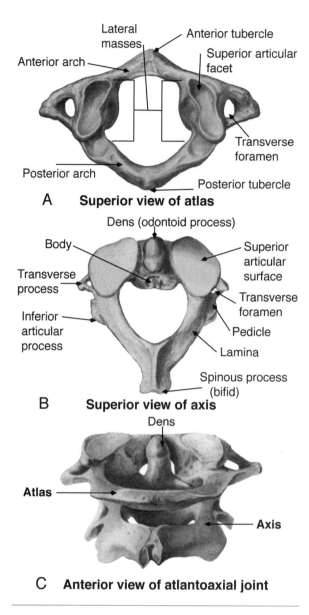

A   **Superior view of atlas**

Lateral masses
Anterior tubercle
Superior articular facet
Anterior arch
Transverse foramen
Posterior arch
Posterior tubercle

B   **Superior view of axis**

Dens (odontoid process)
Body
Superior articular surface
Transverse process
Transverse foramen
Inferior articular process
Pedicle
Lamina
Spinous process (bifid)

C   **Anterior view of atlantoaxial joint**

Dens
Atlas
Axis

FIGURE 3.7   Specialized cervical vertebrae: (A) The atlas and (B) the axis articulate to form (C) the atlanto-axial joint.

the axis, and the joint between C1 and C2 is called the **atlantoaxial joint** (figure 3.7C). It is classified as a pivot joint, allowing about 45° to 50° rotation and giving rise to the "no" movement of the head (Hay and Reid, 1982; Magee, 1997).

The extent of movement allowed at both of the craniovertebral joints is much greater than allowed at the other intervertebral articulations, permitting freer movements of the head but leaving the cervical spine vulnerable for injury. These motions are normally constrained by various ligaments of these craniovertebral joints. However, in trauma or combat, the large ligament of the atlas, which normally separates the dens from the spinal cord, can be ruptured, allowing the dens to be driven into the upper spinal cord or lower brainstem, often resulting in paralysis or death (Moore and Agur, 1995).

Joints Between Thoracic Vertebrae and Ribs

In addition to the intervertebral discs and facet joints between adjacent vertebrae, most thoracic vertebrae join with a rib via two gliding joints termed the costovertebral joint and the costotransverse joint. The **costovertebral joint** (L. *costa*, rib) is formed between the head of a rib and flattened areas (called facets or demi-facets) on the side of the body of the corresponding vertebrae or two adjacent vertebrae and the interposed disc. The **costotransverse joint** is formed between another facet on the distal portion of the transverse processes and a small projection (tubercle) found on each of the first 10 ribs (figure 3.8). These 10 upper ribs progress from their attachment onto the spine laterally and then course anteriorly to attach to the sternum either directly ("true ribs") or indirectly ("false ribs") via a segment of cartilage (the costal cartilages) as seen in figure 3.8A. The lower two rib pairs are shorter—they do not join onto the sternum—and because their lateral ends are free, they are called "floating ribs."

The 12 thoracic vertebrae, 12 ribs (and associated costal cartilage), and sternum make up the **thoracic cage,** or rib cage. This arrangement provides an important protective "cage" for vital structures such as the lungs and heart, as well as stability for upright stance and movement, yet allows for small but important motions of the ribs that accompany breathing. During vigorous inhalation, the ribs are elevated, while during exhalation the ribs return to their normal position. This motion of the lower ribs is referred to as the "bucket handle motion" of the ribs (figure 3.8C), since it is like the motion in which a bucket handle is slightly lifted and lowered. Due

paired **atlanto-occipital** joints. Although these are condyloid joints, their parallel arrangement limits their motion to primarily give rise to the "yes" movement, or nodding movement of the head, allowing about 10° to 20° of flexion and 25° of hyperextension (Hay and Reid, 1982; Magee, 1997). Moderate lateral flexion and very limited rotation are also allowed at this joint (Levangie and Norkin, 2001).

The second cervical vertebra has a unique large, peg-like projection, termed the **dens** (L. tooth) or odontoid process, as seen in figure 3.7B. This process projects superiorly from its body to form a pivot for C1 (upon which the skull sits). Hence C2 is called

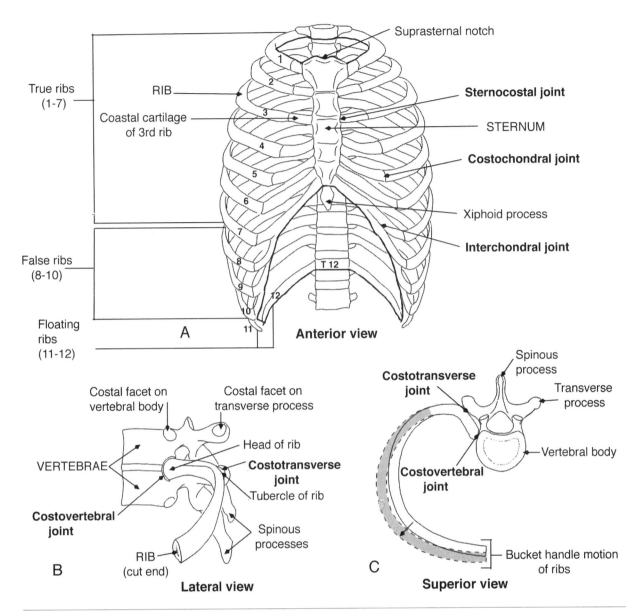

True ribs (1-7)

RIB

Coastal cartilage of 3rd rib

False ribs (8-10)

Floating ribs (11-12)

Suprasternal notch

Sternocostal joint

STERNUM

Costochondral joint

Xiphoid process

Interchondral joint

A   **Anterior view**

Costal facet on vertebral body

Costal facet on transverse process

VERTEBRAE

Costovertebral joint

Head of rib

Costotransverse joint

Tubercle of rib

Spinous processes

RIB (cut end)

B   **Lateral view**

Costotransverse joint

Spinous process

Transverse process

Vertebral body

Costovertebral joint

Bucket handle motion of ribs

C   **Superior view**

FIGURE 3.8   The thoracic cage and selected key joints. (A) Anterior view of key joints, (B) lateral view, and (C) superior view of joints between ribs and vertebrae.

to the shape and orientation of the ribs, elevation creates more of an anterior increase in diameter in the upper ribs and a lateral increase in diameter in the lower ribs.

Lumbosacral Joint

The lower portion of the spine is specialized for transference of weight through the pelvis. The joint between the body of the last lumbar vertebra and rigid sacrum (L5-S1), called the **lumbosacral joint,** is very important for movements of the spine and for the movements of the pelvis relative to the spine (the latter are described in chapter 4). In addition to the regular intervertebral ligaments, this joint receives

further stability from two paired ligaments that span between the transverse processes of the lower lumbar vertebrae and the crest of the ilium (iliolumbar ligament) or sacrum (lumbosacral ligament). However, despite additional ligamental support, due to greater disc thickness and joint surface area there is much greater motion possible at the lumbosacral joint than between the initial lumbar vertebrae. Furthermore, unlike the gradual transitions seen between the other regions of the spine, a sharp angle termed the **lumbosacral angle** occurs at the lumbosacral joint as seen in figure 3.9. This sharp angle increases the tendency for the upper vertebrae to slide forward on the lower vertebrae (shear forces). The greater shear

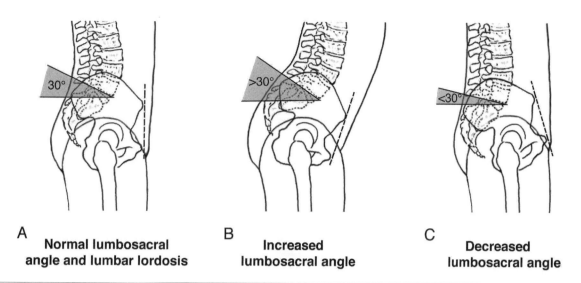

A **Normal lumbosacral angle and lumbar lordosis**

B **Increased lumbosacral angle**

C **Decreased lumbosacral angle**

FIGURE 3.9   The lumbosacral angle (lateral view). (A) Normal, (B) increased, (C) decreased.

and greater motion associated with the lumbosacral joint and lower lumbar spine markedly increase the risk for injury, and approximately 75% (Grabiner, 1989) of all serious back injuries occur at the L4-L5 and L5-S1 levels.

The lateral portions of the sacrum join with the pelvis via the paired **sacroiliac joints.** These joints will be discussed in chapter 4.

Movements of the Vertebral Column

Movements of the vertebral column can be described relative to the spine as a whole or relative to a given motion segment (**segmental movement**). A **motion segment** is composed of two adjacent vertebrae and their related soft tissue, including the interposed intervertebral disc. Segmental movement varies markedly by region (figure 3.10) (White III and Panjabi, 1978), but in general, movements of the vertebral column are more free in the cervical and lumbar region. In contrast, they are more limited (except for rotation) in the thoracic region due to their structural linking to the relatively rigid rib cage.

In terms of specific joint movements, flexion is greatest in the cervical region followed by the lumbar region. It is more limited in the thoracic region due to the presence of the ribs. Extension is most free in the cervical and lumbar regions. It is more limited in the thoracic region due to the longer, vertical spinous processes and the orientation of the thoracic curve (convex posteriorly). Lateral flexion is greatest in the cervical and lumbar regions. It is more limited in the thoracic region due to the ribs. Rotation is free in the upper cervical region (atlantoaxial joint) and the thoracic region. Rotation is more limited in the

lumbar region due to the more vertical orientation of the facet joints that resist such motion. It is helpful to keep these movement ranges in mind when one is analyzing and teaching the desired execution of dance movements. For example, given the large potential extension in the lower lumbar vertebrae and the relatively low amount of extension in the thoracic region, it is easy to see why many dancers excessively arch the low back and do not achieve the desired extension higher in the spine in movements such as port de bras to the back.

While describing movements at individual motion segments is key for research, injury prevention, and rehabilitation, description of movements of the vertebral column as a whole is important for movement analysis and description of the actions of muscles. And although movements between individual vertebrae are relatively small and include only gliding and cartilaginous joints, the summation of all of these small movements produces a considerable range of motion of the spine as a whole, more comparable to that seen with a triaxial joint. Movements of the spine (also termed trunk) include flexion-extension in the sagittal plane, right lateral flexion-left lateral flexion primarily in the frontal plane, and right rotation-left rotation primarily in the transverse plane as seen in figure 3.11.

However, in functional movement, due to various factors, including the presence of the anteroposterior curves of the spine and the facings of the facet joints, movements of the spine often involve small subtle movements in planes in addition to the plane of the primary movement. For example, rotation is generally associated with slight lateral flexion at the segmental level. This consistent linking of motion

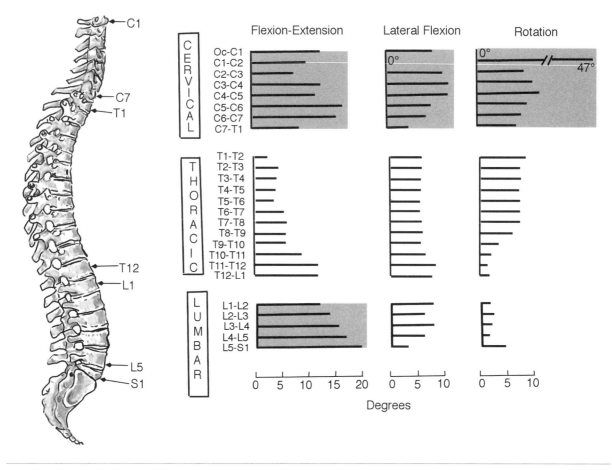

FIGURE 3.10   Composite of segmental movements in different regions of the vertebral column.

Adapted, by permission, from A.A. White and M.M. Panjabi, 1978, "The basic kinematics of the lumbar spine," *Spine* 3: 12-20.

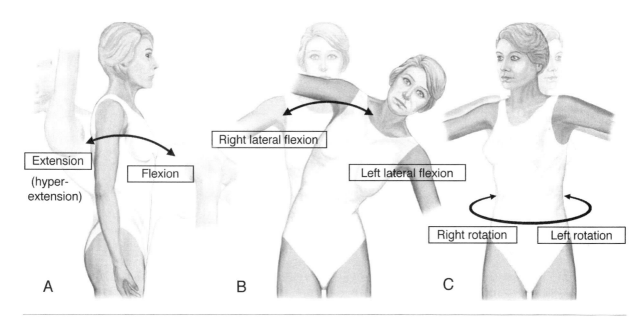

FIGURE 3.11   Movements of the vertebral column. (A) Flexion-extension, (B) right lateral flexion-left lateral flexion, (C) right rotation-left rotation.

around one axis with motion around a different axis is termed **coupling** (Levangie and Norkin, 2001). Skilled dancers often develop a complex array of muscle activation patterns to limit some of this coupling when the dance aesthetics require the look of motion of the spine as a whole in a single plane. For example, some floor work in modern dance utilizes rotation with a "long and lifted spine," with minimal accompanying visible lateral shift or side-bending of portions of the spine.

Muscles

In addition to the many strong ligaments and joint capsules of the vertebral column, many muscles act on the spine. These muscles range from small slips vital for local stabilization to large muscles capable of generating large forces. Given the tremendous number of joints and the complexity of the spine, heightened by the presence of the normal sagittal curvatures, these muscles are vital for moving the spine, stabilizing the spine, and preventing injuries that occur so readily in this region of the body.

Description and Functions of Individual Muscles of the Spine

The back region contains approximately 200 muscles (Rasch and Burke, 1978), including muscles for respiration, moving the upper extremity, and moving the vertebral column. This text will simplify coverage to key muscles for stabilization and movements of the spine, and it will exclude many of the muscles that move the neck and head. The location of these selected spinal muscles has a logical relationship to their actions, with anterior muscles other than the iliopsoas producing spinal flexion, posterior muscles producing spinal extension, and lateral muscles producing lateral flexion. Most anterior and posterior muscles also have secondary actions of spinal rotation and lateral flexion. Many of these muscles attach onto the pelvis and thorax rather than the vertebrae themselves, making their influence on the spine indirect. (See Individual Muscles of the Spine, pp. 82-93.)

Ideal Spinal Alignment and Common Deviations

When one looks from the side, the spine is not a straight column but has four curves as seen in figure 3.1B. The cervical and lumbar curvatures are convex anteriorly, and the thoracic and sacrococcygeal curvatures are convex posteriorly. The thoracic and sacral curvatures are **primary curvatures** that develop during the fetal period and are present at birth (Hall-Craggs, 1985) as seen in figure 3.1A. The thoracic curve is due primarily to the wedged shape of the vertebrae in this region. In contrast, the cervical and lumbar curvatures do not fully develop until after birth and thus are termed **secondary curvatures.** The cervical curve has been conjectured to develop in response to the pull of the neck extensors as the infant begins lifting the head up with sitting and crawling. The lumbar curve is further formed when the child starts standing and walking. When the child stands, the tightness of the iliofemoral ligament and hip flexors (see chapter 4) will tend to tilt the top of the pelvis anteriorly, and the lumbar spine must be extended to keep the torso upright. Unlike the other curves, the lumbar curve also tends to increase during the growth years; an approximate 10° increase occurs between the ages of 7 and 17 (Hall, 1999). The lumbar curve is unique to the human species and is believed to be a specialized adaptation to upright stance and gait (Napier, 1967). The lumbar and sacrococcygeal curvatures tend to be more pronounced in females than in males. In contrast, the thoracic curvature tends to be higher in males than females prior to age 40, and then similar, or in some cases much greater, in females in later years (White III and Panjabi, 1978).

When these sagittal curves are of normal magnitude, their balanced presence contributes to the springlike characteristics of the spine and allows it to withstand greater forces and move more freely than if it were a straight column. However, in some instances, one or more of these curves is excessive, disrupting this balance and placing undue stress on some segments of the spine. Exaggerations of the normal curves in the sagittal plane include cervical lordosis, kyphosis, and lumbar lordosis, while a decrease in the lumbar curve is termed flat back (figure 3.23, p. 94). An abnormal curve occurring primarily in the frontal plane is termed scoliosis. Milder forms of these alignment problems may relate to muscular imbalances and habitual movement patterns, but it is also important to realize that these alignment conditions may be related to more serious underlying pathology and may have a strong genetic basis or psychological basis. Therefore, it is important that the dancer procure a good medical evaluation if any of these conditions are accompanied by pain, appear to be progressing, or are severe in magnitude.

(Text continues on p. 93.)

Individual Muscles of the Spine

Anterior Muscles of the Spine

The anterior muscles of the spine include various muscles that primarily act on the head and neck (sternocleidomastoid, three scaleni, prevertebral group), the abdominal muscles, and the iliopsoas. The abdominal muscles are composed of the paired rectus abdominis, external oblique, internal oblique, and transverse abdominis. The iliopsoas crosses the hip joint, as well as the spine, and only its function relative to the spine will be addressed in this chapter.

Attachments and Primary Actions of Rectus Abdominis

Muscle	Inferior attachment(s)	Superior attachment(s)	Primary action(s)
Rectus abdominis (REK-tus ab-DOM-i-nis)	Crest of pubis of pelvis, pubic symphysis	Cartilages of ribs 5-7	Spinal flexion Spinal lateral flexion (same)

Rectus Abdominis

As its name suggests, the **rectus abdominis** *(rectus,* straight + *abdom,* abdomen) runs up and down, vertically, in the central portion of the abdomen as seen in figure 3.12. The rectus abdominis is a relatively narrow muscle but prominent, and the right and left recti are separated by a tendinous band called the linea alba *(linea,* line + *alba,* white). The muscle fibers are parallel in arrangement and are crossed by three approximately horizontal fibrous bands termed tendinous inscriptions, giving rise to the term "six pack" used to describe highly developed abdominal muscles. The rectus abdominis is located superficially and is encased within a sheath formed by the aponeuroses of the other abdominal muscles as seen in figure 3.21C. The primary action of the rectus abdominis is spinal flexion, and the rectus abdominis is considered the most powerful flexor of the spine. This action of the rectus is used when one curls the torso up from a supine position in floor work or performs "contractions" of the torso in modern or jazz dance. When one

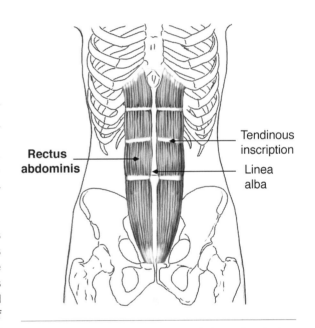

FIGURE 3.12   The rectus abdominis (anterior view).

side of the rectus abdominis contracts alone (**unilateral** contraction), the rectus abdominis can also assist with spinal lateral flexion to the same side. Posturally, the rectus can also work to pull downward on the rib cage, depressing the lower ribs and preventing "rib leading," or to pull upward on the pubic bone, creating a tucked position of the pelvis **(posterior pelvic tilt).**

Palpation: Lying on your back with your knees bent and feet flat on the floor, curl up so that your head and shoulders rise off the floor. The rectus abdominis can be palpated just to the sides of the midline of the abdomen running from the bottom of the sternum (xiphoid process) to the pubic bone (symphysis pubis). Also, run your fingertips along the midline of the abdomen. Dancers who have borne children may occasionally find a crevice between the paired recti abdominis. This separation in the connective tissue—termed **diastasis recti**—can occur from the extreme stresses associated with pregnancy and labor.

Attachments and Primary Actions of External Oblique Abdominal Muscle

Muscle	Lateral attachment(s)	Medial attachment(s)	Primary action(s)
External oblique (o-BLEEK)	Anterolateral aspect of lower 8 ribs	Anterior crest of ilium, crest of pubis, and linea alba	Spinal flexion Spinal lateral flexion (same) Spinal rotation (opposite)

External Oblique Abdominal Muscle (Obliquus Externus Abdominis)

As its name suggests, the **external oblique** (L. *obliquus*, slanting, deviation from the vertical or the horizontal) is the more superficial of the oblique muscles and runs diagonally downward from its lateral attachments toward its more medial attachments. The line of pull of the fibers of this paired muscle can be pictured as forming the letter "V" on the front of the abdomen, with each oblique forming one side of the "V." It's a thin and flat but relatively expansive muscle, covering the abdomen from the rectus abdominis to the latissimus dorsi (figure 3.13). Due to its lateral location and its diagonal line of pull, the external oblique tends to produce spinal lateral flexion to the same side or rotation to the opposite side. With rotation of the spine with the pelvis stationary, it pulls the lateral side of the rib cage downward and medially toward the midline of the trunk such as in twisting the torso. However, when the right and left external obliques contract together (bilateral contraction), they produce spinal flexion and the same type of movements as the rectus abdominis. With their curved position around the side of the abdomen, these muscles are also effectively positioned to help flatten the abdomen, depress the lower rib cage, and maintain appropriate postural positioning of the torso and the pelvis.

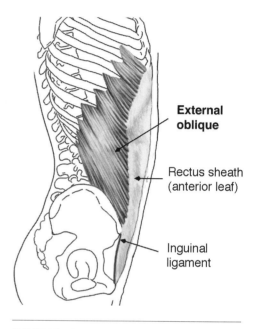

FIGURE 3.13   The external oblique abdominal muscle (lateral view).

Palpation: Curl up about 20° as just described for palpating the rectus abdominis, and then rotate toward the left. You can palpate the contraction of the right external oblique by placing your fingertips below the ribs and about 4 inches (10 centimeters) lateral to the navel (umbilicus).

Attachments and Primary Actions of Internal Oblique Abdominal Muscle

Muscle	Lateral attachment(s)	Medial attachment(s)	Primary action(s)
Internal oblique (o-BLEEK)	Thoracolumbar fascia, anterior 2/3 of iliac crest, lateral inguinal ligament	Ribs 9-12, cartilages of ribs 7-9, and linea alba	Spinal flexion Spinal lateral flexion (same) Spinal rotation (same)

Internal Oblique Abdominal Muscle (Obliquus Internus Abdominis)

As indicated by its name, the **internal oblique** is situated more deeply beneath the external oblique. Like the external oblique it is a very flat muscle, and it forms the intermediate layer of the abdominal muscles. Its upper fibers run diagonally upward in a medial direction from its more lateral lower attachments at approximately a 90° angle to the external oblique muscles as seen in figure 3.14 (its lower fibers run more horizontally). When the internal oblique contracts it can produce lateral flexion to the same side and rotation to the same side such as with side-bending, off-center facings, or spiraling movements of the torso in dance. With rotation with the pelvis stationary, it pulls the medial abdominal area laterally toward the iliac crest and has been shown to demonstrate greater activity in rotation than the external oblique (Ng et al., 2002). In contrast, the external oblique has been shown to exhibit greater activity in lateral flexion than the internal oblique. Bilateral contraction of the right and left internal obliques can produce spinal or trunk flexion and movements like those of the rectus abdominis. Similar to the external obliques, the internal obliques can also help flatten the abdominal wall, pull the lower rib cage down, posteriorly tilt the pelvis, and maintain spinal stability.

Palpation: Because the obliques and transverse abdominis are thin layers of muscle running just superficial or deep to one another, their individual actions cannot be well differentiated. However, when one performs the curl-up with rotation to the left (just described for palpating the external oblique), the tension palpated on the left side of the abdomen, just medial to the front of the crest of the pelvis, is in part due to contraction of the left internal oblique.

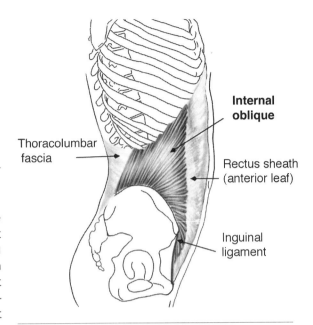

FIGURE 3.14   The internal oblique abdominal muscle (lateral view).

Attachments and Primary Actions of Transverse Abdominis

Muscle	Lateral attachment(s)	Medial attachment(s)	Primary action(s)
Transversus abdominis (trans-VER-sus ab-DOM-i-nis)	Thoracolumbar fascia, anterior 3/4 of iliac crest, lateral inguinal ligament, ribs 7-12 (costal cartilages)	Linea alba, pubis	Constriction of abdominal wall and contents Assists with spinal stabilization

Transverse Abdominis (Transversus Abdominis)

As its name suggests, the **transverse abdominis** (L. *trans,* across + *versus,* to turn + *abdom,* abdomen) runs across the abdominal area in an approximately horizontal manner (figure 3.15). It forms the deepest layer of the abdominal muscles, lying just beneath the internal oblique muscles. Similar to the internal and external obliques, it is a flat muscle, and its muscular fibers are primarily situated at the sides of the abdomen. The anterior aponeuroses of the transverse abdominis fuse with the anterior aponeuroses of the internal and external oblique muscles to form a single tendon (linea alba) that splits centrally to form a sheath, in which the rectus abdominis runs vertically.

In contrast to the other abdominal muscles, the transverse abdominis is considered primarily a postural muscle and a muscle of respiration. With its horizontally directed fibers, it is not capable of producing spinal flexion. Instead, when its muscle

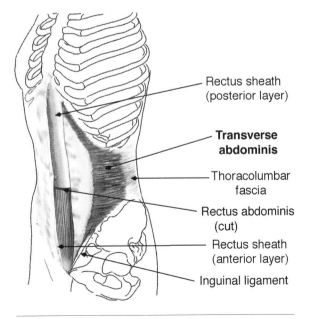

FIGURE 3.15   The transverse abdominis (anterolateral view).

fibers contract, the transverse abdominis compresses the abdominal contents. Hence, it is sometimes referred to as the "corset muscle" because it encloses the abdominal cavity similarly to the way a corset would. The transverse abdominis is used in such actions as forced expiration, coughing, sneezing, speech, laughing, straining, and pulling the abdominal wall in toward the spine. Although in the case of breathing, it appears that the transverse abdominis can be preferentially recruited, the other movements just listed are not effected by the transverse abdominis alone but rather usually also include contraction of the rectus abdominis to a lesser extent and obliques to a greater extent (De Troyer et al., 1990; Floyd and Silver, 1950). The transverse abdominis has also been shown to be particularly important for stabilization of the spine when the arms or legs move and for helping protect the spine during lifting. In dance, the function of the transverse abdominis of "pulling the abdominal wall inward" to help produce the aesthetically desired "flat abdomen" is often emphasized.

Palpation: Place your hand flat against your abdomen, with the heel of the hand below the ribs and above the side of the ilium and the fingers pointing toward the umbilicus. Then, forcibly exhale. Part of the tension felt under your hand is due to contraction of the transverse abdominis.

Attachments and Primary Action of Iliopsoas

Muscle	Proximal attachment(s)	Distal attachment(s)	Primary action(s)
Iliopsoas (il-ee-o-SO-us)			
Psoas major (SO-us)	Transverse processes, bodies, and intervertebral discs of T12-L5	Lesser trochanter of femur	Hip flexion Posture (maintenance of normal lumbar curve)
Iliacus (il-ee-AK-us)	Iliac fossa, crest of ilium, sacrum	Lesser trochanter of femur	Hip flexion

Iliopsoas

The **iliopsoas**—composed of the psoas major and iliacus—is a powerful flexor of the hip, and this function will be further discussed in chapter 4. However, it is important to note that due to its attachment onto the anterior portion of the bodies, discs, and transverse processes of the last thoracic vertebra and entire lumbar spine (T12-L5), the **psoas major** (G. *psoa,* muscles of the loin + great) also can directly influence the lumbar spine, under most conditions producing lumbar extension and lateral flexion during upright standing (see Psoas Paradox on p. 108 for more information). In contrast, the **iliacus** (*iliac,* relating to the ilium) can indirectly affect the curvature of the spine through its extensive attachment on the pelvis (figure 3.16), since pulling the top of the pelvis forward (anterior pelvic tilt) is accompanied by an increase in lumbar extension. Hence, the iliopsoas is believed to be a key for maintaining the normal lumbar curve (Hamilton and Luttgens, 2002; Michele, 1960) during upright

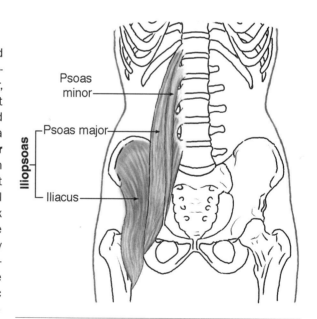

FIGURE 3.16   The iliopsoas (anterior view).

sitting and standing (Basmajian and DeLuca, 1985; Nachemson, 1966), and bilateral tightness can contribute to an excessive lumbar curvature (lumbar hyperlordosis), while excess length and weakness can contribute to an inadequate lumbar curve (flat back posture). Unilateral iliopsoas tightness can produce a lateral curvature of the spine (functional scoliosis) or slight rotations of the spine or pelvis commonly seen in dancers.

Palpation: Sitting on the floor or in a chair, lean forward to relax the abdominal muscles and carefully press your index and middle fingertips deep into the abdomen about 1 inch (2.5 centimeters) medial to the front portion of the top of the iliac crest. Then lift the knee toward the chest (hip flexion) on the same side without leaning back, and you should feel a tightening of the iliopsoas under the more superficial abdominal wall.

Posterior Muscles of the Spine

The muscles located posterior to the spine (the postvertebral muscles) include muscles that primarily act on the neck and head (splenius and suboccipital group) and a large number of paired muscles with the common action of spinal extension. Although many classification schemas exist, this text will use the classification of these spinal extensors into three groups—the erector spinae, semispinalis, and deep posterior spinal group. Within these groups, the muscles are arranged from small slips spanning adjacent vertebrae on the deepest level (deep posterior spinal group) to progressively larger slips with the semispinalis and erector spinae. This arrangement allows for complex fine coordination with the smaller slips and yet large force production with the longer slips.

Attachments and Primary Actions of Erector Spinae

Muscle	Inferior attachment(s)	Superior attachment(s)	Primary action(s)
Spinalis			
Spinalis cervicis (spi-NA-lis ser-VIS-us)	Spinous processes of C7 (sometimes T1-2)	Spinous processes of C2-C4	Spinal extension Spinal lateral flexion (same)
Spinalis thoracis (spi-NA-lis tho-RA-sis)	Spinous processes T11-L2	Spinous processes of upper thoracic vertebrae (T1-4 or T8)	Spinal extension Spinal lateral flexion (same)
Longissimus			
Longissimus capitis (lon-JIS-i-mus kah-PIT-us)	Transverse processes of T1-4 or T5, articular processes of C4 or C5-7	Inferior, lateral skull (mastoid process)	Extension of head Lateral flexion of head and C spine (same) Rotation of head (same)
Longissimus cervicis (lon-JIS-i-mus ser-VIS-us)	Transverse processes of T1-4 or T6	Transverse processes of C2-6	C spinal extension C spinal lateral flexion (same) C spinal rotation (same)
Longissimus thoracis (lon-JIS-i-mus tho-RA-sis)	Lumbar spinous processes, thoracolumbar fascia	Transverse processes of T1-L5, posteromedial portion of lower 10 ribs	Spinal extension Spinal lateral flexion (same) Spinal rotation (same)
Iliocostalis			
Iliocostalis cervicis (il-ee-o-kos-TA-lis ser-VIS-us)	3rd-6th rib angles	Transverse processes of C4-6	Spinal extension Spinal lateral flexion (same) Spinal rotation (same)
Iliocostalis thoracis (il-ee-o-kos-TA-lis tho-RA-sis)	Upper borders of angles of lower 6 ribs	Angles of upper 6 ribs, transverse process of C7	Spinal extension Spinal lateral flexion (same) Spinal rotation (same)
Iliocostalis lumborum (il-ee-o-kos-TA-lis lum-BOR-um)	Spinous processes of T11-L5, posterior sacrum, iliac crest	Inferior border of angles of lower 6 or 7 ribs	Spinal extension Spinal lateral flexion (same) Spinal rotation (same)

Erector Spinae

The **erector spinae** (L. *erector,* to raise or make erect + *spina,* spine) is a paired massive muscle that is the most powerful extensor of the spine. It lies in the trough on each side of the vertebral column. The muscle begins inferiorly as a large mass but soon divides into three approximately vertical columns of muscle. The medial column is called the **spinalis** (*spina,* vertebral column, spine); the intermediate column is called the **longissimus** (*longissimus,* longest); and the lateral column is called the **iliocostalis** (*ilio,* ilium + *cost,* rib). Each column can be further divided into three parts in accordance with its superior attachments as shown in figure 3.17. As can be seen from viewing the attachments of these muscles, they span different regions of the spine and are composed of slips that generally span six to eight vertebral segments. Both the iliocostalis (thoracis and lumborum) and longissimus (thoracis) have attachments onto the ribs in the thoracic region, while the spinalis is more centrally located and spans between vertebrae and associated ligaments only.

Although different components and regions of the erector spinae have slightly different actions, their combined bilateral contraction can produce extension of the spine, the head, or both such as is used when raising the trunk back to vertical from a forward-bent position. When one side contracts, they all can produce lateral flexion to the same side, especially when used in combination with the abdominal muscles. In addition, the longissimus and iliocostalis can produce rotation to the same side for the spine or head such as is used to help twist the torso so that the shoulders face front in an arabesque. The erector spinae also contribute to stability and protection of the spine.

Palpation: While standing, place your fingers flat against the low back with your right fingers just to the right of the low lumbar spinous processes and your left fingers just to the left of the same spinous processes. Slowly flex the trunk forward about 40° and then slowly raise the torso back to vertical. The tension you feel under your fingers when the torso rises is due to contraction of the erector spinae. You can also feel the erector spinae contracting on alternate sides when you walk slowly with your hands in the same position as just described.

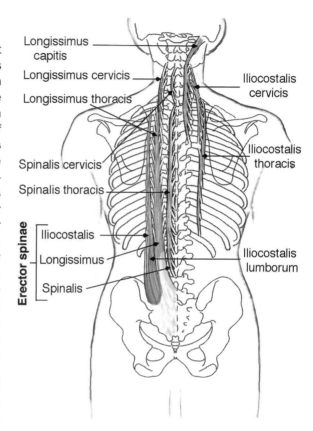

FIGURE 3.17   The erector spinae (posterior view).

Attachments and Primary Actions of Semispinalis

Muscle	Inferior attachment(s)	Superior attachment(s)	Primary action(s)
Semispinalis (sem-ee-spi-NA-lis)			
Semispinalis capitas (kah-PIT-us)	Transverse processes of C7-T7 Articular processes of C4-6	Occipital bone of skull Spinous processes 4-6 Segments above in cervical and upper thoracic regions	Extension of head and C spine Lateral flexion of head and C spine (same) Rotation of head and C spine (opposite)
Semispinalis cervicis (ser-VIS-us)	Transverse processes of T1-6	Spinous processes of C2-5	C and upper T spinal extension C and upper T spinal lateral flexion (same) C and upper T spinal rotation (opposite)
Semispinalis thoracis (tho-RA-sis)	Transverse processes of T6-10	Spinous processes of C6-T4	C and T spinal extension C and T spinal lateral flexion (same) C and T spinal rotation (opposite)

Semispinalis

The **semispinalis** (*semi,* half + *spina,* spine) lies close to the vertebrae beneath the erector spinae. It is divided into three parts in accordance with its superior attachments as seen in figure 3.18. As suggested by their name, these three paired muscles are only located in the thoracic and cervical regions of the spine. Except in the upper region, the muscle fibers span from transverse process to spinous process several vertebrae above, and so their line of pull goes inward and upward from their inferior attachment. In accordance with this line of pull, when one side contracts the action is spinal lateral flexion and rotation to the opposite side. When both sides contract together they can produce extension of the thoracic spine, cervical spine, or the head and are some of the muscles emphasized when trying to strengthen the "upper back." In dance, the semispinalis is used with other spinal extensors to achieve the desired arching of the upper back and a "long and lifted" spine when the torso is vertical.

Palpation: Place the fingers of your right hand flat against the lower neck just to the right of the low cervical spinous processes, and the palm of your left hand against your left temple. Slowly rotate your head to the left. The tension you feel under your fingers when the head rotates is due in part to contraction of the semispinalis (capitis).

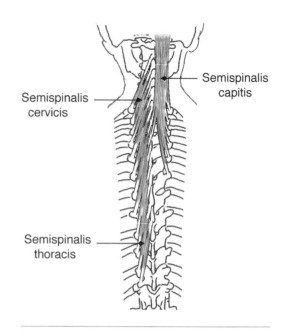

FIGURE 3.18   The semispinalis (posterior view).

Attachments and Primary Actions of Deep Posterior Spinal Group

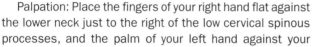

Muscle	Inferior attachment(s)	Superior attachment(s)	Primary action(s)
Interspinales	Spinous processes of C and L vertebrae	Spinous process of vertebra above	Stabilization Local spinal extension
Intertransversales	Primarily transverse processes of C and L vertebrae	Primarily transverse process of vertebra above	Stabilization Local spinal extension Local spinal lateral flexion (same)
Rotatores	Transverse processes of one vertebra, most developed in thoracic region	Junction of laminae and spinous process or transverse process 1-2 vertebrae above	Stabilization Local spinal extension Local spinal lateral flexion (same) Local spinal rotation (opposite)
Multifidus	Sacrum, ilium, transverse processes of T1-T3 and articular processes of C4-C7, most developed in lumbar region	Spinous processes 2-4 vertebrae above from C2-L5	Stabilization Local spinal extension Local spinal lateral flexion (same) Local spinal rotation (opposite)

Deep Posterior Spinal Group

The deep posterior spinal group includes the intertransversales, interspinales, rotatores, and multifidus. These muscles are composed of a series of paired small slips that span one to four vertebrae in various regions of the spine as seen in figure 3.19. In general, the **intertransversales** (*inter,* between) span between transverse processes of adjacent vertebrae, the **interspinales** (*inter,* between) between spinous processes of adjacent vertebrae, and the **rotatores** (L. *rotatio,* to revolve or rotate) and **multifi-**

dus (L. divided into many clefts or segments) between transverse and spinous processes. All of these muscles share the common action of spinal extension when both sides contract. In addition, unilateral contraction of the intertransversales and multifidus can produce small amounts of lateral flexion, while the rotatores and multifidus can produce small amounts of rotation to the opposite side. However, many of these deep muscles have poor mechanical advantage and are believed to be more important for helping stabilize the spine, and helping to control segmental movement, rather than producing the large forces associated with movements of the spine as a whole (Basmajian and DeLuca, 1985; Donisch and Basmajian, 1972; McGill, 2001; Panjabi et al., 1989). These muscles also have higher densities of receptors (muscle spindles); these provide feedback that can be used to detect and monitor precise positions of vertebrae (Moore and Dalley, 1999; Smith, Weiss, and Lehmkuhl, 1996). Due to their deep location, the deep posterior spinal group cannot be readily palpated.

Lateral Muscles of the Spine

There is one paired muscle, the quadratus lumborum, that is located posterolaterally versus anteriorly or posteriorly. This lateral location gives it the unique capacity to produce lateral flexion of the spine without additional movements. The other muscles that can produce lateral flexion are located either anteriorly, and so tend to also cause flexion (the abdominal muscles), or posteriorly, and so tend to also produce extension (spinal extensors).

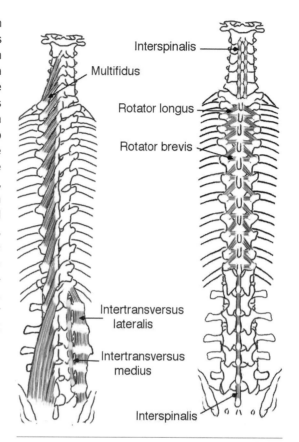

FIGURE 3.19   The deep posterior spinal muscles (posterior view).

Attachments and Primary Actions of the Quadratus Lumborum Muscle

Muscle	Inferior attachment(s)	Superior attachment(s)	Primary action(s)
Quadratus lumborum (kwod-RA-tus lum-BOR-um)	Posterior iliac crest, iliolumbar ligament	12th rib, tips of transverse processes L1-4	Fixes or depresses lower rib Spinal lateral flexion (same) Stabilizes spine and pelvis

Quadratus Lumborum

The **quadratus lumborum** (*quad,* four sided + *lumb,* lumbar region) is a flat muscle located on either side of the spine behind the abdominal cavity in the low back area as shown in figure 3.20. Its fibers run upward from the iliac crest to the lowest rib, with side slips running medially to attach to the top four lumbar vertebrae. When one side of this muscle contracts it can produce lateral flexion of the spine to the same side. Posturally, the quadratus lumborum can help depress the last ribs, stabilize the spine, and keep the pelvis level. This latter function of not allowing one side of the pelvis to drop relative to the rib cage is very crucial on the swing side during walking gait and on the gesture leg during upright dance movements.

Palpation: Sitting in a chair with the upper torso hanging forward, place your fingertips below the last rib and toward the spine (under some of the erector spinae if possible) on the right side. Then, hike the right hip (bring the right iliac crest toward the ribs). The tension you feel is partly due to contraction of the quadratus lumborum.

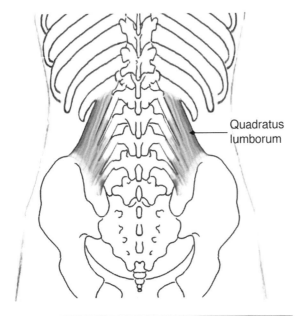

Quadratus
lumborum

FIGURE 3.20   The quadratus lumborum (posterior view).

Summary of Spinal Muscle Attachments and Actions

A summary of the attachments of the spinal muscles is provided in table 3.1, and selected muscles and attachments are shown in figures 3.21, A and B, and 3.22, A and B. From these resources, deduce the line of pull and resultant possible actions of the primary muscles of the spine; check your results by looking at figure 3.21D and figure 3.22C.

TABLE 3.1   Summary of Spinal Muscle Attachments and Primary Actions

Muscle	Origin*	Insertion**	Primary action
Anterior muscles			
Rectus abdominis (REK-tus ab-DOM-i-nis)	Crest of pubis of pelvis, pubic symphysis	Cartilages of ribs 5-7	Spinal flexion Spinal lateral flexion (same)
External oblique (o-BLEEK)	Anterolateral aspect of lower 8 ribs	Anterior crest of ilium, crest of pubis, and linea alba	Spinal flexion Spinal lateral flexion (same) Spinal rotation (opposite)
Internal oblique (o-BLEEK)	Thoracolumbar fascia, anterior 2/3 of iliac crest, lateral inguinal ligament	Ribs 9-12, cartilages of ribs 7-9, and linea alba	Spinal flexion Spinal lateral flexion (same) Spinal rotation (same)
Transversus abdominis (trans-VER-sus ab-DOM-i-nis)	Thoracolumbar fascia, anterior 3/4 of iliac crest, lateral inguinal ligament, ribs 7-12	Linea alba, pubis	Constriction of abdominal wall and contents Assists with spinal stabilization
Iliopsoas (il-ee-o-SO-us)			
Psoas major (SO-us)	Transverse processes, bodies, and intervertebral discs of T12-L5	Lesser trochanter of femur	Hip flexion Posture (maintenance of normal lumbar curve)
Iliacus (il-ee-AK-us)	Iliac fossa, crest of ilium, sacrum	Lesser trochanter of femur	Hip flexion

Muscle	Origin*	Insertion**	Primary action
Posterior muscles			
Erector spinae (e-REK-tor SPEE-nuh): Spinalis			
Spinalis cervicis (spi-NA-lis ser-VIS-us)	Spinous processes of C7 (sometimes T1-2)	Spinous processes of C2-C4	Spinal extension Spinal lateral flexion (same)
Spinalis thoracis (spi-NA-lis tho-RA-sis)	Spinous processes T11-L2	Spinous processes of upper thoracic vertebrae (T1-4 or T8)	Spinal extension Spinal lateral flexion (same)
Erector spinae: Longissimus			
Longissimus capitis (lon-JIS-i-mus kah-PIT-us)	Transverse processes of T1-4 or T5, articular processes of C4 or C5-7	Inferior, lateral skull (mastoid process)	Extension of head Lateral flexion of head and C spine (same) Rotation of head (same)
Longissimus cervicis (lon-JIS-i-mus ser-VIS-us)	Transverse processes of T1-4 or T6	Transverse processes of C2-6	C spinal extension C spinal lateral flexion (same) C spinal rotation (same)
Longissimus thoracis (lon-JIS-i-mus tho-RA-sis)	Lumbar spinous processes, thoracolumbar fascia	Transverse processes of T1-L5, posteromedial portion of lower 10 ribs	Spinal extension Spinal lateral flexion (same) Spinal rotation (same)
Erector spinae: Iliocostalis			
Iliocostalis cervicis (il-ee-o-kos-TA-lis ser-VIS-us)	3rd-6th rib angles	Transverse processes of C4-6	Spinal extension Spinal lateral flexion (same) Spinal rotation (same)
Iliocostalis thoracis (il-ee-o-kos-TA-lis tho-RA-sis)	Upper borders of angles of lower 6 ribs	Angles of upper 6 ribs, transverse process of C7	Spinal extension Spinal lateral flexion (same) Spinal rotation (same)
Iliocostalis lumborum (il-ee-o-kos-TA-lis lum-BOR-um)	Spinous processes of T11-L5, posterior sacrum, iliac crest	Inferior border of angles of lower 6 or 7 ribs	Spinal extension Spinal lateral flexion (same) Spinal rotation (same)
Semispinalis (sem-ee-spi-NA-lis)	Slips of muscles spanning several vertebrae from the transverse processes of C4-T10 to the posterior skull or spinous processes of C2-T4		Extension of head and C spine Lateral flexion of head and C spine (same) Rotation of head and C spine (opposite)
Deep posterior spinal group	1. Spinous process to spinous process (interspinales) 2. Transverse process to transverse process (intertransversales) 3. Transverse process to laminae of vertebra above (rotatores) 4. Generally transverse process to spinous processes above (multifidus)		Stabilization Local spinal extension Local spinal lateral flexion (same) Local spinal rotation (opposite)
Lateral muscles			
Quadratus lumborum (kwod-RA-tus lum-BOR-um)	Posterior iliac crest, iliolumbar ligament	12th rib, tips of transverse processes L1-4	Fixes or depresses lower rib Spinal lateral flexion (same) Stabilizes spine and pelvis

*Inferior, lateral, or proximal attachment for anterior muscles; inferior attachment for posterior and lateral spinal muscles.

**Superior, medial, or distal attachment for anterior muscles; superior attachment for posterior and lateral spinal muscles.

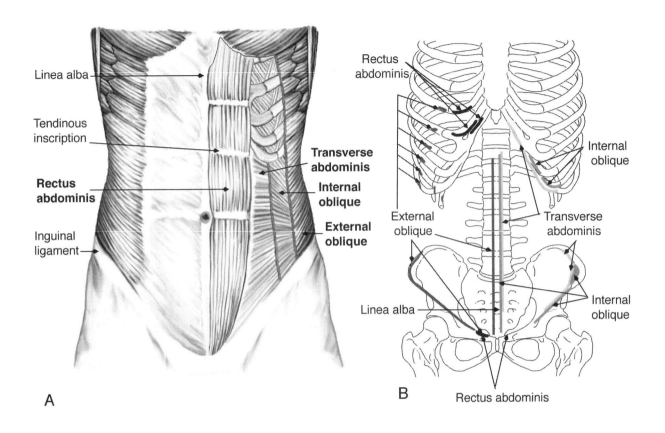

A

B

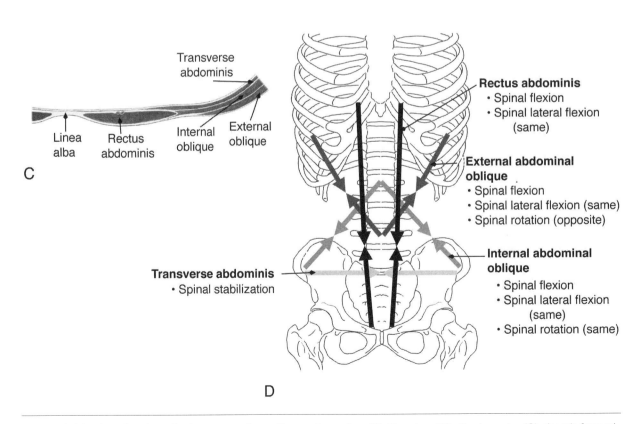

C

Rectus abdominis
- Spinal flexion
- Spinal lateral flexion (same)

External abdominal oblique
- Spinal flexion
- Spinal lateral flexion (same)
- Spinal rotation (opposite)

Internal abdominal oblique
- Spinal flexion
- Spinal lateral flexion (same)
- Spinal rotation (same)

Transverse abdominis
- Spinal stabilization

D

FIGURE 3.21   Anterior view of primary muscles acting on the spine. (A) Muscles, (B) attachments, (C) sheath formed by the aponeuroses of abdominal muscles, (D) line of pull and actions.

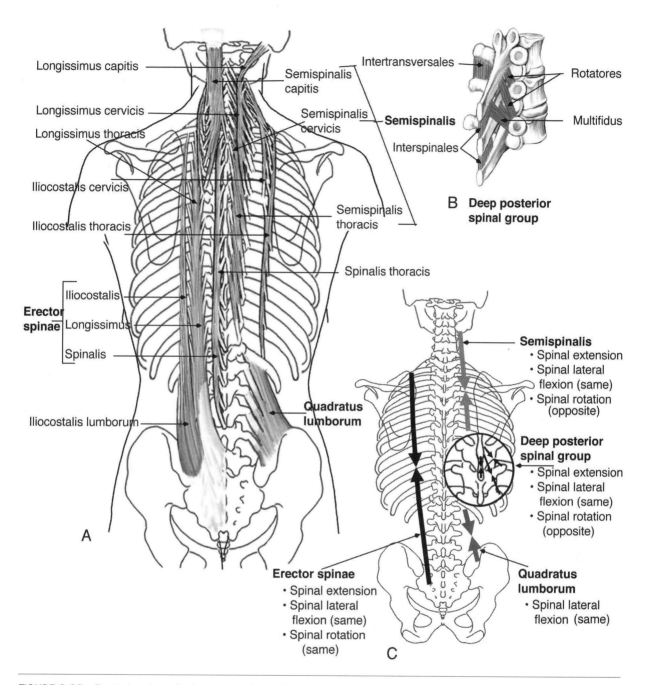

FIGURE 3.22   Posterior view of primary muscles acting on the spine. (A) Muscles and attachments, (B) deep posterior spinal group, (C) line of pull and actions.

Ideal Standing Postural Alignment

Although controversial, this text will consider ideal posture to encompass a balance of these sagittal curves and a positioning of joints so that the body's line of gravity is located in the median plane and runs in front of the thoracic vertebrae and just anterior to or through S2 as seen in figure 3.23A (Hamilton and Luttgens, 2002; Levangie and Norkin, 2001). This gravity line would ideally pass through or close to the centers of key weightbearing joints so that undue joint stress is avoided and minimal muscular contraction is required to maintain the desired positioning.

More specifically, positioning of the line of gravity allows much of the necessary support for the spine to be provided by intervertebral disc pressures and constraints offered by ligaments, fascia, and capsules of the facet joints (Caillet, 1996). Slight additional active support is often provided by low levels of activity of the spinal extensors (particularly the thoracic

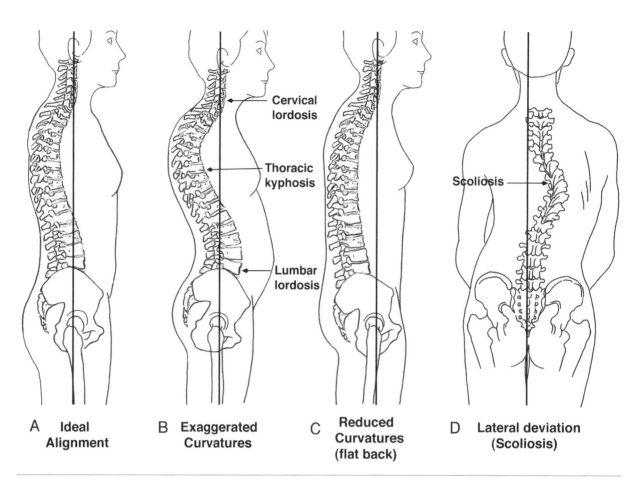

A Ideal Alignment

B Exaggerated Curvatures

C Reduced Curvatures (flat back)

D Lateral deviation (Scoliosis)

Cervical lordosis

Thoracic kyphosis

Lumbar lordosis

Scoliosis

FIGURE 3.23 Curvatures of the spine. (A) Normal; (B) lumbar lordosis, thoracic kyphosis, and cervical lordosis; (C) flat back; (D) scoliosis.

extensors and deep posterior spinal group) and the abdominals (particularly the internal obliques). As the gravity line continues downward, it runs slightly posterior to the axis of the hip joint with the resulting tendency for hip extension (extensor moment) limited by the iliofemoral ligaments (LaBan, Raptou, and Johnson, 1965), and in some cases, slight activity of the iliopsoas muscle (Basmajian and DeLuca, 1985); just anterior to the axis of the knee, with the resulting tendency for the knees to extend (extensor moment) limited by passive constraints (posterior knee capsule and knee ligaments); and just anterior to the ankle axis, generally requiring low levels of activity in the calf muscles (particularly the soleus) to prevent the body from falling forward (Basmajian and DeLuca, 1985; Floyd and Silver, 1950; Nachemson, 1966; Ortengren and Andersson, 1977).

To utilize the concept of ideal postural alignment practically, the vertical gravity line is reflected by a **plumb line,** and surface landmarks on the body are used to reflect where this gravity line would actually run inside the body (Kendall, McCreary, and

Provance, 1993). A plumb line is a cord with a weight (plumb bob) attached to its distal end so that when hung it will provide an absolute vertical line as a reference for measuring deviations. If one viewed a dancer from the side, the plumb line would be aligned with the ankle/foot (just in front of the lateral malleolus, which is the distal end of the fibula). This would serve as the fixed point. Then, with ideal alignment the following external landmarks would all be located right along the plumb line: the lobe of the ear, middle of the tip of the shoulder, middle of the thorax, greater trochanter (projection on lateral femur), just in front of the middle of the knee, and just in front of the lateral malleolus. Any of these landmarks that do not fall upon the plumb line would reflect deviations from ideal alignment. Assuming that the shoulders are not "rolled," having all of these landmarks aligned along the plumb line generally indicates a very basic correct balance of the sagittal spinal curves.

From this lateral view, the positioning of the pelvis should also be noted. With ideal alignment the pelvis is vertical (ASIS in a vertical plane with the pubic symphysis; see chapter 4) rather than tilted forward or backward. This positioning of the pelvis will directly affect spinal alignment, as an anterior pelvic tilt tends to increase the lumbar curve while a posterior pelvic tilt tends to decrease the lumbar curve. Positioning of the spine and pelvis also affects alignment of the lower extremity and can contribute to such alignment deviations as hyperextended knees (genu recurvatum) and rolling in of the feet (pronation), discussed in later chapters of this text.

The body can also be viewed relative to a vertical plumb line from the front or the back. When one views the dancer from behind, the gravity line should bisect the distance between the heels and ideally be in line with the spinous processes of the vertebrae. When viewing from the front, the gravity line should again bisect the distance between the feet and ideally be in line with midline structures such as the pubic symphysis, umbilicus, and nose. These anterior and posterior views provide the opportunity to see asymmetries between right and left sides of the body such as is associated with scoliosis.

Lumbar Hyperlordosis

In the normal upright stance the sacrum tilts anteriorly and inferiorly an average of about 30° (normal lumbosacral angle). This tilt necessitates that the lumbar spine extend (termed lordosis) in order to bring the torso upright (figure 3.23A), giving rise to the normal lumbar curve. However, in some individuals there is an abnormally large lumbar curvature. This postural condition is termed lumbar lordosis (G. *lordosis,* a bending backward), or more accurately **lumbar hyperlordosis** (figure 3.23B). Lumbar hyperlordosis is often accompanied by an increased inclination of the sacrum (increased lumbosacral angle), an anterior pelvic tilt, and sometimes a forward displacement of the torso relative to the ideal posture plumb line.

Lumbar hyperlordosis not only is undesirable from a perspective of the aesthetics of many dance forms but also may increase the risk for low back injury (Goldberg and Boiardo, 1984; Ohlen, Wredmark, and Spangfort, 1989). First, lumbar lordosis increases the tendency for the lower vertebrae to slide forward on the underlying vertebrae (shear forces). For example, inclining the sacrum forward 10° or 20° is associated with an increase in the shear force acting across the lumbosacral joint from 50% of body weight to 65% or 75% of the body weight above this joint, respectively (Hamill and Knutzen, 1995). This increased shear produces extra stress on

many spinal structures, including the portion of the vertebrae (pars interarticularis) commonly involved in stress fractures (spondylolysis). In addition to increased shear, fixed hyperlordosis is associated with greater contraction of the erector spinae (Frankel and Nordin, 1980; Wolf et al., 1979), which may allow low back muscle fatigue and strain to occur more readily. Furthermore, fixed lordosis can interfere with the cyclic loading and unloading of the facet joints necessary for proper cartilage nutrition, which may precipitate early breakdown of this cartilage (Stanish, 1979).

Lumbar hyperlordosis is often prevalent in young dancers and is sometimes exaggerated in an effort to achieve greater turnout. However, at least in ballet, lordosis may decrease with years of training. Dance training encompasses alignment directives that may tend to create straighter cervical, thoracic, and lumbar curvatures. One study of young ballet dancers showed that although lumbar range of motion in extension was higher, the depth of lumbar lordosis was significantly lower in dancers than in age-matched non-dancers (Livanelioglu et al., 1998). Similarly, in another study of ballet dancers, lumbar hyperlordosis was very prevalent in Level 1 dancers but not in Level 6 or advanced/company dancers (Clippinger-Robertson, 1991). In contrast, in higher levels of dance, fatigue posture was prevalent. So, it is important for dancers to realize that having hyperlordosis at one point in training does not mean that this will always be a problem, and care must be taken not to overcorrect and excessively reduce the lumbar curve.

When lumbar hyperlordosis is present, strengthening the abdominal muscles (figure 3.25A and table 3.4 [p. 134]) can often help improve the condition. Posteriorly, the spine forms a bony connection between the rib cage and pelvis. However, in the front, this connection is effected purely by the abdominal musculature. Because of this structure, the strength, resting length, and activation of the abdominal musculature are very critical in determining the distance between the rib cage and pelvis. That distance, in turn, affects the curvature of the lower spine and hence ideal alignment as seen in figure 3.24.

In addition to inadequate abdominal strength, lumbar lordosis may also involve low back and hip flexor (especially the iliopsoas) tightness as seen in figure 3.24A. Excessive lordosis associated with muscle tightness is particularly common during adolescent growth spurts (Micheli, 1983). If this is the case, stretching of the hip flexors (figure 3.25B and table 4.7A [p. 224]) and low back (figure 3.25C and table 3.7, A and B [p. 144]) will also be necessary

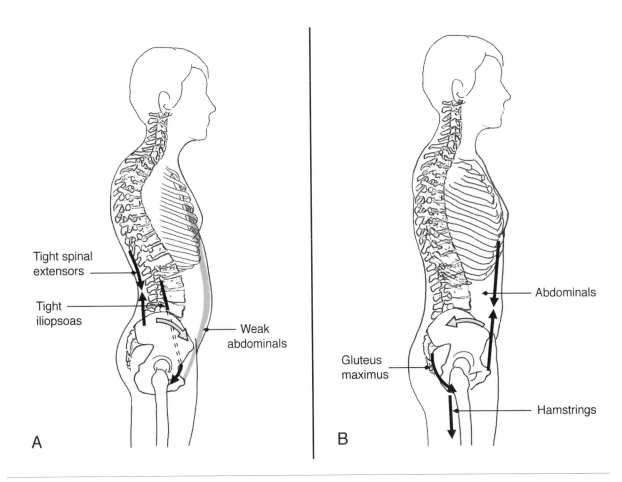

FIGURE 3.24   (A) Lumbar hyperlordosis, (B) contraction of the abdominal muscles to establish the desired neutral position of the pelvis and normal curve of the lumbar spine.

to improve the condition, and little improvement will be seen with just strengthening the abdominal muscles. Testing for range of motion of the hip flexors is recommended (see chapter 4) so that it can be determined whether these muscles are a contributing factor and need to be stretched.

Unfortunately, improving strength and flexibility in key muscles is often not sufficient to correct lumbar hyperlordosis, and working with changing movement patterns is also necessary. Studies suggest that some individuals tend to maintain posture more with the spinal extensors versus the abdominals (Klausen, Nielsen, and Madsen, 1981) and also show more prevalent use of the spinal extensors in movement (Hamliton and Luttgens, 2002). Many dancers with hyperlordosis appear to exhibit excessive back extensor activation, and successful change in this posture for standing and dynamic movement often involves greater co-activation of the abdominal muscles and upper back extensors for correct positioning and spinal stabilization. In an effort to achieve this, cueing dancers to "pull the pubic bone up" (inferior attachment of some of the abdominal

muscles) so that it is in line with the ASIS can help achieve neutral alignment. Overexaggeration of incorrect positions (anterior tilt and posterior tilt), visual cues, and tactile cues are often helpful for "relearning" neutral pelvis and ideal spinal alignment, as the lumbar hyperlordosis posture will feel "normal" and corrections foreign.

Some dancers who have a greater degree of lumbar lordosis or who excessively extend the spine higher up also will tend to displace the lower ribs forward (sometimes termed "rib leading") and may also need to focus on bringing the lower rib cage "down and back." In essence this involves a contraction of the abdominal muscles whereby both superior and inferior attachments move and are brought closer together, shortening the distance between the front of the rib cage and pubic bone. Cueing to knit the front of the pelvis and rib cage closer together while still maintaining a lift along the central plumb line or lift of the upper back can sometimes be effective.

Rehearsal of muscle activation patterns resulting in desired alignment should gradually progress from simple isolation exercises to simple dance skills such

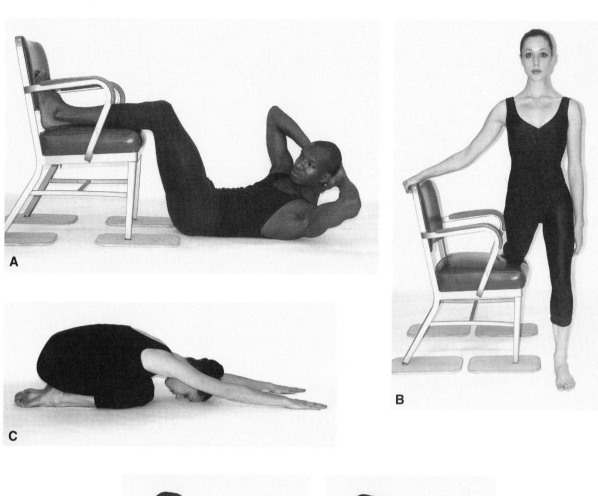

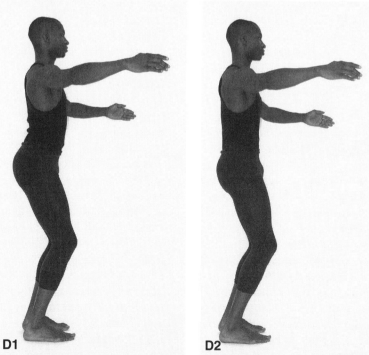

FIGURE 3.25 Correcting functional lumbar lordosis. (A) Strengthening abdominal muscles; (B) stretching hip flexors; (C) stretching low back; and (D) technique: activation of abdominal muscles to maintain neutral lumbopelvic alignment in pliés.

DANCE CUES 3.1

"Pull Up With Your Abs"

The cue to "pull up" or "lift" is often used in conjunction with the abdominal muscles (e.g., "pull up or lift with your abdominals") in response to seeing a dancer that is excessively arching the low back and anteriorly tilting the pelvis. A desired anatomical interpretation of this cue is to contract the abdominal muscles such that the inferior attachment onto the pelvis is the moving end, rotating the pelvis posteriorly and decreasing lumbar hyperlordosis to achieve the desired neutral position of the pelvis and normal curvature of the lumbar spine. However, some dancers misinterpret this cue as one directing them to pull up the superior attachment of the abdominal muscles onto the rib cage, requiring contraction of the thoracic spinal extensors versus abdominal muscles and resulting in "rib leading," or undesired backward movement of the upper back. Dancers can be assisted in achieving the desired intent of "pulling up" by standing with one side to the mirror for visual feedback and using one hand to maintain the lower anterior rib cage in its desired neutral position while the other hand is placed on the low abdomen to encourage the use of the abdominal muscles to lift the pelvis to a neutral position as shown in figure 3.24B.

as pliés (figure 3.25D) and rises to more complex dance movement such as turning and jumping. As strength, flexibility, and kinesthetic awareness improve, the conscious effort required to maintain ideal alignment should decline or disappear. There is evidence that shortened muscles may be more readily recruited in movement patterns (Pitt-Brooke, 1998); so restoring balanced strength and flexibility between the abdominal muscles, spinal extensors, and hip flexors should allow neutral alignment to be achieved more easily.

Kyphosis

Kyphosis (G. humpback) is characterized by an abnormal increase in the thoracic curvature as seen in figure 3.23B. This excessive curvature can be rigid in nature as a consequence of various diseases or structural abnormalities, while in other cases it is more flexible and functional in nature. The latter more functional version is commonly seen in sedentary individuals who sit with slumped posture, adolescents who carry heavy school backpacks, and athletes such as swimmers and weightlifters who have a strength or flexibility imbalance (or both) between anterior and posterior shoulder muscles (discussed in chapter 7) or spinal muscles. Dancers also sometimes exhibit mild kyphosis that is associated with weak upper back extensors or inadequate thoracic extensor activation and the tendency to let the upper back collapse and rest on passive constraints (fatigue posture). This also sometimes occurs in dancers who

perform abdominal work in a small range of motion (tending to create tightness) without stretching the abdominal muscles or balancing abdominal exercises with back extension exercises utilizing a full range of motion. As with lumbar lordosis, postural kyphosis is common in young children and adolescents; about 25% of adolescents have kyphosis-related difficulties (Hall, 1999).

In terms of correction, in normal standing and sitting the gravity line falls in front of the thoracic curve, tending to produce flexion of the thoracic spine (particularly in females with larger breasts). This tendency must be countered by consistent low level activity in the thoracic extensors, such as the longissimus and multifidus muscles of this region (Levangie and Norkin, 2001). Hence, strengthening the upper back extensors and using cues such as "lift the upper back up toward the ceiling" to encourage activation of these muscles are keys for prevention and improvement of kyphosis. However, considering the range of extension is so much lower in the thoracic region than in the lumbar region, the challenge with upper back exercises is to stabilize the low back by firmly pulling up the inferior attachment of the abdominal muscles, while the focus is on the relatively small movement in the upper back. The exercises in figure 3.26 use the back of the chair to help the dancer focus on isolating movement to this upper back region for strengthening (figure 3.26A and table 3.4H [p. 137]), stretching (figure 3.26B), and practicing correct alignment (figure 3.26C). When kyphosis is accompanied by a forward position

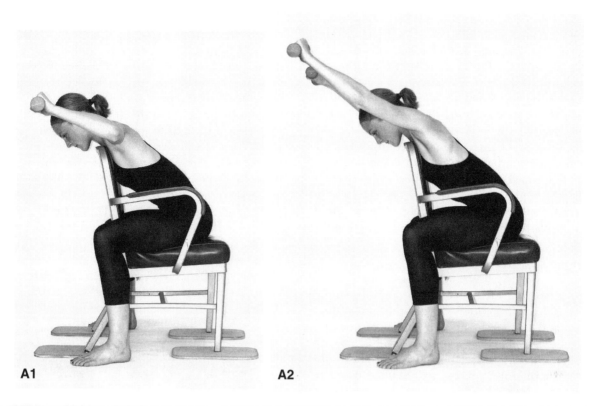

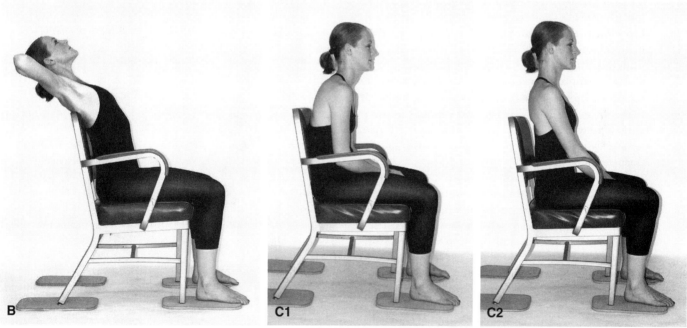

FIGURE 3.26   Improving kyphosis. (A) Strengthening upper back extensors; (B) stretching abdominal muscles and increasing upper back range in extension; (C) technique: thoracic extension while maintaining neutral lumbopelvic alignment.

of the shoulder termed "rolled shoulders," this must also be addressed (chapter 7).

However, if kyphosis is painful or pronounced, it is important to seek a medical evaluation to rule out Scheuermann's disease or other medical conditions. Scheuermann's disease classically develops around puberty and actually involves a wedging of one or more thoracic vertebrae related to abnormal behavior of the epiphyseal plate. The pronounced kyphosis (Dowager's hump) seen with aging (and particularly in postmenopausal women) involves erosion and collapse of the anterior portion of one or more thoracic vertebrae due to osteoporosis. These and other medical conditions produce a structural versus functional kyphosis that requires specific medical treatment.

Kyphosis is often seen in association with other spinal or pelvic deviations. When combined with lumbar lordosis, the resultant postural deviation is termed **kypholordosis.** When combined with a forward displacement of the pelvis, the resultant condition is termed fatigue posture.

Fatigue Posture

Fatigue posture involves a forward displacement of the pelvis relative to the ankle and "plumb line" (Tests and Measurements 3.1) and backward displacement of the torso relative to the pelvis and "plumb line" as seen in figure 3.27A. The posterior torso is frequently kyphotic, and the lumbar curve varies according to the level and degree of posterior displacement of the torso. In contrast to lumbar lordosis posture, fatigue posture classically involves hip joint extension or hyperextension rather than flexion, and generally a posterior rather than anterior tilt of the pelvis. This posture gets its name of fatigue posture from the fact that it involves resting on the ligaments (especially the iliofemoral ligament discussed in chapter 4) for support and thus requires almost no muscular effort for maintenance. Hence, it actually requires less energy to stand with fatigue posture than with ideal posture.

However, sustained use of ligaments for support can be detrimental, while the associated posterior shift of the weight of the trunk alters force transmission in the low back area such that sacroiliac pain may occur. The posterior position of the torso also distorts the normal transfer of weight of the arms and head to the spine and can be associated with upper back and neck fatigue or pain, and a compensatory forward position of the head. The fatigue posture occurs very frequently in mature individuals and in highly trained dancers. For example, in a study of university dance students and another study of adult non-dancers, the average hip marker was found to be anterior to the knee in standing posture (Woodhull, Maltrud, and Mello, 1985; Woodhull-McNeal et al., 1990). Similarly, in a study of young ballet dancers, about half of Level 6 and almost all of the advanced/professional dancers studied displayed fatigue posture with relaxed standing (Clippinger-Robertson, 1991).

This high incidence of fatigue posture in dancers may relate in part to the tendency for many dancers to dramatically increase flexibility in the hip flexors and other soft tissues to allow sufficient hip hyperextension to achieve the desired aesthetic in movements to the back such as arabesques. Since with normal alignment the gravity line falls slightly posterior to the axis of the hip joint, gravity would tend to produce hip hyperextension. However, in the dancer with increased range in this area, the normal passive constraints that would limit this motion would not be operative until much later, allowing excessive posterior tilting of the pelvis and hip hyperextension (e.g., the fatigue posture) unless (a) the iliopsoas is actively used to prevent this, (b) the center of mass of the torso is moved slightly forward to lessen this extension tendency (extension moment), or (c) both forms of correction are used. Another possible explanation is that the lumbar flexion and posterior tilt of

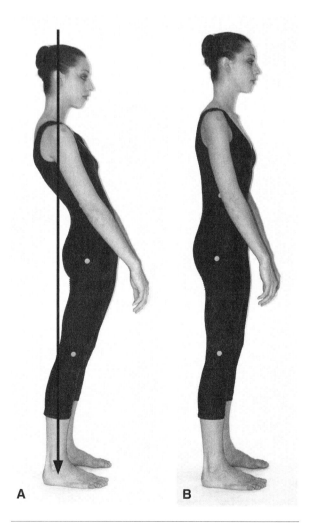

FIGURE 3.27 (A) Fatigue posture; (B) activation of thoracic spinal extensors and hip flexors.

Evaluation of Standing Postural Alignment

Perform the following observations on another dancer or on yourself (with your side to a mirror) using figures 3.23 and 3.27 for reference. Observation will be easier if a bathing suit or leotard and tights are worn. One can devise a plumb line by attaching a piece of string overhead and hanging a plumb bob or some other small weight from this piece of string. The piece of string should be long enough that the weight just clears the floor.

General Observation

Have your partner stand upright with the legs parallel and feet under the hip joints. Apply markers (adhesive dots, small pieces of masking or colored tape) to the landmarks shown in figure 3.27. Situate your partner with her or his side to the plumb line so that it runs through the ankle marker. Note the relationships of the landmarks and the curves of the spine to each other and the plumb line. Attempt to classify this standing alignment, noting the presence of ideal, lumbar hyperlordosis, kyphosis, flat back, or fatigue posture.

Replicate Common Postural Deviations

To help train your eye and understand the differences, have your partner perform the following maneuvers, and note the changes in the spinal curves; changes in the relative positioning of the head, torso, and pelvis; and changes relative to the plumb line.

1. Round and sink backward into his or her upper back to simulate kyphosis.
2. Tilt the top of the pelvis forward and arch the low back to simulate lumbar hyperlordosis.
3. Press the bottom of the pelvis forward and let the upper back relax backward to simulate fatigue posture.
4. Tuck the pelvis slightly, pull the abdominal muscles back against the lumbar spine, and lift the spine upward as much as possible to simulate flat back posture.

Apply to Simple Movement

Repeat the same alignment observation with your partner performing a first position plié and rise (parallel and then turned out). Note if the general postural pattern observed with standing remains or changes.

the pelvis may reflect an effort to stabilize the lumbar spine (McMeeken et al., 2002), which is known to have marked increased mobility in dancers.

The fatigue posture can often be improved with strengthening of the upper back extensors (figure 3.28A and table 3.4H [p. 137]), and sometimes the hip flexors (figure 3.28B and table 4.5, A-C [pp. 213-214]). In some cases abdominal tightness is also a factor, and stretching is advised. When rolled shoulders are involved, this must also be addressed. With some dancers, fatigue posture can actually relate to overcorrection of lumbar lordosis. Performing lots of abdominal exercises in short ranges of motion (e.g., curl-ups) in an effort to correct lumbar lordosis over a long period of time can sometimes lead to the opposite imbalance in which the abdominal muscles

are too tight or strong (or both) relative to the back extensors. This overcorrection can readily be avoided by including stretches for the abdominal muscles or full range of motion abdominal exercises, such as seen in figure 3.28C (and table 3.4C, variation 1 [p. 134]), and spinal extension exercises (table 3.4, I and J [p. 138]), which will dynamically stretch the abdominal muscles, in one's regular routine.

However, as with other postural problems, successful correction of the fatigue posture often requires changing muscle activation patterns and breaking habitual patterns. Since the fatigue posture is a passive posture involving hanging on the ligaments, muscles need to be activated to avoid this posture. Use of the upper back extensors will tend to decrease the exaggerated thoracic curve (kyphosis), while a

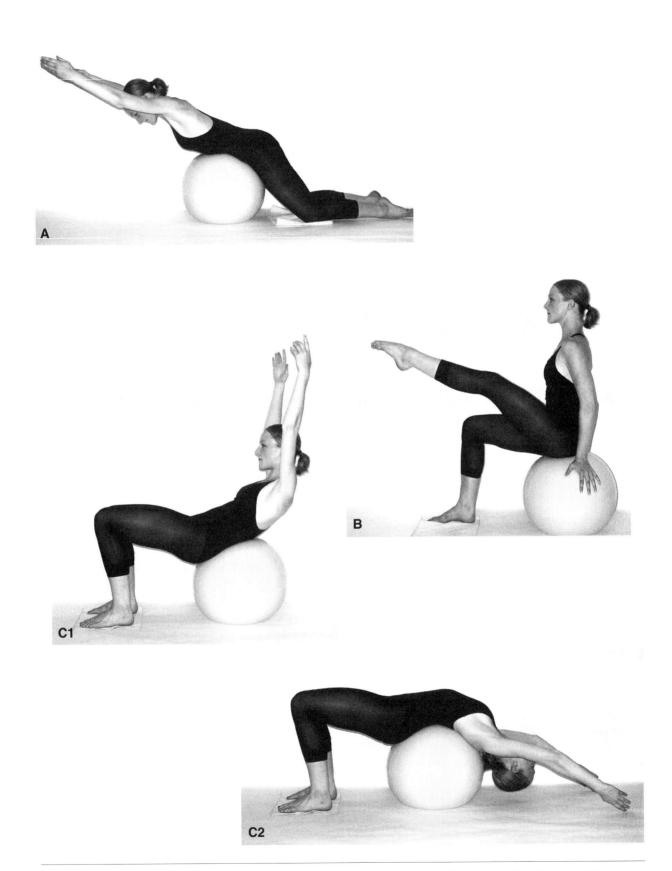

FIGURE 3.28   Improving fatigue posture. (A) Strengthening upper back extensors; (B) strengthening hip flexors if indicated; (C) performing abdominal strengthening incorporating a range in which the abdominals are dynamically stretched.

small co-contraction of the abdominal muscles can be used to bring the torso forward (so that it is more directly over the pelvis) and into alignment along the plumb line. This repositioning of the torso will also lessen the forces (extensor moment) tending to cause the hip hyperextension and posterior tilting of the pelvis associated with the fatigue posture. Cueing to "lift the upper back up and forward," as though there was a string attached to the spine (at a level between the shoulder blades) that is being pulled up on a slight forward diagonal, can often be used to find correct positioning. If slight hip hyperextension is still present, slight activation of the hip flexors (iliopsoas) by cueing to bring the front of the pelvis slightly forward toward the thigh can be used to establish the desired neutral position of the pelvis and hip joint (figure 3.27B).

Cervical Lordosis and Forward Head

An increased curve in the upper back (often associated with kyphosis) can bring the head forward and the eye level down. To reach a horizontal eye level, the upper neck is then brought into extension, resulting in cervical lordosis and an undesired forward positioning of the chin termed **forward head** (Palmer and Epler, 1990) as seen in figure 3.29A. This forward position also moves the center of gravity of the head in front of the line of gravity of the body; and Caillet (1996) estimates that when the head is 3 inches (7.6 centimeters) forward, the weight of the head (approximately 10 pounds or 4.5 kilograms) exerts about 30 pounds (13.6 kilograms) of torque on the cervical spine. This places excessive demands upon the spinal extensors and facet joints.

Over time, this position tends to create a shortening of the cervical extensors; and neck presses (figure 3.29B), in which the chin is brought down and the head is gently pressed back against the hand for 5 seconds, are often recommended for relief. The neck extensors can also be stretched using the hand to gently lengthen the neck by bringing the head "out and forward" on a slight diagonal (figure 3.29C). However, when kyphosis is involved, correcting the kyphosis is essential for correct head positioning. Use of images such as bringing the chin slightly back and imagining "being suspended from just behind the ears" can sometimes help get the desired length in the neck and avoid the tendency for the chin to jut forward (figure 3.29D). However, care must be taken not to excessively stretch or straighten the neck. When X rays are taken, many dancers find that they have lost the natural curve (lordosis) in their cervical spines, and so working with a qualified physical therapist is advisable if this condition is marked.

Flat Back

Flat back posture involves a decreased lumbar curve such that the low back looks flat as seen in figure 3.23C. The flat back posture reduces the normal shock absorbency of the spine and is hypothesized to contribute to disc degeneration. Interestingly, having decreased curvatures of the spine is thought to increase the risk for low back injury (Klausen, Nielsen, and Madsen, 1981; McMeeken et al., 2002), just as having excessive curvatures can increase injury risk. The flat back posture is sometimes seen in dancers who have worked so hard to decrease their excessive lumbar lordosis that they have actually overcorrected and taken out the desired curve in their lumbar spines. It is also likely that the cueing and alignment encouraged in many forms of dance, focusing on "lengthening the spine," tend to decrease the cervical, thoracic, and lumbar curvatures. Whether the extent of curve reduction

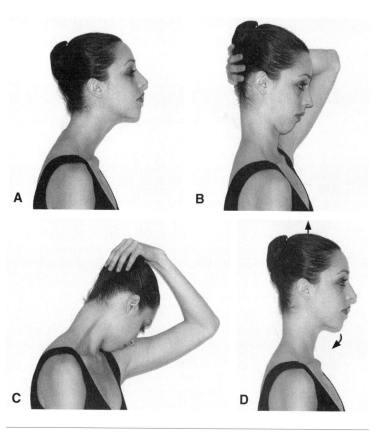

FIGURE 3.29   Improving forward head. (A) Forward head posture; (B) strengthening neck flexors with neck press; (C) stretching neck extensors; (D) technique: chin back with neck lifting up.

associated with such dance training has long-term negative health consequences and whether greater curvatures automatically return when training stops will require investigation.

Correction of flat back posture is controversial, but in some cases may be aided by strengthening the low back extensors as well as the hip flexors (iliopsoas). In other cases this posture is more related to repetitively standing in a passive posture (such as fatigue posture) in which the pelvis is tucked (posterior pelvic tilt), thereby decreasing the lumbar curve. In this case, successful correction will require the use of lumbar supports and a re-education of static and dynamic alignment focusing on restoring a neutral pelvis and associated normal lumbar curve.

Scoliosis

Scoliosis (G. *skoliosis,* crookedness) is characterized by a lateral curvature of the vertebral column in an approximately frontal plane. When one looks from behind the vertebral column, the spine ideally runs approximately straight up and down. It is common to have a very slight right thoracic curve, which has been conjectured to be due to the position of the aorta or handedness (White III and Panjabi, 1978). However, the presence of an appreciable lateral curve or curves of the spine as seen in figure 3.23D is termed scoliosis. Scoliosis can involve a single lateral curve, termed a "C" curve, or multiple curves. When two alternating curves are present the curve is termed an "S" curve as seen in figure 3.30B. The vertebrae involved with the lateral curves also frequently rotate, generally with the spinous processes turning toward the concavity of the abnormal curvature (figure 3.30D). This gives rise to the prominent raised portion of the posterior rib cage ("rib hump") to one side of the spine, often evident in dancers with scoliosis, as shown in figure 3.30C. This rotation also appears to have a very negative impact on spinal mechanics, and current models of scoliosis suggest that scoliosis be visualized as a complex three-dimensional deformity with torsion(s) similar to an elongated helix.

Scoliosis can be divided into two types—nonstructural scoliosis and structural scoliosis. **Nonstructural scoliosis** is reversible and will generally improve when the underlying condition is treated. Examples of underlying conditions include leg length difference, muscle spasms, asymmetrical muscle development, and handedness patterns. In contrast, **structural scoliosis** is generally considered irreversible and involves structural changes both within and between the vertebrae. For example, a vertebra may be asymmetrical as a consequence of having different length pedicles,

different orientation of the transverse processes, or a spinous process that is not centrally located. Surprisingly, about 90% of structural scoliosis occurs with no known cause (Mercier, 1995); this type of scoliosis with no known cause is termed idiopathic scoliosis (G. *idios,* one's own + *pathos,* suffering).

Although the causes of idiopathic scoliosis are poorly understood, there is strong evidence that familial factors play a role; the risk of having scoliosis increases about 10 times if someone in your immediate family has it. Gender also plays a role in terms of incidence and severity; females are 8 times more likely than males to require treatment for scoliosis (Liederbach, Spivak, and Rose, 1997). Activity also can influence scoliosis incidence. Although this influence was originally believed to be linked to muscle imbalances associated with asymmetrical occupations and sports, the elevated incidence of scoliosis in activities considered more symmetrical (e.g., swimming and ballet) suggests this association is more complex than initially believed (Becker, 1986; Sward, 1992).

While the incidence of scoliosis for the general U.S. adolescent population has been estimated to be between 10% and 16% (Akella et al., 1991; Trepman, Walaszek, and Micheli, 1990), studies of female ballet dancers have reported incidences of 24% (Warren et al., 1986), 33% (Hamilton et al., 1997), 40.7% (Akella et al., 1991), and 65% (Molnar and Esterson, 1997). The higher incidence of scoliosis found in dancers may relate to a higher familial incidence; the common recommendation for children with scoliosis to take ballet; a greater prevalence of a taller, more ectomorphic body type; a greater prevalence of increased flexibility or actual hypermobility; the tendency for prolonged growth spurts due to delayed maturation; low estrogen levels associated with delayed maturation and disrupted menstrual cycles (amenorrhea); and inadequate nutrition with suboptimal calcium and vitamin D. Further investigation of causative factors is important so that prevention can be better addressed. Prevalence of scoliosis in dance forms other than ballet warrants further investigation.

Given its high incidence, it is important that dancers and their teachers have a basic understanding of the detection and treatment of scoliosis. Although it may be seen at any age, scoliosis is usually detected clinically between the ages of 10 and 13. Detection often relates to noticing apparent asymmetries or results of screening tests such as the forward bend test (described in Tests and Measurements 3.2) commonly used in schools. Early detection is important because the combination of bracing, therapeutic exercise, and other therapeutic treatments may be able to halt or slow further progression in moderate curves (>25°). Unfortunately, if curves are allowed to progress to about 40° (see figure 3.30A for one method of measurement), very drastic surgery involving spinal fusion along the length of the abnormal curve and various forms of instrumentation to try to stabilize the spine may be recommended (Warren et al., 1986). So, dancers should watch for asymmetries and seek medical evaluation if scoliosis is suspected.

In terms of prevention, dancers should also be careful to carry their dance bags and books in a backpack worn over both shoulders, or if using a single strap over one shoulder, to regularly switch the side on which it is carried. In some cases, using a small bag on wheels that can be pulled with alternate arms may be a better option. Dancers should also regularly perform exercises for trunk stabilization and abdominal and back extensor strength that emphasize rotation (Mooney, Gulick, and Pozos, 2000), while taking extra care to work for symmetry in their stretching exercises, strengthening exercises, and dance technique. If teaching dance, care must be taken to avoid demonstrating on the same side and to avoid consistent one-sided biases in choreography (e.g., always turning one way).

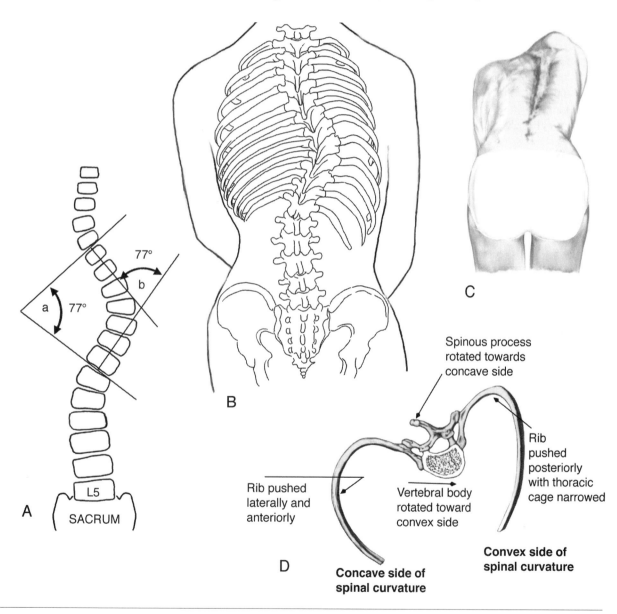

FIGURE 3.30 Scoliosis (posterior view except superior view on D). (A) Cobb method of measuring curvatures, (B) structural scoliosis with widened rib space on convex side and narrowed rib space on concave side of thoracic curvature, (C) visible rib hump with forward bend test, (D) rotation of vertebrae and effect on thoracic cage.

Detection of Scoliosis

Perform the observations and forward bend test on another dancer as described next, using figure 3.30 as a reference. Observation will be easier if female dancers wear a swimsuit top, a halter top, or a backless leotard and if male dancers remove their shirts.

General Observation

Have your partner stand upright with the legs parallel and feet under the hip joints. Viewing your partner from both the front and back, note any apparent asymmetries such as a difference in shoulder height, scapular prominence, unequal height of hands or distance of arms from sides of body, difference in height of one side of the pelvis versus the other, one side of the pelvis rotated farther forward than the other, unequal waistline, or leg length discrepancy. Standing from behind, palpate the spinous processes from the top of the neck to the sacrum and note any apparent lateral curvature or rotation.

Forward Bend Test

Then, observing from directly behind, have your partner very slowly bend forward ("roll down"), starting from the top of the head, and progress downward while the arms hang free by the sides. Look for symmetry of the sides of the trunk at each level of the spine and note whether one side is higher and if there is a "rib hump."

Note: Although helpful, it is important to realize that many factors such as leg length difference and handedness patterns can create asymmetries. However, young dancers with apparent scoliosis are best referred for medical evaluation to determine the basis and magnitude of apparent asymmetries.

Although a well-balanced "S" scoliosis, even if involving large curvatures, does not necessarily preclude a professional dance career, it is associated with an increased risk for stress fractures (Warren et al., 1986) and low back injury. In the experience of the author, even many dancers with low curvatures (especially when accompanied by larger rotations) experience asymmetry in their work. Hence, particular attention should be directed toward avoiding further development of asymmetries, with assistance procured from a qualified physical therapist if needed. Furthermore, attention should be paid to preventative measures for stress factors (including nutritional and hormonal) discussed in chapter 1.

Spinal Mechanics

The fact that the normal spine is comprised of many consecutive segments with alternating curves influences its vulnerability to injury and the actions that muscles can have on it. The abdominals appear to play a particularly key role in protecting the spine via mechanisms still under investigation. One example of how changes in spinal curvature can affect muscles' action is illustrated with the psoas paradox.

Abdominal Contraction for Spinal Protection

The spine can be subjected to tremendous forces during dance and other athletic endeavors. It has been calculated that 2,071 pounds (939 kilograms) of force is imposed on the lumbosacral disc as a person leans forward and lifts a 170-pound (77-kilogram) weight off the ground (Morris, Lucas, and Bresler, 1961). Similarly, a study of selected aerobic dance hip extension exercises (involving motions similar to those utilized in dance) showed that torque values occurring at the lumbar spine were greater than those that are estimated to accompany lifting a 100-pound (45-kilogram) load (Hall and Lindoo, 1985). Such large forces approach or even exceed the forces found to damage discs (Bartelink, 1957) or the bony vertebrae themselves (Eie, 1966) when they are removed from cadavers and studied in a laboratory setting. The fact that apparent damage to the spine does not occur during such rigorous functional activities (despite meeting or exceeding experimental loads that produced damage) suggests that in the living organism, something must serve to protect the spine.

One of the mechanisms that may provide protection for the spine is **intra-abdominal** (L. within the abdomen) **pressure** (IAP). Intra-abdominal pressure is described as the pressure that can be generated if the muscle walls around the abdominal cavity are contracted (abdominal muscles, diaphragm, pelvic floor muscles). The function of IAP was originally described by Bartelink (1957) as that of acting like a fluid ball that resists deformation as soon as the pressure within is raised as seen in figure 3.31A. This was theorized to provide an additional route to help transfer forces from the torso to the pelvis such that an unloading effect estimated to be as high as 30% to 50% is offered to the spine (Morris, Lucas, and Bresler, 1961).

Although this original model has been challenged by recent studies, there is still support for the concept that the abdominal muscles play a role in protecting the spine. One alternate explanation is that the contraction of the abdominal muscles (particularly the transverse abdominis) reduces shear forces by pushing back against the front of the lower spine, resisting lumbar hyperextension and anterior sliding of the vertebrae as seen in figure 3.31B. Another theory is that contraction of the abdominal muscles may help increase stiffness of the trunk so that the spine does not buckle when loads are applied (Hall, 1999). A related theory is that contraction of the abdominal muscles (specifically the transverse abdominis and internal oblique abdominal muscles) and the resultant IAP act by tensioning the thoracolumbar fascia as seen in figure 3.31C. The **thoracolumbar fascia** is a complex structure that can be divided into three layers (Smith, Weiss, and Lehmkuhl, 1996). It has connections to the ribs, vertebrae, sacrum, select posterior ligaments of the spine, and various muscles including the transverse abdominis, internal obliques, erector spinae, multifidus, quadratus lumborum, latissimus dorsi, and gluteus maximus. Due to its posterior attachments onto the spine, this **thoracolumbar fascia tensioning** theory holds that when the thoracolumbar fascia is tightened it tends to produce extension that could assist in movements such as lifting, or at least in stabilizing the spine (Richardson, Hodges, and Hides, 2004), thus decreasing the load on the lumbar spine (Levangie and Norkin, 2001). Still another theory (muscle fusion) holds that contraction of the abdominal muscles has the opposite effect, that is, that it tends to pull the lumbodorsal fascia laterally and to lessen lumbar lordosis, reducing shear and allowing more efficient support of the spine (Plowman, 1992; Saal, 1988b).

Whether IAP, shear reduction, thoracolumbar tensioning, or a combination of these mechanisms is operative, strengthening the abdominals and focusing on using them prior to rigorous movements (such as lifting a partner) should theoretically increase their protective effect for the spine. Studies of IAP have shown the amount of IAP that can be generated is much greater in athletic individuals and elite weightlifters than in slight, nonathletic individuals (Bartelink, 1957; Eie and Wehn, 1962; Grieve, 1978). Studies suggest that the transverse abdominis most importantly, and obliques secondarily, are vital for the generation of IAP (Bartelink, 1957; De Troyer et al., 1990; Grillner, Nilsson, and Thorstensson, 1978; Kumar and Davis, 1978). It appears that the rectus abdominis does not play much of a role in

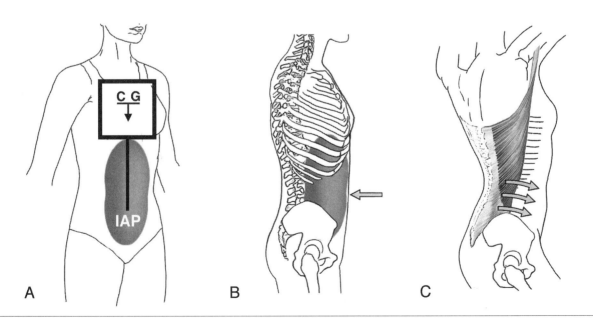

FIGURE 3.31   Potential roles of abdominal muscles in protecting the low back. (A) Original intra-abdominal pressure (IAP) theory, (B) shear reduction theory, (C) thoracolumbar tensioning theory.

intra-abdominal pressure generation, and its role is probably more that of control of movements of the spine. Hence, abdominal strengthening exercises should be selected and cued to emphasize strengthening the transverse and oblique abdominal muscles.

Psoas Paradox

Although the iliopsoas is primarily considered a hip flexor, it can also produce movements of the spine that are influenced by the position of the body. When the spine is in a flexed position, the line of pull of the iliopsoas is generally anterior to the axis of rotation of the lumbar intervertebral joints, and it will tend to produce flexion of the lumbar spine (Levangie and Norkin, 2001). The iliopsoas acts in this function during rope climbing, Graham contractions, and various dance warm-ups performed on the floor that involve swinging the leg forward (hip flexion) with the lumbar spine in flexion. However, in most cases (such as with normal standing) when the lumbar spine is in extension, the line of pull of many of the fibers of the iliopsoas runs posterior to the lumbar intervertebral joints and tends to produce extension (hyperextension) of the lumbar spine. This apparent role reversal from its usual tendency to produce extension of the lumbar spine to being a flexor of the lumbar spine is termed the **psoas paradox.** This general tendency to produce lumbar hyperextension may be desirable in some instances, such as to help maintain the lumbar curve with upright standing. However, there are many other cases, such as when lifting the gesture leg to the front in dance or in double-leg lift abdominal exercises, when it is undesirable, and firm contraction of the abdominal muscles is required to stabilize the proximal attachments of the iliopsoas and prevent the undesired anterior pelvic tilt and spinal hyperextension.

Muscular Analysis of Fundamental Spinal Movements

In analyzing movements of the spine, it is important to realize that they are often linked with movements of the pelvis. This relationship will be discussed in chapter 4. It is also important to realize that the segmental structure of the spine allows different movement capacities in different regions of the spine and allows one part of the spine to move in one direction while another part moves in another direction. However, for purposes of simplicity, it is helpful to first learn movement of the spine as a whole.

To understand what muscles are producing a given movement of the spine, it is essential to appreciate the role of gravity when standing upright. In this upright position, the spine is in a potentially precarious position, and if it is moved in any direction "off center," gravity will tend to make it fall in that direction. Often a slight voluntary concentric contraction is used to initiate movement in a desired direction. Then gravity becomes the primary mover, and muscles with actions opposite to the movement produced by gravity are used to control that movement. To visualize these movements, it is helpful to think of the spine as a flexible column with the muscles acting like guy ropes relative to the spine (Smith, Weiss, and Lehmkuhl, 1996). When the vertebral column is vertical, little or no tension in the guy ropes is required. However, when the vertebral column leans off the vertical, the guy ropes (e.g., muscles) opposite to the direction in which the spine is leaning must contract to control or prevent the falling of the spine in that direction. Muscles of the spine are also often used together (co-contraction) in a coordinated manner to create a stable desired position of the spine. A summary of the muscles capable of producing the fundamental movements of the spine is provided in table 3.2, and an illustration of the fundamental movements of the spine was given in figure 3.11.

Spinal Flexion

Spinal flexion is forward bending in the sagittal plane, tending to bring anterior surfaces of the vertebrae and trunk together. However, because the cervical and lumbar regions curve in the direction of hyperextension (concave posteriorly), flexion of these regions may represent a decrease in extension or a flattening of the curve, without actually necessarily producing a position of flexion of the adjacent vertebrae. It is common in the cervical curve for flexion to reduce the curve to a straight line; and in flexible individuals, the lumbar curve may actually be reversed.

The classic concentric use of the abdominal muscles and other spinal flexors occurs when the spine flexes or the pelvis posteriorly tilts against gravity or another external resistance. When gravity offers the resistance, a supine position of the body allows for effective resistance. For example, in the isometric curl-up (see table 3.4B [p. 134]), the spinal flexors work concentrically on the up-phase to curl the torso. The rectus abdominis and right and left external and internal obliques all act together to produce spinal flexion, while the transverse abdominis ideally aids with pulling the abdominal wall inward. With slow

TABLE 3.2   Fundamental Spinal Movements and the Muscles That Can Produce Them

Spinal movement	Primary muscles	Secondary muscles
Flexion	Rectus abdominis External oblique abdominals Internal oblique abdominals	Iliopsoas*
Extension	Erector spinae	Semispinalis Deep posterior spinal group Iliopsoas
Lateral flexion	Quadratus lumborum External oblique abdominals Internal oblique abdominals Erector spinae	Semispinalis Deep posterior spinal group (intertransversarii and multifidus) Iliopsoas (lumbar lateral flexion)
Rotation	External oblique abdominals Internal oblique abdominals Erector spinae	Semispinalis Deep posterior spinal group (rotatores and multifidus)

*In select circumstances due to the psoas paradox.

movements, the rectus acts alone when the head lifts, and the obliques join in when the shoulders begin to rise. In dance, this type of movement occurs when the dancer is rising from a supine position such as in contractions commonly used in modern and jazz dance.

When standing in an erect position the situation gets more complex. In the standing contraction shown in figure 3.32, the abdominals would still be used rigorously to posteriorly tilt the pelvis, flex the spine, and pull the abdominal wall inward. In addition, a slight co-contraction of the spinal extensors would be required to achieve the desired "lift" of the movement and prevent the upper back from collapsing too far forward. However, if the torso were allowed to round forward such as in a roll-down, the spinal extensors would be the primary muscles working (eccentrically) to control the spinal flexion produced by gravity. In dance, a slight co-contraction of the abdominals is often encouraged to shape the movement, with the head and shoulders staying close to the lower body as the roll-down proceeds.

Spinal Extension

Extension is the return from a position of flexion toward anatomical position or backward bending, in the sagittal plane. When the spine is extended beyond anatomical position the movement can be termed hyperextension. In analysis or description of a movement, we often simply continue to use the term "extension" because the goal is to describe the direction of movement (extension) rather than a position. However, at times, such as in description of a position

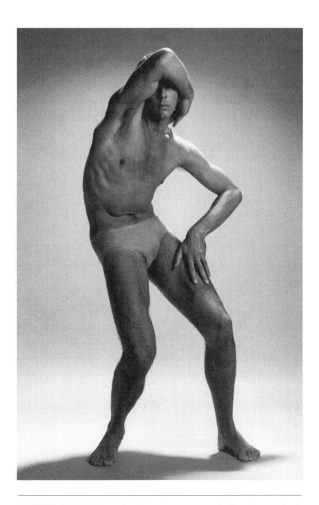

FIGURE 3.32   Sample dance movement showing spinal flexion.

Photo: Roy Blakey. Dancer: Douglas Nielsen in Anna Sokolow's "The Cage The Pond," with Batsheva Dance Company, Tel-Aviv.

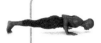

The Role of Gravity in Standing Movements of the Spine

Perform the following movements from a standing position with your feet parallel and about hip-width apart, using figure 3.11 as a reference.

- **Gravity and forward flexion.** Place one hand with the palm on the side of the lumbar spine. Place the other hand on your abdomen. Then, slowly roll down (as if you were going to touch the floor) about halfway. Think about the effect gravity would have during this movement. Explain why you are feeling the muscle contraction you are feeling, and how the abdominal and spinal extensors would operate in this movement.

- **Gravity and spinal extension.** Keeping your hands placed as before, slowly come back up from this position of forward flexion to a vertical position of the spine. What muscles do you feel working? Again, explain the role of the abdominal and spinal extensors in this movement and whether eccentric, concentric, or both types of contractions would be involved. Now, let your torso carefully arch slightly beyond vertical (hyperextension). Explain the influence of gravity with this movement and how it would affect muscle use.

- **Gravity and spinal lateral flexion.** With your hands hanging by your sides, slowly bend the torso to the side. Again, think about the influence of gravity and try to feel and explain what muscles are working on both the down-phase and up-phase of the movement. Include the quadratus lumborum, as well as the abdominal muscles and spinal extensors. Now vary the position of your torso slightly as you bend to the side (torso slightly forward of and then back of a directly side position). How does this influence muscle use?

- **Gravity and spinal rotation.** Lastly, with your hands hanging by your sides, rotate your torso to one side. How is the influence of gravity different in this motion than in the previous motions? How will this influence the contribution and contraction type of the abdominal muscles and spinal extensors?

or a mechanism of injury, it can be helpful to use the term "hyperextension."

The classic concentric use of the spinal extensors occurs when the spine extends or hyperextends against gravity or another external resistance such as in the prone single-arm spine arch (table 3.4I [p. 138]). The erector spinae muscles have been shown to be particularly active during prone extension, with greatest activity in the spinalis, followed by the longissimus, and with the least in the iliocostalis (Basmajian and DeLuca, 1985). The semispinalis and deep posterior spinal group are also active to some degree during prone extension. The latter muscle group is believed to primarily act to help stabilize the spine and adjust motion between individual vertebrae, while the erector spinae provides the primary force for full spine extension.

The spinal extensors are also commonly used concentrically to bring the torso back up toward a vertical position from a position of forward flexion. In dance this use of the extensors is common, such as when the torso is brought from a flexed position

to a vertical or a flat back position in port de bras or center floor warm-ups in modern and jazz dance. The spinal extensors also work very hard to prevent the torso from tilting too far forward and to attempt to maintain a more upright position of the torso when a leg is lifted to the back in an arabesque, back attitude (figure 3.33), or leap.

Spinal Lateral Flexion

Spinal lateral flexion is side-bending in the frontal plane and is termed either right lateral flexion or left lateral flexion. Spinal lateral flexion is named in accordance with the way the side of the upper spine bends with reference to the lower part. So, approximation of the right sides of the vertebrae such as when bending the torso to your right during standing would be termed right lateral flexion. Conversely, approximation of the lateral surfaces of the vertebrae to the left would be termed left lateral flexion. To be consistent with the custom of using a term that describes the direction of the motion, the return to

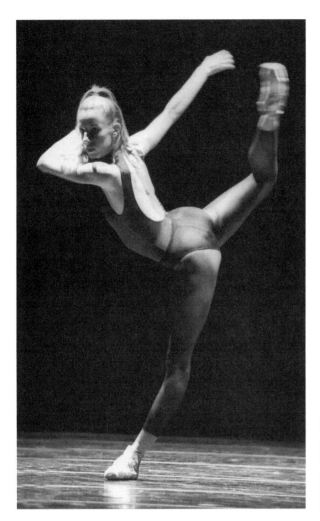

FIGURE 3.33   Sample dance movement showing spinal extension.

© Angela Sterling Photography. Pacific Northwest Ballet dancer Melanie Skinner.

pure lateral flexion occurs there appears to be little action of the rectus abdominis, but when it is combined with slight flexion of the torso, the rectus and oblique co-contract to help produce the motion.

During upright standing, the spinal lateral flexors work whenever the torso is bent to the side. This motion is commonly used in modern and jazz movements and second-position floor or barre stretches in which the torso is bending or reaching to the side as seen in figure 3.34. In the pictured movement, the right lateral flexors initiate the movement. Then once the spine is off center, the left lateral flexors would primarily work to control the motion eccentrically, motivated primarily by gravity once the spine is off center. As with side-lying movements, the specific contribution of the spinal lateral flexors appears to be affected by position of the trunk. However, the oblique muscles appear to be particularly important, with the contribution of the spinal extensors more variable (Basmajian and DeLuca, 1985). For example, one study found greater activity in the

anatomical position from left lateral flexion would be termed right lateral flexion, and vice versa.

The classic concentric use of the spinal lateral flexors occurs when the spine laterally flexes against gravity or resistance such as in side-ups (see table 3.4K [p. 139]). The quadratus lumborum, oblique abdominal muscles, and erector spinae are considered the primary lateral flexors. Note that the external and internal obliques on the same side of the body would be working to produce the same motion (e.g., when lying on your right side, the left external and left internal oblique would both produce the desired left lateral flexion). In some cases, the semispinalis, deep posterior spinal extensors, rectus abdominis, and iliopsoas also assist with the movement. Which muscles contribute to the movement is influenced by the amount of resistance, speed of the motion, and specific positioning of the trunk. For example, when

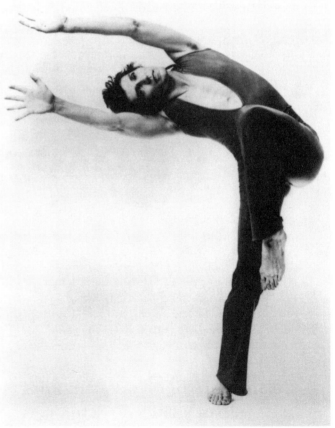

FIGURE 3.34   Sample dance movement showing spinal lateral flexion.

Photo courtesy of Bill Evans. Photographer: Jack Mitchell. Dancer: Bill Evans in "Five Songs."

spinal extensors on the opposite side in the lumbar region but greater activity in the spinal extensors on the same side in the thoracic region (Andersson, Ortengren, and Nachemson, 1977).

Spinal Rotation

Spinal rotation is twisting around the long axis of the spine and, similar to the situation with lateral flexion, is also designated as right or left in accordance with the way the front of the upper spine turns with reference to the lower part. Right rotation is defined as movement of the head or shoulders to the right with respect to a fixed pelvis, or movement of the pelvis to the left with respect to a fixed head or fixed shoulders or upper spine. Return from these positions would be termed left rotation.

Concentric contraction of the spinal rotators is used whenever the head, torso, or pelvis is twisted such as in jazz isolations, spiral movements in modern dance (figure 3.35), and facings in ballet where the front of the torso is rotated relative to the front of the pelvis. For purposes of simplicity, this discussion will be limited to thoracic and lumbar rotation. Performing rotation around the long axis of the spine would be affected primarily by the abdominal obliques and spinal extensor muscles. Theoretically when rotating the torso to the right, the right internal oblique, right longissimus, right iliocostalis, left external oblique, left multifidus, left rotatores, and left semispinalis thoracis muscles would contract to produce the movement. Note that unlike what happens in lateral flexion, the internal and external obliques from opposite sides work together to produce rotation.

While some EMG studies have confirmed this expected activity in the lumbar region (Ortengren and Andersson, 1977), other studies have shown a more complex contribution of muscles than expected, possibly due to the complex interaction of agonists, synergists, antagonists, and stabilizers and the complex lines of pull and multitude of joints crossed by spinal musculature (Basmajian and DeLuca, 1985). Also, as with lateral flexion, positioning of the torso and the relationship of gravity will affect which muscles contribute, as well as the primary site of rotation. For example, when spinal rotation is performed from a vertical standing position, greater rotation tends to occur in the thoracic region. However, when it is performed from a position of hyperextension, a greater amount of rotation tends to occur in the lumbar spine, and the spinal extensors tend to make a larger contribution to the desired rotation. Conversely, when spinal rotation is performed from a position of spinal flexion, greater rotation occurs higher in the spine, and the oblique abdominals tend to be utilized more to produce the rotation. These same concepts apply to strengthening exercises with rotation in a prone position.

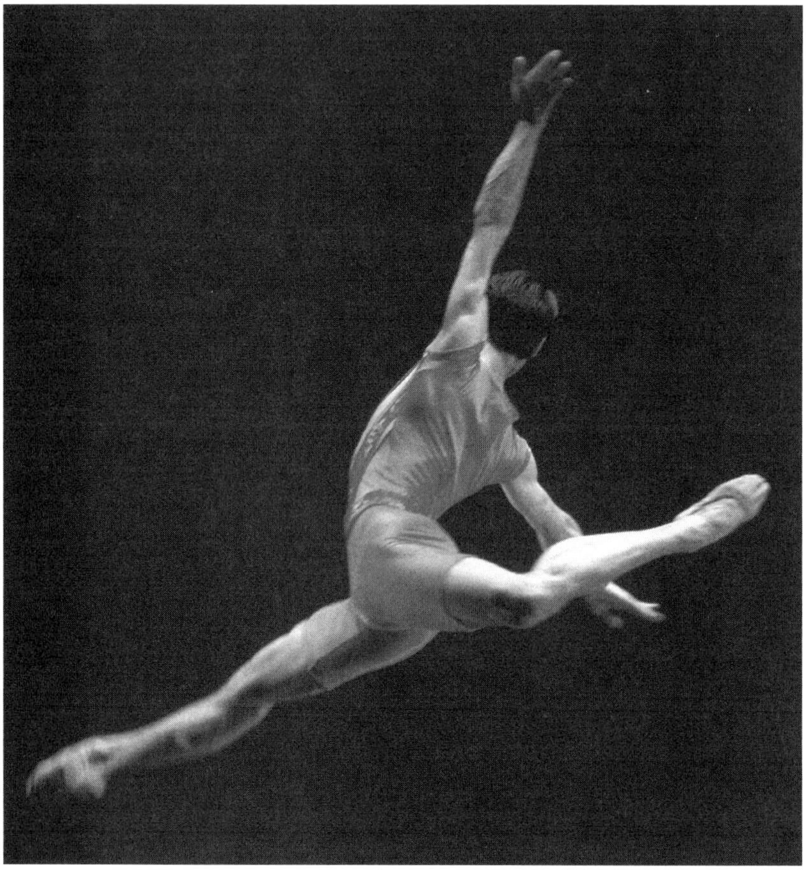

FIGURE 3.35 Sample dance movement showing spinal rotation.
© Angela Sterling Photography. Pacific Northwest Ballet dancer Christophe Maraval.

Key Considerations for the Spine in Whole Body Movement

Due to its central location, coordinated movement between the trunk and limbs is vital to meet movement goals and for injury prevention. Core stability is one important mechanism for protecting the spine and enhancing centered movement.

Core Stability

Core stability (also referred to as trunk stability, lumbopelvic stabilization, and spinal stabilization) can be defined as the development or restoration of neuromuscular aspects of lumbopelvic control vital for protecting the spine from injury or reinjury (Hodges, 2003). Strategies to develop core stability generally utilize two components. One component emphasizes utilizing exercises to improve the muscular strength and endurance of key trunk muscles (muscle capacity). The second component has gained great attention in recent years and focuses on the training of the coordinated use of these key trunk muscles during functional movements (motor control).

As described earlier in this chapter, the vertebral column is very dependent on a balance of the spinal muscles for stability. Unlike some joints such as the hip and knee, which can be "locked" in slight hyperextension to allow the ligaments to provide the primary support, the spine cannot be locked and the anterior-posterior curves of the spine will tend to collapse or buckle due to the effect of gravity if not counterbalanced by appropriate muscles. In fact, an isolated ligamentous spine without muscular support will collapse when less than 5 pounds (2 kilograms) is applied to it (Nachemson, 1966). The torso can be pictured as a cylinder (Nachemson and Morris, 1964), where with ideal alignment muscles located on all sides of the cylinder are balanced so that the torso is "stable," the curves are not exaggerated, and the spine is protected from excessive stress.

Many muscles of the trunk likely play a role in core stabilization, but due to their location the abdominals and back extensors are particularly key. For example, automatic abdominal contraction (transverse abdominis followed by oblique abdominals) prior to quick movements of the arms, and legs, peak vertical forces in walking and running, and landing from jumping has been demonstrated (Grillner, Nilsson, and Thorstensson, 1978; Hodges and Richardson, 1996, 1997). Studies suggest that the central nervous system activates components of the abdominals without our conscious awareness prior to movement of the limbs. This precontraction of the abdominals is believed to aid with trunk stability through the resultant generation of IAP or thoracolumbar fascia tensioning. Similarly, muscles such as the multifidus of the deep posterior spinal group appear to be vital for core stability at the segmental level of the spine. So, well-timed and coordinated contraction of such deep muscles of the spine is believed to be particularly key for stabilizing the spine on a segmental level, while the more superficial trunk muscles that can generate larger forces work to stabilize and control movements of the spine as a whole. Together, these deep and superficial trunk

muscles can be used to lessen or eliminate undesired compensatory trunk movement occurring in response to movements of the limbs and could lessen potentially injurious forces borne by the spine.

Centered Movement

Core stability is also one important aspect of highly skilled movement used by dancers and athletes. In movement forms such as dance, martial arts, and Pilates, use of core stability is one part of desired movement patterns that are often termed "centered" movement. In these movement forms, core stability is often used in a very refined manner to meet aesthetic goals as well as biomechanical goals. For example, in some dance movements, the torso and pelvis are held relatively upright while the arms or legs are used in a variety of movements. Many beginning dancers have difficulty with this coordination, and many visible compensations of the torso leaning front, side, or back are seen. However, as skill progresses, such compensations are minimized such that large range limb movements occur without distorting the desired positioning of the torso. This skill is made more complex in cases where the torso is moved through desired positions off the vertical while the limbs move. For example, the spinal hyperextension accompanying a cambré to the back in ballet, the presentation of the torso in flamenco, a jazz layout, or a spiral arching motion of the torso used in modern all require slightly different use of the abdominals, back extensors, and other trunk muscles to create the desired line and avoid excessive movement of one vertebra relative to another. Achieving and maintaining such desired positions of the torso not only requires strong trunk muscles but also appropriate timing and magnitude of activation of these muscles.

Special Considerations for the Spine in Dance

Various aspects of dance place great demands on the spine. Some areas that are of particular importance in terms of technique and injury prevention are spinal alignment, spinal hyperextension, standing forward flexion, and partnering.

Spinal Alignment in Dance

The standing alignment used at center floor or at the barre in some dance styles is quite similar to the ideal standing alignment previously described. However,

DANCE CUES 3.2

"Lift and Lengthen Your Spine"

The cue to "lift and lengthen your spine" can be interpreted from an anatomical perspective as referring to the use of muscles to counter the tendency of gravity to slightly "collapse" the normal sagittal curves of the spine (A). With well-coordinated contraction of the spinal muscles, the curves can be slightly decreased and the length of the spine very slightly increased. However, the challenge of this cue is that because the curves of the spine go in different directions, a complex co-contraction of muscles in different regions of the spine is necessary to achieve the desired effects. For example, if too much contraction of the abdominal muscles occurs, it will decrease the lumbar curve but increase the thoracic curve, pulling the front of the rib cage too far down and creating a "collapsed" versus "lifted" look. In contrast, if excessive thoracic extension is used, it will tend to bring the shoulders and upper back behind the gravity line and again fail to create the desired "lifted" look.

Sometimes it can be helpful to use supplemental cues, for example the cue of imagining a line of energy starting with the front of the bottom of the pelvis, going under the rib cage (along the front of the spine), and out the top of the head (just behind the middle of the top of the head) as seen in the figure (B). For dancers that still

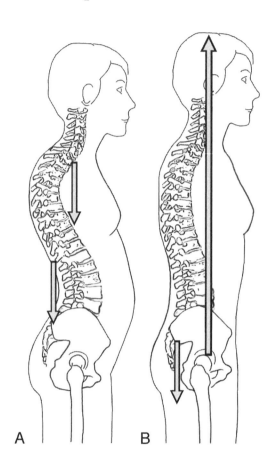

A   B

appear "collapsed" in the chest, thinking of lifting the top of the sternum up toward the ceiling can facilitate desired positioning. For dancers who still tend to shorten the low back (lumbar hyperlordosis), thinking about letting the low back "lengthen" and reach down toward the floor, or imagining having a small weight hanging from the coccyx or having fingertips on the back of the sacrum that pull the sacrum slightly down toward the floor, while still maintaining the "lift" on the front of the body, can be helpful.

because the goal is preparation for movement and an aesthetic of "energy" or "presence" versus relaxed standing, this alignment generally involves more muscle activation. Such greater muscle activation is consistent with many different directives commonly given by dance teachers such as "reach the head up toward the ceiling," "lift the spine toward the ceiling," or "lift and lengthen the spine." But this positioning would still ideally entail spinal curves of appropriate magnitude that are balanced in the sagittal plane and can be thought of as a **neutral base alignment.**

When one is actually dancing, the spine is dynamically changing its position—often in multiple planes that encompass combinations of flexion, lateral flexion, extension, and rotation; but the skilled dancer should be able to quickly reestablish this neutral base alignment when the choreography utilizes an erect position of the torso.

However, some styles of dance may also involve slight differences from this "neutral" base alignment. For example, the aesthetics of some schools of flamenco and ballet may involve greater "lift and arching" of the upper back, while some schools of modern dance prefer slightly anterior positioning of the rib cage. Skilled dancers can learn to achieve these aesthetics while still protecting their low backs with abdominal co-contraction. And as with the neutral base alignment, skilled dancers should be able to quickly reestablish the base alignment of their dance style when demanded by the choreography.

When sitting on the floor as is common in modern and jazz dance, a different challenge for spinal alignment comes into play. Sitting in a relaxed/slumped position as seen in figure 3.36B tends to be associated with as much as 40° of posterior tilting of the pelvis, with a consequent decrease in lumbar lordosis, increase in thoracic kyphosis, and associated increase in intradiscal pressure. It is very easy to assume this position, as it relies on passive support from back ligaments and other soft tissues with little spinal extensor activity. However, using a more erect position during sitting so that a more neutral position of the pelvis is maintained and the weight of the upper body is felt directly over the bottom of the pelvis ("sitz bones" or ischial tuberosities) versus behind, and so that the spinal extensors are used to "lift" the spine and prevent excessive flexion of the lumbar and thoracic regions, will reduce lumbar stress and better achieve the desired dance aesthetic (figure 3.36C). When one is performing floor work in which the knees are extended, it is important to realize that adequate hamstring flexibility will be necessary to allow this more neutral position of the pelvis, and it may be necessary to slightly bend the knees to allow

this positioning in individuals with tight hamstrings (see chapter 4).

In more complex dance movements, spinal alignment becomes much more complicated. However, even though changes in positions are very dynamic, there is still the desire to achieve a given movement without undesired distortion of the spinal curves, or in accordance with the specific positioning dictated by the choreography. For example, when one is performing a side reach, pure lateral flexion involves the torso moving almost directly to the side (figure 3.37A) without the ribs going forward or the bottom of the pelvis going back (figure 3.37B). Such positioning involves a subtle co-contraction of many muscles with appropriate timing and magnitude of force such that both appropriate spinal stabilization and movement are effected in accordance with the goal movement. Such coordination of muscles is one marker of skill in the professional dancer.

Spinal Hyperextension

Hyperextension of the spine tends to make the front part of consecutive vertebrae pull away from each other and the back part of consecutive vertebrae press together. More specifically, hyperextension produces tension on the front of the disc, compression at the back of the disc, and increased pressure within the disc. Hyperextension also creates increased stresses in the posterior portion of the vertebrae; and when it is very forceful or repetitive, the facet joints can become injured or stress fractures to the bone

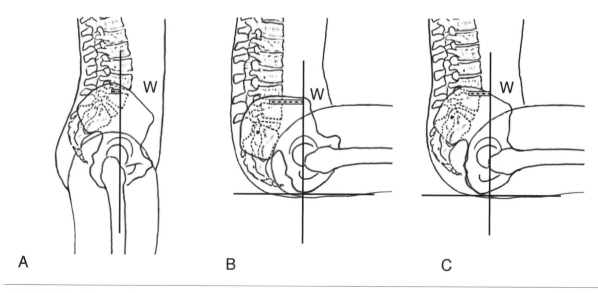

A   B   C

FIGURE 3.36   Changes in the low back with standing and sitting. (A) Normal lumbar curvature with standing, (B) undesired excessive posterior tilt of pelvis and decreased lumbar lordosis with sitting, (C) desired neutral pelvic alignment and less loss of normal lumbar lordosis with sitting.

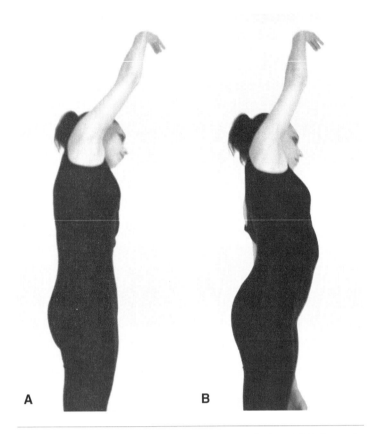

FIGURE 3.37   Spinal alignment during lateral flexion. (A) Balanced muscle co-contraction resulting in desired spinal alignment, (B) inadequate abdominal contraction resulting in undesired spinal alignment.

than the thoracic spine, this technique requires the development of high levels of abdominal and upper back strength, upper back flexibility, and subtle neuromuscular coordination that can take years to develop. Technique cues that can be used to help obtain this arch include (1) imagine arching up and back over a barrel; (2) imagine that someone is lifting you up and back from just below the shoulder blades, and the scapulae become a shelf to support the upper back; (3) think of the spine as a flexible column with the goal to create a continuous long arc rather than allowing the lower portion to collapse and crimp.

Spinal Forward Flexion

Movements involving forward flexion of the spine are very common in modern and jazz dance forms and may relate to the disc injuries more commonly seen in older modern dancers. In contrast to what occurs with hyperextension, with forward flexion the anterior portions of the vertebrae press toward one another and the posterior structures of the spine tend to pull away from one another. This creates compression at the front of the disc and tension at the back of the disc and increases intradiscal pressure. It also creates large stresses on the ligaments that span between adjacent vertebrae posteriorly. Furthermore, during flexion the top vertebrae tends to slide forward as it tilts due to the weight of the trunk. This sliding tendency creates large shear forces. Lastly, muscle activity influences spinal stresses.

In terms of the influence of muscles, the activity of the back extensors initially increases the further the spine bends until about 40 to 50° of spinal flexion (Andersson, Ortengren, and Nachemson, 1977). This is the case because the head and torso are moving farther away from the axis of rotation of the spine (increasing the moment arm of the resistance), and so greater force must be generated by the spinal extensors to eccentrically counter this torque and prevent uncontrolled falling of the torso. This greater force is of concern in terms of straining the back extensors, and muscle endurance has been shown to be adversely affected by greater degrees of flexion. For example, the length of time in which workers were able to maintain a position was reduced from 13 minutes with 20° of forward flexion to 4 minutes with 30° of forward flexion (Soderberg, 1986). The greater force of the back extensors is also

itself can occur (spondylolysis). Activities such as dance that utilize repetitive hyperextension tend to display increased incidence of low back injury, and so an understanding of this movement is important.

Undesired hyperextension can occur statically as part of standing posture (lumbar hyperlordosis) or dynamically in dance movements such as when one is rising from a plié, laterally flexing the spine, jumping, or turning. As just described, an important part of dance training is to develop the desired spinal alignment such that this undesired hyperextension is avoided. However, in other cases such as an arabesque jazz layout or various porte de bras movements involving arching to the back, spinal hyperextension is a necessary component of the dance movement. In such cases, the potential for associated injury can be reduced with appropriate co-contraction of the abdominal muscles and back extensors, so that the amount of hyperextension and shear stress in the low lumbar spine is limited and greater emphasis is placed on arching higher and throughout more of the back (figure 3.38). Since tremendously more hyperextension is naturally allowed in the lumbar

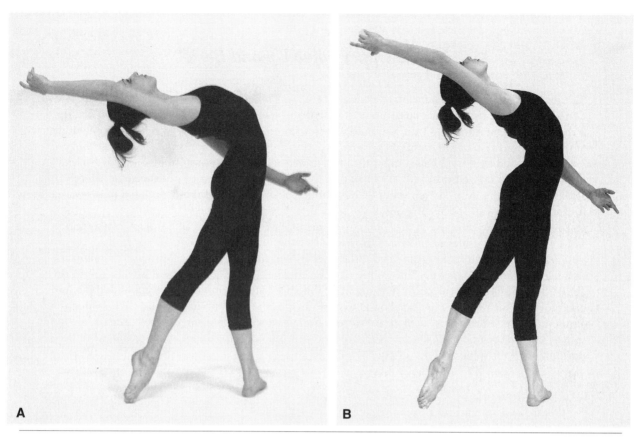

FIGURE 3.38   Specific co-contraction of the abdominal muscles and spinal extensors to limit hyperextension in the low lumbar spine and emphasize upper back extension. (A) Incorrect technique, (B) correct technique.

of concern because of the increased stress it creates within the discs. One study reported that intradiscal pressure at L3 doubled in magnitude with 40° of forward bending (Nachemson, 1981).

A different concern becomes operative with extreme degrees of forward bending. After about 50° of forward bending, the activity of the spinal extensors actually decreases instead of increasing, until at full flexion these muscles are inactive; this is termed the **flexion relaxation phenomenon** (Hall, 1999). In this position of full flexion, the spine is devoid of the stability and protection provided by muscular contraction and relies on passive support from the joint capsules and ligaments, discs, thoracolumbar fascia, and the passive elastic components of the back extensors. This is potentially dangerous for these passive constraints, particularly given that they are susceptible to fatigue. For example, with repetitive loading, discs appear to lessen their ability to absorb shock or withstand forces, and injury can then result from relatively small forces. In addition, the tension in the interspinous ligament associated with full flexion can increase facet joint loading and anterior shear force (Hall, 1999). These observations

have led to recommendations to use full flexion with care and that adding large forces to this vulnerable position such as those associated with percussive toe touching or bounce stretching is not advisable in recreational athletes.

However, many dancers find roll-downs and such inverted positions helpful for developing flexibility, reducing excessive low back tightness, and finding certain neuromuscular connections. One approach is to use such spinal flexion in dance populations prudently (avoiding excessive use in terms of duration of holds or number of consecutive repetitions) when the body is adequately warmed and with careful attention to technique. In terms of technique, potential risks can theoretically be lessened by emphasizing keeping the head close to the torso as the dancer flexes the spine (decreasing the moment arm of the resistance) and by emphasizing tightening the abdominals and pulling them in toward the spine to help reduce shear forces and protect the spine via intra-abdominal pressure or thoracolumbar fascia tensioning. Also, inadequate hamstring flexibility will not allow adequate forward rotation of the pelvis, which occurs after about 45° of spinal flexion (see

"Lift the Upper Spine Up and Back"

The cue to "lift the upper spine up and back" can be interpreted anatomically as focusing on extending the thoracic spine backward without letting the rib cage go forward. Focusing on "pulling up" with the inferior attachment of the abdominal muscles onto the pelvis will help limit anterior tilting of the pelvis and resultant undesired excessive hyperextension in the lower lumbar vertebrae. Then, focusing on arching the mid and upper thoracic spine such that the sternum lifts up and back will help achieve the desired distribution of some of the arch to higher regions of the spine. However, achievement of this desired arch requires very subtle co-contraction of the abdominal muscles and back extensors in very specific regions of the spine.

For example, excessive use of the spinal extensors in the lower thoracic and upper lumbar region will tend to create undesired forward movement of the anterior rib cage. In contrast, excessive stabilization of the rib cage by the abdominal muscles and holding the ribs down will not allow the thoracic spine to hyperextend. Thus, while a consistent "pulling up" of the lower attachment of the abdominal muscles onto the pelvis is maintained, the upper attachment of the rectus abdominis and obliques onto the rib cage must be allowed to move away as the sternum lifts up and back, so that the abdominal muscles are used eccentrically to help control backward movement of the trunk while the spinal extensors (particularly the thoracic) are used concentrically to cooperatively create the desired positioning of the spine as seen in figure 3.38B.

Lumbar-Pelvic Rhythm on p. 183 for more information) and can result in increased stress to the lumbar spine (Hamill and Knutzen, 1995; Plowman, 1992). Dancers with tight hamstrings can modify such a position to reduce back stress by slightly bending the knees or supporting the torso with forearms on the thighs until adequate hamstring flexibility is developed.

Partnering

Partnering other dancers is associated with very large forces, but the potential risk to the spine can be lessened by appropriate spinal and pelvic alignment of the lifter, specific muscle emphasis during lifting, appropriate positioning of the partner, and adequate strength and flexibility in key muscles. In terms of alignment, emphasis on lifting with the legs with the torso more vertical is associated with lower forces borne by the spine than bending the spine forward and "lifting with the back." The intradiscal pressure at L3 has been estimated to be about 382 pounds (173 kilograms) of force when one is picking up a 22-pound (10-kilogram) weight with the back straight and knees bent, versus 427 pounds (194 kilograms) when bending forward with the back (Nachemson, 1981). Considering that another dancer is likely to weigh five or six times more than the weight used in that study, such a change in load to the discs could be

very meaningful. Similarly, the degree of rotation can markedly influence spinal stresses. Some structures of the spine such as the discs are vulnerable to rotation, and most back injuries involve a combination of flexion and rotation or hyperextension and rotation. During lifting of that same 22-pound weight, rotating 20° with the spine flexed 20° increases intradiscal pressure to 472 pounds (214 kilograms) of force. Furthermore, asymmetrical positioning has been shown to negatively affect the ability to lift heavy loads, with losses of 12%, 21%, and 31% at 30°, 60°, and 90° of asymmetry, respectively (Caillet, 1996).

Even more dramatic in determining stresses to the spine is the distance the partner is from the spine. Having a dancer farther away from your body will greatly increase the resistance torque that must be overcome by the shoulder muscles and the bending torque that must be met by the trunk muscles to maintain a stable position. Studies have shown that whether one is lifting with the torso erect or bent forward, the farther the weight is from the body the greater the activity of the spinal extensors and the greater the pressure borne by the discs (White III and Panjabi, 1978). The calculation in one study was that lifting a 100-pound (45-kilogram) weight with the weight about 30 inches (76 centimeters) in front of the fulcrum (L-S disc) and the legs straight would require 1,500 pounds (680 kilograms) of muscle pull and produce 1,600 pounds (726 kilograms) of pressure on the lumbosacral disc (Bradford and Spurling, 1945).

So, to reduce the potential forces borne by the spine, dancers should directly face their partner, bring the partner close to them, keep the torso as vertical as possible, and emphasize lifting by extending the hips and knees rather than the back whenever the choreography allows. One can encourage the latter desired mechanics by suggesting that dancers think of pushing down into the ground with the feet, knees, and hips as they straighten, rather than lifting the back. Also, it is helpful to emphasize looking straight ahead versus down to encourage a more upright position of the spine. Strengthening the hips and knees with exercises such as squats, lunges, or leg presses (chapter 4) will allow a dancer to lift a partner more readily using this upright body alignment.

The dancer should also avoid excessive lumbar lordosis and utilize adequate trunk stabilization when lifting another dancer as shown in figure 3.39. Focusing on firmly tightening the abdominal muscles, pulling the abdominal wall in toward the spine and the ribs down toward the pelvis so that the torso is directly over the pelvis just prior to and during the lift, will help utilize the protective effects of IAP and prevent the large shear forces associated with excessive arching of the back. In addition, balanced co-contraction of the spinal extensors is key for stabilizing the spine and preventing the weight of the partner from pulling the trunk forward. Although the ideal desired position of the lumbar spine at the beginning of a lift is still an area of great controversy (Gracovetsky et al., 1989; Hall, 1999; LaFreniere, 1985; McGill, 2001), there is generally agreement that it should be neutral or just momentarily slightly flexed, with both hyperextension or exaggerated or sustained flexion avoided. Strengthening the abdominal muscles and back extensors and

performing trunk stabilization exercises can improve this aspect of lifting. However, in some cases, excessive arching of the low back and leaning the torso back during lifting are a compensation due to inadequate shoulder flexibility (necessary to allow an overhead position) or inadequate upper extremity strength. In such cases, strengthening and stretching key upper extremity muscles used in partnering can also help protect the back (chapter 7).

While applying the principles just discussed can help reduce the stress to the spine, there are many cases in which the choreography will not allow application of all of them. For example, often choreography requires that the partner be lifted with the

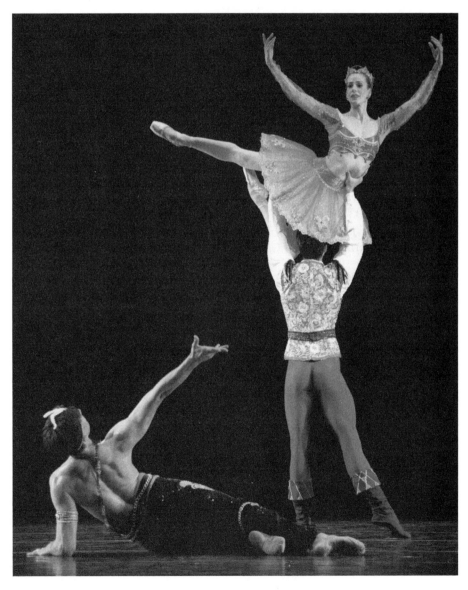

FIGURE 3.39   Maintaining proper spinal alignment and adequate stabilization is key for reducing injury risk during partnering.

© Angela Sterling Photography. Pacific Northwest Ballet dancers Patricia Barker, Stanko Milov, and Casey Herd.

spine bent forward, with the torso twisted, or with the partner moving away from the body. Nevertheless, if the dancer develops adequate strength, utilizes good core stabilization, and applies whichever other principles are relevant, partnering can be performed without injury to the back. In addition, when lifting from a forward flexed position is required, it is desirable not only to emphasize abdominal stabilization but also to focus on keeping the knees slightly bent and using the hip extensors to bring the pelvis under first before extending the knees and spine.

Conditioning Exercises for the Spine

Adequate and balanced muscular strength and flexibility of the spine are essential for correct mechanics, optimal movement, and injury prevention. However, there is tremendous controversy regarding the relative benefit and risk of various trunk exercises, and many of the exercises commonly performed by dancers would be considered contraindicated for recreational athletes or individuals with a history of back problems. Hence, a discussion of general principles related to spinal exercises precedes the discussion of specific conditioning exercises.

General Guidelines for Abdominal Strengthening

Many dancers and other athletes perform abdominal exercises regularly and yet show marked weakness when tested for abdominal strength. In testing of pre-professional ballet dancers using Kendall and McCreary's leg-lowering test, 68% could not maintain a stable pelvis when their legs were lowered beyond 60°, and only 4% could lower their legs all the way to the table while maintaining desired positioning (Molnar and Esterson, 1997). Similarly, the author has found inadequate abdominal strength as evidenced by the curl-up height test, and inability to maintain pelvic stabilization with leg lowering, when testing pre-professional ballet students, performing arts high school dance majors, and university dance majors. This frequent occurrence of low abdominal strength levels is likely due in part to the use of ineffective exercises and formatting. Recommendations follow for improving the gains obtained from abdominal work while keeping injury risk relatively low.

Enhancing Abdominal Exercise Effectiveness

Selection of appropriate exercises, meticulous technique, adequate muscle overload, and proper formatting of exercises can help achieve greater abdominal strength and the development of abdominal use that can more readily be applied to dancing. The following is a discussion of these and other principles that can be used to make many abdominal exercises more effective.

Emphasizing Flexing Spine Versus Hip   Remember that the abdominal muscles work to flex the spine while the hip flexors work to bring the torso closer to the thighs (e.g., hip flexion). Hence, emphasizing sequentially curling (flexing) the torso and keeping the torso as rounded forward as possible (figure 3.40A), versus lifting the torso with a flat back (figure 3.40B), in exercises such as curl-ups can help achieve the desired abdominal emphasis. Cues such as "maintaining a 'C' curve" or "imagining hugging a large ball" can sometimes help achieve this desired use of the abdominal muscles. Excessive use of the hip flexors not only decreases desired overload to the abdominal muscles but also can place undue stress on the spine if the spine is not sufficiently stabilized. For individuals with excessive lumbar lordosis, performing "abdominal" exercises with excessive use of the hip flexors can actually worsen rather than help correct this postural condition.

Keeping Head and Neck in Line   Focus on continuing flexion of the spine through the cervical region, thinking of the head and neck continuing the "C" curve of the lower spine. If one is having difficulty achieving this alignment or is experiencing neck discomfort when performing supine abdominal exercises, it is helpful to try focusing on "softening the chest" (making it slightly concave) and bringing the sternum slightly back and down as if hugging someone, while bringing the chin slightly in toward the chest (as if holding an orange between the chin and chest). If the neck muscles are not strong enough, it may also be necessary to initially use one hand to support the neck. One should avoid pulling on the neck, alternate the arm used for support, and gradually increase the number of repetitions that can be performed without support. It can also be helpful to perform exercises starting from sitting (such as the curl-back shown in table 3.4C [p. 134]), which involves less stress for the neck flexors because the weight of the head is closer to the axis of rotation (shorter moment arm).

Keeping Feet Unrestrained   Keeping the feet free will generally make the abdominal muscles work more and hip flexors work less (Godfrey, Kindig, and Windell, 1977; Guimaraes et al., 1991; Hall, Lee, and Wood, 1990; Lipetz and Gutin, 1970), and so most abdominal work should be done with the

Abdominal Strength and Endurance Tests

Perform the following two tests on another dancer to estimate the strength and endurance of the abdominal muscles.

Curl-Up Height Test (Muscular Strength)

Start with your partner supine with the knees bent to about 90° and the feet resting on the ground (not held down). The elbows are bent with the fingers spread and the tips of the thumbs in contact with the top of the head. Then, keeping the elbows back and in line with the ears, your partner should very slowly curl up as high as possible without using momentum, without letting the elbows come forward, and without letting the feet lift. Cue your partner to round the spine as much as possible (spinal flexion) rather than raise with a flat back. Measure the perpendicular distance from the prominent vertebra at the base of the neck (C7—vertebra prominens) to the ground using a tape measure, as shown in A. The goal is to be able to come all the way up to a sitting position.

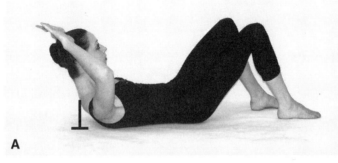

A

Note: Due to differences in spine length and flexibility, the same measured distance will not reflect the exact same angle of trunk flexion from individual to individual. However, this measure will give you an approximate indication of strength (with stronger individuals able to come up higher) and provides a useful tool to monitor improvement in strength within the same individual.

Curl-Up Repetition Test (Muscular Endurance)

Start with your partner supine with the hips and knees bent to 90° and the feet against a wall (B1). The elbows are bent and face forward, and the fingers surround the ears. Cue your partner to curl up

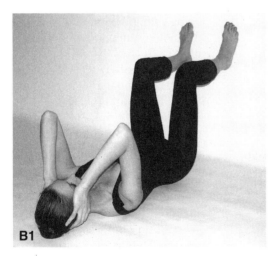

B1

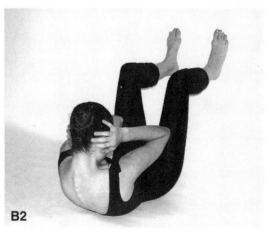

B2

(continued)

TESTS AND MEASUREMENTS 3.3   *(continued)*

and touch the elbows to the mid-thighs in cadence with a metronome or count set at 25 curl-ups per minute for a maximum of 4 minutes (B2) (Sparling, 1997). Count the number of proper curl-ups your partner completes. The count stops as soon as the elbows no longer touch the knees or the dancer is not able to keep up with the count. The dancer may not rest and then begin again. The maximum goal would be 100 repetitions in 4 minutes, but the mean for professional hockey players tested was 50, with 11% of players meeting the endpoint (Quinney, Smith, and Wenger, 1984). Based on some preliminary tests with dancers, this author considers 40 to 59 repetitions "good" and greater than or equal to 60 repetitions "excellent."

Note: Dancers with inadequate strength to touch the elbows to the thighs can cross their arms in front of their chest and touch their forearms to their thighs. Or they can bring their arms down to their sides and place a strip of masking tape just in front of their middle finger and a second strip of masking tape 3 inches (7.6 centimeters) in front of the first strip. With each curl the hands must move forward to touch the second strip of tape (Robertson et al., 1988; Sparling, 1997).

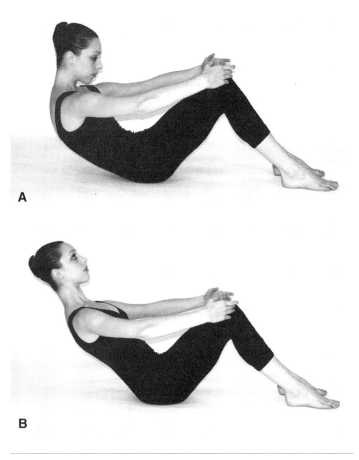

FIGURE 3.40   Technique for abdominal exercises. (A) Correct—emphasis on rounded spine (spinal flexion) with abdominal wall pulled inward; (B) incorrect—flat back with emphasis on using hip flexors to raise torso.

feet free. Dancers who develop high levels of abdominal strength and excellent technique may want to perform one set of an advanced variation with the feet restrained (e.g., under the strap of an incline bench, Reformer, or Cadillac) if spinal flexion can be effectively maintained. However, several sets of exercises should also be done with the feet free.

Pulling Abdominal Wall Inward   When one is performing abdominal exercises, emphasis on pulling the abdominal wall inward toward the spine will help recruit the obliques and transverse abdominis. Remember that the transverse abdominis is not capable of producing spinal flexion and so will not necessarily be recruited with abdominal exercises unless its function of pulling the abdominal wall inward (often termed "hollowing" in dance) is emphasized. One study showed that by using multisensory cueing including verbal cues that emphasized pulling the navel up and against the spine, subjects were able to recruit more transverse abdominis and internal obliques and less hip flexors (iliopsoas) on the down-phase of a curl-up (Miller and Medeiros, 1987). An exaggerated, slow exhalation or quick, forced exhalation can also serve to emphasize greater use of the transverse abdominis (De Troyer et al., 1990). Emphasizing this inward pull of the abdominal muscles is also important for helping develop the aesthetically desired use of the

CONCEPT DEMONSTRATION 3.2

Creating a "C" Curve

Start lying supine with the knees bent to about 90° and the feet resting on the floor. For the first three of the following, place one hand on the back of each thigh and use the hands to help bring the spine into about 20° of flexion.

· **Emphasizing spinal flexion.** While maintaining the back of the sacrum fully in contact with the floor, use your hands to pull the spine into further flexion. First, focus on pulling the bottom of the sternum down and back, and then focus on pulling the bottom of the anterolateral rib cage down and back to further increase spinal flexion, while the hands slightly assist the motion. Then, let go with the hands and focus on keeping the low ribs back and the same angle of spinal flexion without help from the hands.

· **Emphasizing the low abdominal muscles.** While maintaining the upper spine at the same degree of flexion, gently pull the pubic symphysis toward the navel, creating a small "tuck" (posterior pelvic tilt). Let go with the hands, and attempt to maintain the same positioning of the trunk, with the pubic bone and ribs pulling toward each other.

· **Emphasizing the transverse abdominis.** Slowly breathe into the abdomen and push the abdominal wall outward. Then, slowly exhale and pull the abdominal wall inward toward the spine, from the pubic bone to the sternum. Make the whole abdominal surface concave, as if you were wrapping it around a large ball; let go with the hands, and maintain this concave position without hand support. Now, dissociate the muscle contraction from the breathing, focusing on alternately pushing the wall out and pulling it back in while natural, unlinked breathing occurs.

· **Putting it all together.** Beginning from a supine position, pull the pubic bone and ribs toward each other and scoop the abdomen inward as the torso curls up as shown in the figure. If there is difficulty with one element, practice that element alone and then try to put all three elements back together.

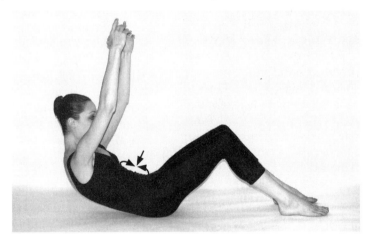

abdominal muscles to aid in keeping the abdomen flatter versus protruding while dancing.

Posterior Pelvic Tilt and Lower Abdominal Emphasis Slightly tilting the top of the pelvis backward so that the pubic bone comes up into a slightly "tucked" position (posterior pelvic tilt), while bringing the bottom of the anterior rib cage slightly down and in,

will produce greater overload to the abdominal muscles by causing shortening of the muscle from both directions. Furthermore, adding a posterior tilt to various abdominal exercises and including other exercises that emphasize moving the inferior attachment of the abdominals on the pelvis, such as the hip lift (Sarti et al., 1996) (table 3.4E [p. 135]) and hanging leg lift (figure 3.44 [p. 130]), can help develop the motor patterns important for correcting lumbar lordosis and creating a neutral pelvis during functional movement and may involve more activation of muscle fibers located lower in some of the abdominal muscle groups.

Adequate Range of Motion   Full sit-ups with the legs straight have been shown to only recruit various abdominal muscles from 20% to 34% of the time (Halpern and Bleck, 1979) and are associated with greater use of the hip flexors (Ricci, Marchetti, and Figura, 1981) and greater stresses to the spine (Axler and McGill, 1997) than curl-ups. Hence, the trend for abdominal work has been to substitute smaller range curl-ups where various abdominal muscles are active 90% to 93% of the time, and there is probably less lumbar stress. However, this trend can be taken too far, such that inadequate range is utilized to provide necessary abdominal overload. In the very beginning phase of the curl-up, the neck flexors and rectus abdominis are primarily working. As the torso curls higher (up to about 40 to 50°) the obliques are recruited and the abdominals work harder (length–tension principle), achieving about 50% of a maximum voluntary contraction with 45° of flexion (Floyd and Silver, 1950; Sheffield, 1962; Soderberg, 1986). After about 50° of spinal flexion, the hip flexors become more primary and activation of the abdominals decreases. Hence, an effort should be made to keep the back of the sacrum in contact with the floor and fully flex the spine (30 to 45°) rather than the common error of either only flexing the spine slightly and barely raising the torso off the ground in the exercise or only flexing the spine slightly and then primarily using the hip flexors to raise the torso further. Using a larger range of spinal flexion is also important for dancers because some dance movements (such as getting up and down from the floor in modern and jazz) incorporate a full range of motion, and strength gains are specific to the range worked, declining markedly the farther away the angle is from that used for strengthening.

Type of Muscle Contraction   One way of working a fuller range of motion in dancers who do not have adequate strength to curl up very high (concentric contraction), as seen in figure 3.41A, is to use isometric or eccentric contractions. For example, after one curls up concentrically, the hands can be used to pull the shoulders up slightly higher (e.g., to flex the spine further). The hands are then released, and either the position is held (isometric contraction) as seen in figure 3.41B and table 3.4B (p. 134) or the torso is slowly lowered back down to the floor (eccentric contraction). Since greater force can be generated with an eccentric or isometric contraction than with a concentric contraction, strength can be developed at a range higher than could be reached with a concentric contraction alone. One can apply this same principle by starting from a sitting position and curling back toward the floor (eccentric contraction) as seen in figure 3.41C and table 3.4C (p. 134). Lower ranges can be held isometrically (to add more overload) and then, initially, the hands can be used to pull on the legs to assist with coming back up to sitting (concentric contraction). As strength increases, use of the hands can be lessened and then discontinued.

Spinal Rotation   Adding rotation to relevant abdominal exercises such as a curl-up will cause greater challenge to the oblique abdominal muscles. When one is performing a straight curl-up, both sides of the external oblique and internal oblique muscles can act with the rectus abdominis. However, when rotation is added, some of the obliques are antagonists to the movement, and only the internal oblique on the same side (ipsilateral) as the direction of movement and the external oblique on the opposite side (contralateral) of the direction of the movement can aid with the movement.

Use of Adequate Overload   To produce desired improvements in muscular strength, the abdominal exercises should be difficult enough that one can perform about 12 repetitions at the most. If more repetitions can be performed, the difficulty should be increased, for example by working in a higher range (up to about 40° or 50°), adding trunk rotation, bringing the feet closer toward the buttocks when they are on the floor (Hall, Lee, and Wood, 1990), bringing the legs up (90° hip and knee flexion) with the lower legs in the air or supported by the seat of a chair or bench (Gutin and Lipetz, 1971), bringing the arms farther away from the navel to increase the moment arm of the resistance (e.g., from by the sides to across the chest, supporting the head, or reaching overhead), or adding external resistance such as dumbbells held in the hands. Furthermore, remember that the effect of gravity on the body is primarily creating the resistance in these exercises. Therefore the body must be appropriately positioned so that the abdominal muscles are having to work against gravity, such as when one is performing a curl-up from a supine position or a side-up from a side-lying position. In contrast, exercises that neglect this principle related to gravity, such as standing full-waist circles or standing reaches, are so ineffective in terms of overload that they are virtually useless for abdominal strengthening.

Recovery   After 6 to 12 repetitions of an appropriate exercise, one should allow recovery of the abdominal muscles for 2 to 3 minutes before performing

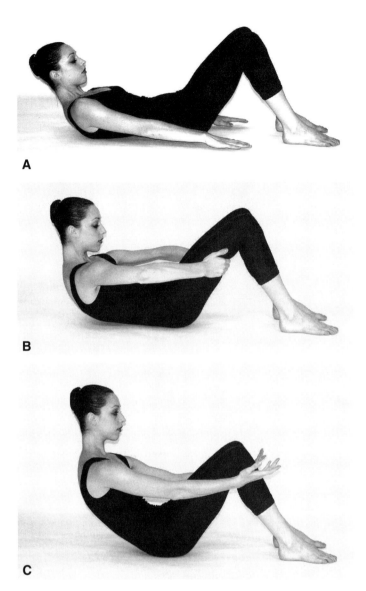

A

B

C

FIGURE 3.41   Using different types of muscle contraction to develop abdominal strength in a greater range of motion. (A) This is the height that can be reached with a concentric contraction. (B) Hands are used to pull up slightly higher; then hands are released, and this higher range is isometrically maintained. (C) Start from sitting and curl back to use an eccentric contraction in a higher range than can be obtained concentrically.

first three sets of abdominal muscle exercises can be performed in a strength format with adequate overload and recovery and the final set performed in an endurance format with lower overload and higher reps.

Stabilization Exercises   Because the abdominal muscles play a very important role as postural stabilizers as well as spinal flexors, some exercise specialists advocate that strengthening the abdominal muscles is not sufficient in itself and recommend the inclusion of exercises that emphasize the abdominal muscles working in an isometric manner to help stabilize the trunk while the upper limbs, lower limbs, or whole body moves. Stabilization exercises generally emphasize co-contraction of trunk muscles including the spinal flexors and extensors while a neutral position of the pelvis (not tucked) and spine (with a normal lumbar lordosis) is maintained. These exercises are designed to emphasize the motor control aspect of developing core stability. Although this is currently a very popular notion, what exercises best develop core stabilization is controversial and will require sound scientific investigation. Furthermore, some of the exercises advocated for stabilization are low in effectiveness for building abdominal strength, and so, in the opinion of the author, should be done in addition to, rather than in place of, traditional abdominal exercises.

An example of a stabilization exercise is the leg reach shown in table 3.4G (p. 136). As skill improves, learning to stabilize the torso while the torso changes its position in space and relationship to gravity is a way to try to foster transfer to more complex movement. For example, side support positions can be performed on the elbows or hands, focusing on keeping the spine and pelvis stable as the body shifts from side, to facedown, to opposite side (figure 3.42A). Similarly, the abdominals can be used to posteriorly tilt the pelvis as the ball is brought toward the shoulders and then to stabilize the spine and pelvis as the ball moves away and the body moves into an extended plank position (kneeling abs, figure 3.42B). This ball exercise can be made more challenging by starting with the feet on the ball and lifting the body with the knees straight to an inverted "V" position (table 3.4F [p. 136]) as the ball moves toward the shoulders. Adding a push-up in either the inverted (figure 3.42C) or plank position can also be useful for developing stabilization skills. Electromyographic

another set of 6 to 12 repetitions of abdominal work. During this recovery time, other muscle groups could be strengthened or stretched. The common practice of performing multiple sets of abdominal exercises immediately following one another generally results in little if any improvement in strength and makes the exercises primarily beneficial for muscular endurance. For the dancer who wants to maximize improvement in both strength and endurance, the

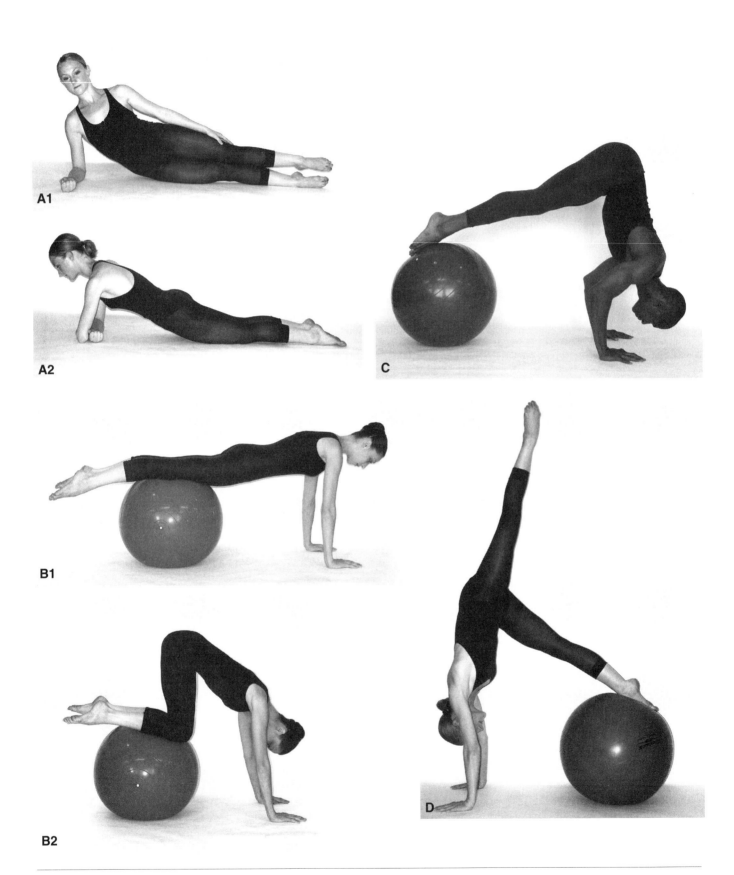

FIGURE 3.42 Sample stabilization exercises. (A) Side support, (B) kneeling abs, (C) inverted "V" and push-up, (D) inverted arabesque.

126

Maintaining a Neutral Lumbar Spine

Start lying supine with the knees bent to about 90° and the feet resting on the floor while one hand rests on the front of the abdomen and the fingertips of the other hand are under the side of the low back region.

• **Emphasizing isometric contraction of the abdominal muscles.** While maintaining the back of the sacrum and thoracic spine in contact with the floor, pull the abdominal wall in toward the front of your spine without letting your pelvis or rib cage move. Your hand should feel the abdominal wall pulling inward without the anterior rib cage and pubic symphysis coming closer together.

• **Emphasizing maintaining a lumbar curve.** When the abdominal muscles contract they will tend to produce lumbar flexion. One approach to maintaining a normal lumbar curve is to try to isolate muscle contraction to the transverse abdominis, whose function is stabilization without trunk flexion. Another approach is to maintain the lumbar curve with co-contraction of the lumbar spinal extensors. Thinking of pulling the front and back of the spine toward each other, or pulling evenly up with the front and back of the pelvis, can encourage co-contraction of the abdominal muscles and spinal extensors. Your fingertips should feel the lumbar area stay lifted versus flattening out.

• **Comparison to a "C" curve.** Contrast this sensation and positioning to that associated with a "C" curve. When creating a "C" curve, note that the lumbar area comes closer to the fingertips, and the contact of the sacrum on the floor shifts upward as the pelvis and ribs come closer together.

studies indicate that moderate abdominal activity is required in push-ups to maintain trunk alignment (Flint and Gudgell, 1965) and that combining two skills requiring abdominal contraction (kneeling abs or inverted "V" and push-up) may help train stabilization in a more functional manner that can more readily transfer to dancers' movements (Lange et al., 2000). As skill increases, one can develop asymmetrical stabilization by adding lifting one leg in the inverted position (figure 3.42D). Due to the associated decrease in stability of the base of support, performing other types of abdominal exercises such as shown in figure 3.41 may also offer greater stabilization benefits than performing exercises on the floor (Stanforth et al., 1998).

Technique and Kinesthetic Awareness Essential to an effective abdominal strengthening program is that proper form not be jeopardized in an attempt to do more repetitions or to do a variation that is too difficult for current levels of strength or skill. One aspect of good form is that exercises should be done in a slow and controlled manner, without undue use of momentum. Another aspect of good form is that the desired specific sequencing of spinal and pelvic movements occurs, with an appropriate magnitude and without undesired compensations. The goal is

not only to improve specific abdominal strength, but also to develop a better kinesthetic awareness of trunk positioning and appropriate muscle activation for stabilization as well as movement. To aid with development of kinesthetic awareness, it is often helpful to utilize external feedback such as that from a mirror, that from a partner, contact of the back relative to the ground, or to use the hand to feel the position of the ribs, pelvis, or protrusion of the abdomen. In time, a new kinesthetic awareness can be developed and utilized in motor programs that will allow for the desired neutral position of the spine with static alignment and appropriate contraction of the abdominal muscles in dynamic movement to protect the spine and achieve the desired dance aesthetic. A summary of the principles just discussed for making abdominal strengthening exercises effective is provided in table 3.3.

Limiting Abdominal Exercise Risk

Many of the principles just discussed for increasing the effectiveness of abdominal exercises also increase the stresses applied to the spine. So, while appropriate for many highly skilled dancers with no back injury history, a less-skilled, less-conditioned, or injured dancer may need to take a more conservative

TABLE 3.3   Summary Guidelines for Effective Abdominal Strengthening

Form	Adequate overload/progression	Format
Pull abdominal wall inward	Increase range of motion	Perform 6-12 repetitions of each exercise (1 set)
Generally utilize a posterior pelvic tilt and pull the front of the lower rib cage down and back	Bring arms further overhead	Perform 3-5 sets (generally perform 1 set each of different abdominal exercises)
Emphasize rounding whole spine and softening chest	Bring feet closer to buttocks	Use variations of sufficient difficulty that muscle failure is approached but correct form is maintained
Use adequate range of motion	Add spinal rotation or lateral flexion	Allow 2-3 minutes recovery between sets of abdominal exercises
Keep feet unrestrained	Add dumbbells in the hands	
Perform slowly with control		

approach such as initially using a smaller range of motion, avoiding rotation, and not using dumbbells. Three other controversial considerations for injury risk include the use of long-lying positions, flexed versus neutral lumbar spine, and long lever arms.

Long-Lying Position   Some exercises in modern and jazz dance floor work, as well as Pilates (e.g., roll-up), involve abdominal work performed supine with the knees straight versus bent—termed the long-lying position. Dancers who have tight hip flexors or marked lumbar lordosis may not be able to assume a long-lying position without excessive arching of the low back and anterior tilting of the pelvis, or at least will be unable to effect the desired posterior pelvic tilt prior to the curl-up or the necessary flattening of the lumbar curve during the curl-up. Bending the knees causes flexion at the hip that slackens the hip flexors and iliofemoral ligament and decreases the lumbar curve. Hence, dancers with these conditions should perform abdominal work with the knees at least slightly bent until adequate hip and low back flexibility is achieved.

Flexed Versus Neutral Lumbar Spine   Flexion of the lumbar spine is associated with an increase in disc pressure. Hence, maintaining the curve in the lumbar spine (neutral spine) is often recommended for patients with disc injury. Due to the associated increase in disc pressure and the desire to dance with a neutral versus tucked position, some exercise specialists also advocate using a neutral versus tucked position during abdominal work in general. However, since the elevation in disc pressure is much less than that occurring with rigorous dance movements, and since lumbar flexion is a natural movement of

the spine that accompanies many daily activities such as leaning forward, the approach generally used by the author for dancers without back pain is to incorporate a slight posterior tilt (with associated lumbar flexion) for greater overload and greater low abdominal activation, as well as to help dancers gain better control of tilting the pelvis, when exercises are being performed for abdominal strength—and generally a neutral position for stabilization exercises. However, there is theoretical support and there are advantages to both approaches.

Long Lever Arms   Exercises in which the legs provide the resistance, such as those in which both legs are raised and lowered while one is lying on the back or supported on the forearms, can produce strain and arching of the low back if inadequate abdominal strength is present as seen in figure 3.43A. Such exercises have regained popularity in recent years because of their inclusion in Pilates mat work and apparatus work. However, it is important to realize that the prime mover for such exercises is actually the hip flexors, while the abdominal muscles act as stabilizers to prevent undesired anterior tilting of the pelvis and further extension in the lumbar spine. Given that several studies have shown these exercises to be relatively low in effectiveness for abdominal strengthening (Flint and Gudgell, 1965; Guimaraes et al., 1991; Lipetz and Gutin, 1970) and that they are considered contraindicated for individuals with weak abdominal muscles (Hamill and Knutzen, 1995), these exercises are better viewed as stabilization exercises that should be used only with appropriate individuals, and they often require modification and a gradual progression. For example, in contrast to many other stabilization exercises in

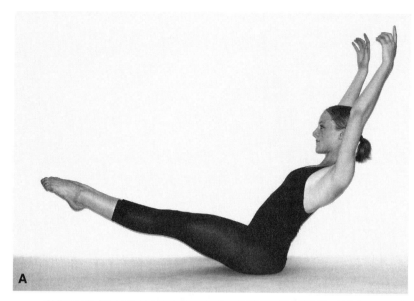

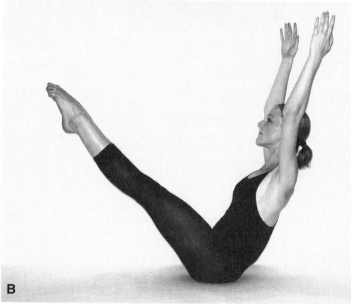

FIGURE 3.43 Long lever arms. (A) Inadequate abdominal stabilization resulting in the iliopsoas pulling the lumbar spine into hyperextension and undesired low back stress, (B) adequate abdominal stabilization with a slight posterior pelvic tilt.

muscles facilitates the ability to stabilize the pelvis.

Similarly, if leg lifts are advanced for highly conditioned dancers to variations where the torso is vertical (at a gym or with the Pilates Cadillac as seen in figure 3.44A), one or both knees should be initially bent to reduce the torque produced by the legs while adequate abdominal stabilization strength and skill are developed. Then, over time, one or both legs can be partially and eventually fully extended, only as long as adequate stabilization of the lumbar spine can be maintained (figure 3.44B). Changing the relationship to gravity such that the moment arm of the resistance (represented by the legs) gets longer as the legs are lifted to 90° (versus shorter as occurs with the supine version) makes the abdominals have to work much harder. Hence, the hanging leg lift (in contrast to supine variations) has been shown to be one of the most effective abdominal exercises for recruiting the obliques as well as the rectus abdominis (Axler and McGill, 1997; Flint and Gudgell, 1965; Guimaraes et al., 1991; Gutin and Lipetz, 1971).

General Guidelines for Back Extensor Strengthening

In the past it was believed that lumbar hyperlordosis posture and much of back injury were due to a strength imbalance, with the abdominal muscles being weaker than the back extensors. Hence, the emphasis was primarily on strengthening the abdominal muscles. However, in recent years this theory has been challenged. There is increasing evidence that many individuals are weak in their back muscles as well as their abdominal muscles (Graves et al., 1990; Pollock et al., 1989; Smidt et al., 1983; Suzuki and Endo, 1983), and the tightness of the low back commonly seen with lumbar hyperlordosis is not necessarily indicative of high strength levels. Furthermore, it has been shown that inadequate spinal extensor strength and endurance can increase the risk for low back injury (Caillet, 1996; Parnianpour et al., 1988) and that both inadequate extensor strength and, particularly, inadequate endurance are commonly present in individuals with low back pain (Chaffin, 1974;

which use of a neutral pelvis is advocated, use of a slight posterior pelvic tilt when one is first learning long lever arm exercises can help ensure that lumbar hyperextension is avoided (figure 3.43B). To further reduce risk, such exercises can initially be performed on the forearms with only one leg extended (table 3.4G [p. 136], leg reach), with the legs pointing up more toward the ceiling or with the knees bent such that the torque produced by the legs will be less, or with the hands or a pillow under the pelvis so that a better angle of attachment for the abdominal

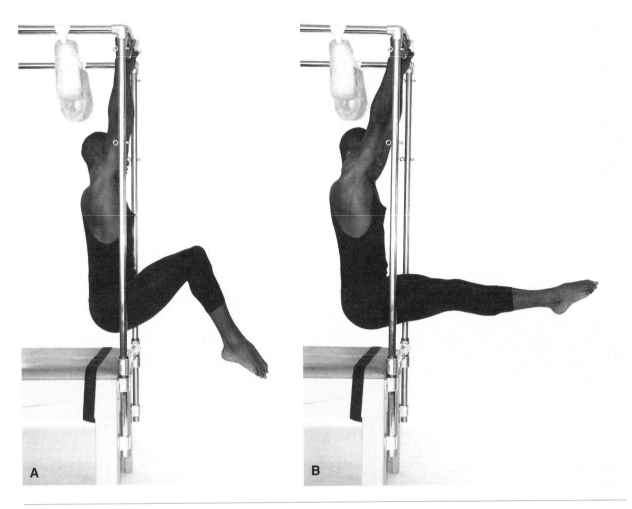

FIGURE 3.44   Hanging leg lift. (A) Modified with knees bent, (B) advanced with knees straight.
CSULB dancer Dwayne Worthington.

Hides et al., 1994; Levangie and Norkin, 2001; Pollock et al., 1989; Roy, DeLuca, and Casavant, 1989).

Conversely, a high level of physical activity has correlated with greater strength of the vertebrae and discs (Porter, Adams, and Hutton, 1989), and several studies have also shown that individuals with good back extensor endurance and better general conditioning have fewer incidences of back problems and less risk of osteoporosis than deconditioned individuals. Similarly, a recent study with university dancers showed a decrease in the number of classes missed due to back pain after participation in a back strengthening program (Welsh et al., 1998). So, there is sufficient basis to indicate that dancers should include strengthening for their back extensors as well as their abdominal muscles. However, a balance with abdominal strengthening is important, as strengthening the back extensors alone has been shown to actually have a negative effect on postural stability (Kollmitzer et al., 2000).

Enhancing Back Extensor Strengthening Effectiveness

As with abdominal exercises, careful selection and performance of back extensor exercises are keys for obtaining potential strength benefits. Many of the principles discussed with the abdominals are also relevant for the back.

Feet Unrestrained and Restrained. As with abdominal exercises, when the feet are restrained the hip muscles can assist the spinal muscles with the movement. Therefore, it is important that some exercises for the spinal extensors be performed without the feet stabilized. However, when the feet are held down by a partner, strap, or bar, most dancers are able to arch the back much higher, and so it provides a way that strength in a higher range of motion can be carefully developed. In addition, when the feet are restrained, the dancer can often more readily focus on using the hip extensors to pull the bottom of the

—— TESTS AND MEASUREMENTS 3.4 ——

Back Extensor Strength Test

Perform the following test on another dancer to estimate the strength of the back extensors. This test should be performed slowly, carefully, after the back is fully warmed up, and only if it is pain free. Dancers with a history of back injury or pain should not perform this test unless approved and supervised by their medical provider.

Back Extension Height Test (Muscular Strength)

Start with your partner prone on a mat with the knees extended and the feet together and resting on the ground. The elbows are bent with the fingers spread and lightly resting on the back of the head. Then, have your partner, with the elbows back behind the ears, very slowly arch up as high as possible without using momentum, without letting the elbows come forward, and without letting the feet lift off the ground. Cue your partner to arch the spine starting from the top of the spine and continuing to the bottom. Measure the perpendicular distance from the indentation at the base of the neck (sternal notch) to the ground using a tape measure as shown in the figure. The goal is to be able to come up to the same height with this active test as the dancer can achieve passively (when using the arms to press against the floor to arch the back). Average back extension test results for performing arts high school dance majors tested by the author were 13 inches (33 centimeters) for female and 12 inches (30 centimeters) for male dancers.

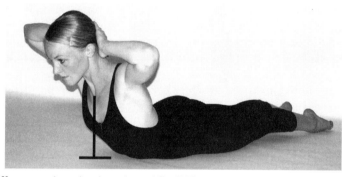

Note: Due to differences in spine length and flexibility, the same measured distance will not reflect the exact same angle of spinal extension from individual to individual. However, this measure will give you an approximate indication of strength (with stronger individuals able to come up higher) and provides a useful tool to monitor improvement in strength within the same individual.

pelvis down to help prevent excessive anterior tilting of the pelvis and reduce excessive hyperextension in the low lumbar area.

Upper Back Emphasis. Given the markedly greater range of hyperextension possible in the lumbar region and the larger cross-sectional area of the spinal extensors in this region, it is easy for back extension exercises to primarily challenge and strengthen the low back region. However, since there are actually different muscles (e.g., the semispinalis) and different slips of muscles in the thoracic region than in the lumbar region, it is important to also include exercises that emphasize strengthening the

upper back. One way to achieve this is to select positions such as sitting (e.g., scarecrow, table 3.4H [p. 137]) or kneeling over a ball (e.g., kneeling scarecrow, table 7.10H [p. 439]) where the abdominals can be used to more readily keep the lumbar spine in slight flexion, as extension higher in the spine is emphasized. However, because the thoracic curve is concave anteriorly, it is important to note that the range of extension will be very small compared to that which occurs in the lumbar spine.

Type of Muscle Contraction. As with the abdominals, the arms can be used (in this case to press down on the ground when prone) to achieve a slightly greater height of the torso (e.g., greater spinal extension) than can be achieved with a concentric contraction. This higher position can be held for several counts (isometric contraction) or followed immediately with a controlled lowering (eccentric contraction) to the prone starting position. However, particular care must be taken not to strain the back extensors by only going a few degrees higher than can be reached concentrically, and starting by only sliding one arm out as the other arm still offers support.

Spinal Rotation. Adding rotation to back extension exercises can add greater overload to the muscles that produce rotation in the desired direction. Furthermore, because there are actually different spinal extensor muscles and slips of muscles in different regions of the spine, rotation in different regions and positions of the spine can actually produce greater challenge to different muscles. For example, pure rotation was found to elicit a marked response in the multifidus and rotatores while the iliocostalis showed greater activity when forward flexion (from standing) was combined with rotation (Basmajian and DeLuca, 1985). In prone or kneeling positions, subtle rotations and stabilizations, similar to those used in dance, can be effected by lifting one arm, one leg, or an arm and a leg at the same time (e.g., prone arabesque, table 3.4N [p. 140]. When on the hands and knees, lifting the opposite arm when one leg is lifted increases the upper erector spinae activity by about 30% (Levangie and Norkin, 2001).

Adequate Overload and Recovery. As with the abdominals, to produce desired improvements in muscular strength, the exercises that are performed should be difficult enough that only about 12 or fewer repetitions can be performed, and a 2- to 3-minute recovery of the spinal extensors should be allowed between sets of back extension exercises. Difficulty can be increased by using a larger range of motion, adding rotation, bringing the arms to the side or overhead versus down by the sides, and adding dumbbells in the hands for resistance. Since the effect of gravity on the body is primarily creating the resistance in many back extensor exercises, appropriate body positioning should be used so that the torso or pelvis is moving against gravity to produce spinal extension, such as when performing prone back extensions (e.g., table 3.4I [p. 138]).

Technique and Kinesthetic Awareness. Performing back extensor exercises in a smooth and controlled versus jerky manner with precise spinal articulation and positioning of the pelvis is essential for effectiveness and safety. Subtle stabilization skills and kinesthetic awareness must be developed to achieve the desired sequential extension of spinal vertebrae rather than having large segments of the spine move as a whole or almost all of the movement occur in the low lumbar spine. Lack of adequate stabilization can make many back exercises potentially injurious rather than therapeutic.

Limiting Back Extensor Exercise Risk

Unfortunately, applying many of the principles that increase effectiveness, such as the addition of rotation and resistance, will also increase the stresses borne by the discs and other spinal structures. So a more conservative approach is often recommended, with particular attention paid to range of motion and stabilization.

Range of Motion. Using a greater range of motion produces more overload through shortening of the muscles and allows for development of strength through a full range of motion. However, greater range of motion will generally require marked spinal hyperextension, which is of concern in terms of injury. Hence, there is still controversy as to how much range of motion should be used in back extension exercises. For dancers with access to a gym (roman chair), exercise ball, bench, or Pilates barrel, this controversy can be avoided by performing back extensions from a position of flexion to just a straight (neutral) spine. And one study showed marked gains in back extensor strength in a flexed to neutral position when training on exercise equipment in a relatively small arc of 36° flexion (Graves et al., 1990). However, because of the prevalent use of marked spinal hyperextension in dance, there is a theoretical basis in terms of functional issues to support using a range of motion in strength training for dances that includes hyperextension. And only studies that have linked back strength to the demands of the job have shown the ability to predict future back injuries (Parnianpour et al., 1988). But to reduce injury risk, hyperextension should only be performed (without medical supervision) if no back discomfort is present, there is no history of back pain or medical contraindication, range is gradually developed over time, and sound technique is employed. One approach is to initially limit hyperextension to about 10 or 20° while focusing on developing abdominal co-contraction/stabilization skills. Then range can be gradually increased as long as appropriate stabilization is used and the movement remains pain free.

Abdominal Co-Contraction. One important aspect of these stabilization skills is utilizing a co-contraction of the abdominals, as discussed under Spinal Hyper-the pubic symphysis into the ball or floor while the navel stays lifted, can make it easier to achieve the desired form as shown in figure 3.45.

Strength Exercises for the Spine

Specific sample strength and stabilization exercises for the spine are provided in table 3.4. The principles just discussed should be applied to performance of these exercises. Exercises should be carefully selected to match each dancer's current level of strength and skill, and a variety of exercises should be used to capture the unique benefits each has to offer. In general, start with pure spinal flexion and spinal extension exercises (in the sagittal plane) with less conditioned dancers, and then add rotation and lateral flexion as strength and stabilization skill develop. An example of a progression for abdominal exercises is provided in table 3.5 on page 142.

In terms of the ratio of abdominal and back extensor exercises that should be used, multiple factors should be considered. Several studies showed that the back extensors made greater improvements in strength (tested isometrically) than other muscles with just one workout per week (Carpenter et al., 1990; Graves et al., 1990; Pollock et al., 1989), suggesting that abdominal exercises should be performed with greater frequency or more sets than extensor exercises.

However, this may change with aging, and performance of more back extension exercises may be necessary to counter the tendency for kyphosis and the decrease in spinal extensor size noted to gradually occur in men over 30 years of age and the decrease in spinal extensor density noted in women in the 40 to 49 age range (Imamura et al., 1983). In addition, static and dynamic alignment should be taken into account, and dancers with excessive hyperlordosis often benefit from greater abdominal work and back extensor exercises that use very low range while emphasizing abdominal co-contraction and stabilization.

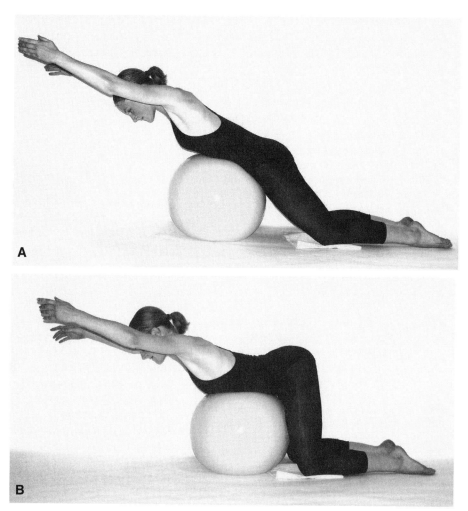

FIGURE 3.45 Upper back extension with co-contraction of abdominal muscles. (A) Adequate stabilization of low lumbar spine, (B) inadequate stabilization of low lumbar spine.

extension (p. 115), to decrease the magnitude of extension and shear in the lowest lumbar vertebral segments. For example, when arching from a prone position, focus on pulling the pubic symphysis up with the lower attachment of the abdominals moving so that the waist is lifted a half inch (1.2 centimeters) from the floor versus pushing into the floor, and maintain this position of the pelvis as the back slightly arches in the thoracic region. If this exercise is progressed to higher ranges of spinal extension, lumbar hyperextension will be necessary, but "pulling up and in" with the lower attachment of the abdominals onto the pelvis (as you allow the upper attachment of the abdominals onto the rib cage to move away) can still help limit anterior pelvic tilting and low back stress. If difficulty in maintaining desired positioning is experienced, performing this exercise with a towel roll under the front of the top of the pelvis, or kneeling with the hips on a ball while focusing on pressing

(Text continues on p. 140.)

TABLE 3.4 Selected Strength Exercises for the Spine

Exercise name (Resistance)	Description (Technique cues)	Progression
Muscle group: Spinal flexors **Muscles emphasized: Abdominals/technique**		
Joint movement: Spinal flexion with posterior pelvic tilting		
A. Pelvic tilt 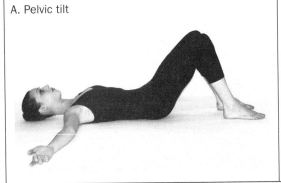	Lie supine with knees bent to about 90° with the feet flat on the ground. Pull pubic bones and lower ribs toward each other, focusing on tilting the top of the pelvis posteriorly so that the lumbar spine flattens against the floor. Hold 8 counts, then return pelvis and ribs to starting position. (Pull whole abdominal wall inward so that it is concave, not protruding.)	1. Increase range. 2. Increase symmetry of upper and lower movement.
Muscle group: Spinal flexors **Muscles emphasized: Abdominals/isometric**		
Joint movement: Spinal flexion with posterior pelvic tilting		
B. Isometric curl-up (Body weight) 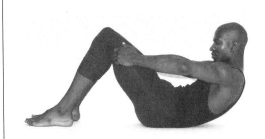	Lie supine with knees bent to about 90°, feet flat on the floor and arms down by sides. Perform a slight posterior pelvic tilt, bring the chin toward the chest, and curl up sequentially until shoulder blades are off the floor. Then, place hands on the outside of the thighs and use them to pull the torso up slightly higher. Release hands, hold for 4 counts, and return torso to starting position. (Keep abdominal wall pulled inward, and avoid letting torso drop down when hands release.)	1. Bring feet closer toward buttocks. 2. Increase hold to 8 counts. 3. Bring arms slowly back overhead (high fifth) and then forward again during the hold. 4. Perform on a diagonal with both hands on the outside of the same distal thigh.
Muscle group: Spinal flexors **Muscles emphasized: Abdominals/eccentric**		
Joint movement: Spinal flexion with posterior pelvic tilting and hip flexion		
C. Curl-back (Body weight) 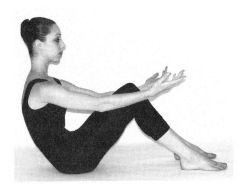	Sit with your knees bent about 90° and feet flat on the floor. Perform a slight posterior pelvic tilt and then curl the torso back down toward the floor. Begin by bringing the sacrum in contact with the floor, then proceed until the back of the waist is in contact with the floor. Hold 4 counts, and slowly curl back up to starting position, using the hands on the thighs to assist on the way up if needed. (Keep spine as flexed as possible throughout the movement.) *Variation 1:* Perform sitting on an exercise ball, starting with the knees bent about 90° and the feet flat on the floor.	1. Increase hold to 8 counts. 2. Bring hands behind head and then forward during hold. 3. Start with the arms in high fifth. 4. Bring knee to chest during hold. 5. Bring knee to chest and then extend knee (développé) during hold.

134

Exercise name (Resistance)	Description (Technique cues)	Progression
Muscle group: Spinal flexors **Muscles emphasized: Abdominals/stabilization and latissimus dorsi**		
Joint movement: Spinal flexion with shoulder extension		
D. Reformer curl-up (Reformer) 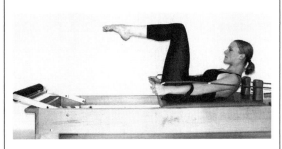	Lie supine with knees flexed just over hip joints, and lower legs parallel to the carriage while the hands are overhead holding straps. Bring arms forward and down (shoulder extension), curl torso up while keeping elbows extended so that straps provide resistance to spinal flexion, pause, bring arms back overhead while torso remains up, and then slowly lower torso to starting position. (Curl torso up as high as strength will allow while still maintaining back of waist in contact with carriage, and avoid letting torso lower down as arms go overhead.)	1. Curl torso higher. 2. Increase springs. 3. Extend knees with feet pointing toward ceiling as arms go overhead.
Muscle group: Spinal flexors **Muscles emphasized: "Lower" abdominals**		
Joint movement: Lumbar spinal flexion with posterior pelvic tilting		
E. Hip lift (Elastic band) 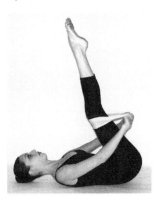	Lie supine with knees slightly bent and directly over the hips while the hands hold a band stretched across the front of the thigh to resist the motion. Perform a posterior pelvic tilt and then continue that movement until the sacrum slowly lifts off the ground and the thighs come closer to the shoulders. Hold 4 counts, and slowly lower the hips back to the starting position. (Emphasize the abdominals by posteriorly tilting the pelvis to produce the lift rather than flexing the hip, and avoid the use of momentum.)	1. Lift pelvis higher. 2. Use a heavier band. 3. Lift the pelvis on a diagonal.

(continued)

TABLE 3.4 Selected Strength Exercises for the Spine *(continued)*

Exercise name (Resistance)	Description (Technique cues)	Progression
Muscle group: Spinal flexors **Muscles emphasized: "Lower" abdominals/stabilization**		
Joint movement: Lumbar spinal flexion with posterior pelvic tilting and hip flexion		
F. Inverted "V" (Exercise ball and body weight)	Support the body weight with the hands on the floor and feet on an exercise ball (plank position) with the pelvis and spine in a neutral position. Perform a posterior pelvic tilt and then lift the hips up toward the ceiling as the feet pull the ball closer toward the hands. Pause, and slowly lower to starting position. (Emphasize keeping abdominal wall pulled inward as hips lift up, and avoid letting the pelvis anteriorly tilt or the low back excessively arch when returning to starting position.)	1. Lift pelvis higher. 2. Add a push-up in plank position. 3. Add a push-up in inverted "V" position. 4. Add lifting one leg up toward the ceiling in inverted "V" position (arabesque).
Muscle group: Spinal flexors **Muscles emphasized: Abdominal stabilization**		
Joint movement: Lumbar spinal flexion with posterior pelvic tilt maintained		
G. Leg reach (Body weight)	Lean back on elbows with knees bent about 90° and feet flat on floor. Perform a slight posterior pelvic tilt, and bring knees to chest one at a time. Then slowly straighten one leg to a height where the foot is about 2 feet (61 centimeters) off the ground while the other knee stays above the hip with the lower leg parallel to the floor. Hold 4 counts, then bring the first knee back in toward the chest. Alternate legs. (Maintain a stable pelvis with abdominals pulled in firmly toward the spine throughout the exercise.)	1. Begin to straighten second knee while the first knee is extended, but only in a range where the pelvis can be kept stationary and the low back does not arch. 2. Fully straighten second knee. 3. Perform with spine slightly flexed and no arm support. 4. Perform with a neutral pelvis.

136

Exercise name (Resistance)	Description (Technique cues)	Progression

Muscle group: Spinal extensors
Muscles emphasized: Upper back extensors

Joint movement: Cervical and thoracic spinal extension

H. Scarecrow (Reformer) 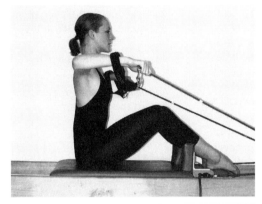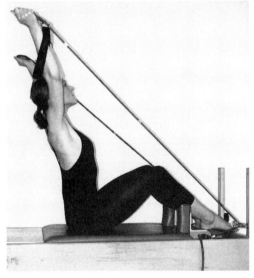	Sit on the carriage with the knees bent and the feet flat on the headrest while the arms are at shoulder height with the elbows extended. Hold the straps in the hands with the palms facing down. Pull the elbows back slightly behind the shoulders, externally rotate at the shoulder so that the palms face front, hyperextend the upper back as the arms reach overhead, pause, and reverse the pattern to slowly return to the starting position. (Keep the pelvis and low lumbar spine stationary, emphasizing movement and muscular work in the upper back. Keep elbows at shoulder height and maintain about 90° of elbow flexion during the shoulder rotation phase.)	1. Increase range of motion of arch in the upper back. 2. Increase spring resistance from very light to light. 3. Add slight rotation of the torso as the arms reach overhead.

(continued)

TABLE 3.4 Selected Strength Exercises for the Spine *(continued)*

Exercise name (Resistance)	Description (Technique cues)	Progression
Muscle group: Spinal extensors **Muscles emphasized: Upper and lower back extensors/stabilization**		
Joint movement: Spinal extension with shoulder flexion		
I. Prone single-arm spine arch (Body weight) 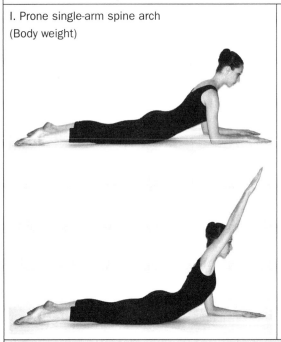	Lie prone on forearms with legs straight and feet together. Use the abdominals to lift the front of the pelvis (ASIS) until a straight line could be drawn through the sides of the shoulder, torso, and pelvis. Then reach one arm forward and upward as the back arches, pause, and return to the starting position. (Keep "pulling up" from the low attachments of the abdominals to limit the degree of anterior tilting of the pelvis as the back arches. Bring the arm to or behind the ear, and focus on "lifting" and arching the upper back first.)	1. Increase range of motion of thoracic spinal extension while still maintaining ASIS off the floor. 2. Add a small dumbbell in the hands. 3. Add slight rotation of the torso toward the raised arm.
Muscle groups: Spinal extensors and shoulder flexors **Muscles emphasized: Back extensors/sequential**		
Joint movement: Spinal extension with shoulder flexion maintained		
J. Spine arch with overhead press (Reformer and bar)	Lie prone with the hips at the edge of the box and heels on the footbar, with the knees bent and a weighted bar in the hands behind the head with the elbows bent. Extend the elbows to reach the bar overhead, extend the knees and hyperextend the spine, pause, and slowly return to the starting position. (Keep "pulling up" with low attachment of abdominals to limit anterior tilting of the pelvis and sequentially extend the spine from upper to lower, working only in a pain-free range.)	1. Gradually increase bar resistance from 1 pound to 5 pounds (0.5-2.25 kilograms).

138

Exercise name (Resistance)	Description (Technique cues)	Progression
Muscle group: Spinal lateral flexors **Muscles emphasized: Oblique abdominals**		
Joint movement: Spinal lateral flexion		
K. Side-up (Body weight) 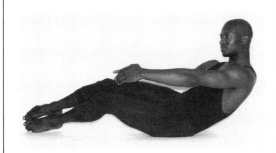	Lie on one side with the knees and hips slightly flexed, then rock the whole body back as a unit such that the knees are about 8 inches (20 centimeters) off the floor. Slightly flex the spine, then sequentially raise head, shoulders, and torso toward the ceiling. Hold 4 counts, then slowly lower to starting position. (Keep abdominal wall pulled inward, and lead with the lower arm such that the spine slightly flexes and rotates as it laterally flexes.) *Variation 1:* Perform on the Pilates Cadillac with the feet under the restraining strap. *Variation 2:* Perform with a "short box" on the Pilates Reformer with the feet under the restraining strap, and increase range of motion by beginning with the torso laterally flexed toward the floor.	1. Increase range of motion. 2. Bring arms overhead and then back when torso is raised. 3. Add dumbbells in hands.
Muscle group: Spinal lateral flexors **Muscles emphasized: Oblique abdominals/stabilization**		
Joint movement: Spinal lateral flexion with shoulder abduction		
L. Side reach (Body weight) 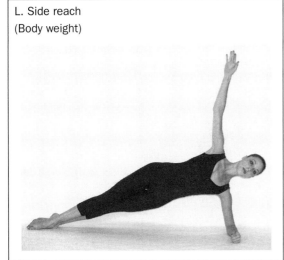	Begin on one side with weight supported on forearm of bottom arm and feet, with top foot in front of bottom foot. Top arm is in line with shoulder. Slowly lower hips toward floor as the arm goes down by the side, and then raise hips toward the ceiling as top arm raises overhead, pause, and return to starting position. (Keep spine/pelvis neutral in the sagittal plane and avoid sticking ribs forward, reach from feet to fingertips when arm goes overhead while maintaining stability of the support shoulder.)	1. Increase range of lowering and raising of hips. 2. Support weight on the hand of the bottom arm (with elbow extended). 3. Perform one time, shift to face-down with two-arm support and do push-up, shift to perform one time on the other side. Repeat series 2-6 times.

(continued)

TABLE 3.4   Selected Strength Exercises for the Spine   *(continued)*

Exercise name (Resistance)	Description (Technique cues)	Progression
Muscle group: Spinal rotators **Muscles emphasized: Oblique abdominals**		
Joint movement: Spinal rotation with flexion		
M. Curl-up with rotation (Body weight) 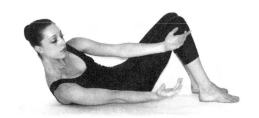	Lie supine with knees bent to about 90° and the feet flat on the floor and the hands behind the head. Then bring the chin to the chest, and sequentially curl up the torso as high as strength allows without letting the back of the waist leave the floor. Bring arms forward, slowly rotate right and then center, then bring hands back behind head, and curl back down to starting position. (Keep the spine flexed as you rotate, and think of bringing the shoulder higher as you rotate.)	1. Rotate right, center, left, center. 2. Bring the arms back behind the head and then forward again when in the rotated position.
Muscle group: Spinal rotators **Muscles emphasized: Spinal extensors**		
Joint movement: Spinal rotation with extension		
N. Prone arabesque (Body weight)	Lie prone with legs extended and arms out to sides. Contract abdominals to lift waist off floor, and raise both arms off the floor in second position as head and upper back lift. Then raise one leg about 6 inches (15.2 centimeters) off the floor, bring the opposite arm overhead, rotate the torso toward the overhead arm, pause, and lower the arm and torso to the starting position. (Keep "pulling up" with lower attachment of the abdominals to limit anterior tilting of the pelvis, and lift the torso slightly higher as the torso rotates.)	1. Raise the torso slightly higher as the arm returns to second position. 2. Add a 1-pound (0.5-kilogram) dumbbell to the hands. 3. Gradually increase the dumbbell from 1 pound to 3 pounds (0.5-1.4 kilograms).

For all abdominal exercises, focus on pulling the abdominal wall inward toward the spine to help strengthen the transverse abdominis. For assymetrical exercises, perform 4-6 repetitions on one side and then 4-6 repetitions on the other side.

In contrast, dancers with fatigue posture or flat back posture need adequate inclusion of back extension exercises with an emphasis on extension in the appropriate spinal region.

Spinal Flexor (Abdominal) Strengthening

As previously described, strong abdominal muscles are believed to be important for preventing lumbar lordosis, generating IAP, stabilizing the spine, and preventing low back injury. In dance, strong abdominal muscles are important for floor work in modern dance such as Graham contractions or "hollowing,"

and for chest lifts used to rise from supine to sitting in jazz dance. The stabilization function of the abdominal muscles is essential for achieving the desired aesthetic in many dance movements.

The first exercise listed in table 3.4, the pelvic tilt, is not very effective for strengthening the abdominal muscles but is included to develop the technique of posteriorly tilting the pelvis that is used as part of many other abdominal exercises. As skill develops, it is no longer necessary to perform the pelvic tilt as a separate exercise; rather it can be included in other, more effective abdominal exercises. The isometric curl-up (table 3.4B) and the curl-back (table 3.4C) are meant to emphasize developing strength in a range higher than one can reach in the up-phase of the curl-up, so that in time the ability to concentrically curl up higher is enhanced. Some examples of progressions are provided, but keep in mind that any of the procedures for increasing overload previously discussed can be used with these exercises. The Reformer curl-up (table 3.4D) uses the straps to provide greater overload and effectiveness. The hip lift (table 3.4E), kneeling abs (figure 3.42B), and inverted "V" (table 3.4F) emphasize lower abdominal use and control of the pelvis essential for correcting lumbar lordosis. The side support (figure 3.42A, p. 126) and leg reach (table 3.4G) emphasize developing strength and skill in spinal stabilization. In all of these exercises it is important to emphasize pulling the abdominal wall in and up toward the spine to challenge the vital transverse abdominis muscles.

Spinal Extensor Strengthening

Strong spinal extensors are very important for stabilizing the spine, bending the torso forward and back when upright, and arching the back. Strong back extensors are also important for preventing undesired forward movement of the torso in movements such as in an arabesque, split jumps, or lifting a dancer overhead. As with the abdominal muscles, a variety of exercises is recommended to provide a wider range of benefits—for example, including exercises that emphasize arching the upper back, the full spine, rotation, and stabilization.

The scarecrow performed sitting on the Reformer (table 3.4H) or sitting in a chair (figure 3.26A, p. 99) emphasize challenging the upper back extensors in a position where it is easier to stabilize the lumbar spine. The thoracic extensors are important posturally to prevent kyphosis and prevent the upper back from falling forward. Furthermore, one study showed that as back extensor fatigue occurs the contribution of the thoracic extensors becomes more prominent (Klausen, Nielsen, and Madsen, 1981). However, in order to target these upper back extensors, the lower attachment of the pelvis must be actively "pulled up" so that the top of the pelvis is not allowed to tilt forward and the lumbar spine is not allowed to excessively hyperextend, while the upper back arches with a very small range of movement (figure 3.45). This is a difficult coordination, and it often requires practice and help from a partner or the use of a mirror to monitor technique. The prone single-arm spine arch (table 3.4I) and spine arch with overhead press (table 3.4J) are designed to combine use of the upper and lower back extensors while focusing on abdominal co-contraction.

Spinal Lateral Flexor Strengthening

Strong spinal lateral flexors are important for floor movements involving rising from a position of lying on the side. They are also used in the side-bending movements of the torso commonly performed in modern and jazz dance. Often when bending the torso to the side, dancers allow the lumbar spine to excessively arch, due to inadequate co-contraction of the abdominal muscles. Hence, side-ups (table 3.4K) are provided that emphasize slight trunk flexion and rotation as the spine is laterally flexing, placing greater emphasis on the obliques. One can also add difficulty to this exercise by focusing on keeping the pelvis stable as the torso laterally rises as high as current strength will allow. Stabilization exercises using side positions such as the side reach (table 3.4L) can also provide challenge to the spinal lateral flexors.

Spinal Rotator Strengthening

Strong spinal rotators are necessary for both stabilization and movement of the spine. Many injuries to the back involve rotation, so it is particularly important to strengthen the muscles involved in rotation and to practice proper mechanics during rotation. Subtle use of the spinal rotator muscles is also involved in asymmetrical movements that include lifting of one leg or arm such as in an arabesque. Grosser use of the rotators is involved in movements in which the torso is twisting relative to the pelvis or the pelvis is twisting relative to the torso, such as in jazz isolations or many warm-up combinations and movement phrases in jazz and modern dance.

Most of the spinal flexors and extensors are also capable of producing rotation. The curl-up with rotation (table 3.4M) challenges the spinal flexors (oblique abdominal muscles) capable of rotation. For effective challenge and to practice sound mechanics, it is important to keep the spine flexed as the torso rotates, rather than let one shoulder drop and the low back flatten or arch. The prone arabesque (table 3.4N) emphasizes strengthening the spinal extensors capable of rotation. Adding lifting one leg to any spinal extension exercise will also produce slight spinal rotation. Adding such rotation increases the challenge and more specifically recruits some of the spinal extensors believed to be commonly injured in lumbosacral strains. Remember that the amount of spinal extension present when rotation is added will influence the region of the spine involved in the rotation and the specific components of the spinal extensors stressed. So, using varied positions will provide more comprehensive strengthening. However, to help protect the spine, it is important that there be a small co-contraction of the abdominal muscles to prevent excessive hyperextension in the low lumbar spine.

Sample Abdominal Exercise Progression

A sample routine for abdominal strength and stability with progressions is provided in table 3.5. However, progressions should only be performed after excellent form has been mastered in easier variations. When harder variations are added, it is often necessary to initially use smaller ranges of motion and lower repetitions so that proper technique can be maintained.

Stretches for the Spine

Very large ranges of motion of the spine are required to achieve the desired aesthetic in many dance forms including ballet, modern, jazz, flamenco, and African

dance. And, for example, while 20° to 30° of spinal hyperextension is considered normal for the general adult population (table 3.6), elite female ballet dancers were found to have an average of 79° (range 60° to 124°) (see figure 3.46) and elite male ballet dancers an average of 65° (range 45° to 93°) of spinal hyperextension (Clippinger-Robertson, 1991). A study of flamenco dancers showed significantly larger range of lumbar extension, lateral flexion (lumbar and thoracic), and rotation (thoracic) than in controls (Bejjani, Halpern, and Pavlidis, 1990). So, stretches in all three planes of motion are recommended for the spine. A discussion of specific selected stretches for the spine follows, and many of these exercises are pictured and further described in table 3.7. For purposes of time economy, stretches for the spine are also commonly combined with stretches for the hip performed standing, sitting on the floor, or at the barre (see chapter 4).

However, as shown in table 3.6, many structures other than muscles offer constraints to spinal

TABLE 3.5 Sample Abdominal Exercise Progression

Exercise name (from table 3.4)	Version of exercise	Repetitions
Level I		
Pelvic tilt	Basic form	6 times
Isometric curl-up	Basic form	6 times . . . 12 times
Curl-back	Basic form	6 times . . . 12 times
Hip lift	Basic form	6 times . . . 12 times
Level II		
Isometric curl-up	Bring feet closer to buttocks	6 times . . . 12 times
Curl-back	Bring arms from low fifth to high fifth, then progress to adding weights in hands	6 times . . . 10 times
Hip lift	Lift pelvis on diagonal toward one shoulder	6 times . . . 10 times
Curl-up with rotation	Basic form	4 times . . . 6 times/side
Leg reach	Basic form	4 times . . . 6 times/side
Level III		
Curl-up with rotation	Rotate right, center, left, center, down	6 times . . . 12 times
Curl-back	With arms in high fifth with weights, bring knee to chest and extend knee	4 times . . . 6 times/side
Side-up	Basic form, then progress to adding weights held across chest	4 times . . . 8 times/side
Inverted "V"	Basic form, then progress to lifting one leg (arabesque)	4 times . . . 4 times/side
Side reach	Basic form, then progress to performing only 1 rep each direction and adding a push-up in the transition	4 times/side . . . 12 total

TABLE 3.6   Normal Range of Motion and Constraints for Fundamental Movements of the Spine

Spine movement (thoracic and lumbar)	Average ranges of joint motion*	Normal passive limiting factors
Flexion	0-80°	Ligaments: posterior spinal ligaments Discs: compression of anterior aspect and tension of posterior aspect Joint capsules: capsules and ligaments of facet joints Muscles: spinal extensors and associated thoracolumbar fascia
Extension	0-30°	Ligament: anterior longitudinal ligament Discs: compression of posterior aspect and tension of anterior aspect Joint capsules: capsules and ligaments of facet joints Muscles: abdominals Bony constraints: overlapping of spinous processes in thoracic region, approximation of facet joints in lumbar region
Lateral flexion	0-35°	Ligaments: contralateral spinal ligaments Discs: compression of ipsilateral portion of disc and tension of contralateral portion of disc Joint capsules: capsules and ligaments of facet joints Muscles: contralateral quadratus lumborum and varying amounts of oblique abdominals and spinal extensors, depending on position of torso Bony constraints: approximation of lower ribs and iliac crest
Rotation	0-45°	Ligaments: costovertebral and perhaps posterior ligaments Discs: tension in annulus fibrosus Joint capsules: capsules of facet joints Muscles: oblique abdominals and spinal extensors, varying with position of torso Bony constraints: facet joints in lumbar region

*From American Academy of Orthopaedic Surgeons (1965).

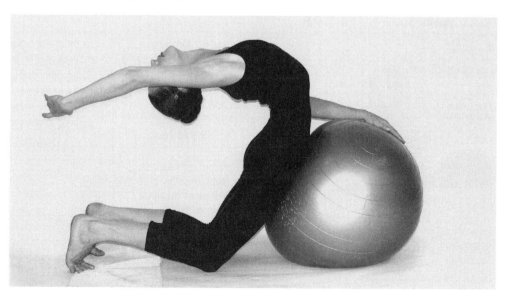

FIGURE 3.46   High range of spinal hyperextension present in some dancers.

TABLE 3.7 Selected Stretches for the Spine

Exercise name	Description (Technique cues)	Progression
Muscle group: Spinal extensors **Muscles emphasized: Lumbar extensors**		
Joint position: Lumbar spinal flexion		
A. Double knee to chest 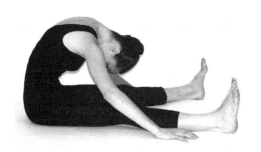	Lie supine with the knees bent and feet flat on the floor. Then use a hand to gently pull one knee and then the other knee toward the chest until a stretch is felt in the low back. (Pull abdominal wall inward, and focus on rounding the lumbar spine.) *Variation 1:* Perform kneeling with the torso resting on thighs and arms overhead (figure 3.25C, p. 97).	1. Bring knees further toward armpits to increase lumbar flexion.
Muscle groups: Spinal extensors and hip extensors **Muscles emphasized: Lumbar extensors and hamstrings (for less flexible dancers)**		
Joint position: Lumbar flexion with hip flexion and knee extension		
B. Sitting forward bend 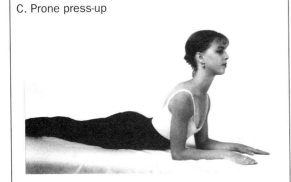	Sit with both legs forward and feet about 2 feet apart (knees may be bent if hamstrings are tight). While keeping pelvis posteriorly tilted, bring head toward floor until stretch is felt in low back. (Emphasize keeping low back rounded—i.e., flexing lumbar spine—vs. flexing at hip joint.) *Variation 1:* Perform sitting in chair with feet on floor and forearms on thighs.	1. Wrap hands around outside of lower legs, and use hands to pull rounded torso closer toward floor.
Muscle group: Abdominals **Muscles emphasized: Rectus abdominis and oblique abdominals**		
Joint position: Spinal hyperextension		
C. Prone press-up	Lie prone, resting on forearms. Then press down with the forearms and sequentially arch spine from head to sacrum. (Keep neck in line with thoracic spine, and "reach" spine out and up using a pain-free range of motion.) *Variation 1:* Perform on exercise ball with hips supported by ball and forearms pressing down on ball (figure 3.47A, p. 148).	1. Bring elbows toward each other until shoulder width apart. 2. Bring elbows back toward waist, and carefully arch higher. 3. Straighten elbows, press with hands, and carefully arch higher.

Exercise name	Description (Technique cues)	Progression

Muscle groups: Abdominals and shoulder extensors
Muscles emphasized: Rectus abdominis, oblique abdominals, and latissimus dorsi

Joint position: Thoracic spinal extension with shoulder flexion

D. Upper back drape 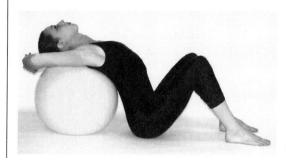	Sit on the floor with knees bent, feet flat on the floor, and the midback resting against an exercise ball. Lace fingertips behind head with elbows bent. Then pull the shoulder blades together and the elbows back, and sequentially arch the thoracic spine from T12 upward. (Pull "low abdominals" in and up to prevent the top of the pelvis from tilting forward, and emphasize arch occurring in upper back with head in line with this arch.) *Variation 1:* Perform sitting in a high-backed chair, and carefully arch the upper back up and over the top of the chair (figure 3.26B, p. 99).	1. Bring sitz bones back, closer to the ball. 2. Extend elbows with hands in line with ears (figure 3.47C, p. 148).

Muscle group: Spinal lateral flexors
Muscles emphasized: Quadratus lumborum and oblique abdominals

Joint position: Spinal lateral flexion

E. Side bend 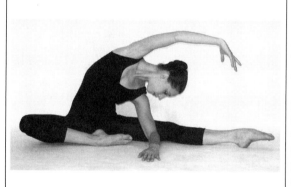	Sit with one knee bent with its side resting on the floor and the other leg extended to the side. Then bend the torso to the side with the lower arm resting on the ground and the top arm reaching toward the outstretched leg. (Reach spine out long as you laterally flex it, and keep both sitz bones firmly in contact with the floor.) *Variation 1:* Perform sitting on the floor with both legs outstretched (second position). *Variation 2:* Perform standing turned out, facing the barre with one leg up on the barre to the side.	1. Reach the hand that was on the floor across the front of the body, and bend the torso further.

(continued)

TABLE 3.7   Selected Stretches for the Spine   (continued)

Exercise name	Description (Technique cues)	Progression
Muscle group: Spinal rotators **Muscles emphasized: Lumbar and thoracic spinal extensors and oblique abdominals**		
Joint position: Spinal rotation		
F. Supine spine twist	Lie supine with one leg outstretched and the other knee bent directly above the hip with the lower leg parallel to the floor. Rotate the spine by using the opposite hand to pull the knee toward the floor while keeping the upper back in place. (Focus on rotating the spine along its length while contracting the abdominals to keep the pelvis slightly tucked and the lower ribs in good alignment with the pelvis.)	1. Bring the knee and upper side of the pelvis further toward the floor without letting the shoulder lift off the floor.

movements, including ligaments, discs, and bony processes. Hence, when one is performing stretches for the back, particular care must be taken that the body is adequately warmed, the stretch is slowly applied without excessive momentum or force, and close attention is paid to proper positioning of the body. It is also important to realize that there is extreme individual variability in spinal motions, some of which is structural in nature. For example, in the elite athletes tested by the author, the range of spinal hyperextension has ranged between 8° (elite male race walker) and 124° (elite female ballet dancer). Thus, it is important to work carefully to increase or maintain the range afforded by one's particular structure rather than trying to forcibly match someone who may have a markedly different structure. Furthermore, when extreme range of motion is present, supplemental stretching outside of class is generally not necessary. Instead, strengthening exercises that work to dynamically maintain range while building strength to support the increased mobility are recommended.

Spinal Extensor (Spinal Flexion) Stretches

Adequate flexibility of the spinal extensors is important for allowing full forward bending of the spine (spinal flexion), for posterior tilting of the pelvis needed for lifting the leg very high to the front, and for prevention of lumbar hyperlordosis posture. The spinal extensors are postural muscles and so often become fatigued and "tight" with dance training, and stretching can help relieve associated soreness and tightness. The double knee to chest stretch (table

3.7A) provides a gentle stretch for the lower back, creating a posterior tilting of the pelvis and a decrease in the lordosis in the lumbar spine. Although it may be too mild for the more flexible dancer to feel a stretch, it offers a position in which the pressure within the intervertebral discs is low and is commonly recommended with low back pain. Similarly, performing this stretch in a kneeling position (figure 3.25C, p. 97), sometimes termed the rest position, can provide relief for tight or fatigued low back extensors.

The sitting forward bend stretch (table 3.7B) provides a more rigorous variation, and a similar position of the spine can also be readily added to stretches for the hamstrings or hip adductors (see chapter 4). However, when performing any of these types of stretches, because the thoracic spine is concave anteriorly and often very flexible, many dancers end up primarily stretching the upper back versus the desired low back area. Maintaining the upper back in extension and pulling the abdominal muscles back toward the spine and keeping a more vertical pelvis while the torso rounds forward can be used as an alternative to achieve a more isolated stretch in the lumbar area.

Spinal Flexor (Spinal Hyperextension) Stretches

Adequate flexibility in the spinal flexors (abdominal muscles) is necessary to allow for the full arching of the back (spinal hyperextension) used in various dance movements. It also appears that having adequate spinal hyperextension range is important for a healthy back, particularly in males (Burton, Tillotson, and Troup, 1989a, 1989b; Klausen, Nielsen, and Madsen, 1981); and a decrease in range in spinal extension has been shown to generally accompany aging in men, but not necessarily in women. However, extreme range (hypermobility) as well as low value (hypomobility) appears to increase the risk for low back trouble. So although spinal flexor stretches are not recommended for dancers who already have high values, they can be useful for dancers who are trying to develop their range or older dancers who are finding a decrease in range.

However, since hyperextension is a classic mechanism for spinal injury, these stretches should be done only if there is no history of lumbar lordosis or low back pain and with particular care, starting with a mild stretch and gradually increasing range over time, always staying in a pain-free range. The prone press-up shown in table 3.7C was selected because arm support will allow for easy control of stretch intensity. As range improves, support can progress to using the hands (with elbows extended) in front of the shoulders, and then further progress through gradually bringing the hands closer toward the shoulders. Range in spine hyperextension can also be improved if one performs this exercise with the hips on an exercise ball (starting with pressing with the elbows and progressing to pressing with the hands against the ball), as seen in figure 3.47A, or uses a gravity-assisted position by lying supine with the back arched over the ball (figure 3.47B).

The upper back drape (table 3.7D) offers a stretch that focuses on improving range in the upper back. One can also add a strength component to the exercise by pressing down with the hands and arching the upper back while attempting to keep the pelvis in a neutral position in a supine rather than sitting position (supine upper back arch, figure 3.47D). Hold this position for 5 seconds, starting with two and gradually progressing over time to six repetitions. Precede and follow this active component with the passive stretch (figure 3.47C) held for 20 to 30 seconds.

Spinal Lateral Flexor Stretches

Adequate flexibility of the lateral flexors is important to allow the spine to bend fully to the side. The side bend (table 3.7E) is an effective stretch that can be performed sitting on the floor or standing with one leg up on the barre. To get full benefits from your stretch, focus on keeping the pelvis level and stationary as the spine arches "up and away" with the ribs lifting "up and over" rather than shifting to the side.

Spinal Rotator Stretches

Adequate flexibility of the spinal rotators is necessary to allow the torso to twist relative to the pelvis, or the pelvis relative to the torso. Dancers are often asymmetric in this motion, and stretching more to the side with less range can help improve symmetry. However, if the genesis of this asymmetry is scoliosis, any stretching or strengthening should be performed under the direction of a qualified physical therapist. The supine spine twist (table 3.7F) is a stretch for the spinal rotators. When performing this stretch, focus on keeping the spine extended and trying to rotate around a central axis without letting the ribs shift to the side.

Back Injuries in Dancers

Because of inherent structural weakness and the great forces it is subjected to from body weight, externally applied forces, and contraction of muscles, the lumbar spine is particularly susceptible to injury. Back injuries appear to have a particularly high incidence in athletics involving 1) weight loading and high compression forces, 2) forceful twists, and 3) activities involving spinal hyperextension, such as competitive swimming (60%), track and field (48%), and weighlifting (40%) (Aggrawal, Kaur, and Kumar, 1979; Mutoh, 1978).

Since dance contains all of these elements, it is not surprising that back injury is prevalent. One study of Broadway dancers found 26% of them sustained an injury to the back or neck during rehearsals while 45% sustained injuries to these areas during the production season (Evans, Evans, and Carvajal, 1996). A study of professional ballet dancers in Sweden found 69% in 1989 and 82% of surveyed dancers in 1995 reported low back pain some time in the previous 12 months (Ramel, Moritz, and Jarnlo, 1999). Another study reports 60% to 80% of ballet and modern dancers had a history of back injuries, while two other surveys involving longer time frames reported incidences of 86% (Clippinger-Robertson, 1985) or higher (Seitsalo et al., 1997). Probably because many dancers sustain multiple injuries and some do not seek medical help for low back pain, the reported percentage of total injuries to the spine is lower than one might suspect from prevalence surveys, often being second only to the ankle-foot region. Some reported percentages of total injuries to the spine were 31% for professional ballet dancers (Garrick and Requa, 1993), 17% for modern dancers (Bronner, Ojofeitimi, and Rose, 2003), 18% for university dance students (Rovere et al., 1983), 20% to 50% for flamenco dancers (Salter-Pedersen and Wilmerding, 1998), and 18% to 34% in Broadway dancers (Evans, Evans, and Carvajal, 1996).

It is also noteworthy that back injuries may require more time off from dancing than some other types of injuries, in some cases requiring dancers to be out

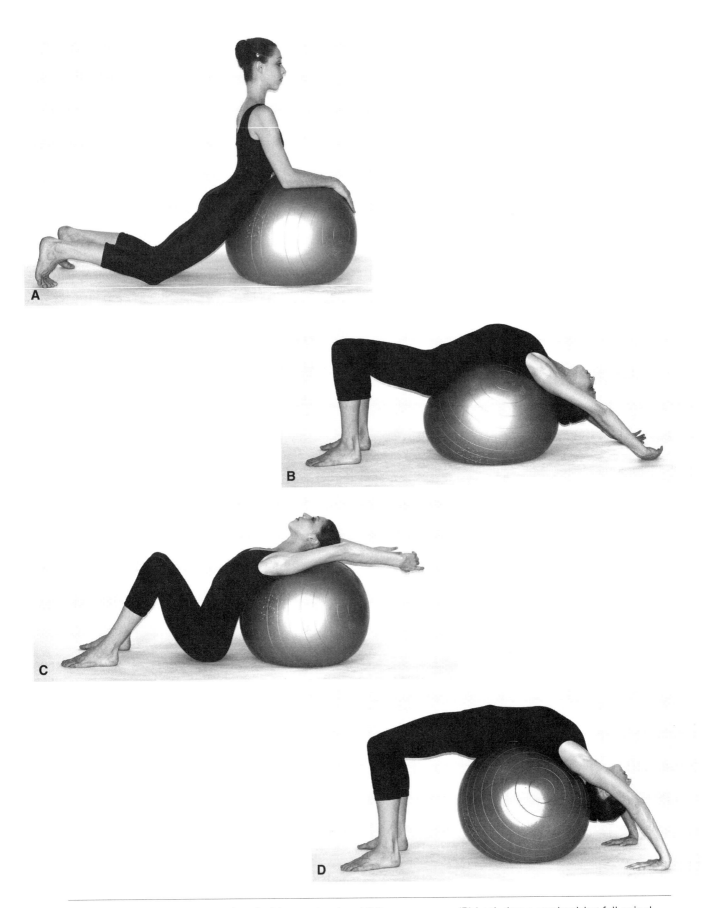

FIGURE 3.47   Increasing range in spinal hyperextension. (A) Torso press-up, (B) back drape emphasizing full spinal passive hyperextension, (C) upper back drape emphasizing increasing range in the upper back, (D) supine upper back arch.

148

for weeks, months, or even a whole year (Micheli, 1983). Furthermore, spinal injury can often result in chronic or recurrent back pain. One survey of adult dancers from various styles found that 17% of all dancers and 23% of dancers with scoliosis reported a history of chronic or recurrent low back pain (Liederbach, Spivak, and Rose, 1997).

Prevention of Back Injuries

Considering the relatively high injury incidence and the potential for a more serious or recurring condition, dancers should take aggressive measures to prevent back injuries. The dancer can reduce injury risk by being adequately warmed up prior to stressful movement; focusing on correct abdominal stabilization and spinal alignment; developing biomechanically sound partnering techniques; developing adequate abdominal, spinal extensor, and upper extremity strength; and developing or maintaining adequate spinal, hip, and shoulder flexibility.

Common Types of Low Back Injuries in Dancers

A few common back injuries will be described here. However, it is important to realize that the same symptom of low back pain can come from numerous very different sources including infections, tumors, rheumatologic conditions such as rheumatoid arthritis, congenital abnormalities, Scheuermann's disease, and chronic and acute injury (Gerbino and Micheli, 1995; Weiker, 1982). Hence, it is emphasized that any dancer who experiences persistent or severe back pain should seek medical help to evaluate and provide appropriate treatment. Self-treatment is particularly ill advised with the back because there are so many causes of low back pain, treatments for one type of injury may aggravate another, and some conditions can have very dire consequences if not properly diagnosed and treated at an early stage.

Lumbosacral Strain or Sprain

Lumbosacral strains or sprains involve excessive stretching and injury to the spinal extensor muscles, ligaments of the spine, or both. Lumbosacral strains often result from extreme movements of the spine involving very forceful concentric contraction, forceful eccentric contraction used to decelerate the torso, mis-timing of a particular movement, or a sudden unexpected exertion during carrying of a heavy object. In the workplace, such injuries often involve muscular overexertion associated with bending and

twisting in an asymmetrical manner (Caillet, 1996). During lifting of heavy weights, or another dancer, small spinal muscles (e.g., deep posterior spinal group) with small moment arms must counterbalance very large external forces with large moment arms, and injury can readily occur. Lumbosacral strains may follow a single trauma, and the dancer may describe the back as "locked" and say that he or she was "unable to move." In other cases, the onset is insidious and results from repetitive stresses of dance training that exceed healing capacity.

Lumbosacral strains are characterized by localized back pain that is relieved by rest and aggravated by activity. Muscle spasm on one or both sides of the spine is often present. Symptoms tend to resolve relatively quickly if there is not more serious underlying pathology such as injury to the disc or bone (Mercier, 1995). Approximately two-thirds of individuals will be relatively symptom free and able to function in work or sport by two weeks (Harvey and Tanner, 1991); 90% of such injuries resolve within two months (Deckey and Weidenbaum, 1997).

Mechanical Low Back Pain

Mechanical low back pain involves a localized aching in the low back region without any well-defined anatomical cause. It is typically associated with lumbar hyperlordosis. Mechanical low back pain commonly occurs in young dancers and is believed to be associated with rapid growth spurts in which tight low back musculature and lumbodorsal fascia, tight hamstrings, tight hip flexors, and weak abdominal muscles often create a temporary imbalance leading to an excessive lumbar curve (Micheli et al., 1999). This hyperlordosis may be present in standing posture or may manifest itself only in dynamic movement such as jumping or partnering. In a study comparing back pain in active teens to that in adults, 26% of teens were diagnosed with mechanical back pain while no adults received this diagnosis (Micheli and Wood, 1995).

Spondylolysis and Spondylolisthesis

Spondylolysis (G. *spondylos,* vertebra + *lysis,* loosening) involves a defect in the weakest region of the lamina located between the superior and inferior articular facets (the pars interarticularis) of the vertebrae, most commonly occurring in the lower lumbar spine (figure 3.48A). Although this condition may be congenital, in many cases the defect is due to a stress fracture. Although other factors come into play, the mechanism for injury is often hyperextension (particularly combined with rotation or axial

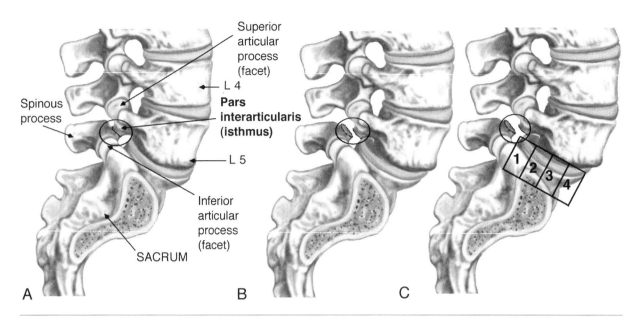

FIGURE 3.48   Spondylolysis and spondylolisthesis (lateral view). (A) Spondylolysis, (B) spondylolisthesis, (C) spondylolisthesis with amount of slippage graded 1 to 4.

loading), and a much higher incidence is found in athletes who are involved in activities requiring repetitive use of such hyperextension such as dancers, gymnasts, weightlifters, football linemen, divers, and figure skaters (Eck and Riley, 2004; Fehlandt and Micheli, 1993; Kotani et al., 1970; Seitsalo et al., 1997; Trepman, Walaszek, and Micheli, 1990). For example, while the incidence of spondylolysis in the general U.S. population is about 5% (Deckey and Weidenbaum, 1997), incidence of spondylolysis was found to be about six times greater (32%) in one study of professional ballet dancers (Seitsalo et al., 1997).

Spondylolysis is of particular concern with young dancers. One study comparing athletic teens to adults with low back pain showed an incidence of spondylolysis of 47% in teens as compared to only 5% in adults (Micheli and Wood, 1995). Some other studies have shown less dramatic, but still markedly increased, incidences of spondylolysis in young athletes and particularly in athletes who participate in sport for more than 15 hours per week (Hall, 1999).

A closely aligned condition to spondylolysis is spondylolisthesis. **Spondylolisthesis** (G. *spondylo*, vertebra + *olisthesis*, slipping) involves an actual sliding forward of one vertebra on the vertebra below, usually secondary to having spondylolysis on both sides (figure 3.48B). It most commonly occurs in the lumbar spine, with L5 slipping on S1 being the most common, followed by L4 slipping on L5 (Weiker, 1982). Spondylolisthesis can be classified according to the amount of forward displacement of the superior vertebra relative to the width of the vertebral body below as seen in figure 3.48C: 1 reflects up to 25% slippage; 2 indicates greater than 25% and up to 50%; 3 reflects greater than 50% and up to 75%; and 4 reflects greater than 75% slippage (Mercier, 1995). Logically, greater slippage is of greater concern in terms of spinal stability, symptoms, prognosis for return to dance, and potential need to stabilize the spine with a surgical procedure.

Symptoms of spondylolysis or spondylolisthesis include low back pain that is often exacerbated by hyperextension, particularly during standing on one leg (such as an arabesque). Tenderness directly on the spine (in contrast to the muscles on the sides of the spine) is often present, and in some cases there may also be radiating pain down the buttocks and leg (sciatica), and tightness in one hamstring. With spondylolisthesis, a "step-off" or "ledge" can sometimes be felt due to the forward displacement of the lumbar spinous process where the vertebra has slid forward.

Although the prevalence of spondylolysis in dancers is high, it is important to be aware that many dancers with spondylolysis or lower grades of spondylolisthesis are able to continue successful dance careers, and some may not even have pain (Deckey and Weidenbaum, 1997; Seitsalo et al., 1997). When traumatic spondylolysis is detected soon after its occurrence, medical treatment including immobilization with antilordotic bracing will often allow healing (Herman, Pizzutillo, and Cavalier, 2003; Micheli, 1983). In other cases, dancers are able to use abdominal co-contraction (Moeller and Rifat, 2001) and technique modification sufficiently to limit shear and symptoms.

Facet Syndrome

While complaints of low back pain with hyperextension (such as the arabesque position) are often associated with spondylolisthesis in the younger dancer, in the older dancer these complaints may be associated with the **facet syndrome** (Drezner and Herring, 2001). The same mechanism of forceful or repetitive hyperextension and rotation places stresses on the facet joint as well as the pars interarticularis. In response, the facet joints and associated structures can become inflamed and undergo degenerative changes (Trepman, Walaszek, and Micheli, 1990). Pain may be localized to the involved side of the low back or may radiate down the lower extremity.

Disc Herniation

The intervertebral disc tends to degenerate with aging and exhibits decreased water content, height, ability to absorb shock, ability to return to normal shape after being deformed, and thickness of the annulus fibrosus (Deckey and Weidenbaum, 1997; Panjabi, Tech, and White III, 1980). These factors all make the annulus fibrosus more vulnerable to damage that can allow the nucleus pulposus to actually extrude out through the annulus fibrosus and into the neural canal, termed **disc herniation,** as seen in figure 3.49. Such disc herniation occurs most frequently in the third or fourth decade of life, when the disc is undergoing the structural changes associated with this marked dehydration (approximately 35% reduction in water content), and the resilient disc under age 30 and the dry, scarred disc over age 50 may be less likely to fragment and displace (Hall, 1999; White III and Panjabi, 1978). Disc herniation most commonly occurs in the posterolateral region of the disc, where the annulus fibrosus is thinner and the posterior longitudinal ligament is weak. Spinal nerves traverse the posterolateral part of the disc, and so herniation

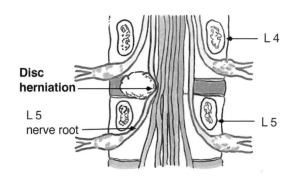

FIGURE 3.49   Herniated intervertebral disc: L4 disc herniation compressing L5 nerve (posterior view with vertebral arch removed).

in this region can readily compress the spinal nerve. Compression of the spinal nerve can lead to pain, numbness, and weakness in areas related to those served by the nerve that is being compressed.

Disc herniation occurs most frequently in the lower lumbar region; 95% of lumbar lesions occur in the discs located between L4 and L5 or L5 and S1 (Mercier, 1995). The mechanism of injury is controversial, but it often involves flexion or hyperextension combined with rotation. As with spondylolysis, sports associated with these mechanisms appear to have a higher incidence of disc degeneration; 75% of retired world-class gymnasts showed signs of disc degeneration (Sward et al., 1991). The intensity of training at a young age may also be a factor, and in gymnasts the incidence of degenerative disc disease rose from 9% to 43% to 63% in pre-elite, elite, and Olympic-level female gymnasts (Gerbino and Micheli, 1995). Early rigorous training, the common use of hyperextension, partnering, and the repetitive use of flexion combined with rotation in modern dance could all potentially increase risk for disc injury in dancers.

The onset of symptoms can be sudden or more vague. One of the primary classic complaints of lumbar disc injury is pain radiating from the back or buttock down the posterior or posterolateral aspect of the thigh, termed **sciatica,** which may be accompanied by weakness or numbness in select areas of the lower extremity (depending on the nerves involved). This pain tends to be exacerbated by coughing, sneezing, the Valsalva maneuver, or prolonged sitting; all of which increase the pressure within the disc. Sitting reduces the lordosis in the lumbar spine, which creates a relative forward shift of the center of gravity (increased moment arm), thus increasing the pressure in the intervertebral discs (figure 3.36 on p. 115). The dancer may lean toward or away from the affected side, a tactic that can increase the space in the appropriate intervertebral foramen and reduce pressure on the compressed nerve root. Tenderness is generally present in the midline of the low back, and spinal muscle spasm is often evident. However, adolescents with disc herniations may sometimes present with back pain and hamstring tightness, but with little of the classic radiating pain or neurologic signs (Deckey and Weidenbaum, 1997).

As with spondylolysis, disc injury does not necessarily mean long-term pain and the inability to dance. First, approximately 25% of healthy adults with no low back pain have evidence of disc herniation (Caillet, 1996); the site of the herniation in relation to the size of the spinal canal and effect on stability of the motion segment may be critical in determining if there is associated pain (Levangie and Norkin, 2001).

Second, there is increased evidence of the ability of the disc to heal, albeit with greater scar tissue and sometimes over as long a time as 12 to 18 months. It appears that disc collagen has a slow turnover, so repair is very slow (Adams and Hutton, 1982). And even some dancers who initially have very debilitating symptoms are able to return to professional dance at a later time. Lastly, it is important to realize that some conditions may mimic disc herniation, such as the piriformis syndrome discussed in chapter 4.

Rehabilitation of Low Back Injuries

Treatment approaches vary and will depend on many factors including the type of injury, severity of symptoms, age of the dancer, and preferred approach of the medical professional. Studies suggest that low back pain will improve in 70% of patients in three weeks and 90% in two months regardless of the type of treatment utilized (White III and Panjabi, 1978). However, in dancers, time is of the essence, and sufficient rehabilitation to prevent further occurrences is vital for professional survival. Hence, working with a skilled physical therapist knowledgeable in the demands of dance is highly recommended.

Initial treatment often involves relative rest, anti-inflammatory medications, modalities, and therapeutic exercise (Weiker, 1982). Note that the term "relative rest" is used, as there has been a shift away from prescribing total bed rest for low back pain (except in the early days with more severe injuries) so that undesired substantial losses in muscle mass, strength, flexibility, and bone density are avoided (Saal, 1988a, 1988b). One study showed about 50% reduction from normal in the size of the sacrospinalis in patients who had been confined to bed for longer than three weeks (Imamura et al., 1983). Modalities such as ice, heat, ultrasound, electrical stimulation, or massage may sometimes be prescribed in an effort to reduce muscle spasm and pain. In some types of injuries, joint mobilization techniques may be utilized to restore normal movement between segments of the spine (Caillet, 1996; Saal, 1988a). Mild activity such as aquatic exercise or walking is also sometimes useful for diminishing pain and muscle spasm and restoring normal physiologic function.

In terms of therapeutic exercise, the controversies and protocols are beyond the scope of this book, but a brief overview of some common principles follows. Many types of low back injury including mechanical low back pain, facet syndrome, spondylolysis and spondylolisthesis, and some types of lumbosacral strains initially emphasize flexion exercises and may be aggravated by adding extension exercises (Drezner

and Herring, 2001). Flexion tends to stretch the thoracolumbar fascia, reduce lumbar lordosis, and lessen anterior shear forces, which can provide relief in cases of mechanical low back pain or spondylolisthesis. Flexion also increases the separation of the pedicles in the lumbar region and decreases compression forces in the facet joints, potentially reducing symptoms when these structures are sources of pain (spondylolysis and facet syndrome). Furthermore, flexion causes a marked increase in the capacity of the spinal canal (Liyang et al., 1989), as well as an increase in the intervertebral foramen width of about 30% (Soderberg, 1986), which can provide relief when pressure to the nerve root is involved. Flexion exercises generally include gentle abdominal strengthening exercises kept in a low range to limit intervertebral disc pressure (e.g., pelvic tilts and small curl-ups), as well as gentle stretches for the spinal extensors (e.g., double knee to chest stretch performed in a supine position) and hamstrings in pain-free ranges. Other anti-lordotic procedures include bracing, placing one foot on a step when standing for extended time, keeping the knees at or slightly higher than hip height when sitting, using the abdominals to help maintain a neutral spinal alignment, avoidance of sleeping on the stomach (sleeping on the side with a pillow between the knees is often recommended for many types of back injury), and avoidance of wearing high-heeled shoes. In terms of dance, when return is permitted, overhead lifting, jumping, and hyperextension are often initially avoided.

Unlike the injuries just discussed, acute disc herniations often respond in an opposite manner and are often aggravated by flexion and given relief with extension exercises (Harvey and Tanner, 1991; Saal, 1988a). Intradiscal pressure increases with spinal flexion, and so curl-up type exercises are often avoided and isometric abdominal or stabilization exercises substituted during initial stages of treatment. Passive hyperextension (such as the prone press-up, table 3.7C) often provides reduction in pain or centralization of pain, and McKenzie extension exercises (McKenzie, 1981) gradually progress from passive to active extension exercises. However, it is important to realize that active hyperextension exercises also cause elevation in disc pressure and should be performed with medical guidance and in a pain-free range. Lying on the back with the legs elevated by pillows or resting on the seat of the chair (figure 3.50) is also often recommended for temporary relief of disc-related back pain (and many other forms of back pain as well). The supine position reduces pressure in the disc, while flexion of the hips and knees reduces potential tension due

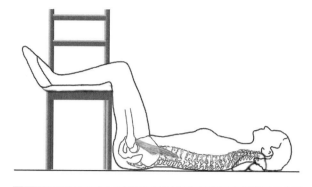

FIGURE 3.50 Rest position often recommended for relief of low back pain.

to the iliopsoas and potential stretch on the sciatic nerve. Recommendations are also often provided for activities of daily living that will tend to preserve the lumbar curve, such as using lumbar supports and avoiding prolonged sitting or flexed postures. In terms of dance, when return is permitted, jumping, lifting, full spinal flexion, flexion with rotation, and extreme hyperextension are often initially avoided and then gradually reintroduced as healing and symptoms allow.

As pain subsides and healing occurs, treatments for different types of injuries become more similar and incorporate the development of balanced strength and flexibility in all of the spinal musculature, development or restoration of adequate flexibility in the spine and hip (particularly in the low back, hip flexors, and hamstrings), correction of any spinal alignment or technique problems, and reestablishment of normal core stabilization. Studies of individuals with chronic low back pain have revealed a delay and disruption of the normal firing pattern of the abdominals prior to movement of the limbs (Hodges and Richardson, 1996), a disruption in the timing and amount of firing of the different sides of the spinal muscles (Grabiner, Koh, and Ghazawi, 1992), very localized wasting of the multifidus thought to be due to neural inhibition (Hides et al., 1994), type II fiber atrophy of the spinal extensors, increased postural sway, and decreased ability to balance in challenging positions (Laskowski, Newcomer-Aney, and Smith, 1997). So, successful rehabilitation appears to require not only adequate strengthening (of sufficient intensity to recruit type II fibers) of the trunk muscles but also restoring of normal stabilization functions and neuromuscular coordination (Richardson, Hodges, and Hides, 2004). It is very important that dancers participate in long-term conditioning that addresses these issues and the specific demands of their dance form and not just stop their exercises when the pain diminishes, as recurrence rates of back pain have

been reported to be about 40% to 60% (Roy and Irvin, 1983).

Upper Back and Neck Injuries in Dancers

While injuries to the spine occur much more frequently in the lumbosacral area in the general population and in ballet, in some dance forms injuries to the upper back and neck can be quite prevalent. A study of professional ballet dancers found that only 9% of injuries to the spine were to the thoracic spine and 16% were to the cervical spine (Garrick and Requa, 1993), while a study of performing arts dance students found that 21% were to the thoracic spine and 10% to the cervical spine but noted that cervical and upper back strains occurred roughly twice as often in modern dancers as they did in ballet dancers (Rovere et al., 1983). An even greater occurrence of upper back and neck injuries was reported in Broadway dancers during the performance season; 29.4% of injuries to the spine involved the upper back and 35.3% the neck (Evans, Evans, and Carvajal, 1996). So, it appears that the different use of the head and neck associated with modern and jazz dance may increase the risk of injury to the upper portion of the spine.

A **strain** of the neck generally involves injuries to the ligaments, tendons, and musculature of the neck. However, many of the injuries that occur in the lumbar region can also occur in the cervical region, including disc herniation, spondylolysis, and spondylolisthesis. With the relatively small vertebrae supporting the relatively large weight of the head, it is not surprising that injuries occur in this region. In a large sample of individuals, cervical disc degeneration was documented in 12% of women and 17% of men in their 20s, and in 89% of women and 86% of men over 60 years of age, often without accompanying pain (Levangie and Norkin, 2001). As with the lumbar spine, the cervical spine is vulnerable to forceful hyperextension or flexion, particularly when combined with rotation. Examples of these motions occur with head isolations and head rolls in jazz and African dance. Dancers training in these dance forms should begin executing such movements with a smaller range of motion until adequate strength and skill are developed.

Another vulnerability for the neck occurs with weighted flexion such as that utilized in the plow or shoulder rolls (back somersaults rolling over one shoulder). Although a controversial area, other low back stretches can be easily substituted for the plow that do not place such large stresses on the neck. Regarding shoulder rolls, such moves should be reserved for more advanced dancers with adequate skill and flexibility so that the weight of the body can be borne primarily on one shoulder and not the neck. Lastly, injury to this area may relate to lifting and overhead use of the arms, and it may involve muscles that stabilize and move the scapulae (chapter 7) as well as muscles that stabilize and move the head and upper spine.

Treatment will vary according to the structures involved and the severity of the injury but often includes anti-inflammatory medications and modalities such as ice massage and mechanical massage (Micheli, 1988). Gentle stretching and movements to maintain range and, later, addition of strengthening exercises (often beginning with isometric and progressing to isotonic) for the upper back extensors and muscles of the shoulder region are often recommended. However, it is important to realize that persistent upper back pain in adolescents may be indicative of Scheuermann's disease, and a prompt medical evaluation is essential.

Summary

The vertebral column houses the vulnerable spinal cord and provides sites for attachments of muscles and ligaments. Its central location makes it particularly important for movement and vulnerable to injury. In an upright position, the vertebral column supports and allows movements of the head, helps support the upper extremity, and provides an important link to the lower extremity via the pelvic girdle. The vertebral column itself consists of 33 vertebrae that are linked (between C2 and S1) by an intervertebral disc between their bodies and gliding joints between their articular processes. Although movement is limited at each joint, together the joints allow relatively large ranges of motion of the spine as a whole, termed flexion, extension, lateral flexion, and rotation. The vertebrae and discs are spanned by numerous strong ligaments that provide stability, and posteriorly by three layers of spinal extensors—the deep posterior spinal group, semispinalis, and erector spinae—which can produce spinal extension, lateral flexion, and rotation. Anteriorly, three of the abdominal muscle groups—rectus abdominis, external obliques, and internal obliques—are capable of producing spinal flexion, lateral flexion, and rotation indirectly through their attachments on the pelvis and thorax. Laterally, the quadratus lumborum gives rise to pure lateral flexion of the spine. In addition to their role in movement, the muscles of the spine are important for posture and provide important stabilization and protection for the spine.

When one analyzes movement of the spine, it is important to take into account the effect of gravity. In the erect position, gravity quickly becomes the primary motive force for many movements, and the muscles with opposite actions to that movement are used eccentrically to control that movement and concentrically to return the trunk back to an upright position. When the position is not erect, the relationship to gravity will again influence what muscles produce and control desired movements. This concept is important for designing effective strengthening exercises for the spine as well as understanding some of the risks inherent in dance and other movements. Unfortunately, back injury is quite prevalent in dance. However, the dancer can markedly reduce injury risk through strengthening the abdominal muscles and spinal extensors, maintaining adequate range of motion in the spine, and utilizing careful technique while still achieving movement aesthetics to minimize inherent risks.

Study Questions and Applications

1. Draw and describe the basic parts of a typical vertebra. How do these parts relate to the spinal cord, spinal nerves, and intervertebral disc?

2. Describe the location of the anterior and posterior longitudinal ligaments and what movements of the spine they primarily limit.

3. Discuss why the lumbosacral joint is particularly vulnerable to injury. Taking these factors into account, list three movements from dance that would put this joint at risk, and state why. How could this risk be diminished?

4. Locate the following muscles or muscle groups on yourself or a partner, and perform actions that these muscles produce as you palpate their contraction: (a) Rectus abdominis, (b) external oblique abdominal muscles, (c) internal oblique abdominal muscles, (d) erector spinae.

5. Observe the normal curves of the spine in the sagittal plane on a skeleton or on an illustration. Describe the direction of these curves at birth and in an adult. Provide the name given when these curves are abnormal, and provide one strength exercise that would be helpful in improving this condition.

6. Define intra-abdominal pressure. How could you maximize its potential protective effects?

7. Perform spinal flexion, extension, and lateral flexion from a standing position. Keeping the influence of gravity in mind, describe which muscle groups would be primarily working with each of these movements on both the up-phase and the down-phase. Then, perform spinal rotation from a standing position. How is the influence of gravity different with this motion?

8. Select a combination used in the warm-up section of a class you teach or take that is oriented toward "warming up the spine." Evaluate it in terms of effectiveness and risk. Is there anything that could be done to improve this warm-up exercise from an anatomical perspective?

9. Describe four things you could do to enhance safety for your low back when partnering another dancer.

10. Carefully perform a flat back position commonly used in jazz and some forms of modern dance. Analyze the torque borne by the lower spine with this position (torque of the resistance) and discuss why "rolling down" with the head close to the spine would alter this torque. If the choreography called for use of a flat back position, what could the dancer do to help decrease the stress to the low back?

11. Do a movement analysis of a double-leg raise, and describe the role of the abdominal muscles, spinal extensors, and hip flexors in this exercise as compared to a curl-up. Discuss the relative benefit and risk of this exercise and how it could be modified to reduce risk. How does the psoas paradox relate to this exercise?

12. Using the curl-up as your basic exercise, provide five variations that would apply the principles discussed for making abdominal strengthening exercises effective. How could these exercises be cued to minimize exercise risk?

13. Perform one exercise for strengthening and one exercise for stretching the spinal extensors. How could a strength exercise be modified to emphasize the upper back versus the lower back? What cues could be used to enhance the safety of back extensor strengthening exercises?

14. Discuss why some common injuries to the spine initially respond better to flexion-based rehabilitation and others more to extension-based rehabilitation.

15. In less trained dancers, jumps are commonly accompanied by a "pumping" motion in which the torso goes back in the up-phase of the jump and forward in the down-phase of the jump. Describe what muscles and cues could be used to try to prevent these undesired movements of the trunk.

CHAPTER FOUR

The Pelvic Girdle and Hip Joint

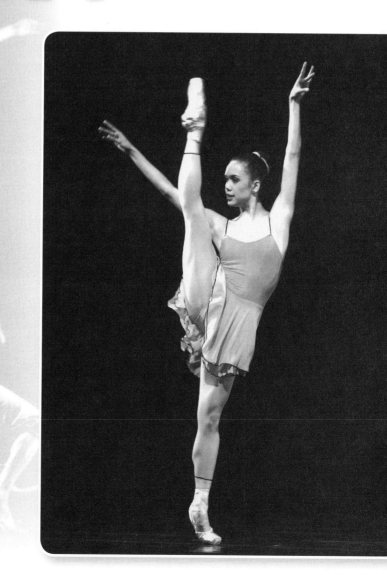

© Angela Sterling Photography. Pacific Northwest Ballet dancer Noelani Pantastico.

In this chapter we turn to structures and movements within the hip region. The two halves of the pelvis form the pelvic girdle. The pelvic girdle provides the very important role of linking the lower limbs to the axial skeleton. The hip joint proper, formed between the femur and pelvis, can be characterized by its exceptional stability essential for withstanding the large forces associated with upright standing and locomotion. However, despite its structural predispositions for stability, the hip joint allows a surprising degree of motion that dancers strive to enhance to a degree rarely seen in other sports. Hip passive and dynamic range of motion is one of the distinguishing landmarks of the elite dancer as exemplified by the movement shown in the photo on page 157. To maximize this potential range without creating injuries, it is particularly important that dancers understand the structure and function of the hip region.

This chapter will present basic anatomy and mechanics of the pelvic girdle and hip joints that influence optimal performance and the vulnerability of this joint to injury. Topics covered will include the following:

- Bones and bony landmarks of the hip region
- Joint structure and movements of the pelvic girdle

- Joint structure and movements of the hip
- Description and functions of individual hip muscles
- Alignment and common deviations of the hip region
- Pelvic and hip mechanics
- Muscular analysis of fundamental hip movements
- Key considerations for the hip in whole body movement
- Special considerations for the hip in dance
- Conditioning exercises for the hip
- Hip injuries in dancers

Bones and Bony Landmarks of the Hip Region

The sides of the pelvis are termed the **os coxae** or os innominatum, and each side is actually made up of three bones—the ilium (L. groin, flank), ischium (G. *ischion*, hip), and pubis (L. *pubes*, the genitals) as seen in figure 4.1—which become fused into a single bone at about 15 or 16 years of age. The **ilium** is a flat

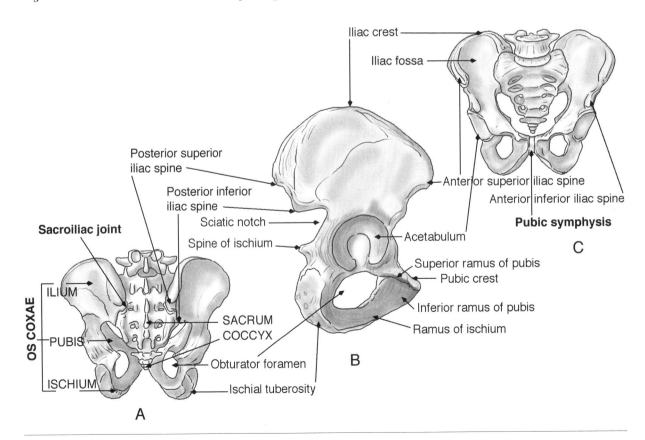

FIGURE 4.1 Bones and bony landmarks of the pelvis. (A) Posterior view, (B) lateral view, (C) anterior view.

bone that is the largest of the three bones. It forms the upper and side "winged" portion of the pelvis. Its internal surface, which is large, smooth, and concave, is termed the **iliac fossa** (L. *fossa,* a trench or ditch) as seen in figure 4.1C. The superior convex border of the ilium is termed the **iliac crest** (L. *crista,* bony ridge) and can be easily palpated below the waist on the sides of the body, running both forward and backward. The top of the iliac crest is generally level with the space between the spines of the fourth and fifth lumbar vertebrae (L4-L5). If the crests are followed in an anterior direction, they begin to curve downward, and the bony prominences that can be felt on the front of the pelvis are called the **anterior superior iliac spines** (L. *spina,* short, sharp process of bone). If the crests are followed in a posterior direction, a rough, broader prominence can be felt—the **posterior superior iliac spines** as seen in figure 4.1A. These landmarks are often abbreviated the **ASIS** and **PSIS,** respectively, and are key for evaluating pelvic symmetry and alignment.

The ischium is an irregular bone that is the strongest of the three bones. It is located in the lower, posterior portion of the pelvis. The most inferior portion of this bone has roughened eminences, upon which we sit, that are termed the **ischial tuberosities** (L. *tuber,* a knob) (figure 4.1B) or "sitz bones." You can easily palpate the tuberosities of the ischium while sitting on a chair by leaning forward and placing the fingers under the bottom of the pelvis from behind. Then, slowly begin to rock your weight back to sit upright, and the tuberosities can be felt pressing down on the fingers. You can also palpate them in a standing position by placing the fingertips at the bottom of the buttocks and slowly leaning the trunk slightly backward and forward. This landmark is key for teaching turnout and pelvic alignment. The ischial tuberosities lie in approximately the same horizontal plane as the lesser trochanters of the femurs.

A thin, flattened portion of the ischium, called the ramus (L. a branch), ascends upward and forward to join with the **inferior ramus** of the pubis as seen in figure 4.1B. The pubis is also an irregular bone, and it is located in the anterior and inferior portion of the pelvis. The thin and flattened **superior ramus** of the pubis ascends to join with the ilium. These rami, as well as other portions of the pubis and ischium, form a large opening in the pelvis termed the **obturator foramen** (L. *foramen,* an aperture). This is the largest foramen in the body. The obturator (L. *obturo,* to occlude an opening) foramen is covered by a membrane, and this membrane and the surrounding bones form attachments for muscles that are key for effecting turnout in dance (the deep outward rotator muscles).

Each os coxae also contains a horseshoe-shaped cavity, composed of elements of the ilium, ischium, and pubis, called the **acetabulum** (L. a shallow vessel or cup), which can be seen in figure 4.1B. Its lower margin is incomplete, and the gap is called the acetabular notch. The spherical proximal end of the femur, called the **head of the femur** (L. *femur,* thigh) and seen in figure 4.2, fits into this hip socket or acetabulum. Distal to the head, the femur tapers to form the **neck of the femur,** which is a common fracture site in older women. This neck angles to join with the long **shaft of the femur.** At this junction, two large bony projections are located. The largest projection faces laterally and is appropriately termed the **greater trochanter** (L. major bony prominence). The smaller projection, located on the medial aspect of the upper femur, is termed the **lesser trochanter** (L. minor bony prominence). The line running between these projections on the front of the femur is termed the **intertrochanteric line** (L. line between trochanters), while the prominent ridge located on the back of the shaft of the femur is termed the **linea aspera** (L. *linea,* line + *asper,* rough), as seen in figure 4.2B.

You can locate the greater trochanter of the femur by placing your thumb on the lateral aspect of the crest of the ilium and reaching down on the thigh with the middle finger. When you internally and externally rotate the leg, you should feel the greater trochanter move beneath the skin. This landmark is useful for evaluating hip mechanics and body alignment. During standing, the tip of the greater trochanter is approximately level with the center of the head of the femur.

When studying the bones that make up the pelvis, it is interesting to note that this is one area of the skeleton where there are marked gender-linked differences necessary to meet the demands of childbearing. The female pelvis is generally broader, roomier, and less vertical than that of a male and has a wider inlet (superior pelvic aperture) and larger outlet (inferior pelvic aperture). The coccyx and sacrum are also situated more posteriorly in women than in men (Mercier, 1995; Moore and Dalley, 1999). In contrast, the pelvis of the male is narrower and deeper.

Joint Structure and Movements of the Pelvic Girdle

The os coxae are firmly joined to the sacrum posteriorly at the sacroiliac joints and anteriorly to each other at the pubic symphysis to form one solid structure, the pelvic girdle. The pelvic girdle provides a link between

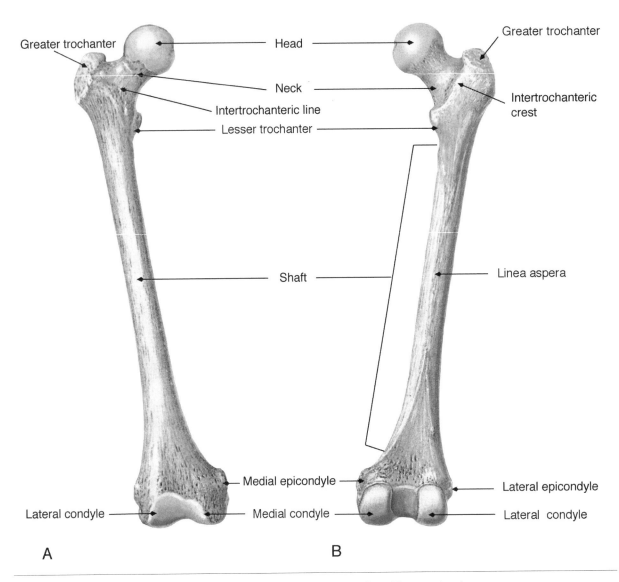

FIGURE 4.2   Bony landmarks of the femur (right femur). (A) Anterior view, (B) posterior view.

the lower limbs and axial skeleton, and the lumbosacral joint is key for describing the movements of the pelvis relative to the axial skeleton. The pelvic girdle also protects and supports vital lower abdominal organs and, in females, the developing fetus.

Pubic Symphysis

The **pubic symphysis** (G. *symphysis,* a growing together) is a cartilaginous joint (figure 4.1C) that is heavily reinforced by ligaments on all sides. Normally this joint only allows slight movement that is important for shock absorbency. However, during pregnancy the width of the cartilage markedly increases and the ligaments become more lax to allow the slight spreading of the os coxae that is associated with pregnancy.

Sacroiliac Joints

The sacroiliac joints (L. *sacrum,* sacred) are formed between paired lateral C-shaped concave articular surfaces of the sacrum and slightly convex articular surfaces of the right and left ilium (figure 4.1A). The paired sacroiliac joints can be palpated just adjacent to each posterior superior iliac spine. The PSIS are at the level of the spine of the second sacral vertebra (S2). These strong joints are complex and evade easy classification, demonstrating characteristics in different regions of cartilaginous, fibrous, and synovial joints (Bechtel, 2001; Chen, Fredericson, and Smuck, 2002; Papadopoulos and Khan, 2004).

The sacroiliac joints are generally quite stable due to the restraints offered by the fibrocartilage and fibrous tissue within the joints, the presence of very strong ligaments that tether the bones together, expansions from surrounding muscles, and the shape of the involved bones (Dujardin et al., 2002; Levangie and Norkin, 2001). Regarding shape, the sacrum sits like a wedge between the two ilia. Because it is wider at the top than the bottom, it will resist the tendency to slide downward produced by the weight of the body from above. In addition, there are interlocking convolutions on the articulating surfaces of the sacrum and ilium that add stability and limit movement in certain directions. However, very small (0.5 to 1.6 millimeters) movements of the sacroiliac joints can occur and are important for normal pelvic mechanics (Chen, Fredericson, and Smuck, 2002). These movements involve a combination of rotation and translation about complex and unclear axes. Unfortunately, as discussed later in this chapter, the sacroiliac joints are a very common site of injury and chronic pain in dancers, particularly older dancers.

Movements of the Pelvic Girdle

The limited movement permitted at the pubic symphysis and sacroiliac joints allows the pelvic girdle to essentially function as a single unit. This arrangement is advantageous in terms of stability and of protective and support functions of the pelvis. However, it is limiting in terms of movement and hence the lower spine, particularly the lumbosacral joint discussed in chapter 3, becomes very important for facilitating positional changes of the pelvis. The movements of the pelvis are termed anterior tilt, posterior tilt, lateral tilt, and rotation. They will be discussed later in the chapter in connection with alignment and are shown in figure 4.15 on page 178.

Joint Structure and Movements of the Hip

In upright posture and movements such as walking or running, the weight of the upper body is transmitted down through the spine and pelvis through one or both rotary hip joints to be supported by the limb or limbs. In addition to withstanding these downward forces of gravity, the hip joint also transmits forces from the ground to the pelvis in these same movements. These important force transmission functions of the hip joint make joint stability and strength a priority. However, while stability is favored, sufficient mobility must be present to facilitate economical locomotor movement and allow for desired positioning of the foot and lower limb in space. The

joint architecture with its unique arrangement of ligaments and multijoint muscles helps the hip meet the bias toward stability, while still allowing adequate mobility.

Hip Joint Classification and Associated Movements

The hip joint, or acetabularfemoral joint, is a ball-and-socket joint formed between the acetabulum and the head of the femur. The acetabulum faces anterolaterally and slightly inferiorly. The head of the femur forms about two-thirds of a sphere and is fully covered by articular cartilage except for a small pit at the top of the head of the femur called the fovea. The head of the femur faces upward and forward relative to its neck, with its convex surface fitting well with the concave surface of the acetabulum. Due to the depth of the socket and the broad surface areas of contact between the articulating bones, joint stability is favored. Approximately 70% of the head of the femur articulates with the acetabulum, in contrast to only 25% contact of the head of the humerus in its socket with the shoulder joint (Hamill and Knutzen, 1995). The hip joint is considered the best example of a ball-and-socket joint in the body.

As with other classic ball-and-socket joints, the hip joint has three degrees of freedom of motion: flexion-extension in the sagittal plane, abduction-adduction in the frontal plane, and external-internal rotation in the transverse plane as seen in figure 4.3. In many dance movements, combinations of these three movement pairs occur. The true axis of motion for the hip joint goes through the center of the femoral head, which can be visually estimated from locating the greater trochanter. However, the neck of the femur serves an important function of increasing the lever arm for the muscles that attach onto the greater trochanter (gluteus maximus, gluteus medius, gluteus minimus, deep outward rotators) so that these muscles can produce markedly greater torque.

Hip Joint Capsule and Key Ligaments

A strong, dense joint capsule encloses the entire hip joint. It attaches from the margin of the acetabulum and runs distally, encasing the neck of the femur like a tube, to attach posteriorly to the distal neck of the femur and anteriorly to the intertrochanteric line. The capsule also has thickened ligamental bands, as shown in figure 4.4, that spiral around the neck of the femur and are named according to the bone from which they originate—the iliofemoral, pubofemoral, and ischiofemoral ligaments. Due to

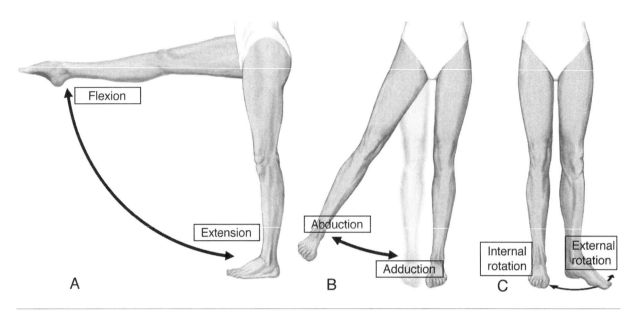

FIGURE 4.3   Movements of the hip joint. (A) Flexion-extension, (B) abduction-adduction, (C) external rotation-internal rotation.

their spiral arrangement, all three ligaments and the capsule become tight with hip extension or posterior tilting of the pelvis, important for providing stability with upright standing (Smith, Weiss, and Lehmkuhl, 1996). Full extension during weight bearing can be considered the close-packed position for the hip joint (Hamill and Knutzen, 1995) in terms of ligamental stability, despite there being greater bony congruence at 90° of hip flexion with slight abduction and external rotation (such as with sitting in a chair). Conversely, all three ligaments become slack with hip flexion, allowing the dancer to have greater range of motion when the hip is not extended. Some additional information about these ligaments follows.

The Iliofemoral Ligament

The **iliofemoral ligament** is located on the front of the hip joint, spiraling inferiorly from the anterior inferior iliac spine of the pelvis to diverge into two bands that attach to the upper and lower portions of the intertrochanteric line, as seen in figure 4.4A. The iliofemoral ligament is sometimes called the "Y" ligament because its appearance resembles an inverted "Y." This ligament is one of the strongest ligaments in the body and plays a very important role in standing posture. In erect stance, the center of gravity generally passes behind the center of rotation of the hip joint and so tends to extend the joint. Because the iliofemoral ligament becomes taut with hip extension, this ligament can passively allow stance to be maintained and prevents the trunk

from falling backward or the head of the femur from displacing anteriorly with little hip muscular activity required.

As well as its postural role, the iliofemoral ligament also serves as a powerful constraint for any movement that involves bringing the leg behind the body such as in a tendu back or an arabesque. Most anatomy texts hold that the iliofemoral ligament limits hip hyperextension to 10° to 20° in the average individual, but many dancers apparently markedly stretch this ligament and the capsule in order to obtain a range of hyperextension as great as 40°. The lateral fibers of the iliofemoral ligament also limit hip external rotation and hip adduction. Due to this restraint to external rotation, some dancers adopt the undesired tactic of anteriorly tilting the pelvis when trying to achieve greater turnout at the hip.

The Pubofemoral Ligament

The **pubofemoral ligament** is located on the anterior and lower portion of the capsule as seen in figure 4.4A. It runs between the pubic bone and an area near the lesser trochanter. Its inferior location makes it particularly effective for limiting hip abduction. It also assists the iliofemoral ligament in limiting hip extension and external rotation.

The Ischiofemoral Ligament

The **ischiofemoral ligament** is located on the posterior side of the hip joint as seen in figure 4.4B and provides protection from posterior displacement of the femur. It spans between a portion of the ischium

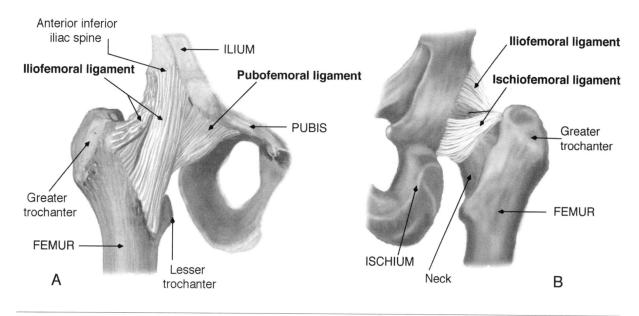

FIGURE 4.4   Key hip joint ligaments (right hip). (A) Anterior view, (B) posterior view.

located just below the acetabulum and the back of the femoral neck. This ligament prevents hip internal rotation and horizontal adduction.

Specialized Structures of the Hip

Various specialized structures and factors are associated with the hip that provide additional joint stability or aid with joint function. These structures include the glenoid labrum and bursae, while suction also makes a significant contribution.

Acetabular Labrum

In addition to the normal articular cartilage present at the hip joint, there is a specialized ring of fibrocartilage situated along the margin of the acetabulum. This rim of fibrocartilage, called the **acetabular labrum** (L. *labrum,* a lip-shaped structure), is considerably thicker at the circumference than at the center, thus increasing the effective depth of the acetabulum and helping to hold the femoral head in place. In addition, by being thicker above and behind, it helps provide cushioning for the top and back of the acetabulum against the large compression forces of the head of the femur during erect stance and movements. Thus, this labrum helps improve joint stability and protects the bone.

Suction

The hip joint has another factor facilitating joint stability. There is a difference in atmospheric pressure in the hip joint such that a vacuum is created

that pulls the head of the femur into the socket. With the depth of the acetabulum, the presence of the acetabular labrum, and the extensive congruency of this joint, suction plays a more prominent role at the hip joint. Even if all the ligaments and muscles are cut, the joint will stay together, and relatively large forces are required to separate the bones as long as the capsule is intact. In adult cadavers, 45 pounds (20 kilograms) of force was required to separate the joint 0.1 inch (3 millimeters), and in healthy adults, 90 pounds (41 kilograms) of force was required to separate the joint even when it was in a loose-packed position (Smith, Weiss, and Lehmkuhl, 1996).

Bursae

Numerous bursae are associated with the hip joint. There are two that more commonly become inflamed in dancers. One is a bursa located over the greater trochanter as seen in figure 4.42 on page 233, which helps protect the soft tissues that cross the back portion of this projection. The other is located between the iliopsoas and the underlying articular capsule.

Muscles

In addition to the strong capsule and ligaments of the hip, there are many strong muscles that cross the hip joint and have a significant stabilizing effect on the joint. Because of their importance in supporting the weight of the body and generating the large forces associated with locomotor movements, these muscles are more massive and stronger than those associated with the upper extremity.

Description and Functions of Individual Hip Muscles

Twenty-two muscles cross the hip joint. However, despite the large number of muscles involved, they are arranged in a logical way that makes remembering their actions easier—the anterior group are all hip flexors, the posterior group are generally hip extensors (except for the deep outward rotators), the lateral group are all hip abductors, and the medial group are all hip adductors. However, although their primary actions are the same, members of these groups may have different secondary actions.

In terms of deducing primary and secondary actions, it is important to keep in mind that since the hip joint has three degrees of freedom of motion, many hip muscles will exert action about all three axes simultaneously. However, one or two actions will often predominate, due to better leverage of the muscle with respect to that axis. For example, the actions of hip flexion and hip adduction predominate with the pectineus, and its contribution to rotation is generally not considered very significant. In addition, some muscles are extensive enough that different portions may have different relationships to a given axis and hence may be capable of a different action. For example, many texts list the upper fibers of the adductor magnus as a flexor and the lower fibers as an extensor. Lastly, remember that as discussed in chapter 2, the action of a muscle may differ with changes in the joint angle due to the shift in the line of pull relative to the axis. For example, the adductor longus aids with early flexion, but its effectiveness decreases continuously until it no longer aids with flexion; and after approximately 70° it actually produces hip extension. Due to this complexity, it is not surprising that many of the secondary actions of hip muscles are still under debate. Many of the controversial secondary actions have been purposely excluded from this text. (See Individual Muscles of the Hip, pp. 165-177.)

Alignment and Common Deviations of the Hip Region

Alignment of the bony segments in the hip region is important in itself and also influences the bony segments above and below the pelvis and hip joint. For example, alignment of the pelvis will influence the spine above and the knee, ankle, and foot below. Three alignment considerations in the hip region that are particularly important are pelvic inclinations or tilts, the angle of femoral inclination, and the angle of femoral torsion.

Pelvic Alignment and Movements

The position of the pelvis can be described as neutral or as having the following deviations: anterior-posterior pelvic tilts, right-left lateral tilts, or right-left rotations. These deviations from neutral can be temporary movements that accompany movements of the spine or femur as described later in this chapter (see Pelvic and Hip Mechanics, p. 181). They can also be small deviations that tend to persist and to be habitual in standing posture or movement, as will be described now. When identifying pelvic alignment or movement, the relative position of bony landmarks such as the iliac crests, ASIS, PSIS, and pubic symphysis are used. *(Text continues on p. 177.)*

DANCE CUES 4.1

"Think of Your Pelvis as a Basin and Avoid Spilling the Contents"

The instruction to "imagine your pelvis is a basin and avoid having the contents spill out by letting it tip" is sometimes used by teachers in an effort to maintain desired alignment of the pelvis. From an anatomical perspective, the directive parallels the concept of a neutral pelvis and avoiding letting the pelvis tilt, particularly in an anterior direction. The problem with this image is that the pelvis is not horizontal but has an angle of inclination. Furthermore, a student who is accustomed to dancing with an anterior pelvic tilt will generally feel that the pelvis is "level." So it is frequently necessary to use tactile or visual cues such as placing the hands on the ASIS and noting when they are vertically aligned relative to the pubic symphysis to identify a neutral position (see Tests and Measurements 4.1, p. 179). Then, the basin or bowl image can often be successfully used to achieve the desired pelvic alignment.

Individual Muscles of the Hip

Anterior Muscles of the Hip

The anterior muscles of the hip include the iliopsoas, rectus femoris, and sartorius. These muscles cross anterior to the axis of the hip joint for flexion-extension and so share the common action of hip flexion used in movements such as walking, running, or leaping.

Attachments and Primary Action of Iliopsoas

Muscle	Proximal attachment(s)	Distal attachment(s)	Primary action(s)
Iliopsoas (il-ee-o-SO-us)			
Psoas major (SO-us)	Transverse processes, bodies, and intervertebral discs of T12-L5	Lesser trochanter of femur	Hip flexion Hip abduction (higher ranges) Posture
Iliacus (il-ee-AK-us)	Iliac fossa, crest of ilium, inner lateral sacrum	Lesser trochanter of femur	Hip flexion Hip abduction (higher ranges)

Iliopsoas

The iliopsoas is actually composed of the psoas major (G. *psoa,* the loins + *major,* the larger) and iliacus (*iliac,* ilium). Since these share a common distal attachment and appear to act together during functional movement, they are frequently referred to together as one muscle, the iliopsoas. The iliopsoas, shown in figure 4.5, is approximately 16 inches (41 centimeters) long (Rasch and Burke, 1978). It runs deep under the abdominal wall from the front of the lower spine and inner portion of the ilium downward to attach onto the medial side of the upper femur at the lesser trochanter. Due to its deep location, it is often difficult for dancers to "feel" or visualize, and careful examination of its attachments on the skeleton is helpful to understand its location and function. The iliopsoas is one of the most powerful muscles in the entire body (Michele, 1960) and can develop a tensile pull in excess of 1,000 pounds (454 kilograms). The iliopsoas has been shown to be the most important muscle for hip flexion above 90°, as evidenced by the inability to lift the thigh above 90° when iliopsoas paralysis is pres-

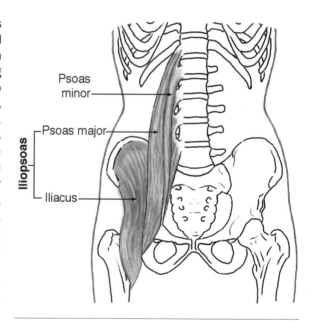

FIGURE 4.5   The iliopsoas muscle (anterior view).

ent (Smith, Weiss, and Lehmkuhl, 1996). It can also assist with hip abduction, particularly at higher ranges. These two latter properties give the iliopsoas key importance for dance movements such as high développés to either the front or side. The potential contribution of the iliopsoas to hip rotation is still under debate, and although it may function as an external rotator when the femur is internally rotated, it appears unlikely to play an important rotation role in other conditions.

Regarding its postural role, the iliopsoas is the only muscle in the human body that has attachments on the spine, pelvis, and femur. Due to these attachments, the iliopsoas is in a unique position not only to produce movement but also to stabilize the hip and effect the positioning of the lumbar spine.

Posturally the iliopsoas plays an important role in preventing the torso from falling backward and may help maintain the lumbar curve. The former role is key when one is performing floor work in modern dance, and many dancers who are unaccustomed to floor work may find themselves getting fatigued and sore in the hip flexors, particularly the iliopsoas. Some also hold that the iliopsoas may play an important role in integrating and coordinating movements between the femur, pelvis, and spine.

Attachments and Primary Actions of Rectus Femoris

Muscle	Proximal attachment(s)	Distal attachment(s)	Primary action(s)
Rectus femoris (REK-tus FEM-o-ris)	Anterior inferior iliac spine Posterior head: just above acetabulum	Tibial tuberosity via patellar tendon	Hip flexion (Knee extension)

Rectus Femoris

The **rectus femoris,** shown in figure 4.6, is one of the four muscles that make up the quadriceps femoris. It is the only member of the group that crosses the hip joint. The other three muscles attach distally relative to the hip joint and act only on the knee. "Rectus" means straight, so as its name implies, the rectus femoris runs straight down the front of the femur or thigh. In addition to its action of flexing the hip, the rectus femoris muscle also extends the knee. Its combined movement of hip flexion and knee extension used with kicking has given rise to its being called the "kicking muscle."

Palpation: Sit in a chair with the left foot crossed over the right ankle. Place your fingertips on the center of the upper portion of your right thigh, and feel the rectus femoris tighten under your fingertips as you attempt to extend your right knee while your left leg prevents this motion.

Sartorius

The **sartorius** is the longest muscle in the body. This slender muscle runs from the front of the pelvis down the thigh obliquely and medially to attach on the inside of the tibia as seen in figure 4.6. In addition to assisting with hip flexion, the sartorius can also abduct and externally rotate the hip. Since this combination of joint motions is used to assume the crossed-legged sitting position on the floor, used by tailors in the past, the sartorius (L. *sartor,* a tailor) is commonly called the "tailor's muscle." These combined motions are also commonly used in dance vocabulary such as a passé. Due to its long, thin composition, the sartorius is designed for speed rather than strength, which may contribute

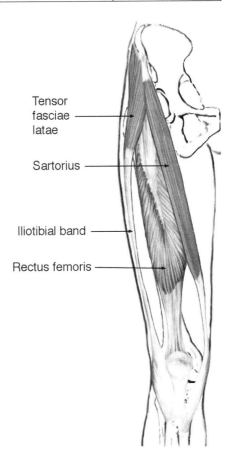

Tensor fasciae latae

Sartorius

Iliotibial band

Rectus femoris

FIGURE 4.6   The rectus femoris, sartorius, and tensor fasciae latae muscles (right hip, anterior view).

Attachments and Primary Actions of Sartorius

Muscle	Proximal attachment(s)	Distal attachment(s)	Primary action(s)
Sartorius (sar-TOR-ee-us)	Anterior superior iliac spine (ASIS) and area just below	Medial surface of upper tibia (pes anserinus)	Hip flexion Hip abduction Hip external rotation (Knee flexion)

to its being a common site of strain in the dancer. The sartorius also can act to produce flexion or internal rotation of the knee, which will be further discussed in chapter 5.

Palpation: While standing on one leg, perform a front attitude (hip flexion and external rotation) with the other leg and then carry this gesture leg to the side. Because the sartorius is the most superficial of the anterior thigh muscles, it can be both seen and easily palpated below and slightly medial to the ASIS. Note that as shown in figure 4.6, an inverted "V" is formed with the sartorius forming the medial ray, the tensor fasciae latae composing the lateral arm, and the rectus femoris lying in between.

Posterior Muscles of the Hip

The posterior muscles of the hip include the gluteus maximus, hamstrings, and deep outward rotators. All three of these muscle groups cross posterior to the axis of the hip joint for flexion-extension, and the gluteus maximus and hamstrings share the common action of hip extension, such as used in a back parallel tendu or in jumping. The hip extensors are well suited for propulsive activity such as jumping and running due to their large cross-sectional area and the power they can generate. However, their ability to produce force is dramatically influenced by the degree of hip flexion, with about twice as much extensor strength present with 90° of hip flexion versus a neutral position of extension (Hamill and Knutzen, 1995). This principle is often utilized by leaning the trunk forward when going up a hill or stairs or in the preparation for a jump. Posturally, these muscles can also play the important role of producing a posterior tilt of the pelvis and countering the tendency for an anterior tilt of the pelvis or forward lean of the torso.

Although the deep outward rotators cross posterior to the flexion-extension axis through the hip, they generally have a very horizontal line of pull. This makes them better suited for effecting hip external rotation and hip horizontal abduction than hip extension.

Gluteus Maximus

The **gluteus maximus** (G. *gloutos,* buttock + *maximus,* largest), shown in figure 4.7, is the largest and most superficial of the buttocks muscles. It forms the roundness of the back of the buttocks. Its large size in humans is thought to be due to the demands of upright stance and locomotion. The gluteus maximus is the most powerful hip extensor and is crucial for movements requiring large forces such as going up stairs, walking up hills, running, and jumping. In addition to hip extension, the gluteus maximus can produce hip external rotation, and the upper fibers can produce hip abduction against resistance. Due to its insertion into the **iliotibial band** or tract, a strong fascia of the lateral thigh that spans between the pelvis and lower leg, the gluteus maximus indirectly also helps support the femur upon the tibia.

Palpation: You can easily palpate the gluteus maximus by placing your fingertips over the back of the buttocks while standing and simply contracting or "setting" the muscle without any joint movement necessary. To elicit a stronger contraction of the muscle, extend and externally rotate the hip by lifting the leg in a back attitude.

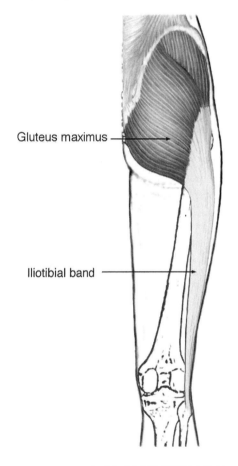

FIGURE 4.7   The gluteus maximus muscle and iliotibial band (right hip, posterior view).

Attachments and Primary Actions of Gluteus Maximus

Muscle	Proximal attachment(s)	Distal attachment(s)	Primary action(s)
Gluteus maximus (GLOO-tee-us MAK-si-mus)	Crest and posterior surface of ilium, posterior surface of sacrum and coccyx	Line on posterior femur between greater trochanter and linea aspera and iliotibial tract	Hip extension Hip external rotation

Hamstrings

The **hamstring** muscle group forms the bulk of the back of the thigh as seen in figure 4.8. This group is composed of three muscles: the **biceps femoris, semitendinosus,** and the deeper **semimembranosus.** Their action of extension comes into play in everyday movements such as standing, walking, and controlling forward motion of the torso. Their function is considered more postural and fine-tuning in contrast to the "power" function of the gluteus maximus. The biceps femoris (*bi,* dual + L. *capus,* head) appears to be particularly active with hip extension and is considered the "workhorse" for hip extension (Hamill and Knutzen, 1995). Because each of the hamstrings inserts distal to the knee, all the hamstrings act as knee flexors as well as hip extensors. The medial hamstrings—semitendinosus (L. *semi,* half + *tendinosus,* tendon) and semimembranosus (L. *semi,* half + *membranosus,* membrane)— insert onto the medial part of the tibia and so can also assist with

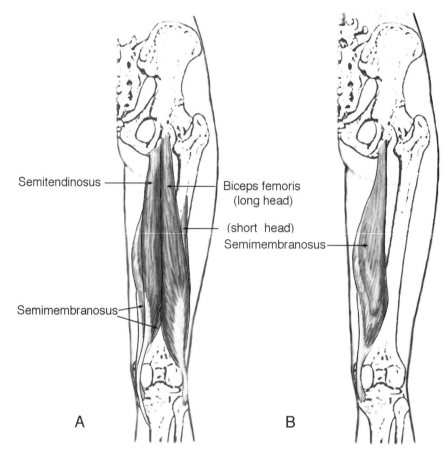

FIGURE 4.8   The hamstring muscles (right hip, posterior view). (A) Superficial view, (B) deeper view.

knee internal rotation or hip internal rotation when the hip and knee are extended. The lateral hamstrings (biceps femoris) insert onto the lateral tibia and fibula and so can also assist with knee external rotation or hip external rotation when the knee and hip are extended.

Palpation: Stand on one leg with your other leg held in a low arabesque position. The hamstrings can be palpated on the lifted leg at the back of your upper thigh, just below the ischial tuberosity. While maintaining the leg in this low arabesque position, internally rotate the leg and lift it slightly higher to the back. The hamstrings and part of the adductor magnus can be felt contracting. Now, place your

Attachments and Primary Actions of Hamstrings

Muscle	Proximal attachment(s)	Distal attachment(s)	Primary action(s)
Hamstrings			
Biceps femoris (BI-seps FEM-o-ris)	Long head: ischial tuberosity Short head: linea aspera of femur	Head of fibula Lateral tibial condyle	Hip extension Hip external rotation (Knee flexion) (Knee external rotation)
Semitendinosus (sem-ee-ten-di-NO-sus)	Ischial tuberosity	Medial surface of upper tibia (pes anserinus)	Hip extension Hip internal rotation (Knee flexion) (Knee internal rotation)
Semimembranosus (sem-ee-mem-brah-NO-sus)	Ischial tuberosity	Medial condyle of tibia	Hip extension Hip internal rotation (Knee flexion) (Knee internal rotation)

fingertips on your buttocks and alternately internally and externally rotate the hip while maintaining the arabesque. Note the decrease in contraction of the gluteus maximus as the leg internally rotates and the increase as the leg is externally rotated.

Deep Outward Rotators

The **deep outward rotators (DOR),** or deep external rotator muscle group, is comprised of the piriformis, obturator internus, obturator externus (*externus,* outside), gemellus inferior, gemellus superior, and quadratus femoris, as seen in figure 4.9, A and B. This group of six small muscles is located deep to the gluteus maximus in the region of the buttocks. The fibers of this muscle group run primarily horizontally, spanning from the inside and outside of the pelvis to the greater trochanter of the femur. The **piriformis** (L. *pirum,* pear), the most superior of the group, is located slightly above the hip joint, and the **quadratus femoris** (L. *quadratus,* square), the most inferior, is located slightly below it. The obturator internus and gemelli are located in the gap between the piriformis and quadratus femoris. As their names suggest, the obturator internus (*internus,* inside) has extensive attachments to the internal surface of the membrane covering the obturator foramen and adjacent areas, while the obturator externus has extensive attachments to the external surface of the obturator membrane and adjacent bones. The **obturator internus** is accompanied above by the **gemellus superior** (L. *geminus,* twin, double + *superior,* above) and below by the **gemellus inferior** (L. *geminus,* twin, double + *inferior,* below) to attach via a common, approximately horizontal, tendon to the greater trochanter; and hence these three muscles are sometimes referred to as a three-headed muscle—the triceps coxae (Moore and Dalley, 1999). The deep outward rotators function as a group to help hold the head of the femur in the acetabulum and can help prevent upward jamming of the femur with hip abduction, making its function very parallel to the rotator cuff's function at the shoulder joint, discussed in chapter 7. However, as their name implies, this group of muscles is particularly known

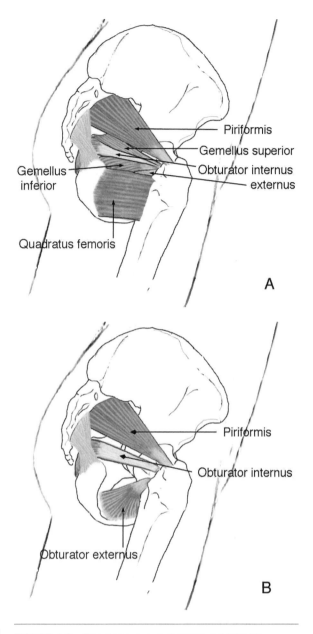

FIGURE 4.9   The deep outward rotators (right hip, posterolateral view). (A) With gluteus maximus removed; (B) deeper view with quadratus femoris, gemellus superior, and gemellus inferior removed.

for its action of hip external rotation. The ability of the group to produce hip external rotation without other major accessory motions makes them key in dance for the production and maintenance of turnout. When the hip is flexed to 90°, some of these muscles are in an effective position to produce hip horizontal abduction, making them important in movements such as a passé and rond de jambe in the air (en l'air) at 90°. Some texts also suggest that the piriformis can assist with hip abduction.

Palpation: Standing on one leg, raise the other leg to the front to a parallel passé (retiré) position. The uppermost of the deep external rotators, the piriformis, can be felt contracting (under the gluteus maximus) several inches above and posterior to the greater trochanter as the leg is brought to the side to a turned-out passé. Then, change positions to standing in parallel first, rock back on the heels, and externally rotate both legs at the hip to achieve a turned-out first position. The lowest of the DOR, the quadratus femoris, can be palpated deeply at the base of the buttocks between the ischial tuberosity and greater trochanter while rotating the legs. The remaining DOR are located between the piriformis and quadratus femoris and can be palpated as a group by placing the fingertips below the piriformis and repetitively externally rotating the hip.

Attachments and Primary Actions of Deep Outward Rotators

Muscle	Proximal attachment(s)	Distal attachment(s)	Primary action(s)
Deep outward rotators			
Piriformis (PIR-i-form-is)	Anterior surface of sacrum, posterior ilium	Superior surface of greater trochanter of femur	Hip external rotation Stabilization of hip joint
Obturator internus (ob-tu-RA-tor in-TER-nus)	Internal surface of obturator foramen and obturator membrane, ischium	Medial surface of greater trochanter of femur	Hip external rotation Stabilization of hip joint
Obturator externus (ob-tu-RA-tor ek-STER-nus)	Rami of pubis and ischium and external surface of obturator membrane	Adjacent to greater trochanter on upper, posterior femur	Hip external rotation Stabilization of hip joint
Gemellus superior (je-ME-lis)	Posterior, lower part of ischium	With obturator internus muscle to medial aspect of greater trochanter of femur	Hip external rotation Stabilization of hip joint
Gemellus inferior (je-ME-lis)	Ischial tuberosity	With obturator internus muscle to medial aspect of greater trochanter of femur	Hip external rotation Stabilization of hip joint
Quadratus femoris (kwod-RA-tus FEM-o-ris)	Lateral ischial tuberosity	The crest between the greater and lesser trochanter on posterior femur	Hip external rotation Stabilization of hip joint

Lateral Muscles of the Hip

The lateral muscles of the hip include the gluteus medius, gluteus minimus, and tensor fasciae latae. They all cross lateral to the axis of the hip joint for abduction-adduction and so share the common action of hip abduction, used in movements such as a parallel side tendu or dégagé. These muscles also play a very important stabilizing role in standing and locomotion. When the weight is on one leg, these muscles act to prevent the pelvis from dropping down on the opposite side or the support femur from excessively adducting ("sitting in the hip").

Attachments and Primary Actions of Gluteus Medius and Minimus Muscles

Muscle	Proximal attachment(s)	Distal attachment(s)	Primary action(s)
Gluteus medius (GLOO-tee-us ME-dee-us)	Outer surface of ilium	Lateral surface of greater trochanter of femur	Hip abduction Hip internal rotation Stabilization of pelvis on femur
Gluteus minimus (GLOO-tee-us MI-ni-mus)	Lower outer surface of ilium	Anterolateral aspect of greater trochanter of femur	Hip abduction Hip internal rotation Stabilization of pelvis on femur

Gluteus Medius and Minimus

The **gluteus medius** (G. *gloutos,* buttock + *medius,* middle) is located on the side of the ilium as shown in figure 4.10A. It provides the rounded contour to the side of the pelvis, although its posterior fibers are covered by the gluteus maximus and its anterior fibers by the tensor fasciae latae. The gluteus medius is the largest of the lateral muscles and is the most fundamental hip abductor, while the gluteus minimus, tensor fasciae latae, and some additional muscles may assist with greater resistance or in specific positions of the joint. The gluteus medius is also a prime mover for hip internal rotation.

The **gluteus minimus** (G. *gloutos,* buttock + L. *minimus,* smallest), as its name implies, is a smaller muscle; it is located deeply, underneath the gluteus medius, in a slightly anterior and inferior position as seen in figure 4.10B. In addition to their role in hip abduction, the anterior fibers of these muscles are key for hip internal rotation, and the posterior fibers assist with extension, at least under some conditions. Their potential contribution to hip flexion or external rotation is still under debate.

Palpation: While standing on one leg, lift the other leg to the side in a parallel position (hip abduction). The gluteus medius can be palpated laterally, below the crest of the ilium and about 2 to 3 inches (5-7.6 centimeters) above the greater trochanter. Since the gluteus minimus lies beneath the gluteus medius, it is difficult to palpate it distinctly from the gluteus medius.

Tensor Fasciae Latae

The **tensor fasciae latae** (*tensor,* to make tense + *fascia,* band + *lata,* wide) is a small muscle located at the front and side of the hip as seen in figure 4.6 on page 166. This muscle is distinct in having no bony distal attachment; rather it inserts into the iliotibial band approximately one-fourth of the way down the outside of the thigh. Its name is derived from the fact that its action is to tighten this fascia, thereby providing important lateral support for the knee joint. At the hip joint, in addition to its role in hip abduction, it assists with hip flexion and hip internal rotation (the latter at least when the hip is flexed).

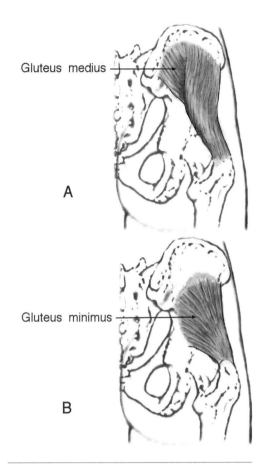

FIGURE 4.10   The gluteus medius and minimus (right hip, posterior view). (A) With gluteus maximus removed, (B) deeper view with gluteus medius removed.

Palpation: Standing on one leg, raise the other leg to the side while maintaining 45° of hip flexion. The tensor fasciae latae can be palpated about 2 inches (5 centimeters) anterior to the greater trochanter.

Attachments and Primary Actions of Tensor Fasciae Latae

Muscle	Proximal attachment(s)	Distal attachment(s)	Primary action(s)
Tensor fasciae latae (TEN-sor FA-she-eh LAT-te)	Anterior outer crest of ilium, lateral aspect of anterior superior iliac spine	Tibia via iliotibial band	Hip abduction Hip flexion Hip internal rotation

Medial Muscles of the Hip (Inner Thigh Muscles)

The medial muscles of the hip include the adductor brevis, adductor longus, adductor magnus, pectineus, and gracilis. These medial muscles are sometimes called the "inner thigh muscles" by dance teachers. Since all of these muscles cross medial to the axis of the hip joint, they all share the common action of hip adduction used in movements such as bringing the leg close to the center of gravity of the body in walking or closing into fifth position in ballet. Posturally, when standing on one leg the hip adductors commonly co-contract with the hip abductors to aid with pelvic stability. The muscle mass of these inner thigh muscles is much larger than the hip abductors or than might be expected given their relationship to gravity in upright stance. One commonly cited explanation for this apparent discrepancy is that each medial muscle has secondary actions, which allow it to contribute widely in activities that do not necessarily involve adduction of the hip. Due to the difficulty in distinguishing individual muscles and the tendency for these muscles to work together in functional movements, palpation will be described for the medial muscles as a group at the end of this section.

Attachments and Primary Actions of Adductor Longus, Brevis, and Magnus

Muscle	Proximal attachment(s)	Distal attachment(s)	Primary action(s)
Adductor longus (ah-DUK-tor LON-gus)	Anterior surface of pubis at crest	Middle third of linea aspera of femur	Hip adduction Hip flexion (lower ranges)
Adductor brevis (ah-DUK-tor BRE-vis)	Inferior ramus of pubis	Superior portion of linea aspera and distal portion of line between lesser trochanter and linea aspera of femur	Hip adduction Hip flexion (lower ranges)
Adductor magnus (ah-DUK-tor MAG-nus)	Inferior rami of pubis and ischium, ischial tuberosity	Linea aspera of femur	Hip adduction Hip extension (lower fibers)

Adductor Longus, Brevis, and Magnus

The **adductor longus** (adduct, move toward midline + L. longus, long) is the most superficial of these three muscles and runs downward from the pubis to the linea aspera along the middle portion of the shaft of the femur as seen in figure 4.11. The **adductor brevis** (adduct, move toward midline + L. brevis, short) is a smaller, deeper muscle that is located above and behind the longus. The **adductor magnus** (adduct, move toward midline + L. magnus, large), as its name implies, is one of the largest muscles in the body, and both its proximal and distal attachments are extensive. Its proximal attachment spans from the front of the pubis to the ischial tuberosity, and its distal attachment spans the length of the shaft of the femur from just below the lesser trochanter to just above the medial epicondyle. The adductor magnus is the deepest of the adductor muscles.

In addition to their action in hip adduction, the medial hip muscles can also play a role in hip flexion and extension. In anatomical position, the adductor longus, brevis, and upper fibers of the magnus lie anterior to the axis for flexion-extension of the hip and so can produce hip flexion. In contrast, the line of pull of the lower fibers of the adductor magnus lies posterior and so can produce hip extension. However, during flexion of the hip, the line of action of these muscles relative to this axis changes. Thus, as flexion proceeds, they become less effective as hip flexors, and between approximately 50° and 70° they become hip extensors (Smith, Weiss, and Lehmkuhl, 1996). There is still much controversy regarding the potential contribution of the hip adductors to rotation, and further research will be required to clarify this issue.

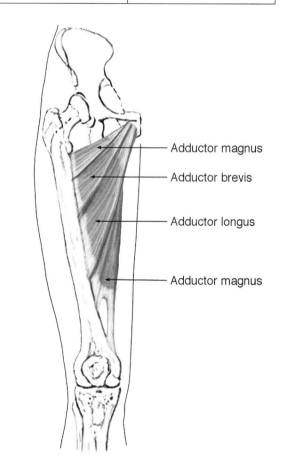

FIGURE 4.11   The adductor longus, adductor brevis, and adductor magnus (right hip, anterior view).

Adductor magnus

Adductor brevis

Adductor longus

Adductor magnus

Attachments and Primary Actions of Pectineus

Muscle	Proximal attachment(s)	Distal attachment(s)	Primary action(s)
Pectineus (pek-TIN-ee-us)	Superior ramus of pubis	Line between lesser trochanter and the linea aspera on the upper shaft of the femur	Hip adduction Hip flexion

Pectineus

The **pectineus** (L. *pectin,* comb), as seen in figure 4.12, is a short, flat muscle located just lateral to the adductor longus and partially covered by the rectus femoris and sartorius. Its proximal attachment is more anterior and superior than the adductor longus or magnus, allowing it to act as a prime mover for hip flexion and hip adduction through a larger range of motion. Due to its combination function as a prime mover for both flexion and adduction and its transitional location, the pectineus is classified in some texts as part of the anterior hip flexor group and in other texts as part of the medial hip adductor group. Its design favors power, and it is used when the hip is vigorously flexed or to lift the thigh to cross it over the other thigh during sitting.

Gracilis

The **gracilis** (L. *gracilis,* slender), as seen in figure 4.12, is a superficial, slender, and long muscle that descends more vertically than the more oblique course of the other medial thigh muscles. It is located the most medially of the inner thigh muscles. In addition to its action of hip adduction, it can contribute to the earlier arc of hip flexion (probably primarily when the knee is extended) and hip internal rotation. It is the only medial muscle of the hip that crosses the knee joint. It attaches onto the medial tibia and can also act in knee flexion and knee internal rotation as discussed in chapter 5.

Palpation of the medial hip muscles: Sit on the floor with the legs separated in a second-position stretch. The adductors can be palpated as a group along the inside of the thigh. Press one leg in isometrically against the hand (hip horizontal adduction) of the same side while using the other hand to palpate the medial muscles. The adductor longus and gracilis are the prominent tendons that you can feel at the top of the inner thigh. The adductor magnus can be palpated along the inside of the middle to lower half of the thigh. Due to its depth, the adductor brevis is difficult to palpate. You can palpate the pectineus just above the adductor longus tendon when lifting that leg over the other as you sit in a chair.

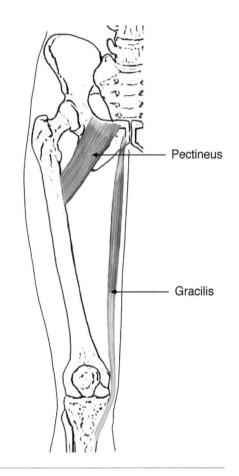

FIGURE 4.12 The pectineus and gracilis (right hip, anterior view).

Attachments and Primary Actions of Gracilis

Muscle	Proximal attachment(s)	Distal attachment(s)	Primary action(s)
Gracilis (grah-SI-lis)	Just below symphysis on pubis, inferior rami of ischium and pubis	Medial surface of upper tibia (pes anserinus)	Hip adduction Hip flexion (Knee flexion)

Summary of Hip Muscle Attachments and Actions

A summary of the attachments of primary hip muscles and their primary actions is provided in table 4.1, and selected muscles and attachments are shown in figures 4.13, A and B, and 4.14, A and B. From these resources, estimate the line of pull of the muscle, deduce its actions, and then check for accuracy by referring to figure 4.13C or 4.14C. Note that the proximal attachment of the iliopsoas is not shown in figure 4.13 but can be approximated from a close examination of figure 4.5 on page 165.

TABLE 4.1   Summary of Attachments and Primary Actions of Hip Muscles

Muscle	Proximal attachment(s)	Distal attachment(s)	Primary action(s)
Anterior muscles			
Iliopsoas (il-ee-o-SO-us)			
Psoas major (SO-us)	Transverse processes, bodies, and intervertebral discs of T12-L5	Lesser trochanter of femur	Hip flexion Hip abduction (higher ranges) Posture
Iliacus (il-ee-AK-us)	Iliac fossa, crest of ilium, inner lateral sacrum	Lesser trochanter of femur	Hip flexion Hip abduction (higher ranges)
Rectus femoris (REK-tus FEM-o-ris)	Anterior inferior iliac spine Posterior head: just above acetabulum	Tibial tuberosity via patellar tendon	Hip flexion (Knee extension)
Sartorius (sar-TOR-ee-us)	Anterior superior iliac spine (ASIS) and area just below	Medial surface of upper tibia (pes anserinus)	Hip flexion Hip abduction Hip external rotation (Knee flexion)
Posterior muscles			
Gluteus maximus (GLOO-tee-us MAK-si-mus)	Crest and posterior surface of ilium, posterior surface of sacrum and coccyx	Line on posterior femur between greater trochanter and linea aspera and iliotibial tract	Hip extension Hip external rotation
Hamstrings			
Biceps femoris (BI-seps FEM-o-ris)	Long head: ischial tuberosity Short head: linea aspera of femur	Head of fibula Lateral tibial condyle	Hip extension Hip external rotation (Knee flexion) (Knee external rotation)
Semitendinosus (sem-ee-ten-di-NO-sus)	Ischial tuberosity	Medial surface of upper tibia (pes anserinus)	Hip extension Hip internal rotation (Knee flexion) (Knee internal rotation)
Semimembranosus (sem-ee-mem-brah-NO-sus)	Ischial tuberosity	Medial condyle of tibia	Hip extension Hip internal rotation (Knee flexion) (Knee internal rotation)

Muscle	Proximal attachment(s)	Distal attachment(s)	Primary action(s)
Posterior muscles (continued)			
Deep outward rotators			
Piriformis (PIR-i-form-is)	Anterior surface of sacrum, posterior ilium	Superior surface of greater trochanter of femur	Hip external rotation Stabilization of hip joint
Obturator internus (ob-tu-RA-tor in-TER-nus)	Internal surface of obturator foramen and obturator membrane, ischium	Medial surface of greater trochanter of femur	Hip external rotation Stabilization of hip joint
Obturator externus (ob-tu-RA-tor ek-STER-nus)	Rami of pubis and ischium and external surface of obturator membrane	Adjacent to greater trochanter on upper, posterior femur	Hip external rotation Stabilization of hip joint
Gemellus superior (je-ME-lis)	Posterior, lower part of ischium	With obturator internus muscle to medial aspect of greater trochanter of femur	Hip external rotation Stabilization of hip joint
Gemellus inferior (je-ME-lis)	Ischial tuberosity	With obturator internus muscle to medial aspect of greater trochanter of femur	Hip external rotation Stabilization of hip joint
Quadratus femoris (kwod-RA-tus FEM-o-ris)	Lateral ischial tuberosity	The crest between the greater and lesser trochanter on posterior femur	Hip external rotation Stabilization of hip joint
Lateral muscles			
Gluteus medius (GLOO-tee-us ME-dee-us)	Outer surface of ilium	Lateral surface of greater trochanter of femur	Hip abduction Hip internal rotation Stabilization of pelvis on femur
Gluteus minimus (GLOO-tee-us MI-ni-mus)	Lower outer surface of ilium	Anterolateral aspect of greater trochanter of femur	Hip abduction Hip internal rotation Stabilization of pelvis on femur
Tensor fasciae latae (TEN-sor FA-she-eh LAT-te)	Anterior outer crest of ilium, lateral aspect of anterior superior iliac spine	Tibia via iliotibial band	Hip abduction Hip flexion Hip internal rotation
Medial muscles			
Adductor longus (ah-DUK-tor LON-gus)	Anterior surface of pubis at crest	Middle third of linea aspera of femur	Hip adduction Hip flexion (lower ranges)
Adductor brevis (ah-DUK-tor BRE-vis)	Inferior ramus of pubis	Superior portion of linea aspera and distal portion of line between lesser trochanter and linea aspera of femur	Hip adduction Hip flexion (lower ranges)

(continued)

TABLE 4.1 Summary of Attachments and Primary Actions of Hip Muscles *(continued)*

Muscle	Proximal attachment(s)	Distal attachment(s)	Primary action(s)
Medial muscles *(continued)*			
Adductor magnus (ah-DUK-tor MAG-nus)	Inferior rami of pubis and ischium, ischial tuberosity	Linea aspera of femur	Hip adduction Hip flexion (lower fibers)
Pectineus (pek-TIN-ee-us)	Superior ramus of pubis	Line between lesser trochanter and the linea aspera on the upper shaft of the femur	Hip adduction Hip flexion
Gracilis (grah-SI-lis)	Just below symphysis on pubis, inferior rami of ischium and pubis	Medial surface of upper tibia (pes anserinus)	Hip adduction Hip flexion (Knee flexion)

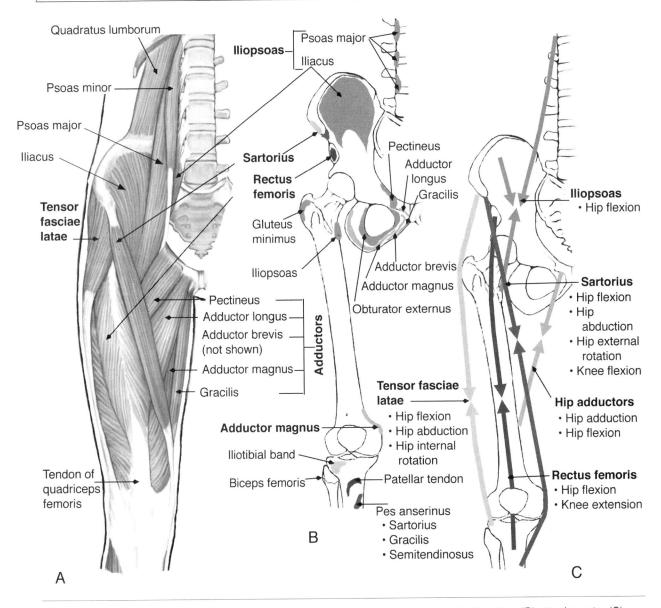

FIGURE 4.13   Anterior view of primary muscles acting on the hip joint (right hip). (A) Muscles, (B) attachments, (C) lines of pull and actions.

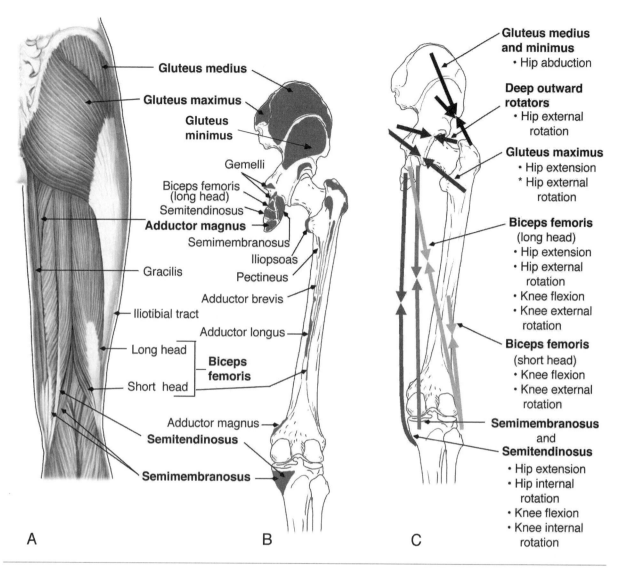

FIGURE 4.14   Posterior view of primary muscles acting on the hip joint (right hip). (A) Muscles, (B) attachments, (C) lines of pull and actions.

This is because bony landmarks are more reflective of the underlying bony structure and generally will provide a more accurate appraisal than body contours.

Neutral Position

During standing in an upright position, an oblique plane through the PSIS of the ilia and the symphysis pubis forms an angle of about 60° relative to the horizontal plane. This angle is termed the **angle of pelvic inclination** (Smith, Weiss, and Lehmkuhl, 1996). This is the **neutral position** of the pelvis and roughly corresponds to a position in which both of the ASIS and the pubic symphysis are in the same frontal plane as seen in figure 4.15A. Since the angle of inclination cannot be determined in a class setting, the vertical alignment of the landmarks is used as an easy method to evaluate pelvic position. A neutral position of the pelvis also takes into account other

planes, such that one ASIS would not be higher or lower or rotated forward or backward relative to the other ASIS.

Anterior and Posterior Pelvic Tilt

Anterior and posterior pelvic tilts are opposite movements of the whole pelvis in the sagittal plane about a mediolateral axis. In an **anterior tilt** (increased inclination), the top of the pelvis rotates forward such that the ASIS are forward relative to the pubic symphysis as seen in figure 4.15B. From a side view, a vertical plane extending from the ASIS would fall in front of the pubic symphysis. In dance this is sometimes referred to as a "released" position of the pelvis.

In a **posterior tilt** or backward tilt (decreased inclination), the top of the pelvis rotates backward such that the ASIS are back relative to the pubic symphysis as

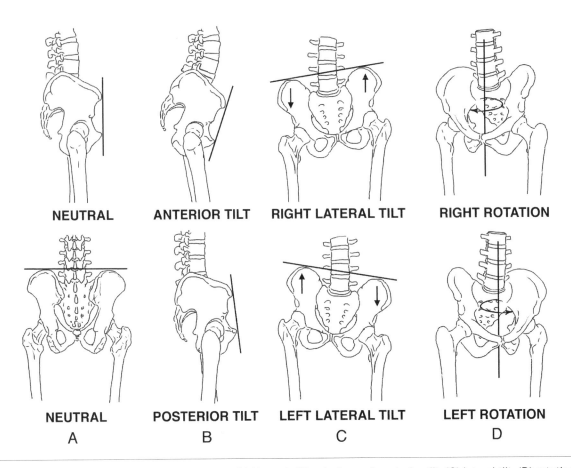

FIGURE 4.15   Pelvic alignment and movement. (A) Neutral, (B) anterior and posterior tilt, (C) lateral tilt, (D) rotation.

seen in figure 4.15B. From a side view, a vertical plane through the ASIS would fall behind the pubic symphysis. In dance this is often referred to as a "tucked" position of the pelvis. Notice that when one is describing an anterior or posterior pelvic tilt the reference is to the top of the pelvis. This is important to remember since the bottom of the pelvis will be moving in the opposite direction.

Lateral Pelvic Tilt

A **lateral tilt** is movement of the whole pelvis in the frontal plane about an anteroposterior axis. It involves a side tilt of the top of the pelvis such that one iliac crest and ASIS drops below the opposite iliac crest and ASIS. So, when viewed from the front, the pelvis is not level, and one ASIS is lower than the other as seen in figure 4.15C; and when viewed from behind, one PSIS is lower than the other. Lateral tilts are named in terms of which side of the pelvis is low, so with a right lateral tilt the iliac crest, ASIS, and PSIS are lower on the right side. Lateral tilt, or pelvic obliquity, is commonly seen in dancers who have one leg shorter than the other or in dancers who have certain types of scoliosis.

Pelvic Rotation

Pelvic rotation is movement of the whole pelvis in the transverse plane about a vertical axis. It involves a rotation of the pelvis such that one ASIS is anterior or posterior to the other ASIS. When viewed from the front or side, one ASIS is in front of the other as seen in figure 4.15D. Pelvic rotation is commonly observed in dancers who have scoliosis that involves rotation in the lumbar region. The rotation is named in terms of the direction toward which the front of the pelvis turns. So, if the left ASIS is behind the right ASIS, this means that the front of the pelvis is rotating to the left, and this is termed left pelvic rotation.

Angle of Femoral Inclination

The **angle of femoral inclination** is an angle formed between the neck of the femur and the shaft of the femur when viewed from the front, as seen in figure 4.16B. It occurs close to, but not strictly in, the frontal plane, since the greater trochanter lies somewhat posterior to the head of the femur. In the newborn this angle is about 150°; it decreases to approximately

TESTS AND MEASUREMENTS 4.1

Pelvic Alignment: Anterior Pelvic Tilt, Posterior Pelvic Tilt, and Neutral

Use figure 4.15 for reference and the procedure described next to learn to identify an anterior pelvic tilt, posterior pelvic tilt, and a neutral pelvis.

1. Stand in parallel first position with your side to a mirror, and place your right index finger on your right ASIS and your left index finger on your left ASIS.

   a. Tilt the top of the pelvis forward to create an anterior pelvic tilt, and note in the mirror that the ASIS are in front of the pubic symphysis.

   b. Tilt the top of the pelvis backward to create a posterior pelvic tilt, and note in the mirror that the ASIS are behind the pubic symphysis.

   c. Tilt the top of the pelvis in the necessary direction to create a neutral pelvis by lining up the ASIS directly above the pubic symphysis, in the same vertical plane.

2. Stand in a parallel first position, and note the alignment of your pelvis. Make any necessary corrections to effect a neutral pelvic alignment.

3. Perform a demi-plié and relevé in parallel and turned-out first positions. Note the alignment of your pelvis throughout the movement and make any necessary adjustments to maintain neutral pelvic alignment. Are there any differences in your pelvic alignment between standing, demi-plié, and relevé in parallel or turned-out positions?

4. Repeat steps 2 and 3 with a partner and, if necessary, help each other to make the necessary adjustments to maintain a neutral pelvic alignment.

5. Now, note if asymmetries exist in relative positioning of your ASIS in the transverse and frontal planes. Place your fingertips on each ASIS, and look at the pelvis from the front. With neutral alignment, the ASIS should be in the same transverse plane; that is, they should appear at the same level or height versus have one lower than the other. They should also be in the same frontal plane versus have one rotated in front of the other.

125° to 130° in the adult and further decreases to about 120° in old age (Levangie and Norkin, 2001; Mercier, 1995). The angle of inclination has an important influence on the mobility and stability of the femur, as well as knee and lower leg alignment. Normally, this inclination helps angle the femur inward so that the center of the knee joint is close to being vertically aligned with the head of the femur and center of motion of the hip joint.

Coxa Vara

When the angle of inclination is abnormally decreased, the condition is called **coxa vara** (*coxa,* hip + L. *varus,* bent inward) as seen in figure 4.16A. This condition decreases the load on the femoral head but increases the load on the neck and increases the risk of fracture of the neck of the femur (Hamill and Knutzen, 1995). Regarding mobility, a decreased angle can decrease the range of hip abduction

but increase the effectiveness of the hip abductors (greater lever arm). Regarding lower leg alignment, with a decreased angle of inclination there is a tendency for the shaft of the femur to slope more inward than normal and to produce a knock-kneed alignment termed **genu valgum** (see chapter 5), in which the knees are medial to the feet during standing in anatomical position.

Coxa Valga

When the angle of inclination is abnormally increased, the condition is called **coxa valga** (*coxa,* hip + L. *valga,* turned outward) as seen in figure 4.16C. This condition increases the load on the femoral head but decreases the load on the neck of the femur. Regarding mobility, an increased angle can increase the range available in hip abduction but reduce the effectiveness of the hip abductors (decreased lever arm). Regarding lower leg alignment,

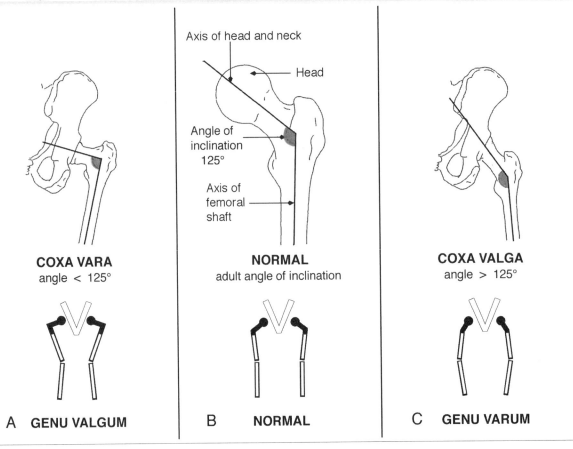

COXA VARA
angle < 125°

NORMAL
adult angle of inclination

COXA VALGA
angle > 125°

A   **GENU VALGUM**

B   **NORMAL**

C   **GENU VARUM**

FIGURE 4.16   Angle of femoral inclination (top row: left hip, anterior view). (A) Coxa vara, (B) normal, (C) coxa valga.

with an increased angle of inclination there is a tendency for the shaft of the femur to run more vertical or even slightly outward and to produce a bow-legged alignment termed **genu varum** (see chapter 5), in which the knees are placed lateral to the feet during standing in anatomical position.

Angle of Femoral Torsion

The **angle of femoral torsion** is the angle of the head and neck of the femur relative to the shaft of the femur and the femoral condyles when viewed from above as seen in figure 4.17. Due to this angle, when one is standing erect with the knees facing directly forward, the center of the head of the femur is not located in the same frontal plane as the tip of the greater trochanter, but rather slightly anterior to the trochanter. In other words, if you place your fingertips on your greater trochanter, the neck of the femur will be angling slightly forward, placing the center of the head of the femur slightly in front of the trochanter. This angle is marked in the newborn, averaging about 35° to 40°, but it decreases with age to an average of approximately 8° to 15° (Bauman, Singson, and Hamilton, 1994; Rasch, 1989). This angle can influence the extent of turnout allowed at the hip and so is important for the dancer to understand.

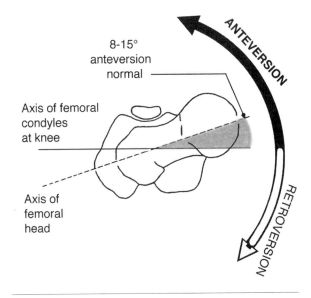

FIGURE 4.17   Angle of femoral torsion (left hip, superior view).

Femoral Anteversion

An abnormal increase in the angle of femoral torsion is termed **femoral anteversion** (turning forward). Excessive femoral anteversion results in greater internal rotation of the femur, which can be responsible for in-toeing, or the tendency to have the toes face inward, as seen in figure 4.18B. When femoral anteversion is excessive, more of the anterior head of the femur becomes uncovered, and internal rotation of the femur is required to better position the head of the femur in the acetabulum (Hamill and Knutzen, 1995). Increased femoral anteversion is also associated with decreased external rotation, probably due to earlier contact between the neck of the femur and the lateral edge of the acetabulum. Due to the restricted external rotation and the tendency for in-toeing, excessive femoral anteversion is considered undesirable for the dancer in professional training, particularly in classical ballet. Femoral anteversion can also negatively impact alignment above and below the hip and is commonly associated with lumbar lordosis, an increased Q angle, and patellar problems (discussed in chapter 5), as well as excessive pronation of the foot (discussed in chapter 6).

Femoral Retroversion

A decrease in the angle of femoral torsion, versus an increase, is termed **femoral retroversion** (turning backward). Femoral retroversion results in greater hip external rotation, which can lead to out-toeing, or the tendency for the feet to face markedly outward as seen in figure 4.18C. Due to the associated increased hip external rotation or turnout, femoral retroversion is considered desirable for dancers in dance forms emphasizing turnout.

Pelvic and Hip Mechanics

Due to the very limited motion allowed at the pubic symphysis and sacroiliac joints, the pelvic girdle primarily acts as a unit, with movement of the pelvis tending to produce movement in the lumbar spine and at both hip joints. In some conditions, linked movements of the pelvis, lumbar spine, and hip joints are encouraged, while in other cases there is an attempt to limit the associated movements in favor of stabilization of one of the segments.

Linked Movements of the Pelvis, Femur, and Lumbar Spine

Movement of the pelvis occurs relative to the spine, primarily at the lumbosacral joint, and relative to the femur at the hip joint. Movements can be initiated from the spine, pelvis, or femur and will tend to produce predictable secondary movements in the other two segments as well. The linked movements that tend to occur will be influenced by whether both ends of the chain are closed, the head is free to move, or the leg/foot is free to move.

Closed-Chain Pelvic Movements

While the terms closed and open kinematic chain are more commonly used for limbs, the concept can also be applied to the pelvis. During erect standing the distal part of the chain becomes fixed (foot). While not structurally fixed, the proximal end of

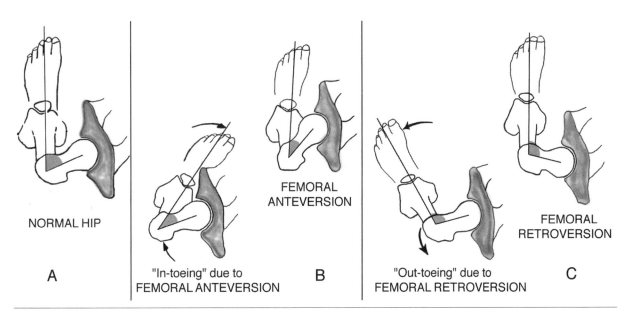

FIGURE 4.18   Angle of femoral torsion and potential influence on lower leg alignment (left hip, superior view). (A) Normal, (B) femoral anteversion and associated in-toeing, (C) femoral retroversion and associated out-toeing.

the chain (head) can become functionally fixed in many movements by the need to keep the head upright and over the base of support (Levangie and Norkin, 2001). When these two conditions exist, movements of the pelvis can be termed **closed-chain pelvic movements,** and they produce predictable movements at the hip joint and lumbar spine. For example, when one is standing erect, if the pelvis tilts anteriorly from its neutral position (figure 4.19A) as seen in figure 4.19B it will produce hip flexion and a compensatory increase in the arch of the lumbar curve (lumbar hyperextension) in order to bring the torso and head back over the pelvis. In contrast, when the pelvis tilts posteriorly as seen in figure 4.19C, it will tend to create hip hyperextension (unless the knees are simultaneously bent) and compensatory decrease in the lumbar curve (lumbar flexion) in order to bring the upper torso and head back over the pelvis. Note that during anterior and posterior pelvic tilts, the movements of the pelvis actually involve "opposite movements" at the lumbosacral and hip joints due to their opposite facings. When the pelvis laterally tilts to the right (with the right side lower than the left), the tilt is accompanied by

slight abduction of the right hip, slight adduction of the left hip, and compensatory left lateral flexion of the lumbosacral joint, resulting in a curve convex to the right. When the pelvis rotates right (with the front of the pelvis rotating to the right without the feet or head moving), this is accompanied by slight external rotation of the left hip, slight internal rotation of the right hip, and compensatory spinal rotation to the left. Left lateral tilt and left rotation of the pelvis are associated with opposite movements to those described for the right.

These linked movements are summarized in table 4.2, and it is important to note that the same linkings tend to occur if the movement is initiated from the spine. For example, arching the low back as in jazz or African dance (lumbar hyperextension) produces an automatic anterior tilt of the pelvis and hip flexion, while flattening the low back (flexion, or decreased lumbar lordosis) as with a contraction is linked to a posterior tilt of the pelvis and extension of the hip. However, in dance, cueing from the pelvis can often produce the desired motion with less stress for the low back. For example, using the cue to reach the bottom of the pelvis down toward the floor and back

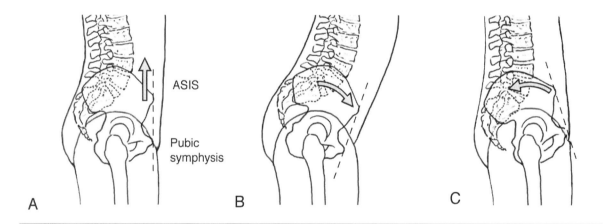

FIGURE 4.19   Closed-chain pelvic movements. (A) Neutral, (B) anterior pelvic tilt, (C) posterior pelvic tilt.

TABLE 4.2   Primary Movements of the Pelvis When Standing With Secondary Movements of the Spine and Hip

Movement of the pelvic girdle	Associated movement of the spine	Associated movement of the hip
Anterior pelvic tilt	Lumbar hyperextension	Hip flexion
Posterior pelvic tilt	Lumbar flexion	Hip extension
Right lateral tilt (right side lower)	Left lateral spinal flexion	Right hip abduction Left hip adduction
Right rotation (front of pelvis rotating right)	Left spinal rotation	Right hip internal rotation Left hip external rotation

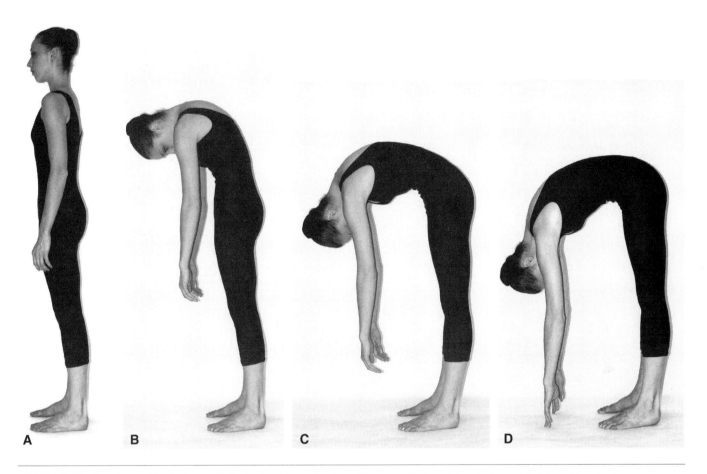

FIGURE 4.20   Lumbar-pelvic rhythm. (A) Neutral pelvis and spine, (B) spinal flexion, (C) anterior pelvic tilt and hip flexion, (D) forward hang.

can produce the desired arch in the low back from the anterior tilt produced by greater contraction of the hip flexors versus contraction of the spinal extensors located in the lumbar region.

Lumbar-Pelvic Rhythm

In contrast to the condition just described, when the distal end of the chain is fixed (feet) by standing but the proximal end of the chain (head) is free to move, linking between the spine, pelvis, and hip is termed the **lumbar-pelvic rhythm.** One important example of the lumbar-pelvic rhythm occurs during bending forward from a standing position and then returning to an upright position (Caillet, 1996). Only about 50° to 70° of spinal flexion (Soderberg, 1986) is possible in most individuals (figure 4.20B), and then additional movement is due to anterior tilting of the pelvis and flexion at the hip joint (figure 4.20, C and D). When this flexion is complete, support of the body weight relies on passive support (flexion relaxation phenomenon). Return from this fully flexed position should reverse

this process used with forward flexion, beginning with extension of the hip joint and posterior tilting of the pelvis, followed by extension of the spine. This return from forward flexion should be a well-coordinated movement; and disruption of this lumbar-pelvic rhythm, such as extending the back too soon or returning in an asymmetrical manner, can increase risk for low back injury.

This movement is commonly used in modern and jazz classes ("roll-downs"); and cues frequently used by teachers to bend the knees slightly and bring the pelvis under, before stacking the spine on the pelvis, can be helpful for encouraging this desired lumbar-pelvic rhythm and reducing low back stress. With forward flexion from a standing position, the ischial tuberosities move backward relative to the hip axis as seen in figure 4.20, A-D; so the hamstrings can pull the ischial tuberosities downward and forward, while the gluteus maximus draws the pelvis back to help return the pelvis to a vertical/neutral position. Starting this return motion with the pelvis delays extension of the spine until the trunk is closer, such that the moment

CONCEPT DEMONSTRATION 4.1

Hip Extensor Function in Posture

The hip extensors can also be palpated in their postural role. Placing one hand below the ischial tuberosity and gluteus maximus and the other hand on one of the buttocks, incline the trunk forward about 45°, and feel the hamstrings and gluteus maximus contract. Then slowly bring the torso to vertical, lean slightly back, and feel the hamstrings and gluteus maximus relax as the center of mass of the torso falls behind the common hip axis.

arm of the resistance (weight of the torso) is less and the stress on the lumbar spine is markedly reduced.

Pelvic-Femoral Rhythm

When extreme ranges of motion are required at the hip joint, movements of the pelvic girdle occur in a different direction and for a different reason, that is, to place the acetabulum in a favorable position to enhance the range through which the leg and foot can be moved. This text will use the term **pelvic-femoral rhythm** to refer to the characteristic linking of these movements of the pelvis to the fundamental movements of the femur at the hip joint as shown in table 4.3. This term was selected to reflect its parallelism to the predictable linking of movements of the scapula with fundamental movements of the humerus at the shoulder joint termed the scapulohumeral rhythm. However, an important difference between these linkings in the upper and lower extremity is that because the pelvis is directly attached to the spine, movements of the pelvis will necessitate movement in the lumbar spine as previously described and listed in table 4.2. In contrast, movements of the scapulae can occur without producing a change in position of the spine.

An example of the pelvic-femoral rhythm entailing linking of a posterior pelvic tilt with hip flexion occurs when one performs a high battement to the front. When the constraints of hamstring flexibility are met, further movement of the leg upward will create a posterior tilt of the pelvis and a decrease in the lordosis (or even flexion) of the lumbar spine. This additional motion of the pelvis and spine will change the facing of the acetabulum more upward, which in turn will allow the leg to go markedly higher relative to the ground. Often, extreme use of this linked motion is not desirable in dance as it will distort desired body alignment, but the specific vocabulary and dance form will dictate the amount of pelvic motion permitted. For example, an extreme posterior pelvic tilt causes flexion of the support knee and spine, distorting the classical desired illusion of a "lifted" and vertically aligned body. However, in jazz or contemporary choreography, a high kick to the front is sometimes purposely performed on élevé with a bent support leg as shown in figure 4.21. This bent knee positioning will allow a marked posterior pelvic tilt so that a much greater height can be achieved with the gesture leg, while extension of the upper spine can be used to limit "dropping back and down" of the torso to within acceptable limits of the choreographer.

While end ranges of hip flexion tend to be linked with a posterior tilt of the pelvis, other movements

TABLE 4.3   Linked Movements of the Pelvis That Accompany Movements of the Femur at the Hip Joint

Movement of the hip joint	Associated movement of the pelvic girdle
Hip flexion	Posterior pelvic tilt
Hip hyperextension	Anterior pelvic tilt
Left hip abduction	Right lateral pelvic tilt (right side lower and left side higher)
Right hip adduction	Right lateral pelvic tilt
Left hip external rotation	Left pelvic rotation
Right hip internal rotation	Left pelvic rotation

of motion in an effort to maximize the height the leg can be lifted. In addition, in strengthening and stretching exercises, there is often an emphasis on limiting initial use of linked pelvic motions so that greater overload can occur to the targeted hip muscle group.

Pelvic Stabilization

While the previous description emphasized the linked movements between the pelvis, spine, and hip joint, there are also many instances in which the emphasis is on keeping the pelvis stationary or on limiting the movements of the pelvis during movements (or certain phases of movements) of either the femur or spine. This process of keeping the pelvis relatively stationary during movement is termed **pelvic stabilization** and can be considered one component of core stabilization. Since the muscles that are used to lift the leg attach onto the pelvis, they will tend to produce movements of the pelvis, lumbar spine, and leg unless the pelvis is stabilized. For example, when the thigh is lifted to the front in an attitude, because the proximal attachments of many of the hip flexors are on the front of the pelvis they will tend to simultaneously create an anterior pelvic tilt and lumbar lordosis, as well as the desired motion of hip flexion. However, other muscles can be used to stabilize the pelvis and prevent these undesired movements of the pelvis and spine so that visible motion is primarily confined to flexion of the thigh at the hip joint.

There are various strategies for achieving the desired stabilization of the pelvis and spine. In the previous chapter, co-activation of the abdominals and back extensors for trunk stabilization was described. Another vital strategy when standing (closed kinematic chain conditions) is co-activation of the abdominals and hamstrings, termed the **abdominal–hamstring force couple.** As seen in figure 4.22, when the limb is fixed such as when standing erect, the proximal attachment of the hamstrings can become the moving end, pulling the ischial tuberosities downward while the lower attachment of the abdominals pulls the pubes upward, both acting to produce a posterior pelvic tilt or prevent an anterior pelvic tilt.

In dance, use of the abdominal–hamstring force couple and other strategies for stabilization of the pelvis are often encouraged when standing on one or both legs so that movement is primarily isolated to the hip joint proper, or at least that movements of the pelvis are limited to an extent allowed by the given dance aesthetic. The refined ability to appropriately time and control movements of the pelvis

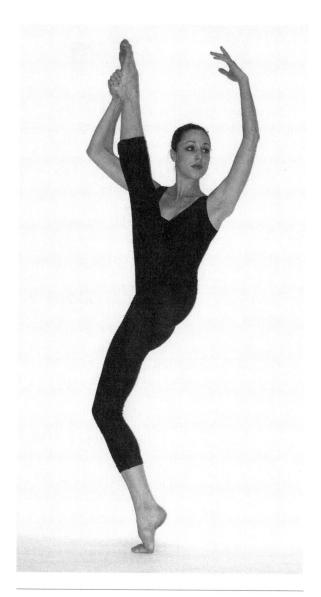

FIGURE 4.21   Performing a front battement with a bent support knee allows for greater use of the pelvic-femoral rhythm to increase leg height.

at the hip joint are linked with pelvic movements as follows. When the thigh is raised backward (hip hyperextension), the pelvis tends to tilt anteriorly; when one thigh is widely abducted or adducted, the pelvis tilts laterally; and when one leg is placed forward and the other backward as in taking a long stride, the pelvis rotates. Associated movements of the lumbar spine can be determined from table 4.2. As previously stated, in dance vocabulary, the timing and extent of these linked movements are often dictated by the aesthetics of the specific school of dance. Frequently, there is an emphasis on minimizing these linked movements in early ranges of motion and reserving their use for the end ranges

DANCE CUES 4.2

"Use the Back of Your Leg"

The instruction to "use more of the back of your leg" is sometimes employed by teachers to encourage greater use of the hamstring muscles when the feet are weight bearing, particularly when the teacher feels that the student is overusing the "front of the legs" (quadriceps femoris). From an anatomical perspective, this directive could be interpreted as encouraging greater use of the abdominal–hamstring force couple. If more stability is established from above, through use of this force couple to help maintain a neutral pelvis and to position the weight of the body appropriately over the support foot/feet (vs. too far back), a dancer could theoretically use less quadriceps contraction to maintain "balance." Another interpretation of this cue relates to emphasizing greater use of the hip extensors versus knee extensors in movements such as pliés, and this emphasis will be discussed in chapter 5.

The problem with this cue is that some dancers do not know how to use "more of the back of the leg"; so substituting more specific cues or performing an exercise to help dancers find these muscles can make the cue more meaningful. For example, thinking of pulling the bottom of the pelvis (ischial tuberosities) down toward the floor until the pelvis is vertically aligned (ASIS and pubic symphysis in same frontal plane) can help some dancers recruit the hamstrings in their force-couple role with the abdominal muscles. Similarly, on the up-phase of the plié, focusing on pressing into the floor with the feet and pulling the sitz bones down and forward to extend the hip joint, before thinking about straightening the knees, can sometimes help dancers feel greater use of the hip extensors. Once a dancer knows how to achieve greater hip extensor activation, the initial cue to use the "back of the leg" or "more hamstrings" can be an effective reminder.

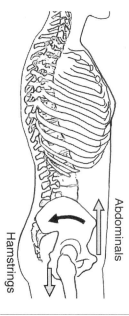

FIGURE 4.22   The abdominal–hamstring force couple. The abdominal muscles pull up on the front of the pelvis while the hamstrings pull down on the back of the pelvis to produce backward rotation of the pelvis (posterior pelvic tilt).

and torso with movements of the limbs is one of the distinguishing factors in dance skill acquisition (Bronner et al., 2000).

Muscular Analysis of Fundamental Hip Movements

As previously described, the hip joint is capable of flexion, extension, abduction, adduction, external rotation, and internal rotation. A summary of the key muscles capable of producing these fundamental movements of the hip can be seen in table 4.4. For purposes of simplicity, initially think of movements in a parallel position. Much of the research related to the actions of muscles has been done with the limbs in parallel (neutral) or almost neutral positions. However, in dance many movements are performed in a turned-out position and so represent combined movements in which the appropriate hip external rotators work with the hip flexors in movements to the front, probably with a combination of hip flexors and hip abductors in movements to the side, and with the hip extensors in movements to the back. Using a turned-out position would likely influence

TABLE 4.4   Fundamental Hip Movements and the Muscles That Can Produce Them

Hip joint movement	Primary muscles	Secondary muscles
Flexion	Iliopsoas Rectus femoris Sartorius	Tensor fasciae latae Adductor longus and brevis (early flexion) Gracilis Pectineus

Extension	Gluteus maximus
	Hamstring muscles:
	    Biceps femoris
	    Semitendinosus
	    Semimembranosus
		Adductor magnus (lower fibers)

Abduction	Gluteus medius Gluteus minimus	Tensor fasciae latae Sartorius Iliopsoas (upper ranges of abduction)
Adduction	Adductor longus Adductor brevis Adductor magnus Gracilis	Pectineus

External rotation	Deep outward rotators:
	    Obturator externus
	    Obturator internus
	    Piriformis
	    Quadratus femoris
	    Gemellus superior
	    Gemellus inferior
	Gluteus maximus
		Sartorius
		Biceps femoris

Internal rotation	Gluteus medius (anterior fibers) Gluteus minimus (anterior fibers)	Tensor fasciae latae Semimembranosus Semitendinosus

the relative activation of the relevant muscle group. For example, performing a turned-out arabesque would theoretically recruit more of the biceps femoris than the medial hamstrings, due to the secondary functions of the medial hamstrings of hip internal rotation. Additional electromyographic (EMG) investigation of basic dance vocabulary in parallel versus turned-out positions would provide valuable insights into relative muscle activation.

Hip Flexion

Hip flexion decreases the angle between the anterior surfaces of the articulating bones. The iliopsoas, rectus femoris, and sartorius are assisted by other hip flexors (table 4.4) to perform their customary action when contracting concentrically against gravity or resistance to lift the femur to the front in knee

to chest, front leg raise, and front développé (table 4.5, A-C, pp. 213-214), or in swinging the leg forward in walking, running, kicking, and many sports. In dance, this type of hip flexion is used whenever the leg is moved to the front such as in a tendu, dégagé, front attitude, front battement, or the front leg of a jump (sissone) as seen in figure 4.23.

The hip flexors are used in their reversal of customary action when they contract concentrically to bring the pelvis or trunk, or both, forward in an anterior pelvic tilt, a sit-up (see figure 2.8 on p. 43), and floor work such as a contraction series in modern or chest lifts in jazz dance. An example of the combined use of movement of the legs and torso is shown in figure 4.24, in which the dancer raises from a flat position on the ground by flexing at the hip and bringing both one thigh and the torso simultaneously together. In contrast to a classic curl-up, the spine is

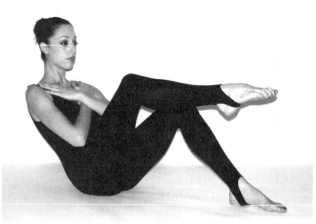

FIGURE 4.24 Hip flexion involving movement of the anterior surface of one femur and the pelvis toward each other.

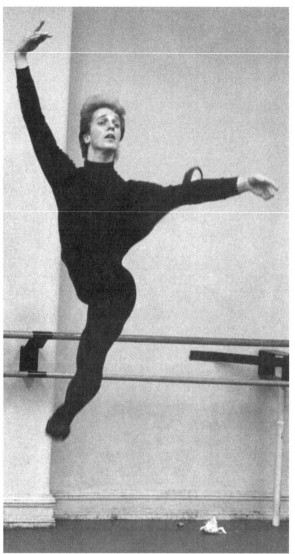

FIGURE 4.23 Sample dance movement showing hip flexion.

Photo courtesy of Myra Armstrong. Dancer: Lorin Johnson with American Ballet Theatre.

kept in a relatively neutral (extended) position, and the trunk moves as a unit about the hip axis versus the sequential flexion of the spine generally used in the curl-up. More dramatic examples of this simultaneous movement of the trunk and thigh occur with "V"-sit or teaser types of movements (previously shown in figure 3.43 on p. 129) in modern, jazz, or Pilates. Such advanced exercises require high strength and skill levels so that abdominal co-contraction can be used to help stabilize the low back and pelvis in order for the hip flexors to bring the thighs and trunk together without undesired and potentially injurious arching of the low back.

However, when hip flexion occurs while the lower limb is weight bearing (closed kinematic chain move-

ments), gravity will tend to create further hip flexion once a small amount of hip flexion is produced. So it is actually the hip extensors that are primarily used eccentrically to control hip flexion and prevent collapse of the body to the ground. Examples of this type of hip flexion occur on the down-phase of a parallel plié, in the landing phase of a parallel jump, or when one brings the trunk forward in a roll-down or to a flat back position.

Hip Extension

Hip extension is a movement in a posterior direction such that the angle between the posterior surfaces of the articulating bones decreases. The hip extensors—the hamstrings and gluteus maximus—perform their customary open kinematic chain action when contracting concentrically against gravity or resistance to move the femur backward in the back leg raise (table 4.5D, p. 214), in the kneeling arabesque (table 4.5E, p. 215), or in running (recovery phase). In dance, one uses this type of hip extension when moving the leg to the back with a leap (back leg), tendu, dégagé, back développé, back attitude, or arabesque penché as seen in figure 4.25.

When the foot remains fixed and in contact with the ground (closed kinematic chain movements), hip extension occurs against gravity when straightening from a flexed position, such as on the up-phase of a squat, plié, or jump or when bringing the trunk back to a vertical position from a flat back position. Concentric hip extension is also used in locomotor movements to bring the weight of the body over the foot, and posturally to create a posterior pelvic tilt, while isometric hip extension is used to maintain

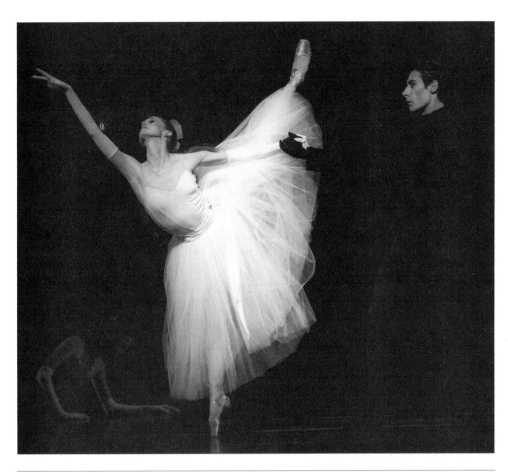

FIGURE 4.25   Sample dance movement showing hip extension.

© Angela Sterling Photography. Pacific Northwest Ballet dancers Louise Nadeau and Christophe Maraval.

cally against gravity or resistance to move the femur sideways in the side leg raise (table 4.5, G and H, pp. 216-217), a side kick in karate, jumping jacks, or side lunges. Examples from dance include parallel movements to the side such as a lateral tilt, extension, tendu, dégagé, or attitude as shown in figure 4.26.

When one foot remains fixed and in contact with the ground (closed kinematic chain movements), concentric hip abduction plays a key role in pulling the side rim of the pelvis closer to the greater trochanter on the weight-bearing side, countering the undesired tendency caused by gravity for the pelvis to drop (laterally tilt) to the opposite side. This function of the hip abductors, called the abductor mechanism (Soderberg, 1986), is important in walking and dancing to allow maintenance of balance and appropriate positioning of the body over the support foot while on one leg. Performing a standing side leg raise (table 4.5H, p. 217) while attempting to maintain a level pelvis with the body weight appropriately positioned over the support foot can be used to develop this important postural function of the hip abductors.

When an individual has dysfunction of the hip abductors, such as gluteus medius weakness, a distinct drop of the pelvis will be seen to the opposite side that the person is unable to correct. This undesired drop of the pelvis is called a positive **Trendelenburg sign.**

an extended hip on the support leg in many dance movements. Bridging (table 4.5F, p. 215) is a conditioning exercise that is aimed at simulating these latter functions of the hip extensors. These closed kinematic chain uses of hip extension are very important in activities of daily living and in dance.

As with other joint movements, when hip extension occurs in the same direction as gravity, the opposite muscle group is generally key in controlling the movement. For example, when the leg is lowered in a controlled manner from being lifted to the front, this type of hip extension involves eccentric contraction of the hip flexors versus the hip extensors.

Hip Abduction

Hip abduction is movement in a sideways direction, such that the angle between the lateral surfaces of the articulating bones decreases. The gluteus medius and minimus are assisted by other hip abductors listed in table 4.4 to perform their customary open kinematic chain action when contracting concentri-

Hip Adduction

Hip adduction is a sideward movement in a medial direction toward the median plane such that the angle between the medial surfaces of the articulating bones decreases. The adductor longus, adductor brevis, adductor magnus, and gracilis are assisted by the pectineus (table 4.4) to perform their customary

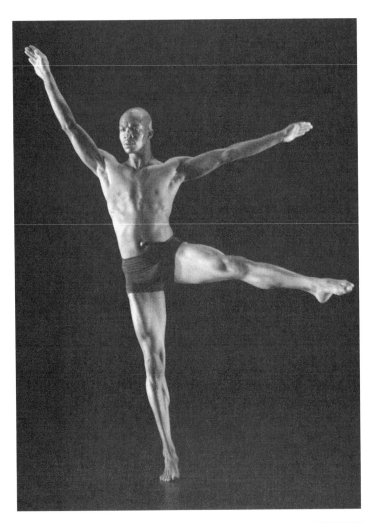

FIGURE 4.26 Sample dance movement showing hip abduction.
Photo courtesy of Patrick Van Osta. CSULB dancer Dwayne Worthington.

legs are brought together from an abducted position, for example on the up-phase of a turned-out plié. Posturally, closed kinematic chain adduction can be used to laterally tilt or side-shift the pelvis relative to the support leg, which is an important mechanism used in locomotion and dance for assisting balance, increasing economy of gait, and helping stabilize the pelvis. This is one of the mechanisms involved in meeting the directive used in dance of "being over your leg."

During upright standing, adduction of the gesture leg will be in the same direction as gravity and so will generally involve use of the antagonist muscles. For example, when the leg is lowered in a controlled manner from being lifted high to the side, eccentric contraction of the hip abductors is used to control the lowering of the leg, at least in the beginning of the lowering.

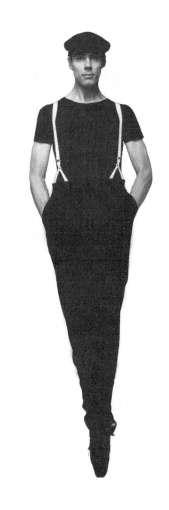

FIGURE 4.27 Sample dance movement showing hip adduction.
Photo: Roy Blakey. Dancer: Douglas Nielsen in "Spirit of Gravity."

open kinematic chain action when contracting concentrically against gravity or resistance to move the femur toward the midline in exercises such as the single leg pull and side leg pull (table 4.5, J and K, p. 218), the frog kick in swimming, and keeping the swinging limb closer to the midline in walking. In functional movement, hip adduction is often combined with slight hip flexion or hip extension to allow the limb to cross the midline without hitting the other limb. Examples of this use of the hip adductors from dance include grapevine-type steps, the final phase of a dégagé when the leg closes into fifth with an "in" emphasis, and the motion of pulling the inner thighs "together and up" at the top of a jump (with or without beats) as shown in figure 4.27.

When the foot remains fixed and in contact with the ground (closed kinematic chain movements), customary hip adduction occurs against gravity as the

The Trendelenburg Test

Use the Trendelenburg test to evaluate the hip abductor mechanism on (1) another dancer and (2) yourself as explained next.

1. Evaluation of another dancer. Have your partner stand on the left leg, with the right hip and knee slightly flexed so that the right foot clears the floor. Kneel behind the dancer, and place your right thumb on the right PSIS and the remaining fingers of the right hand along the right lateral crest of the ilium. Place your left thumb on the left PSIS and the remaining fingers on the left lateral portion of the crest of the ilium. If these matched landmarks appear at the same height, that is, in the same transverse plane, this is a negative Trendelenburg sign (A); if the PSIS or crest of the ilium is markedly lower on the unsupported side, this indicates a positive Trendelenburg sign (B).

2. Self-evaluation. Stand on one leg (with the opposite hip and knee slightly flexed so that the foot is off the ground) in front of a mirror. Place your right index finger on your right ASIS and your left index finger on your left ASIS. If these landmarks appear at the same height, this is a negative Trendelenburg sign, while if the ASIS is markedly lower on the unsupported side, this indicates a positive Trendelenburg sign and suggests that hip abductor weakness is present.

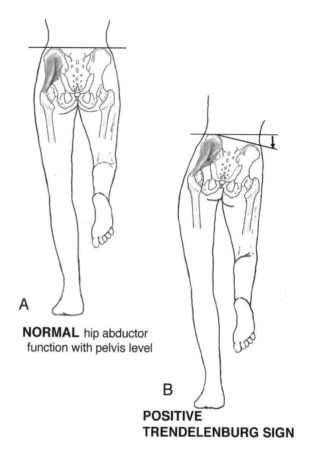

NORMAL hip abductor function with pelvis level

POSITIVE TRENDELENBURG SIGN

Hip External Rotation

Hip external rotation involves lateral rotation of the anterior thigh relative to the pelvis about the mechanical axis of the femur in a transverse plane. Because of the angulation of the neck of the femur, the long axis of rotation is not in the shaft of the femur, but rather medial to it—a line extending between the centers of the hip and knee joints.

The deep outward rotators and gluteus maximus are potentially assisted by other hip external rotators (listed in table 4.4) when contracting concentrically to rotate the legs outward from a parallel first to a turned-out first position or in the prone passé

or prone frog (table 4.5, M and N, pp. 219-220). However, more commonly hip external rotation is combined with other movements of the hip rather than being used in isolation, such as during the swing phase of walking, the frog kick in swimming, or the side leg raise and side leg pull (table 4.5, G [p. 216] and K [p. 218]) variations performed in an externally rotated position. Examples of movements from dance that combine hip extension and external rotation include the back leg of a grand jeté, an arabesque, or a back attitude as shown in figure 4.28. Hip external rotation would also be used in any dance movements performed in a turned-out versus parallel position, and the direction of the

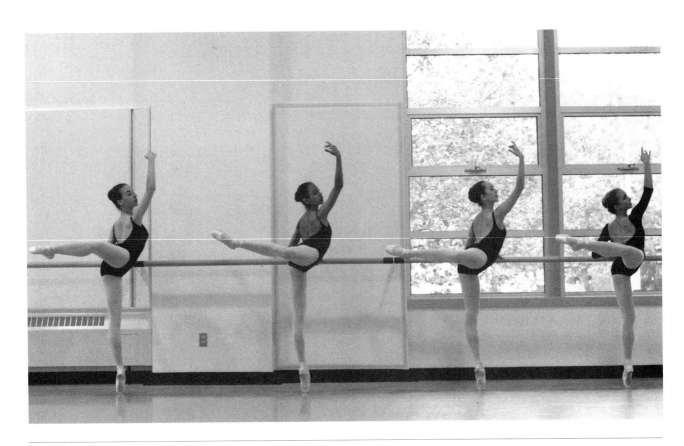

FIGURE 4.28   Sample dance movement showing hip external rotation combined with hip extension.
Photograph by David Cooper. Pacific Northwest Ballet School students.

accompanying movement (e.g., front, side, back) would influence the muscles recruited to produce the desired hip external rotation.

A reversal of the customary action of the hip external rotators can also be used to rotate the pelvis away from a stationary femur. For example, during standing with both legs fixed, rotation of the pelvis to the right will result in internal rotation of the right hip joint and external rotation of the left. This closed kinematic chain rotation is commonly used in throwing, in swinging a baseball bat or tennis racket, and in a golf swing. The mechanism is commonly used in dance for turning, dodging, or change-of-direction movements in which the thrust of the pushing leg turns the pelvis in the desired direction.

Hip Internal Rotation

Hip internal rotation involves medial rotation of the anterior thigh relative to the pelvis about the mechanical axis of the femur in a transverse plane. The anterior fibers of the gluteus medius and gluteus minimus are potentially assisted by other hip internal rotators (listed in table 4.4) when contracting concentrically to rotate the legs inward in the prone

hip internal rotation (table 4.5P, p. 220). However, as with hip external rotation, hip internal rotation is more commonly combined with other hip movements such as on the support leg during the swing phase of walking or in a side kick in karate. Examples of movements from dance include the use of an internally rotated position with side lunges or other stylized movements in jazz or contemporary dance (figure 4.29). Additionally, a quick internal rotation of the thigh (with the knee bent) immediately preceding hip external rotation in a turned-out side développé is sometimes used as a teaching tool for helping students to learn to isolate rotation of the femur in the hip joint without undesired rotation of the pelvis.

A reversal of the customary action of the hip internal rotators can be used to rotate the pelvis toward a stationary femur. This closed kinematic chain internal rotation is used in walking and running, in which the pelvis rotates toward the support leg as the other leg swings forward, functioning to increase stride length. In throwing, striking, and some dance movements, the initial plant of the forward foot places the forward thigh in lateral rotation. However, as the athlete comes forward over the foot,

Key Considerations for the Hip in Whole Body Movement

Many forms of dance utilize movements that demand very large range of motion of the hip. Comprehension of principles relating to multijoint muscles is important for understanding what limits such movements and what conditioning exercises could be used to enhance performance of such dance movements. Furthermore, when weight bearing, the hip must withstand very large loads, making this joint vulnerable to degenerative changes.

Actions of Multijoint Muscles

Many of the muscles of the hip are multijoint muscles, including the psoas major, rectus femoris, gracilis, sartorius, tensor fasciae latae, biceps femoris, semitendinosus, and semimembranosus. To understand the resultant action that occurs when multijoint muscles contract, it is helpful to keep the following concepts in mind that were previously discussed in chapter 2.

First, remember that a multijoint muscle has the tendency to cause movement at all of the joints it crosses, unless a joint is stabilized by other muscles or outside forces. Since these muscles of the hip are attached to the pelvis, contraction will result in accompanying pelvic motions unless the pelvis is purposely stabilized.

Second, remember that motion at one joint alters muscle length, which in turn affects the muscle's ability to produce force or to be stretched across the other joint(s) it crosses. For example, the rectus femoris is more effective as a hip flexor if the knee is bent versus straight, because having it stretched across the knee allows the muscle to work at a favorable length to avoid active insufficiency. In regard to range of motion, greater hip flexion is also allowed if the knee is flexed versus straight, as knee flexion slackens the hamstring muscle across the knee joint, allowing more range in flexion to occur at the hip joint before passive insufficiency occurs.

Third, a multijoint muscle usually does not exert equal effect at all of its joints, but rather has better leverage at one joint than the other(s) and so has its primary action at that joint. For example, the rectus femoris is more efficient as a knee extensor than as a hip flexor, and the sartorius is more effective as a hip flexor than as a knee flexor. This difference in effectiveness is important for achieving the desired movement outcome when many muscles simultaneously contract.

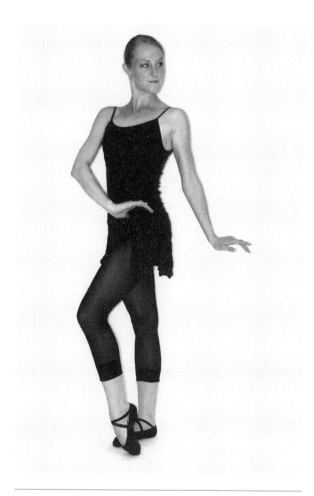

FIGURE 4.29 Sample dance movement showing hip internal rotation.
Sacramento Ballet dancer Merett Miller.

the pelvis is rotated toward the support leg, resulting in hip internal rotation on the front leg.

Hip Horizontal Abduction and Adduction

In dance, some movements such as rond de jambe en l'air occur with the hip flexed to 90°. As discussed in chapter 1, such movements are termed horizontal abduction and adduction. When these movements are performed, the hip flexors, hip abductors, or hip extensors are used to maintain the height of the femur (depending on whether the leg is front, side, or back), while various muscles located medially and anteriorly (adductor longus, adductor brevis, adductor magnus, and pectineus) act to pull the leg toward the midline for horizontal adduction, and various muscles located posteriorly and laterally (gluteus medius, gluteus minimus, gluteus maximus, and DOR) act to pull the leg away from the midline for horizontal abduction (Hall, 1999; Kreighbaum and Barthels, 1996).

Compressive Loads on the Hip Joint

The hip joint is required to bear body weight during upright standing and the support phases of movements such as walking and running. During standing with the weight evenly distributed between the two feet, each hip joint must support one-half of the weight of the body segments above the hip, or about one-third of total body weight (Hall, 1999). However, during standing on one leg, that hip must now support the total weight of the head, arms, and trunk, as well as the weight of the opposite leg, or about 85% of total body weight (Smith, Weiss, and Lehmkuhl, 1996). In addition, the load actually borne by each hip is significantly greater than just body weight during movement due to the additional compression produced by contraction of the strong muscles of the hip and impact forces translated upward from the foot. So, during walking and jogging, compressive loads on the hip can range from three to five and a half times body weight (Hall, 1999) and with activities such as stair climbing may reach seven times body weight (Levangie and Norkin, 2001). Hip loading can also be markedly increased by the wearing of hard-soled shoes, hard heel strikes during locomotion, and carrying a load (as in partnering). The high loads borne by the hip make it vulnerable to degenerative changes that can lead to having total hip replacements in dancers at younger ages than one would expect or hope.

Special Considerations for the Hip in Dance

Varied movements, often encompassing a large range of motion at the hip joint, requiring complex coordination between movements of the pelvis and femur, and utilizing multiple planes, are essential for meeting the aesthetics of dance. Examples of such movements include the roll-down, flat back positions, and many movements employing turnout such as extensions and the arabesque.

Roll-Down

When first learning a roll-down, some dancers make the error of emphasizing flexion of the hip too early, before adequate flexion of the spine has occurred. This increases the torque from the weight of the torso and often is accompanied by shifting the pelvis back in an attempt to counterbalance this torque and prevent the dancer from falling forward (figure 4.30A). However, to achieve the desired dance aesthetic and lessen low back and knee stress, the dancer should apply the lumbar-pelvic rhythm, first utilizing the abdominal–hamstring force couple to maintain a neutral pelvis while motion is isolated to spinal flexion. During this motion the dancer should focus on sequentially flexing the spine from the top down and keeping the head as close to the torso and pelvis as possible. When spinal flexion is complete, focusing on rotating the pelvis about the femur, with the head of the femur staying in place as much as possible and the ischial tuberosities rapidly going up toward the ceiling, will help achieve the aesthetic and desired positioning of the pelvis closer to being over the ankle joint (figure 4.30B).

Flat Back Positions

Jazz and some modern classes also frequently use flat back positions (figure 4.31A). In contrast to roll-downs, these positions actually primarily involve hip flexion (not spinal flexion) while contraction of the spinal extensors is used to prevent undesired flexion of the spine. Strong contraction of the hamstring muscles is required (eccentrically) to control the flexion of the hip, and when muscles are not adequately warmed or when forceful bouncing is added to these positions, hamstring strains can occur. Furthermore, in this flat back position, the moment arm is very large for the spine, and so large forces are imposed on the spine. To reduce injury risk, it is recommended that when these positions are used, the hamstrings and spinal extensors be first adequately warmed up, the use of large bounces and momentum be avoided, and students be cued to use firm abdominal co-contraction to help reduce spinal stress and avoid lumbar hyperextension. For dancers having difficulty effectively activating this latter abdominal co-contraction, it may be helpful to practice from a kneeling position with the chest supported on a ball (to reduce the moment of the resistance). First, carefully allow the abdominals to relax and the low back to arch (figure 4.31B). Then contract the abdominals to achieve the desired flat back position (figure 4.31C). As skill develops, this position can then be tried standing without the ball, requiring well-coordinated co-contraction of the abdominals, back extensors, and hip extensors. If needed, the fingertips can be placed on a wall or barre to reduce the resistance from the weight of the torso.

Some dance sequences combine flat back positions with roll-downs. These combinations can be helpful for developing spinal articulation; coordinated movements between the spine, pelvis, and

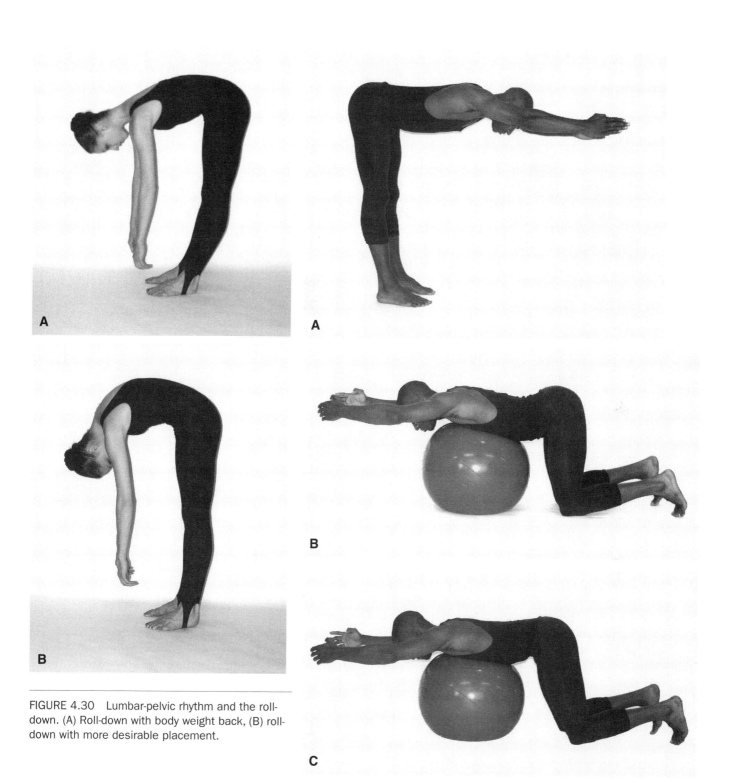

FIGURE 4.30 Lumbar-pelvic rhythm and the roll-down. (A) Roll-down with body weight back, (B) roll-down with more desirable placement.

FIGURE 4.31 Flat back position. (A) Standing with co-contraction of abdominals and back extensors, (B) kneeling with inadequate abdominal contraction, (C) kneeling with adequate abdominal contraction.

femur; and the awareness of neutral, flexed, and hyperextended positions of the spine. However, the principles previously discussed should be applied to enhance technique and reduce spinal stress.

Turnout

The use of external rotation of the hip is an important element of classical ballet and many other dance forms, and many dancers are concerned about how much turnout their bodies possess. The extent of hip external rotation, or turnout, possible for a dancer is primarily determined by bony, ligamental, and muscular factors. Bony factors include the depth and shape of the hip socket (acetabulum). A more shallow acetabulum that faces more laterally is generally considered to favor external rotation, while a deeper socket that faces more anteriorly can lessen the extent of external rotation permitted. The angle of the shaft of the femur relative to the neck of the femur also affects the extent of turnout possible. As described earlier in this chapter, individuals with less anteversion or more retroversion tend to have greater external rotation. Curvature and length of the femoral neck may also affect mobility. A neck that is more concave and longer will tend to facilitate abduction and lateral rotation, while a shorter, less concave neck will lessen the potential end ranges of these motions, due to contact with the edge of the acetabulum.

The joint capsule and its associated ligaments can also affect potential hip external rotation. The capsule and certain ligaments, particularly the ilio-femoral ligament, become taut with hip external rotation. Hence, if they are more extensible they will allow greater turnout. Similarly, adequate extensibility of key muscles, including the hip internal rotators and adductors, will allow the range permitted by the bony and ligamental constraints to be realized. The relative contribution of, and the magnitude of change possible in, each of these constraints is an area of controversy. It has been theorized that early training may be able to actually affect bony constraints, allowing for a molding of femoral torsion up to about age 11 or 12 (Brown and Micheli, 1998; Sammarco, 1983), but that after this age, improvements in passive turnout would be due to stretching of soft tissue constraints (capsule, ligaments, and muscles). Although an earlier study suggested changes in femoral torsion in favor of retroversion with elite ballet dancers who began training prior to 10 years of age (Miller et al., 1975), the failure in a recent study to find greater retroversion in elite ballet dancers (Bauman, Singson, and Hamilton, 1994)

and the observation that measurement of passive hip external rotation appeared to increase markedly following participation in class (Garrick and Requa, 1994) suggest that the greater external hip rotation seen in the average dancer may be due more to soft tissue constraints than bony changes.

Various screening tests can be utilized to estimate the passive hip external rotation present in a dancer, and the results will vary markedly in accordance with the measurement techniques used. However, studies agree that ballet dancers exhibit significantly greater passive and active hip external rotation than non-dancers; and some studies also showed lower levels of hip internal rotation, with even lower levels of internal rotation in male versus female ballet dancers (DiTullio et al., 1989; Garrick and Requa, 1994; Hamilton et al., 1992; Khan et al., 1997).

Some orthopedic surgeons hold that a minimum of 60° of hip external rotation should be present by 15 years of age in a dancer who wishes to pursue a career in classical ballet (Brown and Micheli, 1998; Thomasen, 1982). Measurements performed by the author showed the average hip external rotation of elite advanced/professional ballet dancers to be 59.9°. The technique for measurement, used on dancers who had just warmed up, involved a prone position with moderate force applied while an assistant stabilized the hip such that the endpoint was reached at which any additional rotation was of the pelvis and not the femur. Use of protocols with less manual assistance, or with the knees touching (hip adduction) versus hip-width apart (neutral), would reveal lower values. Another study of elite professional ballet dancers showed average hip external rotation of 52° for both men and women (Hamilton et al., 1992).

While using an exact measure as a screening factor is probably unwise due to diverse results, the complex relationship between passive and active use of turnout, and the controversy regarding the extent to which turnout can change with training, the concept is still germane that a ballet dancer with very limited hip external rotation will likely have difficulty achieving the required aesthetic without undue stress and injury (Garrick and Requa, 1994; Hamilton et al., 1992) and will be more prone to dropout from professional training (Hamilton et al., 1997). In many other dance forms including modern, jazz, and tap, the aesthetic does not dictate as extreme a lateral facing of the feet, and there is likely more tolerance for lower values of hip external rotation. One study showed that when asked to adopt a comfortable turned-out first position, modern dancers' mean position was 29° less turned out than the mean for ballet dancers (Trepman et al., 1994).

Screening Test for Hip Turnout

A test is shown for measuring passive hip external rotation. While the dancer is in a prone position with one knee in 90° flexion, the examiner places one hand on the lower leg of the bent knee and externally rotates the hip while the pelvis remains in a neutral position with both ASIS in contact with the table as seen in the picture. For a more accurate measurement, care must be taken to emphasize movement from the hip and avoid motion at the knee or pelvis. For example, allowing the pelvis to anteriorly tilt will slacken the hip joint capsule and iliofemoral ligament and give a falsely high measure of external rotation. Using an assistant to prevent one side of the pelvis from lifting (pelvic rotation) and to prevent an anterior pelvic tilt is helpful.

The axis of the goniometer is placed over the patellar tendon, the stationary arm vertical and the movable arm along the middle of the lower leg. A reading of 0° refers to the position in which the lower leg and foot are facing straight up toward the ceiling, 45° to the position in which the lower leg is halfway toward the table; 90° would be the theoretical position if the knee faced directly to the side with the lower leg lying flat on the table. If a goniometer is not available, one can estimate the range by visually dividing the 0°-to-90° arc in half, then further dividing each half in thirds, and approximating the degrees of motion.

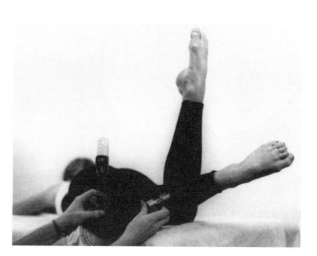

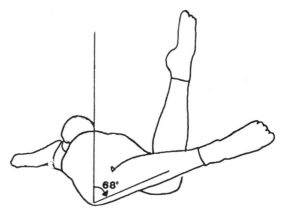

In addition to the results of these passive hip external rotation tests being useful for comparison with dance norms, they can also be helpful for better understanding a given dancer's potential turnout. For example, in some cases the test will confirm a dancer's or teacher's impression that turnout is relatively low, while in other cases results suggest that there is potential turnout that is not being fully realized in the technique class. This latter discrepancy is seen because in actual movement, in contrast to passive measurement of hip rotation, adequate strength and appropriate activation patterns in key muscles including the DOR are also important to allow utilization of the dancer's potential turnout.

In the author's experience, few dancers use their full potential hip external rotation; and specific flexibility exercises, strength exercises, and focus on technique can allow most dancers to markedly increase their use of turnout. A sample stretch is shown in figure 4.32A. This modified prone frog stretch allows the pelvis to remain neutral while the dancer focuses on externally rotating the legs at the hip and reaching the knees to the side. The abdominals should be firmly contracted to maintain a neutral pelvis, and the dancer should focus on pressing the bottom of the pelvis (ischium) slightly down and forward to achieve the desired stretch and avoid undesired anterior tilting of the pelvis. When performing the

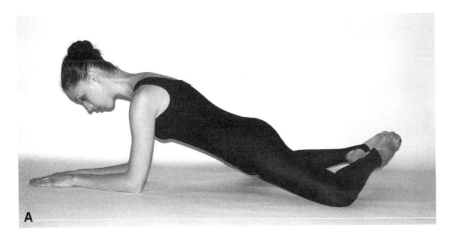

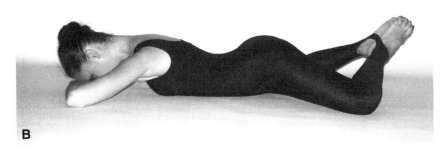

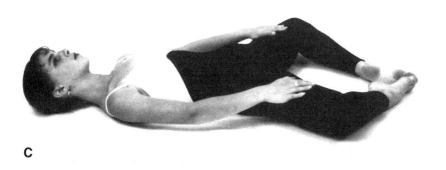

FIGURE 4.32   Sample stretches for improving turnout. (A) Modified prone frog stretch, (B) classic prone frog stretch with incorrect body positioning, (C) supine frog stretch.

hands on the thighs can be used to carefully apply a stretch.

A sample strength exercise for improving turnout is shown in figure 4.33A and later described in table 4.5M (prone passé, variation 1, p. 219). However, as with stretches, specific exercise technique is essential. Here, it is necessary to focus on using and strengthening the lower DOR rather than the gluteus maximus. Due to the ability of the DOR to produce hip external rotation in such a variety of positions and with limited other joint actions, these muscles are essential for effecting turnout in dance movement. In essence, they are able to produce turnout while leaving the dancer free to move in whatever direction is dictated by the choreo-graphy. Focusing on rotating (1) "lower," at the bottom of the buttocks, (2) deeper below the gluteus maximus, and (3) more specifically but less forcibly can often help activate the DOR more than the gluteus maximus. In addition, thinking of bringing the greater trochanter back toward the ischium, and palpating with the fingers to be sure that the quadratus femoris is contracting in this area, can help achieve the desired specific muscle activation. If the dancer has difficulty adequately activating the DOR or experiences knee discomfort, hip external rotation can also be performed side-lying with the band just above the knee (figure 4.33B) or prone on a ball (figure 4.33C, described in table 4.5N on p. 220).

classic prone frog stretch (figure 4.32B), many dancers make the error of anteriorly tilting the pelvis, which slackens the structures that are the target of the stretch and can put undesired stress on the low back and knees. The other common error of trying to force the feet down to the floor in this position can also place potentially injurious stress on the knees and is counter to the goal of enhancing external rotation at the hip versus the knee. For dancers who are tighter and who experience knee or hip discomfort even when performing the modified prone frog stretch, the supine frog stretch (figure 4.32C) provides a gentler alternative where gravity and gentle application of the

This use and maintenance of turnout is important not only for meeting the aesthetics of classical ballet and various other dance forms but also for injury prevention. Failure to maintain turnout at the hip and excessive twisting from the knee down are believed to be a contributing factor to many injuries of the knee, shin, ankle, and foot.

Influence of Turnout on Muscle Activation

When dancers work in a position of marked hip external rotation, the line of pull of many of the muscles of the hip is dramatically changed. How

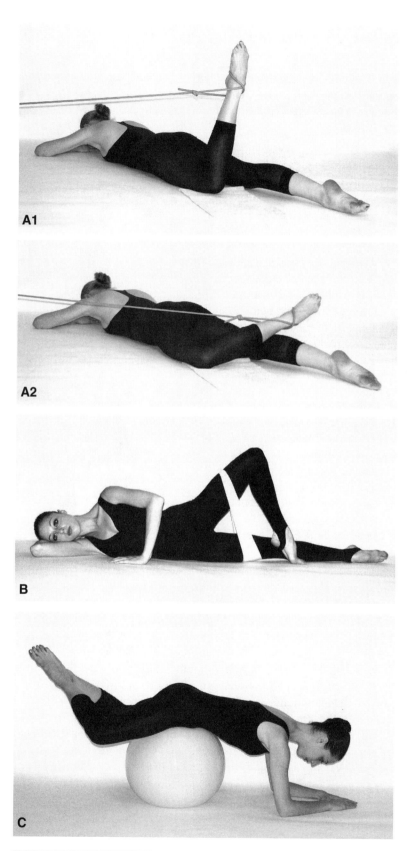

A1

A2

B

C

FIGURE 4.33   Strength exercises for the turnout muscles. (A) Prone passé with tubing, (B) side-lying passé with band, (C) prone frog on ball.

much and in what manner this influences muscle use is an area that needs further investigation. For example, looking at the line of pull on skeletal models, one would theorize that this position of external rotation would place the hip adductors in a more key role in movement execution during standing (closed kinematic chain movements). In a second-position grand plié, for instance, the motion occurs closer to a frontal plane rather than in a sagittal plane. This would place the hip adductors in a position to work concentrically on the rise to help bring the legs back together (hip adduction) and eccentrically on the lowering phase to control the separation of the legs. The knee extensors (quadriceps femoris) would still be required to produce knee extension on the up-phase and to control knee flexion on the down-phase of the plié, but their use could be de-emphasized if greater focus was placed on the motion at the hip. This concept that using turned-out positions enhances recruitment of the hip adductor muscles was given preliminary support by findings that highly skilled ballet and modern dancers without patellofemoral pain showed recruitment of the hip adductors when performing second-position grand pliés. Furthermore, standing in first position showed sustained hip adductor activity in some dancers, and use of images to enhance hip external rotation was accompanied by increased hip adductor activation in some dancers (Clippinger-Robertson, 1984).

However, the variability of use of adductors seen between dancers suggests that use of the hip adductors is likely a learned activation achieved by some dancers in line with the cues and aesthetics of some schools of dance. This conjecture is also given support by another study that found only 58% of the dancers studied utilized the hip adductors in the rising phase of the demi-plié (Trepman et al., 1994). Furthermore, in the author's experience, when using exercises like the wall plié to help dancers direct their knees more

Selective Muscle Focus in the Wall Plié

Stand in second position turned out with the upper back (at the level of the shoulder blades) and posterior side of the sacrum against the wall, while the heels are a few inches away from the wall in line with the greater trochanter.

· **Emphasizing use of the DOR muscles.** Place the fingertips deep, just lateral to the ischial tuberosities at the sides of the base of the buttocks. Perform a demi-plié, and at the bottom of the plié purposely let the knees drop inside the feet (A). Then, while maintaining the same depth of plié, use the low DOR muscles located under your fingertips to externally rotate the femur at the hip joint and pull the knees back over the feet (B). Repeat this motion of letting the knees fall in and pulling them back out several times until easy conscious control of the DOR is established. Next, perform a second-position grand plié slowly, focusing on using the DOR to maintain hip external rotation and guide the knees as directly side as possible on both the down- and up-phase of the plié. Study of an anatomical model of the 22 hip muscles showed a 1.5-centimeter or more decrease in length of the estimated line of pull in the gluteus maximus, hamstrings, and all 6 deep outward rotators when replicating this second-position plié performed correctly with the "knees side" versus "dropped forward" (Clippinger-Robertson, 1984). However, when normalizing this change in the axial line of pull of these muscles relative to their "length" when standing in second position, a 54% change was seen in the quadratus femoris, 52% in the gemellus inferior, and 46% in the gemellus superior compared to much smaller percentage changes in other muscles, such as 12% for the gluteus maximus and 5% for the hamstrings. This dramatic percentage change in length in these rotator muscles provides indirect evidence for their vital role in establishing and maintaining appropriate positioning of the greater trochanter for optimal turnout.

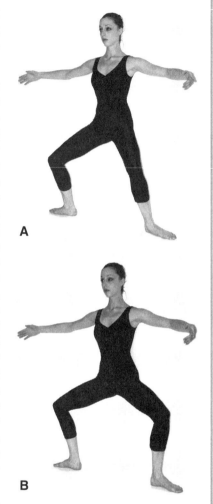

A

B

· **Emphasizing use of the inner thigh muscles.** Place the hands on the insides of the thighs. On the up-phase of the plié, focus on rotating the thighs at the hip joint, emphasizing the DOR and at the same time pulling the "inner thighs together and up" (concentric contraction of the hip adductors). Gently squeeze your "inner thighs" together and against your hands to feel the hip adductors contracting under your fingers, and try to gain better control of activation of these muscles. On the down-phase of the plié, focus on externally rotating the thighs at the hip joint and then "reaching the knees as far to the side as possible" with the pelvis going straight down toward the floor (eccentric contraction of the hip adductors).

· **Influencing muscle use by forward trunk inclination.** Lean the trunk forward by flexing at the hip, and notice any change in the muscles being used. Some dancers feel greater use of the quadriceps in this position and have difficulty utilizing the hip adductors. Maintaining a vertical (neutral) position of the pelvis can be helpful for utilizing the DOR and hip adductors, at least when one is first learning to emphasize activation of these muscles.

· **Applying this muscle focus to class.** Step a few inches away from the wall, and repeat the plié, trying to maintain a vertical pelvis, use of the lower DOR, and use of the hip adductors. To transfer a new muscle activation emphasis to class, it is often helpful to key in to a kinesthetic sensation or develop an image that will allow for quick access. For example, if a dancer tends to lean the torso forward at the base of the plié and excessively use the quadriceps, it may be helpful to think of sliding down the wall as the knees reach to the side. In contrast, if a dancer tends to lose rotation on the up-phase of the plié, focusing on the back of the leg "wrapping to the inside and lifting up" as the knees straighten may be helpful.

to the side, dancers will often describe a very intense sensation related to the use of the hip adductors and make a comment that now they understand what their teachers wanted when cueing them to use more of their "inner thighs." Additional research using EMG is needed to clarify the specific use of muscles desired to achieve the aesthetic and biomechanical goals of specific dance forms and schools. However, care must be taken to not consider "average values" obtained from dancers necessarily "optimal."

Extensions to the Front

Many dancers seek to improve the height they can lift their leg to the front in movements like extensions. This presents a challenge because many of the muscles that effectively contribute to hip flexion in lower ranges (e.g., adductor longus, adductor brevis, upper fibers of adductor magnus, and gracilis) are no longer able to aid with flexion past 50° to 70°, and other muscles such as the rectus femoris lose their

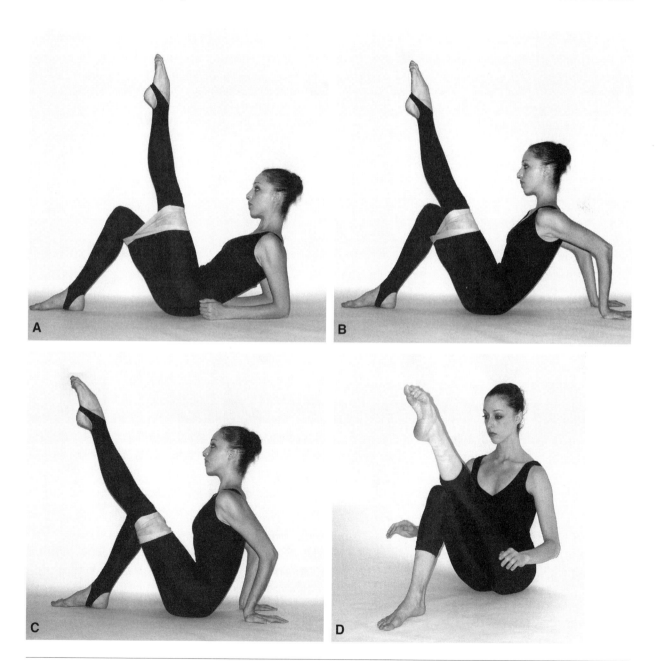

FIGURE 4.34 Sample strength exercise for improving front développés and extensions. (A) Front développé on elbows, (B) front développé with hands back, (C) front développé with hands back and torso more vertical, (D) front développé with torso vertical against a wall and no hand support.

ability to produce force due to active insufficiency. However, the iliopsoas can still produce effective force in this range, but many dancers appear to not have adequate strength or sufficient ability to activate this muscle and mistakenly believe that they cannot achieve high extensions. But regular performance of strengthening exercises with an emphasis on learning to better activate the iliopsoas and a focus on overloading the muscles in a high range of hip flexion can markedly improve the height of front extensions.

A sample strength exercise is provided in figure 4.34 and described in table 4.5C (variation 1, p. 214). The front développé performed on the elbows (figure 4.34A) is often the easiest position from which to work on greater recruitment of the iliopsoas. However, as improvements are made in strength and activation, moving the torso to a more vertical position (figure 4.34, B and C) and eventually performing it with the torso vertical, the back against the wall with limited lumbar flexion, and no hands for support (figure 4.34D) will provide greater challenge to the hip flexors and better replicate the demands of dance.

Additionally, progressing to performing développés and extensions in a standing position will better replicate functional demands and enhance transfer to the technique class. Additional leg height can be developed when standing by applying the principle that greater force can be generated by a muscle with an eccentric, then isometric, then concentric contraction (chapter 2). Practically, this means that the leg can be maintained at or lowered from a greater height than the height to which the leg can be lifted with a concentric contraction. An example of an exercise applying this principle involves raising the leg to the front as high as possible with the knee straight (concentric contraction), using the hand to raise the leg about 10° to 20° higher (figure 4.35A), and then slowly letting go with the hands and holding the position for

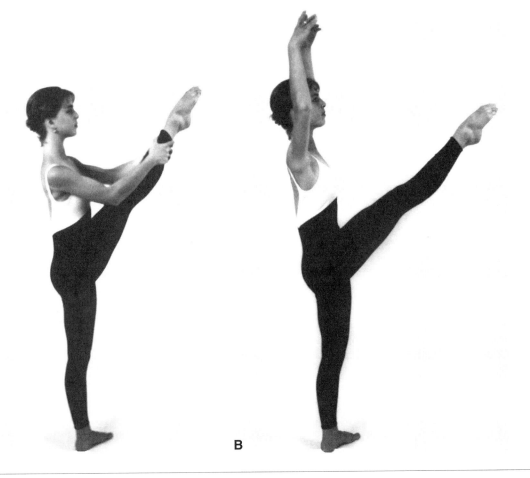

A   B

FIGURE 4.35   Functional exercise for improving front extensions. (A) Using the hands to raise the leg slightly higher than can be achieved with a concentric contraction, and (B) slowly lowering the leg to the height that can be achieved with a concentric contraction.

Iliopsoas Emphasis in the Front Développé

Perform the following exercises to try to develop a better awareness of and ability to activate the iliopsoas. After performing the exercise on one side, repeat the same sequence with the other leg. When good iliopsoas control has been achieved, greater strength benefits can be obtained by adding resistance from a band (figure 4.34 and table 4.5A, p. 213), ankle cuff (table 4.5B, p. 213), or springs (table 4.5C, p. 214).

· **Emphasizing use of the iliopsoas with the knee bent.** Sitting on the floor with the right leg crossed over the left and the torso rounded forward, press the fingertips of the right hand in about 1 inch (2.5 centimeters) medial to the ASIS, and feel the iliopsoas contracting under the abdominal wall as the right knee is lifted toward the chest. Repeat this motion of lifting and lowering the knee until more awareness of the iliopsoas is established. Next, try to consciously contract the iliopsoas isometrically and then concentrically to lift the leg.

· **Emphasizing use of the iliopsoas with a développé.** Return to the starting position, and after the right knee has been lifted, extend the knee slowly without letting the knee drop down; then bring the leg to the front, and lift it higher three times with the knee straight; finally return to the starting position. Use of the rectus femoris can be decreased by using a position in which the knee is bent, but the challenge is to continue contracting the iliopsoas to keep the thigh close to the chest (e.g., maintain the same angle of hip flexion) as the quadriceps femoris is used to straighten the knee. This is an important skill to learn because the rectus femoris is already shortened across the hip and will reach a position of active insufficiency as it is also shortened across the knee, tending to make the leg drop in height unless adequate contraction of the iliopsoas is used to maintain hip flexion. Initially using a slightly tucked position (increasing the mechanical advantage of the iliopsoas), palpating the iliopsoas, and using this feedback to make sure that it is continuing to work as the knee straightens, as well as concentrating on continuing to bring the thigh slightly closer to the chest as the knee extends, can help with the desired iliopsoas focus.

· **Emphasizing use of the iliopsoas with the knee straight.** Sitting with one leg to the front, raise the leg, keeping the knee straight. First perform this movement with an emphasis on the quadriceps femoris by firmly "pulling the kneecap up toward the hip" and thinking of lifting the leg from the knee. Then, when you reach a height where you feel discomfort and cannot raise the leg higher, think of reaching the leg out, slightly tuck the pelvis, and focus on lifting the leg with the iliopsoas. Optimally, greater height of the leg with less sense of effort will be achieved.

· **Applying this muscle focus to class.** Some dancers can key in to the sensation of the iliopsoas contracting and easily use that for feedback to transfer iliopsoas emphasis to other movements in class. However, other dancers have little sensation associated with the iliopsoas, but rather just feel that it is easier to lift the leg and that there is less sensation of discomfort in the rectus femoris and other hip flexors. Images such as (1) folding the thigh into the chest before extending the knee in développé or (2) lifting the thigh with a string, pulling from just below the crease in the front of the thigh to the front of the lower spine, can sometimes be helpful.

4 counts (isometric contraction) or taking 4 counts to slowly lower the leg about 10° to 20° (eccentric contraction; figure 4.35B) to the level that can be achieved concentrically. A variation on this approach is to raise the leg to the front as high as possible with the knee straight (concentric contraction), bend the knee to decrease the moment of the resistance, raise the leg about 10° to 20° higher, slowly extend the knee

as straight as possible without dropping the height of the knee or creating a sense of excessive muscle strain at the hip (table 4.5B, p. 213), and hold this position for 4 counts (isometric contraction) or take 4 counts to slowly lower the leg (eccentric contraction).

In addition to hip flexor strength and iliopsoas activation, the height to which the leg can be lifted can be influenced by hamstring flexibility. When the knee is straight, the hamstrings are stretched across the back of both the hip and knee, and hip flexion can proceed passively only as far as extensibility of the hamstrings will allow. A screening test can be utilized to evaluate hamstring flexibility (Tests and Measurements 4.4). If hamstring flexibility is low, emphasis should be placed on stretching the hamstrings (table 4.7, C and D, p. 225) as well as strengthening the hip flexors. If hamstring flexibility is high, this suggests that the limiting factor is more hip flexor strength and perhaps more specific activation of the iliopsoas.

When lifting the leg to the front in a turned-out versus parallel position, another consideration comes into play. Many dancers have difficulty maintaining external rotation as leg height is increased. This is logical for two reasons. First, the DOR become less effective in their ability to produce external rotation, and the upper DOR (the piriformis) may actually switch its function to become an internal rotator in high ranges of hip flexion (Smith, Weiss, and Lehmkuhl, 1996). Second, the anterior fibers of the gluteus medius, gluteus minimus, and tensor fasciae latae increase their leverage for hip internal rotation as the hip is flexed. So, while when the hip is in extension the maximum torque for internal and external rotation is about equal in the general population, when the hip is flexed the maximum torque generated by the hip internal rotators is increased about three times. To counter this problem, it is important that dancers develop greater strength in the hip external rotators and specifically in the lower DOR that are still in a position to produce hip external rotation. Focusing on bringing the greater trochanter "down and under" can often help achieve the desired activation of the quadratus femoris.

Extensions to the Side

Extensions to the side are one of the measures of skill used for selection of dancers in the professional ballet arena (figure 4.36), and many dancers strive to increase their height. The use of turnout in this position produces a unique situation in which the anterior surface of the thigh is moving in a frontal versus sagittal plane, a hybrid between hip flexion and hip abduction. Although research will be necessary for better understanding of the interplay of muscles in this action, EMG studies and study of the line of pull of the muscle suggest that the iliopsoas as well as the hip abductors are key in higher ranges of hip abduction. As hip abduction progresses, the distal iliopsoas slides over to the lateral side of the center of rotation of the hip joint and is thus positioned to be capable of producing hip abduction.

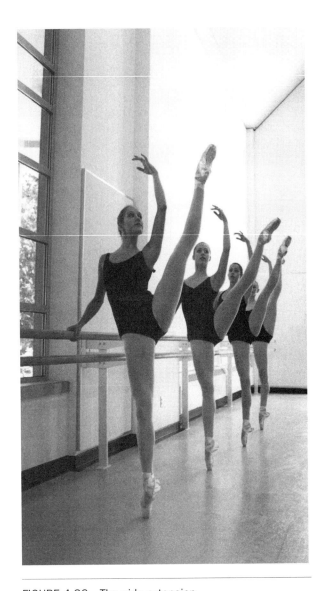

FIGURE 4.36   The side extension.
Photograph by Rex Tranter. Pacific Northwest Ballet School students.

Hence, strengthening the hip flexors and developing greater activation of the iliopsoas as just described with extensions to the front can improve movements such as extensions to the side.

In addition, proper mechanics play a fundamental role in optimizing leg height. When the thigh is kept parallel or in medial rotation, range of motion is limited to about 45° abduction in general populations, probably due to impingement of the greater trochanter on the superior rim of the acetabulum and nearby ilium. However, if the leg is externally rotated such that the greater trochanter rotates inferiorly, it will no longer impinge, and the range of hip abduction is tremendously increased. So, greater external rotation will allow a greater range of hip abduction to be achieved (Kushner et al., 1990), and use of this

TESTS AND MEASUREMENTS 4.4

Screening Test for Hamstring Flexibility

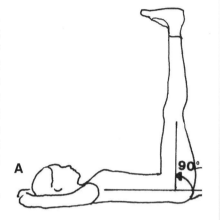

A test is shown for measuring passive flexibility of the hamstrings. While the dancer is in a supine position, one leg is gently brought toward the chest with the knee straight (hip flexion) by the examiner as the other leg remains straight down (B). For a more precise test for hamstring length, the pelvis is maintained in a neutral position while the leg is raised to a point of slight resistance but no pain; for a more functional test of hip flexion, slight posterior tilting of the pelvis is allowed only to the point where the back of the lower leg still maintains contact with the table. This latter approach allows the pelvic-femoral rhythm normally associated with marked hip flexion, such as used in front développés or grand battements in dance class.

The axis of the goniometer is placed on the greater trochanter, the stationary arm horizontally along the side of the trunk and the movable arm along the outer thigh. A reading of 0° refers to the position when the leg is lying flat on the table, 90° when the leg is going straight up toward the ceiling (A), and greater than 90° when the leg comes closer to the chest as shown in B. While 90° is considered normal range in general populations, the average value for functional hip flexion for elite advanced/professional female ballet dancers was shown to be 150° (Clippinger-Robertson, 1991). If a goniometer is not available, one can estimate the range by visually dividing the upper arc in thirds (A) and approximating the degrees of motion.

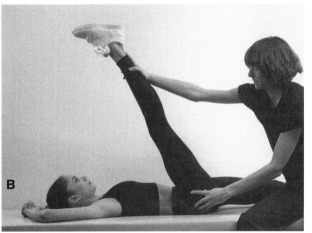

external rotation can also allow the leg to be placed farther to the side and the hips to be more level as seen in figure 4.37B. Many schools of dance allow the normally linked lateral tilt of the pelvis to occur in the later stages of the movement to achieve greater height of the leg as shown in figure 4.36, while other schools limit the amount of lateral pelvic tilt.

Whatever the aesthetic of the end position, the initial stages of the movement should focus on keeping the hips more level rather than excessively laterally tilting the pelvis, as seen in figure 4.37A, and maximally rotating and "dropping" the greater trochanter so that optimal range and placement of the gesture leg can be achieved as seen in figure 4.37, B and C. So, adequate strength and activation of specific external rotator muscles as well as the iliopsoas are important for achieving the desired height and aesthetics in side extensions. The side leg raise with

an ankle weight (figure 4.38A and table 4.5G, p. 216) or band (figure 4.38B and table 4.5G, variation 2, p. 216) are exercises designed to help the dancer focus on the technique of fully rotating the femur as the leg is being lifted. As described with extensions to the front, as strength and desired activation patterns improve, progression of strength exercises to include a more vertical position of the torso, and eventually standing, will help with transfer of desired improvements in leg height and technique to class. When progressing from side-lying (with an ankle weight) to a sitting or standing position, lifting the leg above 90° is now opposed (due to the differing relationship to gravity) versus assisted by gravity, and most dancers will not have the strength to raise the leg close to the height achieved side-lying. Initially, using the hand to help find the desired drop of the greater trochanter and maintain the desired height of the

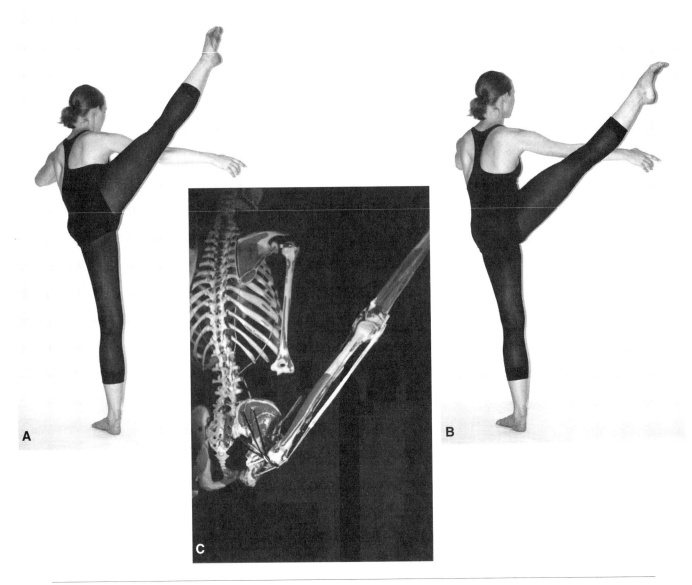

FIGURE 4.37   Side développé. (A) With hip excessively lifted, (B) more desired hip placement with trochanter close to sitz bones on dancer and (C) on skeleton.

thigh as the knee is extended (figure 4.38C) can be useful. To help build necessary strength to eventually be able to achieve this height without use of the hand, similar procedures to those described for standing front développés can be used. For example, the hand can be used to help lift the leg with the knee bent as shown in figure 4.38C, and then the hand is slowly released as the position is maintained for 4 counts. As strength improves, this exercise can be progressed to extending the knee after the hand is released. The focus should be on using the DOR to maintain the turnout at the hip and the iliopsoas to maintain the height of the knee, and only extending the knee as far as possible without letting the knee drop in height

or without undue sense of muscle strain at the hip. Rotator disks can also be added to focus on use of the DOR to maintain turnout on the support leg while developing height of the gesture leg.

In addition to the specific desired active contraction of prime movers, passive constraints offered by antagonist muscles also influence how high the leg can be brought to the side. Because the stretch across the hip is not as direct for the hamstrings when the leg is to the side versus front, the hamstrings will generally not limit range as soon but still are critical in determining how high the leg can be raised. The hip adductors also are critical in determining how far to the side and high the leg can be brought. So, if adequate range is

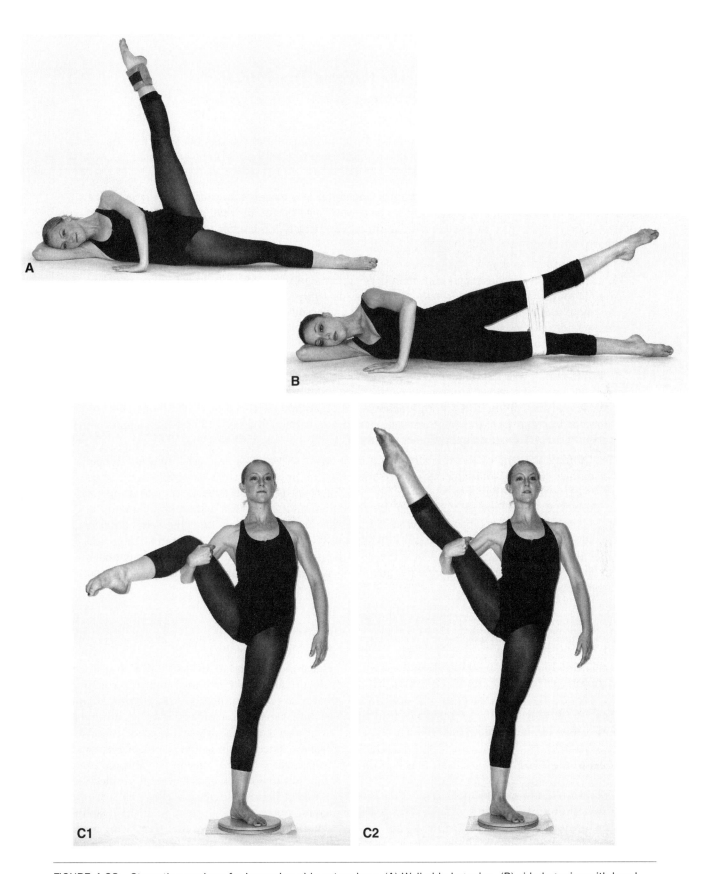

FIGURE 4.38   Strength exercises for improving side extensions. (A) Wall side leg raise, (B) side leg raise with band, (C) standing side développé assisted by the arm.

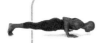

Dropping the Greater Trochanter Toward the Sitz Bones in the Side Développé

Perform the following exercises on both sides to try to develop a better awareness of the desired movement of the greater trochanter that can markedly increase the height of the gesture leg, as well as to help bring the leg more to the side.

· **Observing the excursion of the greater trochanter in a passé.** With your partner lying on the left side with the top leg in a parallel passé, place your fingertips on the right greater trochanter and right ischial tuberosity (sitz bones), and note the movement of the greater trochanter as the leg is brought into a turned-out passé (retiré).

· **Increasing the drop of the greater trochanter.** When performing this turned-out passé, many dancers primarily use horizontal abduction to bring the leg to the side and do not utilize sufficient external rotation of the femur. To help your partner find this rotation, support the weight of the leg and rotate the thigh internally and externally, emphasizing the external rotation and the drop of the greater trochanter toward the ischial tuberosity. Remember that rotation occurs about the mechanical axis of the femur, and so the knee should just pivot in place as the thigh rotates. With this addition of rotation, the greater trochanter should come down much closer to the ischial tuberosity (figure 4.37C) than with pure horizontal abduction. After your partner has experienced the desired position passively, he or she should try to produce the same drop of the trochanter by actively contracting the lower muscles of the DOR. Dance teachers sometimes aptly describe this important distinction of rotation by instructing students to imagine turning a door knob (rotation of the femur) versus just opening the door (horizontal abduction of the thigh).

· **Utilizing the drop of the trochanter in a développé.** As the knee is raised from retiré, help your partner externally rotate the femur further so that the trochanter stays dropped and the knee goes slightly backward (as if to bring it behind the shoulder) before the knee extends to complete the développé. Then, have your partner lift the hip (laterally tilt the pelvis) and internally rotate the leg, and note how the leg drops and comes forward. Now, have your partner bring the pelvis down to almost a neutral position, externally rotate the femur, and with one hand on your partner's hip and the other hand just below their knee, help them rotate further by bringing the greater trochanter back and down; note that this movement of the greater trochanter allows greater elevation of the leg and a more open second position.

not present, stretching the hip adductors and hamstrings as shown in table 4.7, C-F (pp. 225-226) can also improve leg height and lessen the effort required to lift the leg by decreasing the internal resistance from the opposing muscles that must be overcome.

Extensions to the Back

Proper execution of movements to the back such as an extension, attitude, or arabesque is also key for progression in technical level in various forms of dance, and it offers a complex kinesiological challenge. The amount of movement possible at the hip in a backward direction is much more limited than to the front or side. In the average individual, hip hyper-

extension is limited to 10° to 15° due to constraints from the anterior ligaments, joint capsule, and in some cases the hip flexors. Although elite dancers may have two or three times this range, bringing the gesture leg to a position where it is horizontal to the ground will necessitate an anterior tilt of the pelvis and compensatory hyperextension of the spine to bring the upper torso back to the vertical position. Many schools of dance also allow some pelvic rotation to increase leg height, with rotation of the torso in the opposite direction to keep the torso facing forward. However, the extent and timing of these movements of the pelvis and spine have important implications for achieving the desired aesthetic and for the stresses borne by the lumbar spine (see figure 4.39).

DANCE CUES 4.3

"Lift From Under the Leg"

For performance of extensions or grand battements to the side, teachers sometimes cue students to "lift from under the leg" or "use the hamstrings to lift the leg, not the quads." This cue is not consistent with current anatomical knowledge, and substituting an alternative cue is recommended. The action of the hamstrings is hip extension, not hip flexion, and so they would pull the leg down, not lift it up, in battements. However, the underlying aim of this cue, to achieve greater height of the leg with less "effort," particularly with less contraction of the quadriceps, can be addressed anatomically from several perspectives. First, the reference to the sensation of the hamstrings working may relate to its potential action at the knee versus the hip. When the knee hyperextends, the line of pull of the hamstrings now crosses anterior to the axis of the knee joint, and so the hamstrings can produce further hyperextension or be used to maintain hyperextension of the knee rather than the normal action of knee flexion. So, some dancers with hyperextended knees may use the distal attachment of the hamstrings to maintain the knee in hyperextension in a battement. Theoretically, this could allow less use of the quadriceps femoris to maintain a straight (actually hyperextended) position of the knee. However, these actions would be relative to the knee joint, and the hip flexors would still be necessary to lift the thigh.

A second interpretation of the intent of this cue relates to feeling the greater trochanter dropping "back and under" just prior to emphasizing the use of the iliopsoas to lift the leg to the side. This function can be thought of as parallel to the SIT (subscapularis, infraspinatus, teres minor) force couple acting on the shoulder that will be discussed in chapter 7. When the hip is in an extended position, because of its attachments, contraction of the gluteus medius will tend to pull the greater trochanter upward (large stabilizing component as discussed in chapter 2). However, some of the inferior muscles of the hip deep outward rotators are in a position to act to counter this upward pull and facilitate the desired rotary motion of the shaft of the femur in abduction and prevent bony impingement of the greater trochanter, allowing the leg to be lifted much higher. So, alternative cues aimed at achieving the desired drop of the greater trochanter or "wrapping the side of the thigh under" just prior to the lift of the leg would better represent the desired mechanics.

To optimize height of the leg with less stress to the lumbar spine, the following considerations can be helpful. (1) Maximize external rotation of the femur with the lower DOR muscles rather than rotate the pelvis ("open the hip") during the first part of the movement. (2) Think of "reaching the leg out," stretching across the front of the hip and utilizing the full possible range of hip hyperextension, rather than immediately anteriorly tilting the pelvis as the leg lifts. (3) Focus on "lifting the leg from the knee" to encourage more use of the hamstrings to try to increase hip extension range and the height of the leg. (4) When full range of hip hyperextension is reached and the pelvis must tilt anteriorly, "pull the lower abdominal area up and in" and "lift the upper back" to lessen the shear stress in the lower lumbar area and better distribute the necessary hyperextension throughout more of the spine as described in chapter 3. (5) Delay the pelvic rotation, and limit the extent in accordance with the aesthetic of the school of dance so that the

contribution of hip external rotation and hip hyperextension can be emphasized, with less low lumbar spinal hyperextension and pelvic rotation required to achieve a horizontal leg height.

In addition to focusing on technique, strengthening the hip extensors and back extensors can enhance leg height in movements of the leg to the back. Since it is the hip extensors that lift the leg, strengthening the hip extensors in a range similar to the range of these motions and with an emphasis on using the hamstrings should be a focus. However, as the leg is lifted, the pelvis and torso will rotate forward unless the back extensors are used to bring the torso back up toward an upright position. Hence, strengthening the back extensors is also key. Sample strength exercises for improving the arabesque are provided in figure 4.40. The kneeling arabesque with a band (shown in figure 4.40A and described in table 4.5E, variation 1, p. 215) provides an effective exercise to focus on developing strength and awareness of using the hamstrings while

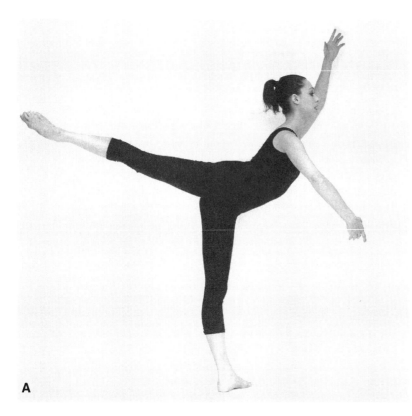

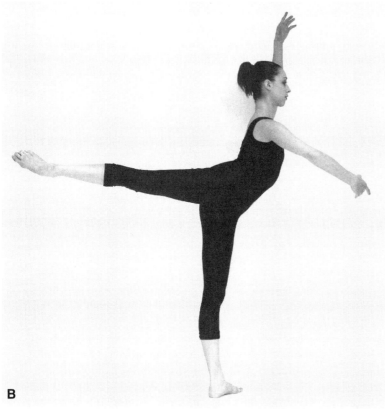

FIGURE 4.39   The arabesque with (A) excessive pelvis rotation and inadequate abdominal co-contraction and (B) more desired hip hyperextension and coordinated use of the abdominal muscles and back extensors.

keeping the pelvis stable. The back leg raise on the ball (figure 4.40B and table 4.5D, variation 2, p. 214) allows the dancer to work on lifting the leg higher while coordinating the associated slight anterior pelvic tilt and lumbar hyperextension. Tactile feedback from the ball can help the dancer focus on keeping both ASIS in contact with the ball initially while emphasizing use of the hamstring to maximize hip hyperextension. After full hip hyperextension is achieved, feedback from the ball can help the dancer focus on co-contracting the abdominals and back extensors as the pelvis slightly anteriorly tilts and the ASIS on the side of the gesture leg raises off the ball slightly to facilitate pelvic rotation and greater height of the gesture leg. The standing back leg raise (figure 4.40C and table 4.5D, progression 2, p. 214) represents a more functional exercise designed to transfer gains to dance performance. Similar procedures to those described for standing front and side développés can be used to develop height of the gesture leg. For example, the hand can be used to help lift the leg slightly higher to the back with the knee bent and then the hand slowly released as the position is maintained for 4 counts. Again, a rotator disk can be used to focus on maintaining turnout on the support leg while improving height and technique of the gesture leg.

Other exercises for strengthening the back extensors presented in chapter 3 would also be helpful for improving movements like the arabesque. One study showed that strengthening the spinal extensors increased the height of the arabesque by 3.6° (Welsh et al., 1998). University dancers participating in a class taught by the author for 14 weeks—incorporating exercises for back extensor strength, hip extensor strength, hip flexor flexibility, and technique focus—increased the average height of the gesture foot by approximately 8 inches (20 centimeters). However, as previously discussed, exercises that involve spinal hyperextension carry a high risk and should be performed only by dancers without a history of low back problems, in a pain-free range, with

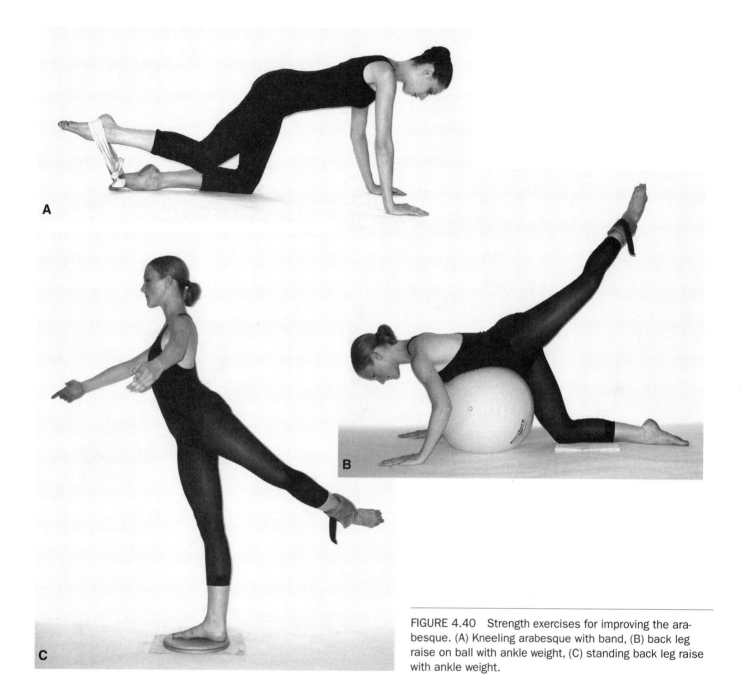

FIGURE 4.40 Strength exercises for improving the arabesque. (A) Kneeling arabesque with band, (B) back leg raise on ball with ankle weight, (C) standing back leg raise with ankle weight.

initial supervision, and with meticulous technique including co-contraction of the abdominal muscles to lessen lumbosacral stress.

While technique and specific strength are key, the height the leg can be lifted, the aesthetics of the movement, and the stress to the back are also markedly influenced by hip flexor flexibility. A screening test can be utilized to evaluate hip flexor flexibility (Tests and Measurements 4.5). If hip flexor flexibility is low, emphasis should be placed on stretching the hip flexors (table 4.7, A-C, pp. 224-225) as well as strengthening the hip and back extensors. If hip

flexor flexibility (hip hyperextension range) is high, this suggests that strength and technique should be a greater focus.

Conditioning Exercises for the Hip

Adequate strength and flexibility of the muscles crossing the hip are important for performance of demanding movements such as jumps, battements, and split leaps. However, when performing hip

TESTS AND MEASUREMENTS 4.5

Screening Test for Hip Flexor Flexibility

A test is shown for measuring passive flexibility of the hip flexors. For some dancers, the constraints will also be the hip ligaments and joint capsule. With the dancer in a supine position with one hip over the edge of the table, one knee is bent and held at the chest to help maintain a neutral pelvis while the examiner uses one hand on the other knee to help bring the leg toward the floor and the hip into hyperextension as shown in B. For a more precise test of the hip hyperextension range, the movement must be isolated to the hip versus the lumbosacral joint, and the pelvis should not be allowed to anteriorly tilt.

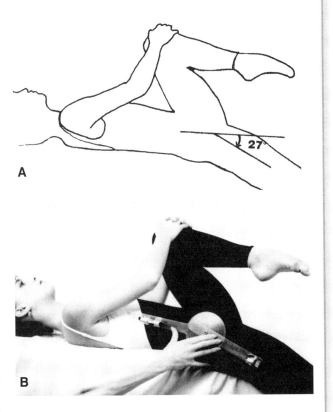

The axis of the goniometer is placed on the greater trochanter, the stationary arm horizontally along the side of the trunk and the movable arm along the outer thigh. A reading of 0° refers to the position when the thigh is horizontal; negative degrees would indicate that the thigh is angled up from the horizontal; and positive degrees would indicate that the thigh is angled down toward the floor relative to the horizontal. While 15° is considered normal range in general populations, the average value for hip hyperextension for elite advanced/professional female ballet dancers was shown to be 27° (Clippinger-Robertson, 1991). Again, this is an area of a lot of variability between dancers, and even within this elite group a range from 6° to 47° was recorded. If a goniometer is not available, one can estimate the range by visually locating the position where the femur would be one-third of the way toward the floor (30°) and dividing that arc in thirds.

conditioning exercises, it is important to remember that due to the previously described attachments of the hip muscles, particular attention needs to be paid to using the abdominals and other necessary muscles to maintain a stable pelvis and spine. To avoid redundancy, this need for lumbopelvic stabilization has not been listed under technique cues for all the exercises in tables 4.5 and 4.7, but it is essential for exercise effectiveness and safety.

Strength Exercises for the Hip

Supplemental hip strengthening is particularly important for the dancer because dance requires strength to hold the limbs in high ranges of motion that are not utilized in activities of daily living. For example, walking only utilizes about 40° of hip flexion and 12° of hip abduction (Hamill and Knutzen, 1995), inadequate to develop the strength to raise the leg above 90° desired in key dance vocabulary such as front or side extensions. The dancer might selectively choose to strengthen one or two areas in order to improve a specific movement. However, for the more advanced dancer, the ideal program should be balanced and designed to include exercises for each of the key muscle groups of the hip: the hip flexors, extensors, abductors, adductors, external rotators, and probably the internal rotators.

(Text continues on p. 221.)

TABLE 4.5   Selected Strength Exercises for the Hip

Exercise name (Resistance)	Description (Technique cues)	Progression
Muscle group: Hip flexors **Muscles emphasized: Iliopsoas**		
Joint movement: Hip flexion with knee flexion maintained		
A. Knee to chest (Elastic band) *Variation 2*	Lean back on the elbows with both knees bent and a band looped above the knees. Bring one knee toward the same shoulder, pause, and return to the starting position as the other knee stays in place. (Maintain a slight posterior pelvic tilt, and emphasize using the iliopsoas versus the rectus femoris.) *Variation 1:* Perform sitting in a chair with the hips at the front edge of the chair, the torso resting back against the back of the chair, and the pelvis in a slight posterior tilt. *Variation 2:* After bringing the knee to the chest, extend it without letting the knee move away from your body.	1. Perform sitting with a slight tuck and resting back on the hands (figure 4.34B, p. 201). 2. Perform sitting with vertical torso and pelvis more neutral (figure 4.34D, p. 201).
Muscle groups: Hip flexors and knee extensors **Muscles emphasized: Iliopsoas and quadriceps femoris**		
Joint movement: Hip flexion with knee extension		
B. Sitting 2-arc front leg raise (Body weight)	Sit leaning back on your hands with one knee bent with the foot on the ground while the other leg is extended to the front. Raise the extended leg as high as you can with good form, pause, bend the knee slightly, raise the leg slightly higher with the knee bent, extend the knee at this higher arc, pause, and slowly lower the leg to the starting position. (Use the quadriceps femoris for knee extension, but emphasize using the iliopsoas for hip flexion. Avoid letting the angle of hip flexion change as the knee extends at the top of the movement.) *Variation 1:* Perform turned out, but if using a weight cuff place it close to the knee rather than at the ankle.	1. Increase the height the leg is raised. 2. Bring the torso to a more vertical position and the lumbar spine more neutral. 3. Perform sitting with the torso vertical and the back against a wall. 4. Add an ankle weight. 5. Perform standing.

(continued)

TABLE 4.5   **Selected Strength Exercises for the Hip**   *(continued)*

Exercise name (Resistance)	Description (Technique cues)	Progression
Muscle group: Hip flexors **Muscles emphasized: Iliopsoas**		
Joint movement: Hip flexion with knee extension		
C. Front développé (Reformer) 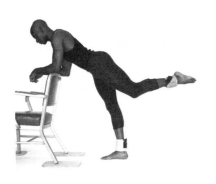	Lean back on the elbows with one knee bent with the foot on the carriage and the other knee bent with the strap above the knee. Bring the knee with the strap closer to the chest, extend the knee, bend the knee while bringing it closer to the shoulder, and then lower it to the starting position. (Focus on using the iliopsoas, and avoid letting the knee lower as it is extended.) *Variation 1:* Perform in the same body position only with a band looped just above the knees.	1. Increase springs. 2. Sit with weight back on hands. 3. Bring the torso to a more vertical position with the pelvis more neutral.
Muscle group: Hip extensors **Muscles emphasized: Hamstrings**		
Joint movement: Hip extension with knee flexion maintained		
D. Back leg raise (Ankle weight)	Lean forward with your arms resting on a barre or the back of a chair and a weight on each ankle. Bring one leg back, slightly bend the knee, and then raise the leg higher up until it is approximately parallel to the floor. (Keep the knee slightly bent as the leg lifts, and focus on using the hamstrings. Use the abdominals to keep the low back from excessively arching.) *Variation 1:* Perform turned out. *Variation 2:* Perform prone with the hips resting on a ball, box, or bench (figure 4.40B, p. 211).	1. Maintain the end position with the leg, and carefully raise the torso up toward a vertical position, co-contracting the abdominals and back extensors. 2. Perform standing with the torso more vertical and without arm support (figure 4.40C, p. 211). 3. Extend the knee at the top of the movement.

Exercise name (Resistance)	Description (Technique cues)	Progression

Muscle group: Hip extensors
Muscles emphasized: Hamstrings

Joint movement: Hip extension with knee extension

E. Kneeling arabesque (Reformer) 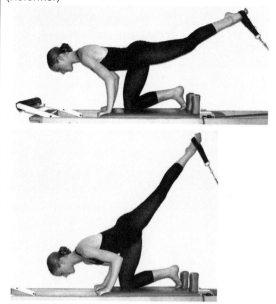	Kneel on the Reformer, facing the footbar, with one foot against the shoulder rest and the other leg back with the strap on the foot and the knee slightly bent. Slowly raise the leg with the strap, gradually extend the knee, pause, and then lower the leg to the starting position. Keep the hands in contact with the front of the carriage, and allow the torso to tilt forward as the leg raises. (Focus on using the hamstrings to "lift the knee," and use the abdominals to avoid arching the low back.) *Variation 1:* Perform in the same body position with a band looped around one foot or ankle and the other foot (figure 4.40A, p. 211).	1. Increase springs. 2. Increase the height the leg is raised.

Muscle group: Hip extensors
Muscles emphasized: Hamstrings/abdominal–hamstring force couple

Joint movement: Hip extension with knee flexion

F. Bridging (Body weight on ball) 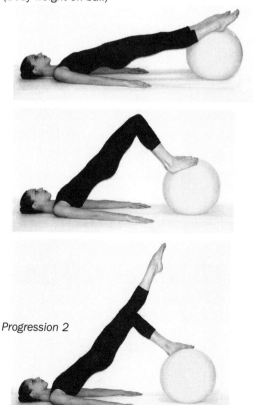 *Progression 2*	Lie on your back with both heels on the top of a ball with your knees extended. Posteriorly tilt the pelvis, and raise the pelvis to attempt to form a straight line along the side of the knee, pelvis, and shoulder. Then bend the knees to about 90° (bringing the ball toward the buttocks), pause, straighten the knees (bringing the ball away), and slowly lower the trunk to the starting position. (Emphasize pressing down with the heels and lifting from the bottom of the pelvis. Keep the pelvis in line as the knees bend and straighten, and avoid letting the low back arch or the knees hyperextend.)	1. Add a 4-count hold in the bent-knee position. 2. Lift one leg off during the hold. 3. Carefully perform with one heel on the ball and the other leg extended in the air, starting and ending with the knee slightly flexed versus straight. Begin with a very small range of motion and only if no knee discomfort is experienced.

(continued)

TABLE 4.5   Selected Strength Exercises for the Hip   *(continued)*

Exercise name (Resistance)	Description (Technique cues)	Progression
Muscle groups: Hip abductors and hip external rotators **Muscles emphasized: Gluteus medius, iliopsoas, and DOR**		
Joint movement: Hip abduction with external rotation		
G. Side leg raise (Ankle weight)	Lie on your side with your back against a wall and both hips externally rotated, with the knees extended and an ankle weight on the top leg. Raise the top leg, pause, and then lower to the starting position. (Focus on keeping the hips level in the early range of the motion and bringing the greater trochanter of the femur back and down toward the ischial tuberosity as the leg is raised. In higher ranges, only allow as much lateral tilt of the pelvis as necessary and lift your waist off the floor to help limit the tilt. Maintain as much turnout as possible as the leg lowers, and keep the sacrum, midback, and little toe of the gesture leg in contact with the wall throughout the exercise.) *Variation 1:* Perform with both legs parallel to emphasize the hip abductors alone. (Focus on keeping the pelvis level initially by reaching the upper iliac crest away toward your feet while thinking of lifting the waist off the floor by bringing the lower iliac crest toward the lower ribs. Emphasize movement of the femur to achieve full hip abduction. Stop at a range before marked lateral tilt of the pelvis is necessary— generally 45° to 60° abduction when parallel.) *Variation 2:* Perform with a band looped above the knees in parallel or turned out (figure 4.38B, p. 207).	1. Raise top leg higher while still maintaining good form. 2. Increase the turnout achieved and maintained. 3. Increase ankle weight.

Exercise name (Resistance)	Description (Technique cues)	Progression

Muscle group: Hip abductors
Muscles emphasized: Gluteus medius/stabilization

Joint movement: Hip abduction

H. Standing side leg raise (Ankle weight) 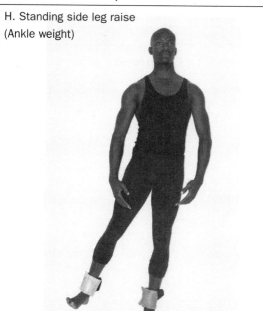	Stand in parallel with an ankle cuff on one leg. Raise the leg with the weight, pause, and then return to the starting position. (Focus initially on keeping the pelvis level and then minimizing the lateral pelvic tilt as the leg raises higher. Keep the weight of the body over the support leg without "sitting in the hip.") *Variation 1:* Perform turned out.	1. Increase ankle weight. 2. Increase height to which the leg is raised.

Muscle groups: Hip abductors, hip flexors, and hip external rotators
Muscles emphasized: Iliopsoas and DOR

Joint movements: Hip abduction and external rotation with knee extension

I. Side développé (Reformer) 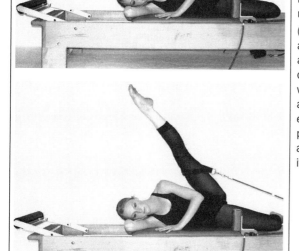	Lie on your side with your head toward the footbar, one leg between the shoulder rests, and the other leg with the knee bent and the strap above the knee. Bring the top knee up toward the top shoulder, slowly extend the knee, pause, bend the knee, and return to the starting position. (Focus on using maximum turnout and bringing the trochanter back and down, with the knee going as directly to the side as possible while the pelvis initially stays almost level versus laterally tilted; emphasize using the iliopsoas to pull the thigh toward the shoulder, and avoid letting the knee lower as it straightens.)	1. Increase springs. 2. Shorten straps. 3. Increase height to which the knee is raised.

(continued)

TABLE 4.5 Selected Strength Exercises for the Hip *(continued)*

Exercise name (Resistance)	Description (Technique cues)	Progression
Muscle group: Hip adductors **Muscles emphasized: Hip adductors/stabilization**		
Joint movement: Hip adduction		
J. Single leg pull (Ankle weight) 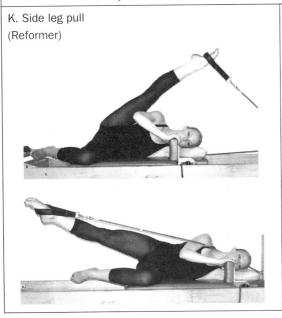	Lie on one side with both legs extended, the top leg up on the seat of a chair and an ankle weight on the lower leg. Raise the lower leg up toward the top leg, pause, and return to the starting position. (Keep directly on the side of the hip, and avoid rocking forward or backward.) *Variation 1:* Perform standing in first position with surgical tubing or a wall pulley providing resistance from the side, in opposition to hip adduction. *Variation 2:* Perform lying on the side or standing with the legs turned out.	1. Increase weight. 2. Use a taller chair or support for the top leg.
Muscle groups: Hip adductors and hip external rotators **Muscles emphasized: Adductor magnus and DOR/ROM**		
Joint movement: Hip adduction with external rotation		
K. Side leg pull (Reformer)	Lie on your side with your head toward the straps, one arm between the shoulder rests, the lower knee bent, and the other leg overhead with the knee extended and the back strap on the foot. Pull the top leg down in line with the middle of the footbar, pause, and then return to the starting position. (Focus on turning out and pulling down with the back of the inner thigh; avoid letting the leg move forward; emphasize dropping the greater trochanter down as the leg raises back to its overhead position.)	1. Increase springs. 2. Shorten straps. 3. Increase height to which the leg is raised.

Exercise name (Resistance)	Description (Technique cues)	Progression
Muscle group: Hip adductors **Muscles emphasized: Hip adductors and lower DOR/ROM**		
Joint movement: Hip horizontal adduction with external rotation		
L. Wall "V" (Ankle weights) 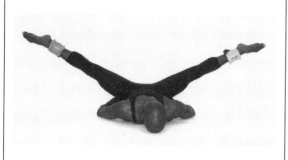	Lie supine with your buttocks against a wall, with the legs turned out and extended up toward the ceiling and weight cuffs on the ankles. Simultaneously bring both legs away from each other and toward the floor, pause, and then bring the legs back together to the starting position. (Lower the legs in a very slow and controlled manner, and attempt to keep the little toes in contact with the wall throughout the exercise. Avoid hyperextending the knees.) *Variation 1:* Perform with both legs parallel.	1. Increase ankle weights. 2. Bring legs further to the side.
Muscle group: Hip external rotators **Muscles emphasized: DOR**		
Joint movement: Hip external rotation with knee flexion maintained		
M. Prone passé (Reformer) 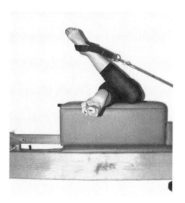	Lie prone crosswise to the long box on the Reformer with the hands on the floor and the knee just past the edge of the box. Bend the knee that is closest to the straps to about 90°, and place the strap around the foot. Start with the hip slightly internally rotated, and then slowly rotate from the hip to bring the knee outward and the foot toward the back of the extended knee. Pause, and return to the starting position. (Emphasize rotating from the hip with the leg moving as a unit, and avoid letting the lower leg twist at the knee. Maintain the knee at 90° flexion, as well as a neutral pelvis with both ASIS in contact with the box.) *Variation 1:* Perform prone on the floor with a figure 8 loop of elastic tubing around the ankle and foot of the bent knee, with the other end of the tubing secured directly to the side that would oppose the movement (figure 4.33A, p. 199).	1. Increase range of external rotation while still maintaining a neutral pelvis. 2. Increase springs. 3. Shorten straps.

(continued)

TABLE 4.5 Selected Strength Exercises for the Hip *(continued)*

Exercise name (Resistance)	Description (Technique cues)	Progression
Muscle group: Hip external rotators **Muscles emphasized: DOR**		
Joint movement: Hip external rotation with horizontal abduction		
N. Prone frog (Body weight on ball) 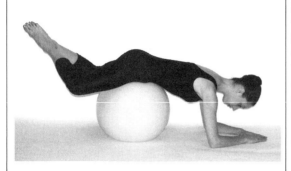	Lie prone with the hips on a ball, the forearms on the floor, and the feet together with the knees bent and out to the sides. Press the feet together, externally rotate both hips, lift the knees toward the ceiling, pause, and then return to the starting position. (Focus on using the lower DOR to rotate the hips and then reach the knees out, around, and up; avoid lifting the feet first or twisting the knees.) *Variation 1:* Perform on a Pilates ladder barrel.	1. Raise the knees slightly higher. 2. After the knees are lifted, extend both knees, keeping the heels together. Focus on lifting the heels as the knees extend and bend.
Muscle groups: Hip external rotators and hip abductors **Muscles emphasized: DOR**		
Joint movement: Hip external rotation with abduction		
O. Hip rotation on elbows (Elastic band) 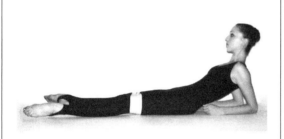	Lean back on your elbows with both knees extended and a band looped above the knees. Simultaneously bring both legs to the side, externally rotate both legs, bring both legs further to the side, pause, and then return to the starting position. (Focus on using the lower DOR at the base of the buttocks to externally rotate femurs and increase the turnout as the legs go further to the side.)	1. Bring legs further to the side. 2. Make the band loop smaller. 3. Use a heavier band.
Muscle group: Hip internal rotators **Muscles emphasized: Gluteus medius and gluteus minimus**		
Joint movement: Hip internal rotation with knee flexion maintained		
P. Prone hip internal rotation (Reformer) 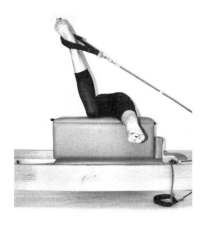	The same as exercise M, only with one strap on the foot farthest from the strap and moving in the opposite direction; that is, starting with the hip slightly externally rotated and internally rotating from the hip such that the knee faces inward and the foot of the bent knee moves away from the extended knee. Pause, and return to the starting position. *Variation 1:* Perform prone on the floor with a figure 8 loop of elastic tubing around the ankle and foot of the bent knee, with the other end of the tubing secured directly to the side that would oppose the movement.	1. Increase range of internal rotation while still maintaining a neutral pelvis. 2. Increase springs. 3. Shorten straps.

Sample strength exercises for the hip are provided in table 4.5, and a brief description of their importance follows. Because many of the muscles of the hip also cross the knee, additional exercises that also strengthen the hip are described with the knee in chapter 5.

Hip Flexor Strengthening

Adequate strength in the hip flexors, and particularly in the iliopsoas, is important for high movements to the front and side such as développés and extensions. One study showed an improvement of extensions to the side (à la seconde) averaging about 6 inches (15 centimeters) following six weeks of hip flexor strengthening emphasizing use of the iliopsoas (Grossman and Wilmerding, 2000). Similarly, the author found average increases of 6 inches for front extensions and 5 inches (13 centimeters) for side extensions following a 14-week class incorporating hip strengthening, stretching, and technique exercises.

The knee to chest (table 4.5A) and front développé (table 4.5C) are hip flexor strengthening exercises designed to focus on use of the iliopsoas through the use of a range of hip flexion greater than 90°, initial use of a posterior pelvic tilt, and the initial use of a flexed knee as discussed earlier in this chapter. However, as strength and the ability to recruit the iliopsoas are developed, exercises should progress to extending the knee after the hip is flexed, performing hip flexion with the knee initially extended (sitting 2 arc front leg raise, table 4.5B), using a neutral pelvis, and bringing the torso to vertical or standing to better replicate the functional demands required in dance class and performance. It may also help to review the procedure given for palpating the iliopsoas and then focus on trying to feel the iliopsoas contract under your fingertips during each of these exercises.

Hip Extensor Strengthening

Developing sufficient strength in the hip extensors is important to allow the leg to be lifted high to the back as in a back attitude or arabesque. To achieve maximum range and the desired dance aesthetic, particular emphasis should be placed on using the hamstrings. The back leg raise (table 4.5D) and kneeling arabesque (table 4.5E) were designed with this goal in mind. Use the hamstrings to bend the knee slightly, and then focus on using these same muscles to lift the leg "from the knee" up toward the ceiling and higher than the pelvis.

Adequate strength and appropriate recruitment of the hip extensors are also important for propulsive movements such as jumping and closed-chain movements such as pliés, or standing on one leg at the barre or center floor. Bridging (table 4.5F) is designed to help with this latter postural goal by encouraging use of the abdominal–hamstring force couple. The abdominal muscles are used to stabilize the pelvis, while the hamstrings are used to pull the ischial tuberosities downward and lift the pelvis via hip extension. Other useful strengthening exercises that more closely mimic the demands of jumping include squats and lunges described in the chapter on the knee (chapter 5), as well as jumping drills described in the chapter on the ankle and foot (chapter 6).

Hip Abductor Strengthening

Strengthening the hip abductors is key for achieving adequate height in movements to the side such as a développé or extension. Elite ballet dancers have been shown to have significantly greater hip abductor strength than normal (Hamilton et al., 1992), providing support for the importance of this muscle group for ballet. The side leg raise (table 4.5G) and side développé (table 4.5I) are designed to help improve the height the leg can be lifted. Strengthening the hip abductors is also important for side-to-side motion and stability during standing on one leg. The standing side leg raise (table 4.5H) is designed to emphasize this latter stability on the support leg.

Hip Adductor Strengthening

Strength exercises for the hip adductors are important for muscle balance relative to the often stronger hip abductors, and a study of professional ice hockey players found a 17-fold greater risk for hip adductor strains if hip adductor strength were less than 80% of abductor strength (Tyler et al., 2001). Strength exercises for the hip adductors are also important for optimal placement of the pelvis when standing on one leg and to help achieve the use of these "inner thigh muscles" in turned-out positions encouraged by many schools of dance. The single leg pull (table 4.5J) is designed to encourage use of the adductors in the final phase of closing into and standing in first or fifth position. The side leg pull (figure 4.5K) utilizes a large range of motion so that both dynamic flexibility and strength are encouraged and pelvic stabilization is challenged. The wall "V" (figure 4.5L) is an alternative for dancers who do not have access to the equipment required by the side leg pull. The wall "V" actually involves horizontal adduction versus pure hip adduction. However, it was included because it offers the advantage of working in a large range of motion.

Hip External Rotator Strengthening

Developing specific strength and activation of the hip external rotators can help dancers realize and maintain their full potential turnout. The prone passé (table 4.5M) is designed to emphasize strengthening the DOR with larger range of motion of the femur. Care must be taken that the knee is stabilized with appropriate muscles and that the rotation is occurring from the hip and not at the knee. The prone frog (table 4.5N) incorporates a smaller motion of the femur and is helpful for encouraging maintenance of turnout, such as when holding one leg in passé during a pirouette. This exercise can also be helpful for dancers who feel that they are excessively using the front of the thigh (sartorius) for rotation, since the slight horizontal abduction against gravity utilized in this exercise will encourage activation of the desired deep outward rotator muscles.

Strengthening and specific use of the hip external rotators can also be encouraged through addition of external rotation to the other hip movements of flexion, extension, abduction, and adduction. For example, hip rotation on elbows (table 4.5O) combines hip abduction with hip external rotation. Many of the other exercises as just described and included in table 4.5 can also have hip external rotation added to them. This approach will allow strengthening of the rotators in a specific manner that will tend to enhance particular movements mimicked by the exercises. Furthermore, many of these exercises can incorporate hip external rotation with the knee extended, a valuable alternative for any dancer who experiences knee discomfort in exercises in which the knee is bent, such as the prone passé.

Hip Internal Rotator Strengthening

Inclusion of strengthening exercises for the hip internal rotators is an area of controversy. One approach is to selectively work the external rotators, to purposely create an imbalance that will favor the maintenance of turnout and help prevent the common technique error of letting the knee fall medial to the foot. Another approach is to include at least some internal rotation out of concern that selectively strengthening the external rotators without the internal rotators may predispose dancers to certain types of injuries. Further research will be necessary to clarify this controversy. Prone hip internal rotation (table 4.5P) is an exercise for the internal rotators that can be easily performed after prone passé by just switching the strap or tubing to the other foot.

Stretches for the Hip

Extreme range of motion at the hip is essential to achieve the desired dance aesthetic. Table 4.6 provides the normal range of motion for non-dancers in each of the primary movements of the hip, and selected average values for elite dancers are also provided to demonstrate the need for ranges tremendously higher than seen in non-dance populations. Since the passive limits to many hip movements (as shown in table 4.6) are muscular in nature, consistent stretching can yield dramatic improvements in range of motion. Stretching of the hamstrings, hip flexors, and hip adductors is particularly important for achieving dance aesthetics. Sample flexibility exercises for these and other hip muscle groups are provided in table 4.7, and a brief description of the importance of these exercises follows. Dancers who utilize turned-out positions in their dance forms should perform these stretches with the targeted leg turned out as well as parallel.

Hip Flexor Stretches

Adequate hip flexor flexibility is critical for allowing proper technique when working the leg behind the body (i.e., hip hyperextension), and inadequate flexibility will tend to limit the height the leg can be raised and necessitate the undesired technique errors of excessive and premature lumbar hyperextension, anterior pelvic tilting, or "opening the hip" (i.e., pelvic rotation) in an effort to achieve desired height of the back leg. For example, a dancer with tight hip flexors that allow only 5° of hip hyperextension will not even be able to perform a tendu to the back or walk (requires 10° of hip hyperextension) without tilting the pelvis forward or arching the low back. In contrast, a dancer with 30° of hip hyperextension would be able to raise the leg a third of the way to horizontal without an anterior pelvic tilt or compensatory hyperextension of the spine.

Given this association with hip hyperextension, it is not surprising that in a study of non-dancers, low mobility in hip extension showed the highest correlation with low back pain (Mellin, 1988). Hence, it is important that hip flexor range be evaluated (see Tests and Measurements 4.5, p. 212) and that daily stretching be made a priority in dancers who are limited by this constraint. However, angles beyond about 20° of hyperextension are often limited by extensibility of the joint capsule and ligaments as well as the hip flexors. Hence, stretches should be done carefully, with the body adequately warmed up and with a slow application of a low to moderate stretch in a pain-free range.

TABLE 4.6 Normal Range of Motion and Constraints for Fundamental Movements of the Hip (Non-Dance Populations)

Hip joint movement	Normal range of motion*	Normal passive limiting factors
Flexion	0-120° (knee flexed) 0-80° (knee extended)**	Soft tissue: apposition of thigh on abdomen Muscle: hamstring group
Extension	0-15°**	Joint capsule: anterior portion Ligaments: iliofemoral and pubofemoral Muscle: iliopsoas
Abduction	0-45°	Joint capsule: inferior portion Ligaments: pubofemoral, ischiofemoral, and lower iliofemoral Muscles: hip adductors
Adduction	0-30°	Soft tissue: apposition of thighs With opposite hip in abduction or flexion: *Joint capsule:* superior portion *Ligaments:* upper iliofemoral and ischiofemoral, iliotibial band *Muscles:* hip abductors
External rotation	0-45°	Joint capsule: anterior portion Ligaments: iliofemoral and pubofemoral Muscles: internal rotators and others depending on joint position
Internal rotation	0-40°** 0-45°	Joint capsule: posterior portion Ligament: ischiofemoral Muscles: external rotators

*From American Academy of Orthopaedic Surgeons (1965).
**From Gerhardt and Rippstein (1990).

The low lunge stretch (table 4.7A) is a stretch for the hip flexors that can easily be performed after class. However, if the dancer has difficulty feeling the stretch or keeping the pelvis from tilting forward, try the chair lunge stretch (table 4.7B). Performing this stretch on a chair makes it easier to keep the pelvis more upright without a balance challenge and with less flexion of the front knee. As flexibility improves, the low lunge stretch can be advanced by extending the back knee (progression 1) or going into a split from the low lunge stretch (progression 2). The split stretch is actually a compound stretch, challenging multiple muscle groups including the hamstrings on the front leg and the hip flexors in the back leg.

Hip Extensor Stretches (Hamstrings)

Extreme hamstring flexibility is a necessity for achieving the aesthetic goals of the skilled dancer and for successful execution of movements such as a split (front leg), split leap, penché (support leg), and high kick to the front. Furthermore, hamstring flexibility allowing greater than 90° of hip flexion is necessary for allowing the desired upright (neutral) position of the pelvis in floor work or floor stretches where the knees are straight. If less than this range is present, the dancer will display a posterior pelvic tilt accompanied by flexion of the lumbar spine, and use of the hip flexors will be required to keep the torso from falling backward in such positions. Adequate and balanced hamstring flexibility may also help prevent hamstring strains and low back pain, particularly in male adolescents (Mellin, 1988; Mierau, Cassidy, and Yong-Hing, 1989).

Both the supine hamstring stretch and sitting hamstring stretch use this combination of hip flexion and knee extension to apply an effective stretch to the hamstrings. The supine hamstring stretch (table 4.7C) uses a position in which the back is supported to more closely replicate the position needed for standing hip flexion with a vertical torso. The sitting hamstring stretch (table 4.7D) incorporates stretching both the low back and hamstrings and is more similar to the position needed in "roll-downs" commonly used in modern and jazz classes.

TABLE 4.7 Selected Stretches for the Hip

Exercise name (Method of stretch)	Description (Technique cues)	Progression
Muscle group: Hip flexors **Muscles emphasized: Iliopsoas**		
Joint position: Hip hyperextension		
A. Low lunge stretch (Static)	Assume a lunge position with weight on the front foot, with the knee bent to 90° and weight on the lower back leg. Then slide the back leg back until a stretch is felt across the front of the back hip. (Keep the front knee directly over the front ankle, and keep both ASIS facing directly front while focusing on pressing the bottom of the pelvis forward.) *Variation 1:* Perform with the back leg turned out. *Variation 2:* After reaching the lunge stretch position, use the hands to support the body weight, and slide the front leg forward as far as your flexibility will allow or until in a split position. This combines a hip flexor stretch on the back leg with a hip extensor (e.g., hamstrings) stretch on the front leg.	1. After reaching the stretch position, bring the toes under (metatarsophalangeal extension) to help support the body weight, and extend the back knee. 2. After reaching the stretch position, place the hands on the front thigh, and arch the torso up and back while trying to keep the pelvis as vertical as possible.
Muscle group: Hip flexors **Muscles emphasized: Iliopsoas**		
Joint position: Hip hyperextension with knee flexion		
B. Chair lunge stretch (Static)	Place one knee on a chair seat with the other leg in front of the side of the chair. Bend the front knee until a stretch is felt across the front of the back hip. (Use one hand on the back of the chair to help keep the torso upright, not forward, while using the abdominals to effect a posterior pelvic tilt as the bottom of the pelvis is pressed forward.) *Variation 1:* Perform with the back knee turned out. *Variation 2:* Perform standing, grasping the foot of the back leg with the hand and using it to pull the knee back and up until a stretch is felt across the front of the hip.	1. Move the foot on the ground further forward. 2. Carefully add an upper back arch.

Exercise name (Method of stretch)	Description (Technique cues)	Progression

Muscle group: Hip extensors
Muscles emphasized: Hamstrings

Joint position: Hip flexion with knee extension

| C. Supine hamstring stretch (Static) 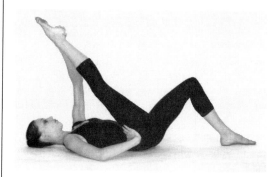 | Lie on the back with one knee bent with the foot on the ground and the other knee extended. Use the hands to bring the extended leg up toward the chest until a stretch is felt at the back of the thigh. (Focus on flexing at the hip rather than the spine and keeping the back of the lower sacrum in contact with the floor.) *Variation 1:* PNF—While in this stretch position, contract the hamstrings by attempting to lower the top leg back toward the ground (i.e., hip extension) as the arms resist the motion. *Variation 2:* Perform static or PNF variation with the extended leg turned out. *Variation 3:* Perform the stretch, carrying the extended leg to the side to include a stretch of the hip adductors as well as the hamstrings. | 1. Bring the top leg closer to the chest. 2. Perform with the lower leg resting on the floor with the knee extended. |

Muscle group: Hip extensors
Muscles emphasized: Hamstrings and low back extensors

Joint position: Hip flexion with knee extension and lumbar flexion

| D. Sitting hamstring stretch (Static) 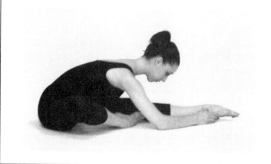 | Sit with one knee bent to the side and the other leg forward with the knee extended. Lean forward from the hip until a stretch is felt on the back of the extended leg. (Pull the pelvis back on the side of the outstretched leg, and turn the torso so that it leans directly over the outstretched leg; emphasize flexing the hip joint rather than just the spine.) *Variation 1:* Perform with the extended leg turned out. | 1. Grasp foot or lower leg with the hands, and use them to pull the torso forward and down over the extended leg. 2. Perform with both legs extended to the front. 3. Perform with both legs extended to the front with one ankle crossed over the top of the other ankle. |

(continued)

TABLE 4.7 **Selected Stretches for the Hip** *(continued)*

Exercise name (Method of stretch)	Description (Technique cues)	Progression
Muscle groups: Hip adductors and hip extensors **Muscles emphasized: Hip adductors, hamstrings, and hip internal rotators**		
Joint position: Hip abduction with external rotation		
E. Side développé stretch (Static)	Lie on one side with the bottom leg extended and the top leg flexed at the hip and knee, with both hips externally rotated. Grasp the foot or lower calf of the upper leg with the hand of the upper arm, and use it to pull the knee close to the top shoulder and then to help extend the knee. Hold this final position with both knees extended. (Focus on bringing the greater trochanter back and down as the leg is extended.) *Variation 1:* PNF—Add PNF by using the top arm to resist knee flexion. *Variation 2:* Perform the original stretch lying on your back instead of your side.	1. Bring the upper leg closer to the top shoulder. 2. Perform the stretch standing instead of side-lying.
Muscle group: Hip adductors **Muscles exmphasized: Hip adductors and hamstrings**		
Joint position: Hip horizontal abduction with hip flexion		
F. Second-position stretch (Static)	Spread the legs away from each other to the sides with the knees slightly bent (or straight, in accordance with current flexibility), and then lean the torso forward at the hips until a stretch is felt along the inner thighs. (Bring the ischial tuberosities back, and reach the torso forward while the knees stay facing directly up toward the ceiling.) *Variation 1:* Perform lying on the back with the legs going to the side slightly above hip height in either a parallel or turned-out position. *Variation 2:* PNF—Add PNF to either variation by placing the hands against the inner thighs to resist bringing the legs together. *Variation 3:* Perform lying on the back with the feet against a wall and the back of the legs resting on the ground as they are spread away from each other.	1. Open the legs further to the sides. 2. Perform with both knees straight and feet against a wall to help spread legs further to the side.

Exercise name (Method of stretch)	Description (Technique cues)	Progression

Muscle group: Hip abductors
Muscles emphasized: Tensor fasciae latae and associated iliotibial band, gluteus medius, and gluteus minimus

Joint position: Hip adduction with slight hip flexion

Exercise name (Method of stretch)	Description (Technique cues)	Progression
G. Side-lying hip abductor stretch (Static) 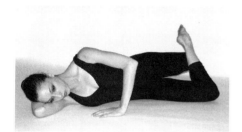	Lie on your side with the top hip extended, with the knee flexed to about 90° and the bottom hip flexed with the knee bent and ankle just above the outside of the top knee. Use the foot of the bottom leg to press the top knee down toward the floor until a stretch is felt on the top hip or outer thigh. (Focus on pulling the lateral iliac crest of the upper leg up toward the lateral rib cage and avoid letting it tilt laterally downward as the top knee is pressed downward.) *Variation 1:* Perform at the edge of a table or bench with the top knee straight and the top leg angled off the table so that it can be stretched below the tabletop. *Variation 2:* Have a partner stabilize the top hip with one hand and gently adduct the top leg with the other hand until a gentle to moderate stretch is felt.	1. Bring the knee further down toward the floor without allowing the pelvis to laterally tilt.

Muscle group: Hip external rotators
Muscles emphasized: DOR

Joint position: Hip horizontal adduction

Exercise name (Method of stretch)	Description (Technique cues)	Progression
H. Knee across body stretch (Static) 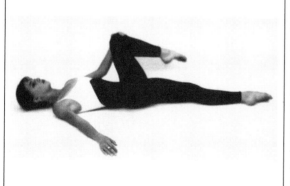	Lie on your back with one leg extended on the floor and the other leg flexed at the hip and knee. Place the opposite hand on the bent knee and use it to pull the knee across the body and slightly up toward the opposite shoulder until a stretch is felt on the side of the buttocks. (Focus on keeping the trunk stable and avoid letting the pelvis, back, or shoulders rotate off the floor as the knee is pulled across the body.) *Variation 1:* Move the knee up slightly and then down slightly before bringing it across the body to focus on stretching different components of the hip deep outward rotators and to find an angle with which the pinching sensation in the hip that some dancers experience can be avoided.	1. Bring the knee further across the body.

(continued)

TABLE 4.7   Selected Stretches for the Hip   *(continued)*

Exercise name (Method of stretch)	Description (Technique cues)	Progression
Muscle group: Hip external rotators **Muscles emphasized: DOR**		
Joint position: Hip internal rotation		
I. Knees-in stretch (Static) 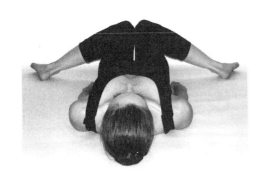	Lie on your back with your feet spread about 2 1/2 feet (76 centimeters) apart and knees bent to approximately 90°. Bring your knees together and toward the floor by rotating the upper legs inward at the hip joint until a stretch is felt along the lower side of the hips and in the buttocks area. (Emphasize moving the whole upper and lower leg together from the hip, allowing the feet to spread away from each other without twisting the knees.)	1. Spread the feet further apart, and use the hands to gently press on the top of the thigh to increase internal rotation at the hip.
Muscle groups: Hip internal rotators* and hip adductors **Muscles emphasized: Hip adductors**		
Joint position: Hip external rotation with horizontal abduction		
J. Frog stretch (Static) 	Sit with both knees bent and facing to the sides, with the soles of the feet together. Use the forearms to gently press the knees toward the floor until a stretch is felt along the inner thighs. (Focus on leaning forward at the hips and externally rotating the hips as the knees are pressed toward the floor.) *Variation 1:* Perform lying on the back (figure 4.32C, p. 198). *Variation 2:* PNF—Add PNF to either variation by using the forearms or hands to resist bringing the knees up and toward each other. *Variation 3:* Have a partner place their hands just above the knees and carefully apply a stretch to variation 1.	1. Bring the knees closer to the floor. 2. When the knees are within 3 inches (7.6 centimeters) of the floor, progress to the modified prone frog stretch if no knee discomfort is experienced (figure 4.32A, p. 198).

*Constraints to external rotation can include the joint capsule, ligaments, and muscles.

To isolate the stretch more to the hamstrings, perform it with a flat back position; and to emphasize stretching the low back, emphasize rounding the back forward. Sitting hamstring stretches require range of the hamstrings of greater than 90° to allow the weight of the torso to produce desired hip flexion when the torso is brought forward. Dancers with inadequate ham-string flexibility should slightly bend the knees and can place a mat or towel roll under the ischial tuberosities to facilitate desired positioning of the body.

Hip Adductor Stretches

Adequate adductor flexibility is essential for allowing the leg to be raised to the side to a desired height and to allow the dancer to work with the legs more directly to the side when using turned-out positions. Adequate flexibility as well as strength in the hip adductors may help prevent the common occurrence in dance of adductor or "groin" strains.

The side développé stretch (table 4.7E) is a compound stretch, stretching the adductors and hamstrings in a turned-out position, with the goal of improving turned-out movements to the side such as développés, extensions, and battements. In contrast, when the second-position stretch (table 4.7F) is done with the knees slightly bent, it isolates the stretch more to the hip adductors and slackens the stretch on the hamstrings. This stretch is designed to try to "open up the hips" to allow the legs to be worked more directly to the side, particularly in movements where the femur is approximately horizontal such as a passé, rond de jambe in the air, or Russian split. If this stretch is performed with the knees straight, the gracilis and hamstring muscles also will potentially be stretched.

Hip Abductor Stretches

Improved flexibility in the hip abductors does not have as clear an association with dance movement goals as seen with the hamstrings and hip adductors. Instead, the rationale for stretching these muscles is to reduce the risk for injuries involving lateral hip and knee pain that have been theorized to relate to hip abductor tightness.

The side-lying hip abductor stretch (table 4.7G) is designed to stretch the hip abductors, but meticulous form is necessary for the stretch to be effective. The dancer must pull the iliac crest of the top hip up toward the waist to stabilize the proximal attachment of the hip abductors so that a stretch will be produced when the thigh is pressed down, that is, adducted. If care is not taken, the pelvis will tend to laterally tilt (downward on the top hip), lessening the stretch. As described under the variations, this exercise can also be done with the knee straight over the edge of a table.

Hip External Rotator Stretches

As with the hip abductors, increased flexibility in the hip external rotators is not directly linked with a specific enhancement of dance technique. However, with the extensive use of the externally rotated position in ballet, some dancers exhibit increased range in external rotation and decreased range in internal rotation (Hamilton et al., 1992; Khan et al., 1997). Some medical professionals conjecture that such a pattern may predispose dancers to hip injuries such as the piriformis syndrome and that stretching

the hip external rotators may serve a role in injury prevention.

The knee across body stretch (table 4.7H) is commonly recommended to stretch the piriformis and other deep outward rotator muscles. For this stretch to be effective, particular care must be taken to keep the pelvis flat on the ground so that the medial attachments of the DOR are held stationary as the lateral attachments onto the greater trochanter move away to produce a stretch as the femur is brought across the body. The knees-in stretch (table 4.7I) is probably less effective but offers an alternative for dancers who experience pinching of the hip flexors in the knee across body stretch.

Stretches for the Hip Internal Rotators and Improving Turnout

Many dancers desire to increase hip external rotation; but as previously discussed, the constraints are more complex than just the hip internal rotators and the extent of improvement less marked, and long-term consequences of stretching on joint health are controversial. So, until additional information is available, it is advisable that such stretches be done particularly carefully, when the body is warm and with a slow, gentle application of force in a pain-free range.

The frog stretch (table 4.7J) is designed to try to enhance turnout when the hip is flexed such as in a front attitude. The supine version replicates the position needed more in movements to the side such as a passé (figure 4.32C, p. 198). In this position it is sometimes difficult to apply sufficient stretch with your own hands, and using a partner to very slowly and carefully apply a stretch can be helpful. More flexible dancers can perform the modified prone frog stretch (figure 4.32A, p. 198) if adequate stabilization of the trunk can be maintained and no knee discomfort is experienced.

Hip Injuries in Dancers

The hip joint is designed for stability with a relatively deep articular socket, relatively large contact areas between the adjacent femur and acetabulum of the pelvis, and very strong ligaments and joint capsule. Hence, hip dislocation or ligamental injury is rare. However, due to the large stresses translated through the hip region and poor nutritional status of many dancers, stress fractures do sometimes occur. More frequently, though, it is the muscles and related structures that become injured.

Studies have reported that in ballet dancers 5.8%, 8.6%, and 11% and in modern dancers 4%

of total injuries were to the hip and pelvis (Quirk, 1983; Schafle, Requa, and Garrick, 1990). A survey of modern dancers reported 11.3% of total injuries were to the hip, with an additional 4.8% to the hamstrings (Solomon and Micheli, 1986). The lower incidence of dancer injuries reported for the hip, in contrast to some other regions of the body, is likely due in part to the marked structural stability present at this joint. However, many dancers experience minor musculotendinous problems at the hip for which they often do not seek medical treatment.

Prevention of Hip Injuries

Due to the common involvement of the muscles in injury, regular strengthening and stretching of the hip muscles, as well as sport-specific training (Emery and Meeuwisse, 2001), are important for preventing injuries. Strengthening exercises should ideally be very dance specific, for example incorporating the high angles of movement utilized in dance movements as well as muscles needed to promote optimal technique. Dancers should resist the temptation to neglect proper technique in order to gain greater height of the leg. Poor habits can result in inappropriate development of muscles and undue stresses, which over time could precipitate injury. Performing an adequate warm-up prior to stretching, rehearsal, or performance can theoretically help prevent injuries. Increasing the body's internal temperature will allow a muscle to stretch further and absorb greater forces before it is injured (Safran et al., 1988; Taylor et al., 1990; Warren, Lehmann, and Koblanski, 1971, 1976).

Common Types of Hip Injuries in Dancers

A description of selected hip injuries that involve the bone, muscle, or tendon follows. Some types of injuries to the hip can have grave consequences if ignored and not properly treated. Furthermore, there are many other serious injuries that can cause symptoms similar to those described in this section, including tumors, infections, referred pain from the lumbosacral spine or pelvic viscera, and injury to the growth plate or growth centers where tendons attach. Hence, dancers are encouraged to obtain medical treatment if hip pain is persistent or severe.

Stress Fractures

Stress fractures can occur at various sites in the pelvis and femur, including the pubic ramus, femoral neck, and femoral shaft. Factors that may increase

the risk for sustaining stress fractures in the pelvis and femur include high-intensity training, changing to a harder training surface, athletic amenorrhea, poor nutrition, osteoporosis, external rotation of the hip beyond 65°, coxa vara, and muscle fatigue with resultant loss of shock absorption (Lacroix, 2000; Lieberman and Harwin, 1997; Ruane and Rossi, 1998; Teitz, 2000).

Symptoms will vary according to the site of the stress fracture, but they may include pain in the groin, thigh, or knee that is worsened with weight bearing. Initially, pain may increase at the beginning of class, decrease during class, and increase again after class (Lieberman and Harwin, 1997; Sammarco, 1987). Although this pain will often subside with rest or layoffs, it will return as soon as dancing is resumed. Pain is often produced with a passé position or with hopping on the affected side (Clement et al., 1993), and limitation of or pain with hip internal rotation is common.

Treatment will vary according to the severity of the stress fracture but often involves reduction of weight bearing sufficiently to be pain free. Crutches may be required and dancing is often temporarily discontinued. When symptoms subside, exercise in the water, followed by non-weight-bearing floor barre and exercises on the Pilates Reformer, is often a helpful adjunct to other traditional strength and flexibility programs. Stress fractures are serious injuries, and Sammarco (1987) states that a minimum of two months and sometimes as much as six months is required before the dancer is able to return to class. Furthermore, if appropriate treatment is not obtained, pain will tend to dramatically increase with very serious potential consequences, including complete bone fractures necessitating surgical treatment and prolonged disability.

Hip Fractures in the Elderly

Although not a problem with young dancers, in older individuals with osteoporosis, the large compressive forces borne by the hip during locomotion can result in fractures of the femoral neck. This is a very problematic fracture due to instability of the fracture site, the limited ability to form new bone, and close approximation of important blood vessels that can be readily injured by the fracture (Moore and Dalley, 1999). Fracture of the hip occurs with a startling frequency, particularly in females over the age of 45 years. Osteoporosis has been estimated to be responsible for 200,000 hip fractures per year; approximately 40,000 of these hip fractures result in death due to complications, making hip fractures a leading cause of death in older individuals in the

United States (Rasch, 1989). Regular physical activity and aggressive measures to prevent osteoporosis can reduce risk for this serious problem.

Osteoarthritis

The large forces borne by the hip can also result in damage to the joint cartilage instead of the bone. **Osteoarthritis** involves a progressive thinning and wearing away of the articular cartilage of the hip joint and associated inflammation. Osteoarthritis of the hip joint is frequently associated with dull, aching pain in the groin, outer thigh, or buttocks that is worse in the morning and gets better with light activity. However, this pain is classically aggravated by vigorous activity and relieved with rest. When the condition worsens, resting no longer relieves the hip or groin pain, which may also occur at night. Loss of hip range of motion, particularly hip internal rotation, is characteristic. Shortening of the hip flexors (contractures) also often occurs, negatively affecting the ability to stand or walk with desired pelvic mechanics and adding stress to the low back.

Treatment often involves activity modification and regular gentle exercise such as swimming, water aerobics, or cycling for strengthening of the hip musculature and maintaining range of motion without excessive joint loading (Browning, 2001). Various medications aimed at reducing pain, diminishing joint inflammation, promoting cartilage healing, or restoring the normal joint protective function of synovial fluid may be used by the attending physician (Marshall and Waddell, 2000). While current methods of early treatment probably cannot reverse osteoarthritis, they can reduce pain and slow the progression. When severe degeneration and pain exist, the orthopedic surgeon may recommend total hip replacement surgery.

The young age at which some dancers, and particularly male dancers, have had total hip replacements is very alarming. It is essential that further research be conducted to clarify contributing factors and possible interventions that can be used to reduce the risk of osteoarthritis for dancers.

Hip Muscle Strains

Muscle strain is one of the most common athletic injuries of the pelvis and hip. Various muscles can be involved, including the hamstrings, adductor longus, gracilis, sartorius, rectus femoris, and iliopsoas—with the hamstrings being most commonly involved. Multijoint muscles appear to be particularly susceptible to being strained. The mechanism of injury most often relates to movements in which the involved muscle is being either passively stretched or working eccentrically, such as with split stretches, large kicks to the front, split leaps, and flat back bounces. Strains can also occur with repetitive movements in which the muscle becomes fatigued such as with running, or with sudden forceful muscle contractions such as with the takeoff in sprinting or leaping.

Factors that have been theorized to increase the risk for muscle strains include inadequate strength, imbalanced strength between right and left sides (Burkett, 1970), imbalanced strength with antagonists, muscle fatigue, electrolyte imbalance, inadequate flexibility (Jonhagen, Nemeth, and Eriksson, 1994; Liemohn, 1978), inadequate warm-up (Dorman, 1971; Ekstrand and Gillquist, 1982; Safran et al., 1988; Warren, Lehmann, and Koblanski, 1971, 1976), and poor coordination and technique (Lacroix, 2000; Lieberman and Harwin, 1997). Furthermore, it is believed that these factors can interact to further increase injury risk (Worrell, 1994). So, for example, a dancer who is inadequately hydrated and has inadequate flexibility is more likely to sustain a strain than a dancer with just one of these factors. However, there are many studies with conflicting results, and additional dance-specific research is needed to better develop preventive measures.

Muscle strains tend to exhibit tenderness over the specific area of injury, and in some cases swelling and muscle spasm may be evident. Pain can generally be produced with stretch as well as with forceful contraction of the involved muscle. With skeletally immature dancers, it is also important to realize that the attachment of the muscle onto the bone is often less strong than the muscle or tendon itself, and thus an avulsion fracture may occur where the muscle is actually pulled off from this attachment site (Lieberman and Harwin, 1997).

Treatment will vary dramatically according to the degree of strain, but often it initially includes relative rest, anti-inflammatory medication, physical therapy modalities, and modification of activity to be pain free. In milder strains, extra warm-up of the area prior to class, use of a pain-free range during class (e.g., limiting the height of the leg to the front with a hamstring strain), and use of ice following class to decrease the inflammatory response may be recommended. With more severe strains, dance may have to be temporarily restricted; and when tolerated, swimming, stationary cycling, or a pool barre may be utilized to allow movement and slight conditioning in a pain-free manner.

As acute symptoms decline, institution of a progressive flexibility and strengthening program for the involved muscle is usually recommended. The strengthening exercises are often advanced from isometric to concentric, to eccentric, to functional exercises as tolerated (Jonhagen, Nemeth, and Eriksson, 1994; Worrell, 1994). This latter functional strengthening step is sometimes neglected by dancers and is essential to prevent the common tendency for strains to reoccur or become chronic (Best and Garrett, 1996; Garett, Califf, and Bassett III, 1984; Safran et al., 1988).

Iliopsoas Tendinitis

Because the iliopsoas is of primary importance during lifting of the leg above 90° to both the front and side, this muscle is used in a demanding and repetitive way in ballet and various other dance forms. Considering these demands, it is not surprising that the iliopsoas is a common site of injury in dancers. In addition to being strained, the tendon of the iliopsoas can also become inflamed; this condition is termed **iliopsoas tendinitis.** The iliopsoas tendon is believed to be particularly vulnerable when the hip is flexed, abducted, and externally rotated as when the dancer performs a développé or battement in second. This commonly used position has been theorized to cause the tendon to turn in a "U" as it passes beneath the inguinal ligament, such that it can readily become irritated (Sammarco, 1987).

Iliopsoas tendinitis occurs more frequently in females and is characterized by crepitus, pain, and stiffness in the groin area. As with other forms of tendinitis, pain is often present at the beginning, lessens during, and then increases after class or rehearsal. Pain is often also exacerbated by lifting the leg to a high level to the front or side.

Treatment commonly includes anti-inflammatory medicine, careful hip flexor stretching, and technique evaluation with correction if needed. In some cases, this condition is associated with "hiking" the hip and inadequate use of external rotation during movements such as développés. Strengthening of the iliopsoas and DOR while correcting technique can often help decrease symptoms and aid recovery.

The Snapping Hip Syndrome

Some dancers experience a snapping sound, or clunk, classically occurring when returning the leg to first or fifth position from a développé or extension to the side, and in some cases from a développé or extension to the front. This snapping is prevalent in dancers, and in one study of ballet dancers it accounted for almost half of the hip injuries seen (Quirk, 1983).

Various theories have been suggested regarding the mechanism of this snap, but one study provides strong evidence that the mechanism is likely the iliopsoas tendon snapping over the femoral head and hip capsule (Jacobson and Allen, 1990). This theory is further supported by anatomical studies that show that when the femur is externally rotated, the head of the femur is directed forward with the iliopsoas tendon crossing the head of the femur laterally (Caillet, 1996). However, when the femur is rotated inward, the iliopsoas tendon moves medially over the head of the femur and capsule and can produce a snap, click, or clunk. This snapping associated with the iliopsoas tendon is termed **internal snapping hip** (Schaberg, Harper, and Allen, 1984).

Treatment may include anti-inflammatory medication, stretching of the hip flexors, and correction of related dance technique. In the author's experience, this click often occurs when the dancer is failing to maintain full hip external rotation as the leg is lowered. Strengthening the hip external rotators, abductors, and iliopsoas while working on technique to maintain turnout and minimize letting the femur rotate inward as the leg is lowered can be useful in alleviating the snapping.

There is also another version of the snapping hip syndrome that involves the iliotibial band's movement over the greater trochanter as seen in figure 4.41. This lateral and more superficial version is called **external snapping hip.** In certain movements, one can palpate a snap by placing the fingers over the greater trochanter, and in some cases this snap can also be heard. This snap commonly accompanies ronds de jambe, standing on one leg and shifting the pelvis toward that leg, and landing from a leap. During landing from a leap, as the tensor fasciae latae muscle contracts to help stabilize the pelvis, its associated band of fascia may snap forward from behind the trochanter and jerk the pelvis into flexion (Sammarco, 1987). The dancer often reports a sensation of the hip slipping out of place.

Factors that have been suggested to increase the risk of external snapping hip include a wide pelvis, prominent trochanter, ligamental laxity, weakness of the hip abductors, "sitting" in the hip, and tightness of the iliotibial band (Khan et al., 1995; Lieberman and Harwin, 1997; Mercier, 1995; Reid et al., 1987; Teitz, 2000). In dancers, a prevalence of the last factor, iliotibial band tightness and associated low values of hip adduction, has been found. However, a study of runners found significant weakness of the hip abductors in the affected limb and reported 92% of the affected runners were pain free after a 6-week rehabilitation program that emphasized strengthening and stretching of the hip abductors (Fredericson, Guillet, and DeBenedictis, 2000).

Hence, treatment of external snapping hip should include stretching the hip abductors and iliotibial

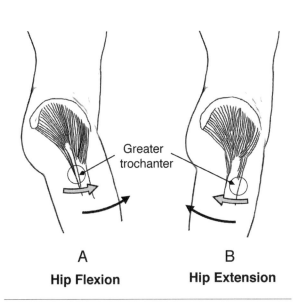

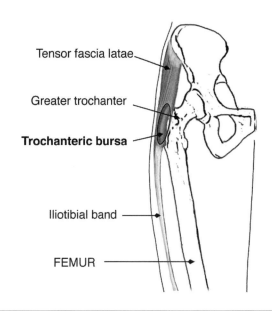

FIGURE 4.41   Snapping hip (right hip, lateral view). The iliotibial band snaps (A) forward with hip flexion and (B) backward when the hip extends.

FIGURE 4.42   Trochanteric bursitis includes inflammation of the bursa located superficial to the greater trochanter and deep to the iliotibial band (right hip, anterior view).

band and strengthening the hip abductors. Anti-inflammatory medication is sometimes prescribed. In the author's experience, the snapping often occurs when the dancer excessively shifts the pelvis laterally relative to the support leg and fails to maintain turnout on the support leg. Hence, strengthening the deep outward rotators, hip abductors, and hip adductors and applying use of these muscles to maintain full turnout with the pelvis appropriately positioned over the support foot will often be helpful for successful reduction of snapping and pain.

Trochanteric Bursitis

Sometimes independently or in association with external snapping hip, the bursa that lies over the greater trochanter and beneath the iliotibial band—the trochanteric bursa—becomes inflamed. When this bursa becomes inflamed and swollen it is readily further irritated by compression or movement of the overlying iliotibial band as seen in figure 4.42. Occasionally, calcium is deposited within the inflamed bursa. In dance, the mechanism of injury is theorized to be overuse from factors such as unbalanced pressures from dancing on a raked stage or alignment problems such as scoliosis, pelvic rotations, leg length differences, or excessive foot pronation on one side that cause weight to be unevenly borne by the legs. Tightness of the iliotibial band, a wide pelvis, inadequate hip abductor strength, and technique errors such as "sitting in the hip" may also

increase injury risk (Desiderio, 1988; Lieberman and Harwin, 1997).

Pain is generally present along the side of the hip, and palpation over the greater trochanter usually reveals localized tenderness and in some cases crepitus. Pain can often be reproduced if the dancer lies on the affected side or if the leg is passively or actively adducted across the midline of the body (Teitz, 2000). As with the external snapping hip, this pain is often exacerbated by rond de jambe or in landing on one leg from a leap or jump.

Treatment may include anti-inflammatory medication, heat application prior to class and ice after class, stretching of the iliotibial band, strengthening of the hip abductors, and working on dance technique to avoid excessive lateral tilt (Trendelenburg sign) or lateral shift of the pelvis. In some cases, aspiration of the fluid from the bursa and corticosteroid injection may be medically prescribed (Sammarco, 1987). If such conservative measures fail, recent research suggests that the gluteus medius tendon may be torn (Kagan II, 1999); this tear is similar to rotator cuff tears seen at the shoulder and discussed in chapter 7.

Piriformis Syndrome

Pain in the buttocks with or without pain radiating down the back of the ipsilateral thigh may be due to the **piriformis syndrome.** Spasm of the piriformis muscle, one of the DOR of the hip, can compress

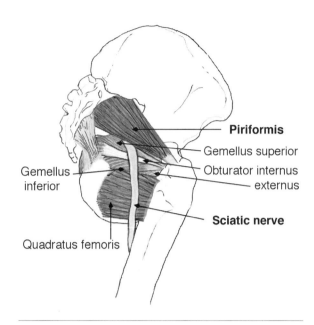

Piriformis

Gemellus superior

Obturator internus

externus

Sciatic nerve

Gemellus inferior

Quadratus femoris

FIGURE 4.43 Piriformis syndrome. Spasm of the piriformis muscle can create compression of the sciatic nerve (right hip, posterolateral view).

the adjacent sciatic nerve as seen in figure 4.43 and can produce the radiating symptoms characteristic of more serious back injury (Papadopoulos and Khan, 2004; Rich and McKeag, 1992). This condition occurs quite frequently in dancers, and possible reasons include the extensive use of external rotation with associated increased risk of strain, tightness, or imbalance with internal rotator strength and flexibility. It may also relate to technique issues (excessive activation of the upper DOR and insufficient use of the lower DOR in turnout) and posture (frequently seen with fatigue posture and dancers who "push" their pelvis forward to try to achieve greater turnout). A common association of piriformis spasm with sacroiliac dysfunction has also been noted, and piriformis syndrome occurs much more frequently in females than males.

Localized tenderness and muscle spasm are often present in the mid-buttocks region (area of the piriformis muscle). A dull aching pain in this same area often occurs after dancing and with extended sitting. Weakness of the hip abductors and tightness of the hamstrings (on the affected side) are commonly associated with this condition.

Treatment often initially emphasizes anti-inflammatory medicine and reducing muscle spasm. Ultrasound, passive stretching of the piriformis muscle, or use of ice massage or FluoriMethane spray while the muscle is stretched can sometimes provide relief (Roy and Irvin, 1983). Later, a balanced strength and flexibility program for both the external and internal

rotators, strengthening of the hip abductors, and correction of any related technique or alignment problems can be helpful. In an unresponsive case, a physician may elect to use an injection of an anesthetic and corticosteroid (Honorio et al., 2003).

Sacroiliac Inflammation and Dysfunction

The sacroiliac joints undergo great stresses as forces are translated to and from the torso and lower extremities. Injury can include ligaments, muscles, or neural structures related to the sacroiliac joints (Chen, Fredericson, and Smuck, 2002). In other cases, the problem is believed to be due to an actual disruption of normal motion of these joints termed **sacroiliac dysfunction.** Slight motion does exist in the sacroiliac joints, with translatory (0.1-1.6 millimeters) and angular movement (0.8-3.9°) occurring in predictable patterns along various axes (Sturesson, Selvik, and Uden, 1989). In some instances the os coxae can get wedged and "lock," most commonly with an anterior displacement of the os coxae on the sacrum (DonTigny, 1990). With exaggerated lumbar lordosis or spinal hyperextension or hip hyperextension, the os coxae will tend to move anterior on the sacrum. Since the sacrum is wider anteriorly, the os coxae may wedge and lock.

Due to differences in pelvic structure and hormones associated with pregnancy and menstruation, sacroiliac motion is markedly greater in females versus males, and sacroiliac problems are more prevalent in women than men (Colliton, 1999). In fact, it has been reported that 30% of males have fused sacroiliac joints (Hamill and Knutzen, 1995). Furthermore, with men, sacroiliac motion tends to decrease with aging, while with women the motion tends to increase (Smith, Weiss, and Lehmkuhl, 1996). Various mechanisms for sacroiliac injury have been described, including falling on the buttocks or hip, weightlifting or partnering, a sudden twisting motion, leaning forward, repetitive standing on one leg, and excessive lumbar lordosis.

Pain is often present posteriorly, over one or both sacroiliac joints. Sharp twinges of pain often occur with certain movements, and this association has been used to develop various pain provocation tests that can be helpful for distinguishing sacroiliac inflammation from other sources of pain (Young, Aprill, and Laslett, 2003). In some cases pain is also experienced in the buttocks, posterior thigh, or groin. When sacroiliac dysfunction is involved, limitation of range in specific motions of the hip is often present. For example, with anterior displacement of an os coxa, dancers will often say that their range in extensions to the front and side on the affected side is markedly reduced and that the hip feels "jammed." With anterior displacement, pain is often aggravated by movements that tend to bring the os coxae forward such as an arabesque. Weakness of the gluteus medius and tightness of the piriformis muscle are also frequently present, both of which tend to increase the stress on the sacroiliac joints and perpetuate the problem.

Treatment will vary according to the structures involved and type of displacement, if present. For example, with anterior displacement stretches in flexion, abdominal strengthening, and avoidance of hyperextension (such as accompanying a high arabesque) may be initially indicated, whereas with posterior displacement, back extensor strengthening and avoidance of flexion (such as accompanying curl-ups) may be initially indicated. In general, restoration of hip abductor strength and pelvic stabilization are key (Barclay and Vega, 2004), and reduction of piriformis and other muscle spasms are often also a focus. Gentle joint mobilization techniques, a sacroiliac belt to aid with stabilization, and correction of biomechanical factors such as true leg length difference with a heel lift are also sometimes prescribed. In select cases, physicians may utilize a corticosteroid injection for patients who do not respond to a comprehensive rehabilitation program (Chen, Fredericson, and Smuck, 2002).

Summary

The os coxae are joined anteriorly at the pubic symphysis and posteriorly indirectly via the sacroiliac joints to form the pelvic girdle. The pelvic girdle serves as a link between the torso and the lower limbs, and movements of the pelvis termed anterior pelvic tilt, posterior pelvic tilt, lateral tilt, and rotation help it move in coordination with the spine and femur via closed kinematic chain pelvic movements, the lumbar-pelvic rhythm, and the pelvic-femoral rhythm. When the lower limb is weight bearing, many of the muscles that classically move the limbs now serve key functions for creating the desired movements or stabilization of the pelvis. For example, the abdominal–hamstring force couple can help maintain a neutral pelvis in the sagittal plane, and the abductor mechanism prevents undesired lateral tilt of the pelvis in the frontal plane.

The hip joint is a ball-and-socket joint formed between the head of the femur and the acetabulum, and the angle of the neck of the femur relative to the shaft of the femur—femoral inclination and femoral torsion—influences potential hip range of motion and lower limb alignment. In general, the design of the hip favors stability through the depth of the acetabulum, extensive contact of articulating bones, a strong joint capsule and ligaments, and many large and powerful muscles that cross the hip joint. The joint capsule and iliofemoral and pubofemoral ligaments limit hip external rotation, hip extension, and posterior tilting of the pelvis and play an important role in helping passively maintain upright posture with less muscular contraction needed. Many of the 22 muscles that cross the hip joint have multiple actions at the hip joint, and some also have actions at the spine and knee. These muscles are important for movements of the lower limbs in all directions. Because the weight and length of these levers are so great, marked strength is required in key muscles to move these limbs through space in the extreme range of motion and with a specific aesthetic demanded by the dance form. Adequate flexibility is also essential to achieve these large-range open kinematic chain motions. Supplemental strength and flexibility exercises can help dancers achieve their performance goals, as well as help reduce injury risk.

Study Questions and Applications

1. Examine closely the location of the iliofemoral ligament in figure 4.4. Using the human skeleton model or your own body, review its functions and describe whether the following movements will make it taut or slack: (a) Anterior pelvic tilt, (b) posterior pelvic tilt, (c) hip external rotation.

2. Draw the following muscles on a skeletal chart, and use an arrow to indicate the line of pull of each muscle. Then, next to each muscle, list its actions. (a) Iliopsoas, (b) rectus femoris, (c) sartorius, (d) gluteus maximus, (e) hamstrings, (f) deep outward rotators (as a group), (g) tensor fasciae latae, (h) gluteus medius and minimus (as a group), (i) hip adductors (as a group).

3. Locate the muscles or muscle groups listed in question 2 on your body, perform actions that these muscles produce, and palpate their contraction.

4. Using figures 4.17 and 4.18 as a reference, identify the angle of femoral torsion on a femur from a disarticulated skeleton and examine how changing that angle would influence turnout and facing of the knees.

5. Working with a partner, demonstrate the fundamental movements of the pelvis (hip flexion, extension, abduction, adduction, external rotation, and internal rotation) on the partner, including both of the following: (a) where the pelvis is stationary and the thigh moves and (b) where the thigh is stationary and the pelvis moves.

6. Working with a partner, have the partner lie supine with both legs extended, and then measure the degree of hip flexion present on one side with the knee extended versus bent. Explain the difference and what could be done to make the two values more similar.

7. Using a skeletal model, evaluate how standing in a turned-out position would change the line of pull of the hip flexors, hip abductors, hip extensors, and hip adductors. Postulate how this might change muscle use in a second-position plié and in a side extension.

8. Analyze "lifting the hip" when performing a passé in terms of motions at the spine, lumbosacral joint, and hip joint proper. What muscle action could correct this undesired action? What dance cues could be used to try to achieve this correction for the dancer?

9. How does the abductor mechanism relate to standing on one leg in dance and the common errors of "sitting in the hip" or "hiking the hip"?

10. Demonstrate one exercise for strengthening and one exercise for stretching the following muscle groups: (a) hip flexors, (b) hip extensors, (c) hip abductors, (d) hip adductors, (e) hip external rotators.

11. When strengthening or stretching the hip extensors, how could one emphasize the hamstrings versus the gluteus maximus? When strengthening the iliopsoas, how could one emphasize the iliopsoas versus rectus femoris?

12. A dancer wishes to improve the height she can raise her leg to the side.

    a. Analyze this movement focusing on the hip of the gesture leg, including the joint movements, muscle groups, and sample muscles of the hip.

    b. Describe factors that would influence the degree of pelvic and spinal lateral tilt accompanying the motion of raising the leg.

    c. Identify appropriate strength and flexibility exercises that could be used to increase the height of the leg and how they could help. Provide three cues that could be utilized to try to implement the desired hip mechanics and technique.

CHAPTER FIVE

The Knee and Patellofemoral Joints

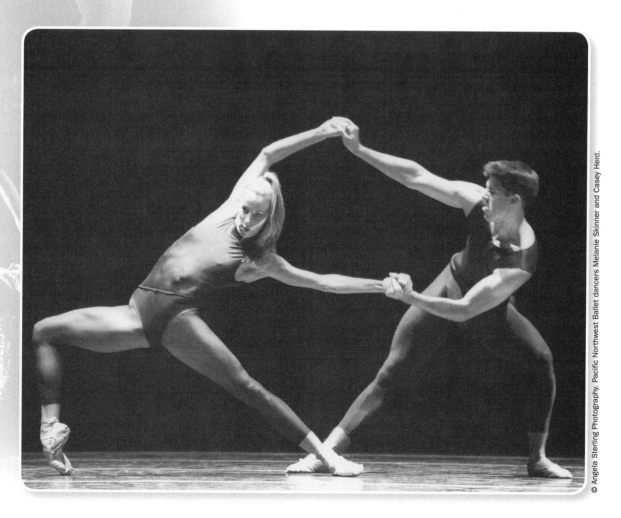

© Angela Sterling Photography. Pacific Northwest Ballet dancers Melanie Skinner and Casey Herd.

This chapter will consider the knee joint and the closely related patellofemoral joint. The knee is the largest articulation in the body, and it is exposed to tremendous stresses due to its location between the very long upright bones of the lower extremity. The knee must accept, transfer, and dissipate large forces from above, due to body weight and the effects of gravity, and below, from the impact associated with weight-bearing movements. Whenever the knee is bent while standing, gravity will tend to make it bend further, and the photo on page 237 exemplifies the skilled contraction of antigravity muscles required to prevent the body from collapsing and achieve the desired positioning of the knee. Although the associated patellofemoral joint, located just above the front of the knee joint proper, contributes additional stability to the tibiofemoral joint, it also must withstand very large forces. Both of these joints are vulnerable to twisting motions, making good alignment and technique during dance particularly important.

This chapter will present basic anatomy and mechanics of the knee and patellofemoral joints that influence optimal performance and the vulnerability of this joint to injury. Topics covered will include the following:

- Bones and bony landmarks of the knee region
- Joint structure and movements of the knee
- Description and functions of individual knee muscles
- Knee alignment and common deviations
- Knee mechanics
- Structure and movements of the patellofemoral joint
- Patellofemoral alignment and the Q angle
- Patellofemoral mechanics
- Muscular analysis of fundamental knee movements
- Key considerations for the knee in whole body movement
- Special considerations for the knee in dance
- Conditioning exercises for the knee
- Knee injuries in dancers

Bones and Bony Landmarks of the Knee Region

The femur, tibia, and patella are all bones that take part in the knee joints and patellofemoral joints. Recall from chapter 1 that the upper leg, or thigh bone, is termed the femur; the primary weight-bearing bone of the lower leg is termed the tibia; and the kneecap is termed the patella. The distal end of the femur is expanded with two enlargements termed the **medial** and **lateral condyles** as shown in figure 5.1. These condyles contain the smooth articular surfaces that rest on the upper tibia to form the knee joint proper. You can palpate a portion of the femoral condyles by bending your knee to 90° and then pressing your fingertips on the sides of the lower portion of the patella. To help locate these articular surfaces, repetitively slightly bend and straighten your knee from this 90° position and feel the condyles move under your fingertips. These condyles also bear prominent projections to the sides that are termed the **medial** and **lateral epicondyles.** You can locate the epicondyles by sliding your hand down your thigh toward the knee and finding the widest point of the knee, at the distal portion of the femur. On the front of the femur, between the condyles, sits a smooth, shallow, concave surface that cannot be palpated. It is termed the **femoral groove,** and it articulates with the patella. Posteriorly, a deeper indentation separates the medial and lateral condyles and is termed the **intercondylar fossa** (L. *inter,* between + *condylar,* condyles + *fossa,* trench), or intercondylar notch (figure 5.1B).

The proximal end of the tibia is also expanded and contains two condyles, again termed the medial and lateral condyles. In contrast to what occurs with the femur, the superior surfaces of these condyles are relatively flat or slightly concave versus rounded, and hence this upper surface is called the **tibial plateau.** On this superior surface of the tibia in between the flattened tibial condyles is a roughened area termed the **anterior** and **posterior intercondylar areas** that contains two small peaks or projections termed the **intercondylar eminence** (L. prominence). The intercondylar eminence serves as an attachment site for ligaments and helps stabilize the tibia and femur during weight bearing. On the anterior tibia, approximately 1/2 inch (1.3 centimeters) from its proximal end are a roughened area and projection called the **tibial tuberosity** (L. *tuberosus,* lump), or tibial tubercle. You can easily palpate this tuberosity by running your finger down the middle of the kneecap and along the patellar tendon until you feel a bump on the tibia: This is the tibial tuberosity.

The patella is approximately triangular in shape with its narrow apex projecting downward and termed the **inferior pole** of the patella. The upper, flatter edge of the patella is called the **superior border,** and the side edges are called the **medial** and **lateral borders.** The undersurface of the patella bears angled surfaces termed **facets,** which articulate with the underlying femur.

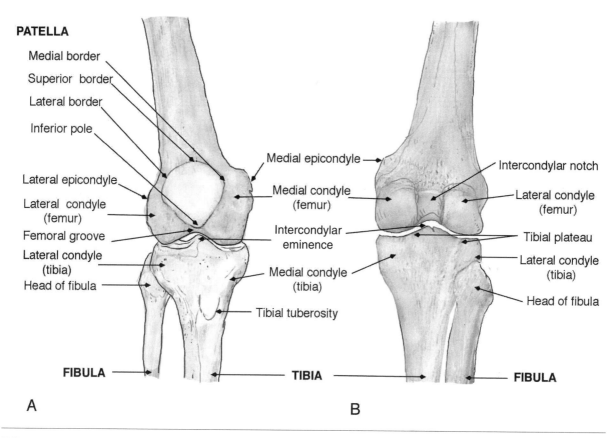

PATELLA
- Medial border
- Superior border
- Lateral border
- Inferior pole
- Lateral epicondyle
- Lateral condyle (femur)
- Femoral groove
- Lateral condyle (tibia)
- Head of fibula

- Medial epicondyle
- Medial condyle (femur)
- Intercondylar eminence
- Medial condyle (tibia)
- Tibial tuberosity

- Intercondylar notch
- Lateral condyle (femur)
- Tibial plateau
- Lateral condyle (tibia)
- Head of fibula

FIBULA   **TIBIA**   **FIBULA**

A   B

FIGURE 5.1   Bones and bony landmarks of the knee region (right knee). (A) Anterior view, (B) posterior view.

Joint Structure and Movements of the Knee

The knee is very complex in its structure and function and is thought to have evolved from three separate joints. Although there is only one joint cavity, the following three articulations are present.

1. Between the medial condyle of the femur and the slightly concave medial plateau of the tibia

2. Between the lateral condyle of the femur and the slightly concave lateral plateau of the tibia

3. Between the backside of the kneecap and the underlying surface on the anterior femur, the femoral groove

The first two articulations between the femoral condyles and tibia compose the **tibiofemoral joint,** or what is commonly referred to as the knee joint. As with other synovial joints, the articular surfaces are covered by articular cartilage that reduces friction and aids with the distribution and absorption of forces. The third articulation is named the patellofemoral joint and will be discussed in a later section of this chapter.

Knee Joint Classification and Associated Movements

The tibiofemoral joint is a modified hinge joint, and its primary joint motions are flexion (or bending) of the knee and extension (or straightening) of the knee (see figure 5.2). In addition, its motion also incorporates slight internal and external rotation, and hence it is termed a "modified" hinge joint.

Knee Joint Capsule and Ligaments

The knee joint is surrounded by an extensive and irregular joint capsule lined with the largest synovial membrane found in the body (Hamill and Knutzen, 1995). In 20% to 60% of people, this membrane contains a permanent fold, termed a **plica** (L. a fold), that sometimes becomes inflamed. The stability offered by this joint capsule is reinforced by numerous strong ligaments. More than at any other joint in the body, the ligaments are essential to stabilize and guide the relative movements of the bones coming together to form the joint (Magee, 1997). However, these ligaments are arranged such that ligamentous stability is not constant (Kreighbaum and Barthels,

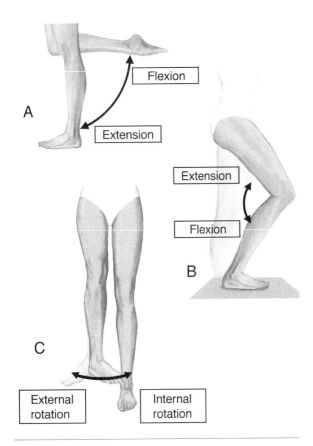

FIGURE 5.2   Movements of the knee joint. (A) Open kinematic chain flexion-extension, (B) closed kinematic chain flexion-extension, (C) external rotation-internal rotation.

1996). Instead, key ligaments are taut to favor stability when the knee is extended, while key ligaments are slack to favor mobility when the knee is flexed.

Four knee ligaments that are particularly important are the paired collateral ligaments and the paired cruciate ligaments. As seen in figure 5.3, the collateral ligaments run longitudinally on each side of the knee, while the paired cruciate ligaments are located within the knee joint.

Medial Collateral Ligament (Tibial Collateral Ligament)

The collateral (side by side) ligament located on the inside of the knee joint is called the **medial collateral ligament** (MCL) or tibial collateral ligament (see figure 5.3). This ligament is composed of two layers, a superficial and a deep layer (Magee, 1997). The superficial layer is a broad, flat, membranous band that joins the medial condyles of the femur and tibia. The deep layer of this ligament runs inferiorly from its proximal attachment on the medial condyle of the femur and merges with the joint capsule and with the capsular fibers that attach the margins of the medial meniscus to the edge of the tibial condyle

(coronary ligaments). Although the medial collateral ligament is stronger than its lateral counterpart (the lateral collateral ligament), it is much more frequently injured.

The medial collateral ligament becomes taut with knee extension and external rotation. It is key for medial stability of the knee and is the principal restraint to forces that tend to open up the inside of the knee, termed **valgus stress** (L. *valgus,* turned outward). At 25° to 30° of knee flexion, almost 80% of the valgus stress to the knee is supported by the medial collateral ligament (Besier, Lloyd, Cochrane, and Ackland, 2001). This valgus type of stress can occur in dance when the knee is allowed to fall inward relative to the foot, for example in a poorly performed plié. The medial collateral ligament also is a key restraint for external rotation of the tibia whether the knee is flexed or extended (Levangie and Norkin, 2001). This may contribute to the vulnerability of the medial collateral ligament to injury in dancers.

Lateral Collateral Ligament (Fibular Collateral Ligament)

The collateral ligament located on the outside of the knee joint is called the **lateral collateral liga-**

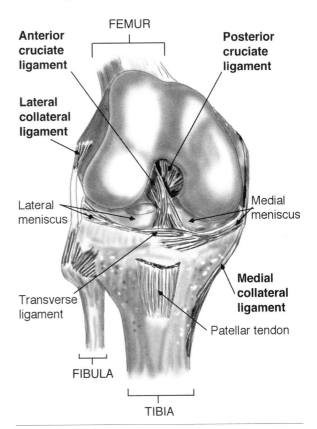

FIGURE 5.3   Key knee ligaments and the menisci (right knee, anterior view).

ment (LCL) or fibular collateral ligament. The lateral collateral ligament is cordlike in shape and joins the lateral condyle of the femur with the head of the fibula. It becomes taut with knee extension. This ligament helps provide lateral stability to the knee and is the primary constraint to forces that tend to open up the lateral aspect of the knee, termed **varus stress** (L. *varus*, bent inward). It has been estimated that the lateral collateral ligament supports close to 70% of the varus stress applied to the knee (Besier, Lloyd, Cochrane, and Ackland, 2001). An example of this varus stress would occur if the dancer were to sit with the lower legs crossed with the feet resting on the inside of the knees, such as is done in the yoga lotus position. Dynamically, varus stress would occur in lateral movements and crossover movements like a grapevine.

The lateral collateral ligament may also assist the medial collateral ligament and other structures in limiting external rotation of the tibia, particularly at about 35° of knee flexion (Levangie and Norkin, 2001). Both of the collateral ligaments slacken with knee flexion, and lessening of these constraints is vital for allowing functional rotation of the tibia used in movements such as pivoting.

Anterior Cruciate Ligament

The cruciate ligaments (L. *cruciatus*, shaped like a cross) are strong, cordlike ligaments that internally join the tibia and femur. These ligaments derive their name from the fact that they cross within the knee joint. The **anterior cruciate ligament** (ACL) runs from the anterior intercondylar area of the tibia upward and backward and outward to insert onto the inner and back part of the lateral femoral condyle. As could be postulated from its attachments, this ligament is important for preventing anterior displacement of the tibia relative to the femur, or posterior displacement of the femur relative to the tibia; and it has been estimated that the ACL is responsible for 85% of the force that restrains anterior displacement of the tibia (Irrgang, 1993). The ACL also has secondary functions of helping to control rotation of the knee (Diduch, Scuderi, and Scott, 1997), varus and valgus stresses, and hyperextension when the knee is fully extended (Caillet, 1996; Magee, 1997). The rotary restraints offered by the cruciates are important for normal functioning of the locking mechanism of the knee, discussed later in this chapter. Functionally, the anterior cruciate plays a particularly key role when large forces or deceleration is involved as with jumping, lowering the body down to the floor, or quick changes of direction in dance. This ligament is essential for joint integrity, and its loss critically affects stability and alters the normal mechanics of the knee.

Posterior Cruciate Ligament

The **posterior cruciate ligament (PCL)** runs from the posterior intercondylar area of the tibia upward, forward, and inward to attach to the outer and front part of the medial femoral condyle. The posterior cruciate is key in preventing posterior displacement of the tibia relative to the femur or anterior displacement of the femur relative to the tibia. It is easiest to remember the functions of the cruciate ligaments relative to the tibia; that is, the anterior cruciate prevents anterior displacement of the tibia while the posterior cruciate prevents posterior displacement of the tibia. The posterior cruciate has been estimated to provide 95% of the total restraining force to posterior movement of the tibia, termed "posterior drawer" (Butler, Noyes, and Grood, 1980). Unlike what occurs with the knee ligaments previously discussed, a majority of the posterior cruciate ligament appears to become taut with knee flexion versus extension, and some authors hold that it is the key stabilizer of the knee when the knee is not extended. During early knee flexion, the posterior cruciate ligament becomes taut when the tibia displaces posteriorly and then becomes the fulcrum about which further knee flexion occurs (Caillet, 1996). Large forces have been shown to be borne by this ligament when deep knee flexion is performed, such as in a parallel squat (Escamilla, 2001). However, the posterior cruciate ligament is 20% to 50% greater in cross-sectional area, up to 50% stronger (Diduch, Scuderi, and Scott, 1997), and less commonly injured than the anterior cruciate.

Ligamental Stress Tests

Simple ligamental stress tests that are performed by physicians are shown in Tests and Measurements 5.1 to illustrate the key function of the primary ligaments just discussed. The presence of abnormal or pathologic motion suggests that the ligament serving as a primary constraint to that motion is injured. Many more complex tests are also classically performed that utilize multiplane motions and incorporate rotation to further evaluate functional stability of the knee.

Specialized Structures of the Knee

Various specialized structures are associated with the knee that provide additional joint stability and aid with knee function. These structures include the menisci, bursae, and iliotibial band.

Selected Orthopedic Stress Tests for the Knee

Selected tests are shown that are commonly performed by physicians to test the stability of the knee and evaluate ligamental injury. Consider each test in terms of the restraints offered by a normal, intact ligament and the excessive motion that would be allowed if injury occurred. In A, the hands are positioned to apply a valgus stress to a slightly bent knee to evaluate the integrity of the medial collateral ligament. When the medial collateral ligament is torn, excessive "opening up" of the inside of the knee is evident. In B, the hands are positioned to apply a varus stress to evaluate the integrity of the lateral collateral ligament. When the lateral collateral ligament is severely torn, excessive "opening up" of the outside of the knee may occur. In C, the hands are positioned to pull the tibia forward to evaluate the integrity of the anterior cruciate ligament (ACL). When the ACL is torn, excessive anterior displacement of the tibia relative to the femur is evident. In D, the hands are positioned to carefully press the tibia backward to evaluate the integrity of the posterior cruciate ligament. When the posterior cruciate ligament is torn, excessive posterior displacement of the tibia occurs; and even before the posterior pressure is applied, the tibia will appear farther back than normal ("posterior sag") as evidenced by a concavity beneath the patella.

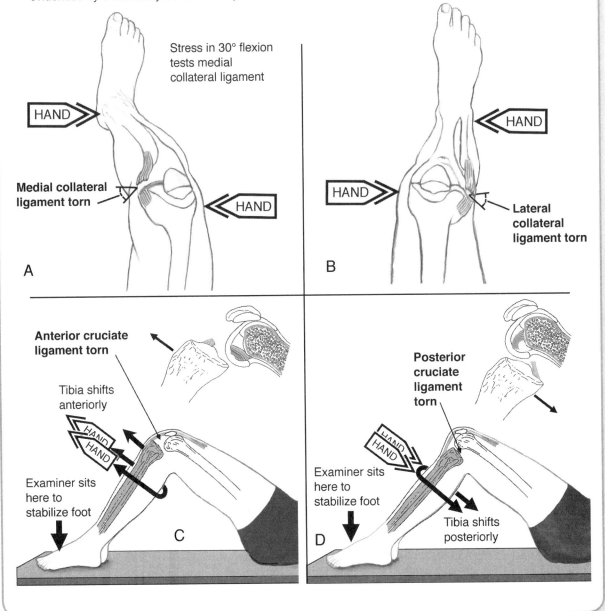

The Menisci

The **menisci** (G. *meniskos,* crescent)—the **medial meniscus** and **lateral meniscus**—are two fibrocartilage discs that sit on the tibial plateau and form the articular surface for the respective medial and lateral condyles of the femur as seen in figure 5.4. These menisci are thicker around their perimeter than centrally, and so form a kind of collar that aids in joint integrity by increasing the depth and fit of the articulation. The inferior surfaces of the menisci are flat to contour to the tibial plateaus, whereas the superior surfaces are concave to conform to the shape of the femoral condyles. By helping to overcome the difference in contour between the articulating femoral condyles and tibial condyles, and providing more surface area of contact between these bones, the menisci also help absorb shock, decrease frictional wear, and facilitate knee movements. Furthermore, due to the properties of cartilage (viscoelastic properties), when they are loaded they further increase the contact area and decrease joint stresses—approximately doubling the contact area in the joint and bearing as much as 45% of the total load absorbed by the knee (Hall, 1999; Hamill and Knutzen, 1995; Soderberg, 1986). Moreover, the further separation of the joint surfaces they provide allows for greater lubrication of the joint, and a 20% increase in friction has been demonstrated to occur with removal of the meniscus. The vital importance of the menisci is evidenced by the tendency for early degenerative changes in knees where a meniscus has been surgically removed due to injury.

The medial meniscus is larger in circumference than the lateral and is "C" shaped, barely forming a semicircle. The lateral meniscus is more "O" shaped, almost forming a complete circle, except where it attaches to the intercondylar area. The medial and lateral menisci are joined to each other anteriorly via the transverse ligament. The menisci are joined to the tibia anteriorly at the anterior intercondylar area, posteriorly at the posterior intercondylar area, and by vertical fibers of the coronary ligaments along their periphery to the edges of the tibial condyles. The inner borders, superior surface, and inferior surface of the menisci are free. The medial meniscus is also securely attached to the medial collateral ligament and one of the medial hamstring muscles (the semimembranosus), making the medial meniscus less freely movable than the lateral. During knee flexion, the menisci move posteriorly with the femur, with the more movable lateral meniscus traveling approximately twice as far (0.4 vs. 0.2 inches [11 vs. 5 millimeters]) as the medial (Dye and Vaupel, 2000). During knee extension, the menisci move anteriorly with the femur. Perhaps partly due to its firmer attachments and more restricted movement, the medial meniscus is much more frequently injured than the lateral meniscus (Caillet, 1996).

Bursae

More than 20 bursae are commonly present around the knee joint (Hamill and Knutzen, 1995). For example, as illustrated in figure 5.5, one bursa lies beneath the distal tendons of a group of muscles key for medial

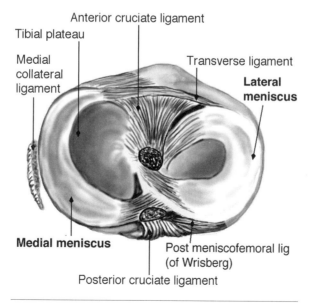

FIGURE 5.4   The menisci and selected associated structures (right knee, superior view).

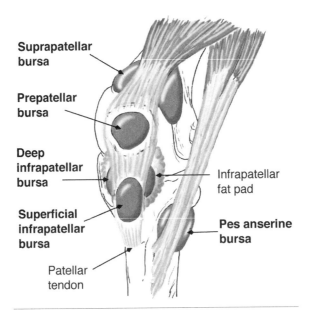

Suprapatellar
bursa

Prepatellar
bursa

Deep
infrapatellar
bursa

Superficial
infrapatellar
bursa

Patellar
tendon

Infrapatellar
fat pad

Pes anserine
bursa

FIGURE 5.5   Selected bursae of the knee (right knee,
anteromedial view).

rotation of the tibia (pes anserine bursa). Anteriorly, bursae lie between the anterior surface of the patella and the overlying skin (prepatellar bursa), as well as underneath (deep infrapatellar bursa) and in front of (superficial infrapatellar bursa) the patellar tendon. With the use of floor work in dance, some of these bursae can readily become inflamed (bursitis).

Iliotibial Band

Recall that the iliotibial band is a fascial band that begins superiorly at the ilium and runs down the side of the thigh to attach to the lateral condyle of the femur, the posterior femur, the patella, and the lateral condyle of the tibia. The tensor fasciae latae, described in the previous chapter on the hip, inserts into this band (figure 4.6, p. 166). When the tensor fasciae latae contracts, it tightens the iliotibial band, which makes this band's function similar to that of a dynamic ligament of the knee. Due to the anterior attachments of some of its fibers, some hold that the iliotibial band can act as a knee extensor when the knee is slightly flexed (0° to 30° knee flexion), but then it acts as a flexor of the knee when the knee is flexed greater than 40° (Dye and Vaupel, 2000). Although controversial, the tensor fasciae latae via the iliotibial band may also assist with external rotation of the tibia or knee (Smith, Weiss, and Lehmkuhl, 1996). The iliotibial band is unique to humans and appears to be a unique adaptation to the demands of erect posture, providing key lateral support to the knee as well as the hip.

Muscles

In addition to the vital ligaments of the knee, various additional muscles that cross the knee provide additional stability to this joint. Some of these muscles, particularly the quadriceps femoris, have also been shown to serve as important shock absorbers that play a significant role in protecting the knee from early degenerative changes.

Description and Functions of Individual Knee Muscles

Twelve muscles cross the knee joint and aid the ligaments with providing stability, as well as give rise to the movements of the knee. The most important muscular support is provided by the quadriceps complex anteriorly and the hamstrings posteriorly. Slight lateral support is also offered by the lateral hamstring muscle, the biceps femoris. Slight medial support is provided by one of the medial hamstring members, the semitendinosus, as well as by other members of the pes anserinus (sartorius and gracilis). A more detailed description of these muscles can be found in Individual Muscles of the Knee on pages 245-250 and 251. Note that many of these muscles cross multiple joints and also can produce movement at the hip or ankle as well as the knee.

Individual Muscles of the Knee

Anterior Muscles of the Knee

The anterior muscles of the knee are the quadriceps femoris group. Because the knee flexes in the opposite direction (with the distal segment moving posteriorly vs. anteriorly) to many of the other synovial joints, anterior muscles of the knee produce extension of the knee. This is in contrast to the spine, hip, shoulder, elbow, wrist, and fingers, where concentric contraction of anterior muscles from anatomical position produces flexion at their respective joints.

Attachments and Primary Actions of the Quadriceps Femoris

Muscle	Proximal attachment(s)	Distal attachment(s)	Primary action(s)
Quadriceps femoris (KWOD-ri-seps FEM-o-ris)			
Rectus femoris (REK-tus FEM-o-ris)	Anterior inferior iliac spine Posterior head: just above acetabulum	Tibial tuberosity via patellar tendon	Knee extension (Hip flexion)
Vastus medialis (VAS-tus me-dee-A-lis)	Medial and posterior surfaces of femur	Quadriceps femoris tendon and medial border of patella	Knee extension
Vastus intermedius (VAS-tus in-ter-ME-dee-us)	Anterior and lateral aspects of femur	Quadriceps femoris tendon and superior border of patella	Knee extension
Vastus lateralis (VAS-tus lat-er-A-lis)	Upper lateral and posterior surfaces of femur	Quadriceps femoris tendon and lateral border of patella	Knee extension

Quadriceps Femoris

The **quadriceps femoris** group is located on the front of the thigh, and as its name indicates (L. *quattuor,* four + *capus,* head), it is composed of four muscles: the **rectus femoris** (L. *rectus,* straight + *femoris,* femur) **vastus lateralis** (L. lateral great muscle), **vastus intermedius** (L. intermediate great muscle), and **vastus medialis** (L. medial great muscle). The rectus femoris, seen in figure 5.6A, is the only one of this muscle group that crosses the hip joint, and its function as a flexor of the hip was discussed in chapter 4. The remaining quadriceps, the three vasti muscles (L. *vastus,* great) seen in figure 5.6B, originate from the femur and so can produce joint movement only at the knee, not the hip. As their names suggest, the vastus medialis is the most medially located of the vasti, and the lateralis is the most laterally located. The vastus intermedius lies between these two muscles and underneath the rectus femoris. The tendons of all four of the quadriceps muscles converge to form the quadriceps femoris tendon. The quadriceps femoris tendon attaches to the superior patella, and the patella is then attached to the tuberosity of the tibia via the patellar tendon. Hence, although the quadriceps converge onto the patella, the continuing attachment of the patella onto the tibia allows the quadriceps femoris group to act as powerful extensors of the knee.

All of the quadriceps act as prime movers to produce knee extension such as in a frappé or maintain knee extension such as in the gesture leg during a rond de jambe. When the knee is in weight-bearing positions, gravity tends to produce knee flexion, and the quadriceps play a key antigravity function in movements such as pliés, walking, running, and jumping. Given this antigravity function, it is not surprising that the quadriceps are one of the strongest muscle groups in the body. They are capable of generating greater than 1,000 pounds (454 kilograms) of force (Hamill and Knutzen, 1995; Smith, Weiss, and Lehmkuhl, 1996).

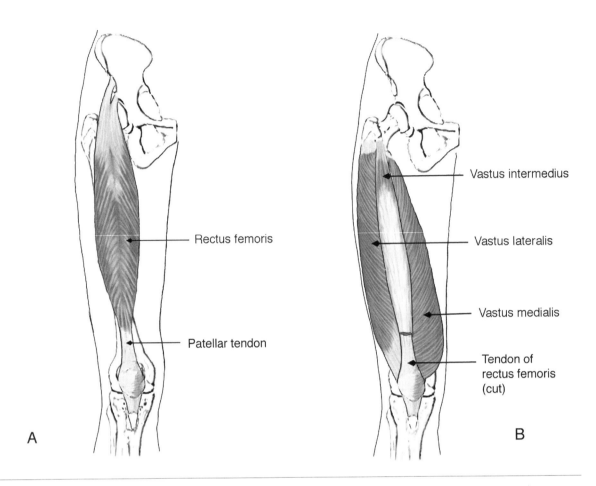

FIGURE 5.6   The quadriceps femoris (right knee, anterior view). (A) Rectus femoris, (B) the three vasti muscles.

Palpation: You can palpate the rectus femoris running down the middle of the front of the thigh. You can palpate the vastus intermedius under the rectus when you approach from the medial or lateral side. The vastus lateralis can be palpated laterally to the rectus, from just below the greater trochanter down to the patella. The distal portion of the vastus medialis can easily be palpated medial to the rectus femoris along the lower third of the thigh. If you place the palm of your hand on the upper thigh in a sitting position, you can feel the whole quadriceps femoris group contracting under your hand if you raise the leg to the front with the knee bent (hip flexion) and then extend the knee as you would with a parallel front développé.

Posterior Muscles of the Knee

The posterior muscles of the knee are the hamstrings, popliteus, and gastrocnemius. The hamstrings and gastrocnemius are multijoint muscles, while the popliteus only crosses and acts on the knee joint.

Hamstrings

As described in the preceding chapter on the hip, the hamstrings—the biceps femoris, semitendinosus, and semimembranosus—originate from the ischial tuberosity of the pelvis (figure 5.7A) and the posterior femur (figure 5.7B) and attach distally below the knee on the tibia and fibula. All three of the hamstrings act to produce knee flexion and can help prevent knee hyperextension. In addition, they can contribute to rotary movements of the knee. The semitendinosus (L. *semi,* half + *tendinosus,* tendon) and semimembranosus (L. *semi,* half + *membranosus,* membrane) insert medially on the tibia and so

Attachments and Primary Actions of Hamstring Muscles

Muscle	Proximal attachment(s)	Distal attachment(s)	Primary action(s)
Hamstrings			
Biceps femoris (BI-seps FEM-o-ris)	Long head: ischial tuberosity Short head: linea aspera of femur	Head of fibula Lateral tibial condyle	Knee flexion Knee external rotation (Hip extension) (Hip external rotation)
Semitendinosus (sem-ee-ten-di-NO-sus)	Ischial tuberosity	Medial surface of upper tibia (pes anserinus)	Knee flexion Knee internal rotation (Hip extension) (Hip internal rotation)
Semimembranosus (sem-ee-mem-brah-NO-sus)	Ischial tuberosity	Medial condyle of tibia	Knee flexion Knee internal rotation (Hip extension) (Hip internal rotation)

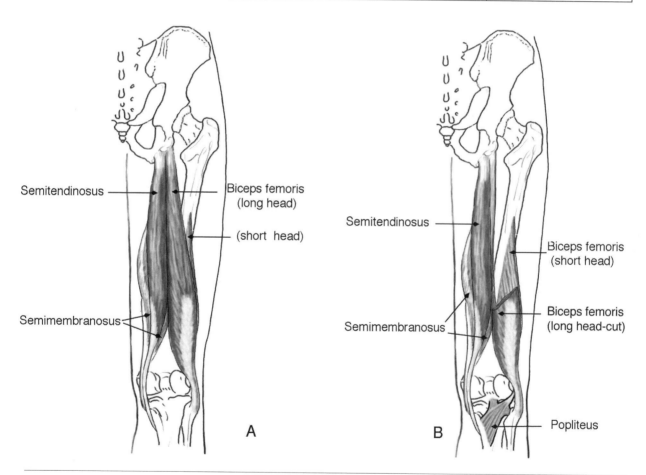

FIGURE 5.7   The hamstrings and popliteus muscles (right knee, posterior view). (A) Superficial view of hamstrings, (B) popliteus and long head cut to show short head of biceps femoris.

cause slight medial rotation of the tibia or knee. In contrast, the biceps femoris (*bi*, dual + L. *capus*, head) inserts laterally on the fibula and tibia and so its action is slight external rotation of the tibia or knee. In dance forms utilizing turnout, slight use of the biceps femoris is often encouraged to help continue the turnout, primarily effected at the hip, through the lower leg.

Palpation: Stand on your left leg with the ball of your right foot about 10 inches (25 centimeters) behind the left foot and the right knee bent. In this position the biceps femoris can be palpated on the right leg along the lateral posterior thigh, with the tendon easily palpated immediately proximal to the back of the knee. The semitendinosus tendon can also be palpated immediately proximal to the back of the knee, only on the medial side of the posterior thigh. The semimembranosus can be palpated on either side of the semitendinosus tendon. Flexing the knee by lifting the foot off the floor, with your hand placed just above the knee joint (posteriorly), allows you to feel the hamstrings contracting and makes the tendons more prominent.

Attachments and Primary Actions of the Popliteus

Muscle	Proximal attachment(s)	Distal attachment(s)	Primary action(s)
Popliteus (pop-LIT-ee-us)	Tripartite tendon: 1. Lateral femoral condyle 2. Head of fibula 3. Posterior aspect of lateral meniscus	Medial posterior aspect of upper tibia	External rotation of femur (when foot fixed) Internal rotation of tibia (when foot free) "Unlocking" knee

Popliteus

The **popliteus** is a small muscle running behind the knee, as shown in figure 5.7B, that is key for knee joint stability and proper mechanics. It is the most deeply located muscle in this region, lying close to the knee joint capsule. It attaches proximally to the lateral femoral condyle, lateral meniscus, and fibula, and distally to the posteromedial aspect of the tibia. When the tibia is fixed such as during weight bearing, the popliteus (L. *poples*, ham/posterior knee) acts to externally rotate the femur and also withdraws the lateral meniscus at the beginning of knee flexion. When the knee is straight, this external rotation function is important to unlock the knee and allow flexion to proceed. In open versus closed kinematic chain conditions when the tibia is free, such as when one performs a circling motion of the foot in the air (rond de jambe en l'air), the femur acts as the fixed segment and the popliteus acts on the tibia versus the femur, producing internal rotation of the tibia.

Palpation: Because of its deep location and because it is covered by the plantaris and lateral head of the gastrocnemius, the popliteus cannot be readily palpated.

Gastrocnemius and Plantaris

The gastrocnemius and plantaris are more fully described in chapter 6 with the ankle and foot (figure 6.15, p. 313). The **plantaris** (L. relating to the sole of the foot) can act as a weak assistant to knee flexion. The **gastrocnemius** (G. *gaster*, belly + *kneme*, leg) originates above the femoral condyles and inserts into the calcaneus via the Achilles tendon. In non-weight-bearing positions, such as a back attitude, the gastrocnemius may assist with knee flexion. However, when the foot is fixed and the knee is in strong extension, such as when functioning as the support leg during movements at the barre or center floor, the gastrocnemius may reverse its role and pull down and back on the femoral condyles and help maintain knee extension versus producing knee flexion.

Additional Secondary Muscles of the Knee

The sartorius and gracilis are biarticular muscles whose primary function at the hip was discussed in chapter 4, but they also cross and can act on the knee joint. They insert on the medial aspect of the proximal tibia in combination with the semitendinosus. The tendinous expansions of these three muscles where they attach onto the medial tibia are referred to as the **pes anserinus** (L. *pes*, foot + *anser*, goose) as seen in figure 5.8. The sartorius and gracilis aid the medial hamstrings with knee flexion and internal rotation of the tibia or knee. However, depending on the specific insertion of the muscle, when the knee is in full extension or hyperextension, the line of pull may pass anterior to the knee axis such that it reverses its function to being an extensor of the knee (Basmajian and DeLuca, 1985). This may be one mechanism that dancers use for helping maintain extension of the knee with less quadriceps activation when raising the leg to the front.

Summary of Knee Muscle Attachments and Actions

A summary of the attachments of the muscles that cross the knee is provided in table 5.1, and some of the more primary of these muscles and their attachments are shown in figures 5.9, A and B, and 5.10, A and B. From these resources, deduce the line of pull and resultant possible actions of the primary muscles of the knee, and then check for accuracy by referring to figures 5.9C and 5.10C.

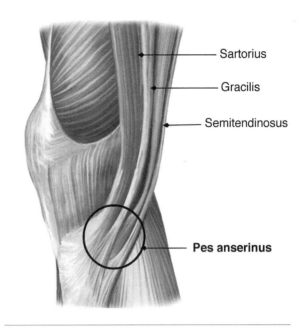

FIGURE 5.8   Pes anserinus (right knee, medial view).

TABLE 5.1   Summary of Attachments and Primary Actions* of Knee Muscles

Muscle	Proximal attachment(s)	Distal attachment(s)	Primary action(s)
Anterior muscles			
Quadriceps femoris (KWOD-ri-seps FEM-o-ris)			
Rectus femoris (REK-tus FEM-o-ris)	Anterior inferior iliac spine Posterior head: just above acetabulum	Tibial tuberosity via patellar tendon	Knee extension (Hip flexion)
Vastus medialis (VAS-tus me-dee-A-lis)	Medial and posterior surfaces of femur	Quadriceps femoris tendon and medial border of patella	Knee extension
Vastus intermedius (VAS-tus in-ter-ME-dee-us)	Anterior and lateral aspects of femur	Quadriceps femoris tendon and superior border of patella	Knee extension
Vastus lateralis (VAS-tus lat-er-A-lis)	Upper lateral and posterior surfaces of femur	Quadriceps femoris tendon and lateral border of patella	Knee extension
Posterior muscles			
Hamstrings			
Biceps femoris (BI-seps FEM-o-ris)	Long head: ischial tuberosity Short head: linea aspera of femur	Head of fibula Lateral tibial condyle	Knee flexion Knee external rotation (Hip extension) (Hip external rotation)
Semitendinosus (sem-ee-ten-di-NO-sus)	Ischial tuberosity	Medial surface of upper tibia (pes anserinus)	Knee flexion Knee internal rotation (Hip extension) (Hip internal rotation)

(continued)

TABLE 5.1 **Summary of Attachments and Primary Actions* of Knee Muscles** (continued)

Muscle	Proximal attachment(s)	Distal attachment(s)	Primary action(s)
Posterior muscles (continued)			
Hamstrings (continued)			
Semimembranosus (sem-ee-mem-brah-NO-sus)	Ischial tuberosity	Medial condyle of tibia	Knee flexion Knee internal rotation (Hip extension) (Hip internal rotation)
Popliteus (pop-LIT-ee-us)	Tripartite tendon: 1. Lateral femoral condyle 2. Head of fibula 3. Posterior aspect of lateral meniscus	Medial posterior aspect of upper tibia	External rotation of femur (when foot fixed) Internal rotation of tibia (when foot free) "Unlocking" knee
Additional secondary muscles			
Gracilis	Just below symphysis on pubis, inferior rami of ischium and pubis	Medial surface of upper tibia (pes anserinus)	Knee flexion (Hip adduction) (Hip flexion)
Sartorius	Anterior superior iliac spine (ASIS) and area just below	Medial surface of upper tibia (pes anserinus)	Knee flexion (Hip flexion) (Hip abduction) (Hip external rotation)
Tensor fasciae latae	Anterior outer crest of ilium, lateral aspect of anterior superior iliac spine	Tibia via iliotibial band	Lateral support of knee (Terminal knee extension) (Knee external rotation) (Hip abduction) (Hip flexion) (Hip internal rotation)
Gastrocnemius	Medial and lateral femoral condyles	Calcaneus (foot) via Achilles tendon	Knee flexion (Ankle plantar flexion)

*Special circumstances for action or action at other joints given in parentheses

Knee Alignment and Common Deviations

Knee alignment can be evaluated relative to the frontal, sagittal, or transverse plane. Appropriate alignment of the bones involved in the knee joint can have important implications in terms of how stresses are borne and the resultant injury predispositions, as well as for one's ability to meet the performance and aesthetic demands of dance. Common alignment deviations include valgus angulation, genu recurvatum, and tibial torsion.

Valgus Angulation

As discussed in chapter 4, when one views the legs from the front or back, the shafts of the femur are not totally vertical but rather angle slightly inward, with the knees more medial than either the femoral head or greater trochanter. Due to this femoral obliquity in the frontal plane, it is normal for the tibia to angle outward slightly relative to the femur. This angulation functions to help establish an approximately vertical positioning of the tibia, desirable for transfer of body weight. The angle between the femur and tibia, which opens out laterally, is termed a valgus angle or **valgus angulation.** In adults, an angle of about 170° to 174° is considered normal (Magee, 1997; Smith, Weiss, and Lehmkuhl, 1996), and such a normal alignment of the tibia relative to the femur is termed **genu rectum** (L. *genu*, knee + *rectus*, straight) as seen in figure 5.11A.

Genu Valgum

However, in some cases this relative lateral deviation of the tibia is exaggerated and the angle between the

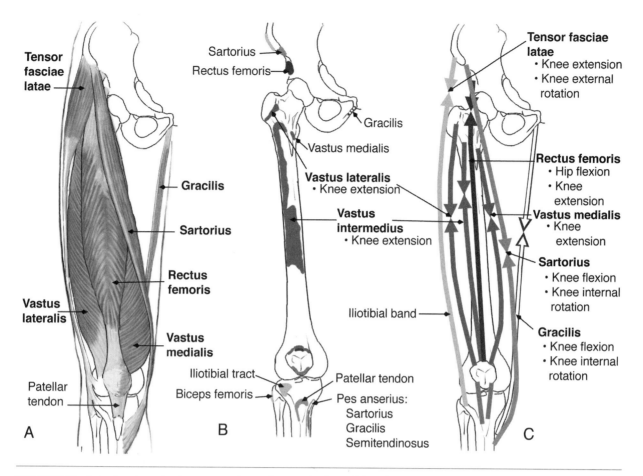

FIGURE 5.9   Anterior view of primary muscles acting on the knee joint (right knee). (A) Muscles, (B) attachments, (C) lines of pull and actions.

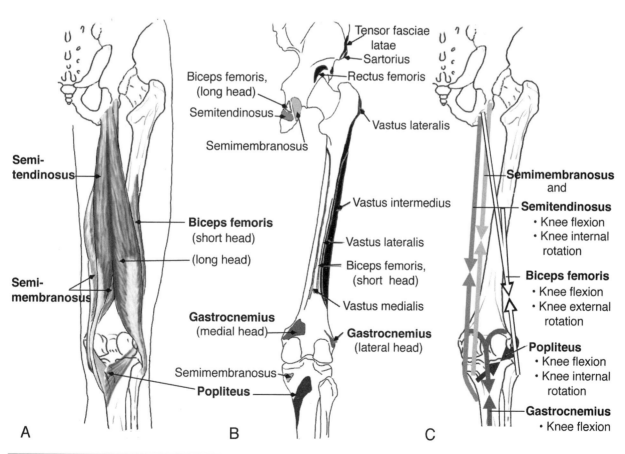

FIGURE 5.10   Posterior view of primary muscles acting on the knee joint (right knee). (A) Muscles, (B) attachments, (C) lines of pull and actions.

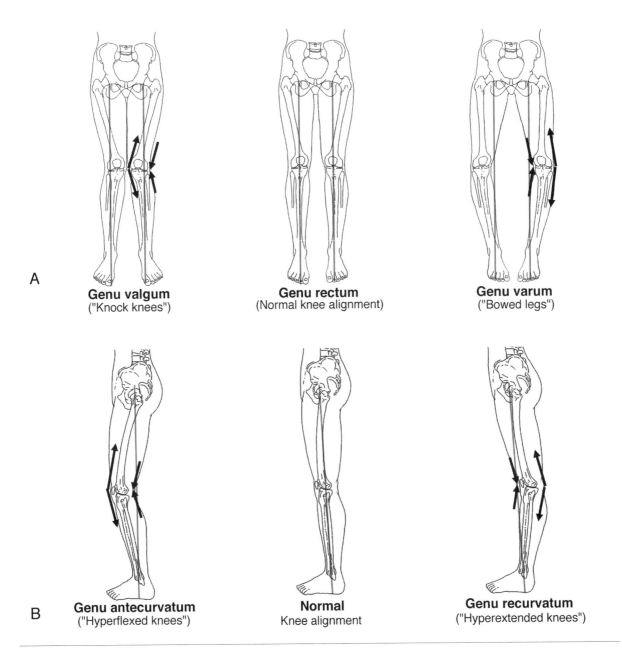

FIGURE 5.11   Knee alignment. (A) Anterior view, (B) lateral view.

tibia and femur is considerably less than 170°. This condition is termed **genu valgum,** or "knock-knees." In such a case, when a dancer stands with the feet parallel and the knees touching, the feet cannot touch and remain separated. To help remember this terminology, associate the "l" in valgum with the "l" in lateral. So, in genu va*l*gum, the tibia angles laterally relative to the femur (figure 5.11A). You can also remember this terminology by thinking that with genu val*gum*, a piece of sticky *gum* is holding the knees together while the tibia angles laterally. A distance of 3.5 inches (9-10 centimeters) or more between the ankles is considered excessive by Magee

(1997). This alignment of the knee is of concern in terms of aesthetics, the resultant increased load on the lateral meniscus and increased tension on the medial collateral ligament, negatively impacting alignment of the patella, and the commonly associated "rolling in" (excessive pronation) of the foot. Orthopedic evaluation of 40 elite ballet students showed no cases of genu valgum (Hamilton et al., 1997). One could postulate that this lack of occurrence was due to dropout from injury or screening out due to aesthetic considerations, or that ballet training tends to alter this knee alignment. Further investigation of this issue would be valuable.

Genu Varum

When the angle between the tibia and femur gets larger and approaches 180°, or the angle of the tibia relative to the femur actually opens medially versus laterally, the condition is termed **genu varum,** or "bowed legs." In such a case, when a dancer stands in a parallel position with the feet touching, there is space between the knees. If two or more fingers fit between the knees when the ankles are touching, this is considered evidence of genu va*rum.* You can remember this terminology by imagining that a barrel of *rum* is being held between the knees, making the legs bow. In addition to involving the angle of the femur relative to the tibia, this condition often involves an actual lateral bowing of the femur or tibia itself (or of both) (figure 5.11A). This positioning is of concern in terms of aesthetics, the resultant increased load on the medial meniscus and increased tension on the lateral collateral ligament, and the associated tendency to "roll out" (excessive supination). However, a high prevalence of genu varum has been noted in elite athletes, and it is interesting that orthopedic evaluation of 40 elite ballet students revealed that 46% demonstrated genu varum (Hamilton et al., 1997). So, although extreme genu varum may be detrimental, a small amount appears to be aesthetically acceptable, as evidenced by its presence in elite dancers. Its potential implications for injury risk will require additional study.

Genu Recurvatum

When one views the knees from the side, the knees can appear slightly bent, straight (extended), or hyperextended as seen in figure 5.11B. When the knees are hyperextended, this is termed **genu recurvatum** (L. *genu,* knee + *re-curvus,* bent back), or "back-knee," as the knees curve backward predominantly in the sagittal plane. Genu recurvatum is more common in females than males, and more common in individuals of any gender with generalized joint laxity ("hypermobility"). In the dance arena, hyperextended knees are sometimes wrongly attributed to excessive strength and use of the quadriceps femoris. However, since this hyperextension actually is often associated with attempting to maintain stability by "hanging" on ligamental constraints versus using muscular control, knee hyperextension is actually associated with less activity of the quadriceps than in subjects who stand with the knees slightly bent (Basmajian and DeLuca, 1985) and is often associated with weak quadriceps (Scioscia, Giffin, and Fu, 2001).

TESTS AND MEASUREMENTS 5.2

Knee Alignment: Valgus Angulation

Perform the following observations, and use figure 5.11 as a reference to identify your valgus angulation.

1. Stand facing a mirror with your feet parallel and approximately hip-width apart. Observe the relationship between the hip, knee, and ankle joints. Due to the slight inward angulation of the femur, with normal valgus angulation the tibia should angle out just slightly relative to the femur so that an angle is formed between these bones of about 170°. Note whether your angle seems less than, greater than, or about equal to 170°.

2. Now, move your feet together so that the inner borders touch, and note the position of your knees. With normal alignment, the knees also are approximately touching. However, if when standing in this position you can see space between your knees, this is suggestive of the presence of genu varum, or "bowed legs."

3. In contrast, if you are unable to bring your feet together because your knees make contact well before the inner borders of your feet can touch, this is suggestive of the presence of genu valgum, or "knock-knees."

4. After identifying the alignment of your knees, slowly move the pelvis between positions of anterior tilt, neutral, and posterior tilt, and note if and how they influence your knee alignment.

A slight amount of knee hyperextension is considered desirable in some dance aesthetics such as classical ballet. However, excessive hyperextension can be of concern from an injury perspective. One approach to meet both biomechanical and aesthetic conditions is to limit the amount of knee hyperextension when the leg is weight bearing and reserve use of a mildly hyperextended knee for the non-weight-bearing gesture leg when aesthetics dictate the "hyperextended line."

For dancers, a knee that does not fully extend and appears bent is also of concern from an aesthetic perspective. This condition is termed **genu antecurvatum** (L. *genu*, knee + *ante-curvus,* forward curve) or "hyperflexed knees" (figure 5.11B). Careful evaluation by a dance medicine physician is essential to determine how much of this limitation is structural versus soft tissue or neuromuscular in nature, as well as whether it is azppropriate to carefully stretch the knee to facilitate full extension. In many cases, desired changes can be achieved with a very careful but consistent stretching program, combined with dance technique modification.

Tibial Torsion

When one views the knee from the front, malalignment of the knee can also be seen predominantly in the transverse plane, as evidenced by inward or outward facing of the knee relative to the hip joint, ankle joint, or both. This transverse rotation can be due to malalignment of related joints (e.g., femoral torsion) or rotation along the length of the bones themselves. If the distal end of the tibia faces medially or excessively laterally when the distal end of the femur faces directly forward, the malalignment is termed **tibial torsion.** One can picture outward or **external tibial torsion** by imagining that the upper tibia and tibial tuberosity stay facing front while the lower tibia is rotated externally so that it is facing slightly toward the side as seen in figure 5.34B (p. 290). In this situation, the foot will be pointing outward relative to the knee. Some dancers exhibit marked external tibial torsion, and this bony alignment offers an advantage for achieving a more turned-out position with the feet without creating undesired torsion at the knee. Conversely, with inward or **internal tibial torsion,** the feet point straight ahead or toward each other when the patellae face forward. When standing, most people exhibit a slight external tibial torsion, which increases from approximately 5° at birth to an average of about 15° at skeletal maturity (Luke and Micheli, 2000). Tibial torsion has important impli-

cations for ankle and foot mechanics, as well as the knee, and will be readdressed in chapter 6.

Knee Mechanics

The mechanics of the knee joint are more complex than is the case for other true hinge joints, primarily due to two factors. First, flexion and extension at the tibiofemoral joint do not involve simple movement around one axis but rather incorporate rolling and gliding with a shifting axis at different degrees of flexion. Second, small amounts of transverse rotation also accompany flexion and extension.

Knee Flexion and Extension

The knee joint motions of flexion and extension occur primarily in the sagittal plane between the condyles of the femur and tibia. The movements of the femoral condyles relative to a fixed tibia (closed kinematic chain) can be compared to that of a bicycle wheel, with the femoral condyles rolling backward and forward upon the tibial condyles like a bicycle wheel on the road as seen in figure 5.12A. In addition, the femoral condyles glide or slide over the tibial condyles similarly to a bicycle wheel when it skids. This latter sliding motion is necessary to keep the femur positioned over the tibial condyles. For example, when the femoral condyles roll backward during flexion (such as during the descent of a first-position parallel plié), the femur would roll off the back of the tibia (figure 5.12A) without an anterior sliding motion that occurs after about 25° of flexion (figure 5.12B) to offset the backward motion associated with rolling (Levangie and Norkin, 2001). The opposite occurs in extension (such as in rising from the plié), with the femoral condyles first rolling forward and then sliding backward to offset the forward motion associated with rolling (figure 5.12C). So, this simultaneous use of rolling and sliding allows for the desired surfaces of the femur to stay in contact during flexion and extension and prevents excessive relative movement of the associated bones that could jeopardize joint integrity.

Knee Rotation

Although the primary motions at the knee joint are flexion and extension, the fact that the two condyles at the distal end of the femur are different in size and shape and are not quite parallel necessitates slight transverse rotation. The degree of rotation permitted varies with the degree of knee flexion and is strongly

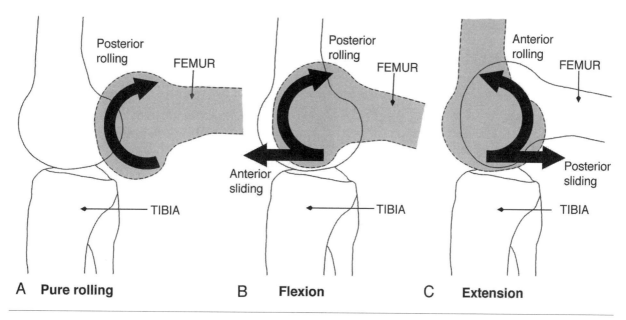

FIGURE 5.12   Motions of the femoral condyles on a fixed tibia (right knee, medial view). (A) Posterior rolling accompanying knee flexion, (B) anterior sliding to offset backward motion of femur during flexion, (C) anterior rolling with posterior sliding to offset forward motion of femur during knee extension.

influenced by ligaments. As previously described, when the knee is extended, key ligaments are relatively taut, and little or no rotation of the tibia relative to the femur is allowed. However, when the knee is bent, the collateral ligaments are more slack, and 20° to 30° of internal and 30° to 45° of external rotation of the tibia are possible (Magee, 1997; Rasch, 1989).

The increased rotation permitted as the knee bends enhances movement possibilities. For example, this rotation is critical for permitting the body to turn when the foot is in contact with the ground from a position of kneeling, squatting, sitting, or standing. It would be very difficult and cumbersome to change direction if this rotation at the knee were not available, and the rotation is vital for quick changes in direction such as a pivot when running or dancing. In non-weight-bearing conditions, this rotation allows the foot to turn, as when one climbs a pole, performs inside ankle kicks in soccer, or "presents the heel" in ballet.

The Locking Mechanism of the Knee

The linking of rotation with the final 20° of knee extension has particular importance for posture and knee stability and is termed the "locking mechanism" of the knee (Hamill and Knutzen, 1995). This automatic mechanism is thought to relate to the restraints offered by the cruciate ligament and the shape of the surfaces articulating at the knee joint. In terms of the latter, the medial femoral condyle projects extensively both longitudinally and medially. This downward pro-

jection of the medial condyle is necessary to compensate for the lateral-to-medial obliquity of the femoral shaft as it progresses distally, allowing the knee joint to be more parallel to the floor than if the condyles were the same size and shape. Due to this difference in size, when the knee extends in a standing position (closed kinematic chain), the excursion of the lateral condyle is completed (close packed) while that of the medial remains uncompleted. In essence, all of the articulating surface has been used on the lateral side, while leaving about a half inch (1.3 centimeters) on the medial side. To use the remaining articular surface on the medial side and reach full extension (close-packed position), the medial femoral condyle continues to roll and slide, producing internal rotation of the femur relative to the tibia as shown in figure 5.13B. The extent of this rotation is small, approximately 5° to 7° (Soderberg, 1986), though significant. This final rotation that creates a congruous position of both condyles of the femur relative to the menisci and underlying tibia is termed the **locking mechanism** or "screw-home" movement of the knee.

This locking mechanism of the knee is an energy-efficient mechanism that allows individuals to maintain the knee in extension over prolonged periods of standing without requiring muscular contraction, as the knee cannot flex without the knee's first being "unlocked." To bend the knee, the reverse process occurs in which the popliteus muscle works to externally rotate the femur relative to the tibia, thereby unlocking the knee and allowing flexion to occur.

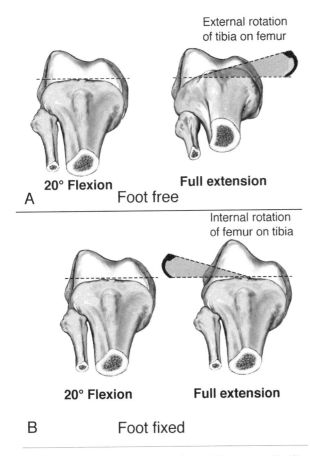

External rotation of tibia on femur

20° Flexion   **Full extension**

A   **Foot free**

Internal rotation of femur on tibia

20° Flexion   **Full extension**

B   **Foot fixed**

FIGURE 5.13   Locking mechanism of the knee with (A) closed kinematic chain and (B) open kinematic chain movements.

When the knee is not weight bearing, such as when the knee is extended in the air in a kick or développé, the tibia is no longer fixed and is now the most easily moved segment. Hence, the rotation occurs primarily in the tibia relative to the femur rather than in the femur relative to the tibia. In this condition the close-packed position of the condyles is achieved through external rotation of the tibia relative to the femur as shown in figure 5.13A, rather than the internal rotation of the femur seen in weight-bearing conditions. This external rotation of the tibia generally occurs during the last 20° to 30° of knee extension. This natural mechanics of the knee is sometimes emphasized when dancers straighten the knee to enhance the look of turnout.

Structure and Movements of the Patellofemoral Joint

As described in chapter 1, the patella is formed within the tendon of the quadriceps femoris muscle group and is the largest sesamoid bone found in the human body. Recall that the quadriceps muscle complex inserts into the superior border of the patella, and the inferior pole of the patella is joined to the tibial tuberosity via the patellar ligament or patellar tendon as seen in figure 5.14A. Some texts refer to this band as the patellar ligament since it attaches bone to bone, while others term it a tendon because functionally it is a tendon, being composed of fibers continuous with those of the quadriceps tendon. The patella is located slightly above and in front of the knee joint proper as seen in figure 5.14B, and the facets located on its posterior surface articulate with the slightly concave femoral groove, or patellar groove, as shown in figure 5.14, C and D; this articulation is termed the **patellofemoral joint.**

Functions of the Patella

As with other sesamoid bones, the patella increases the ability of the muscle within which it is located to produce effective force or torque. The patella serves to increase the moment arm, that is, the perpendicular distance of the line of action of the quadriceps femoris from the axis of rotation of the knee joint (figure 5.15B). Since torque is determined by the force generated by the muscle *times* the perpendicular distance from the line of pull of the muscle to the axis of rotation (chapter 2), the same force of contraction of the quadriceps will result in greater torque than if a patella were not present and the quadriceps ran closer to the middle of the knee joint (figure 5.15C). Decreases in quadriceps torque of up to 49% have been found when the patella has been surgically removed (Levangie and Norkin, 2001). The patella also serves to centralize the divergent pulls of the four muscles of the quadriceps femoris complex, serves as a retainer to help prevent the femur from sliding off the tibia anteriorly, and allows for a better distribution of compression stresses on the femur by increasing the surface area of contact. A reduction of compression stresses is further facilitated by the fact that the undersurface of the patella is lined with thick articular cartilage that deforms under load in such a way as to distribute forces over an even greater contact area. The smooth properties of this cartilage also allow transmission of quadriceps force around an angle during knee flexion, minimizing the losses due to friction. These latter functions are critical for preventing injury to the quadriceps tendon, since tendons are not designed to withstand either large compressive forces or high friction.

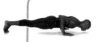

CONCEPT DEMONSTRATION 5.1

The Locking Mechanism of the Knee

Perform the following observations and refer to figure 5.13 to clarify the locking mechanism of the knee.

- **Demonstrate the rotation of the tibia accompanying knee extension in an open kinematic chain movement.** While sitting at the edge of a table with the knees bent to 90°, use a pen to mark an "x" on the midpoint of your patella and another "x" on your tibial tuberosity on your left side. Slowly extend your left knee. Note the movement of the tibial tuberosity relative to the mark over your patella. Redraw the tibial mark with the knee in full extension, and note that it has moved laterally, demonstrating the slight external rotation of the tibia relative to the femur that occurs in the final phases of knee extension with the foot free as shown in the figures.

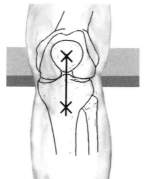

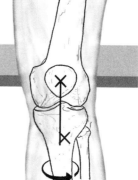

Knee extended

Tibial tuberosity lateral to mid-patella

90° Knee flexion

Tibial tuberosity vertically aligned with medial half of patella

Foot free

External rotation of tibia

- **Demonstrate the rotation of the femur accompanying knee extension in a closed kinematic chain movement.** Stand in first-position parallel and bend the knees about 30°. From this position of slight flexion, slowly straighten your knees, and again note the relative change of your tibial tubercle and mid-patella. The mid-patella mark should now be located more medially, demonstrating the slight internal rotation of the femur relative to the tibia that occurs in the terminal phases of knee extension when the foot is fixed.

Movements of the Patella

During flexion and extension of the knee joint proper, the patella undergoes a complex gliding movement that includes movements up and down with very slight medial, lateral, and rotational components. This leads some authors to consider this a synovial, modified plane joint (Magee, 1997), while others do not consider it a true joint. The kneecap remains at a relatively constant distance from the tibia because of the patellar tendon. Thus, the change of position of the patella occurs in relation to the femur; the patella slides down during flexion and up during extension within the femoral groove. An excursion of the patella on the femoral condyles of approximately 2 3/4 inches (7 centimeters) occurs from extension to full flexion (Frankel and Nordin, 1980). As this excursion proceeds, there is also a continuous transition in contact surface size and location that has important implications for potential cartilage injury.

Connective Tissue Constraints

In addition to being anchored to the tibia by the patellar tendon below, the patella is further stabilized by various other connective tissue structures as seen in figure 5.14A. For example, lateral extensions from the quadriceps tendons (termed patellar ligaments) and fibrous expansions of the vasti and iliotibial band (medial and lateral patellar retinaculum) also provide lateral and medial stability for the patella and are key in preventing the patella from coming out of its groove (patellar subluxations or dislocations).

Muscles of the Patellofemoral Joint

Since the quadriceps femoris directly attaches to the patella, adequate and balanced strength of its components is essential for stability and proper movement of the patella. Other muscles, including the pes anserinus group and hamstrings, can affect the patella less directly. The interplay of these muscles

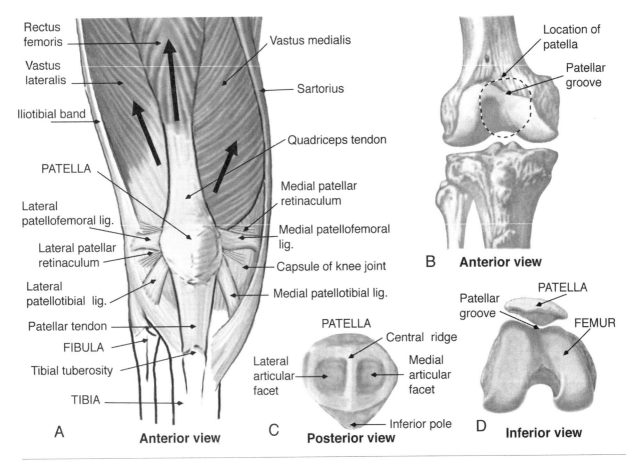

FIGURE 5.14   The patellofemoral joint (right knee). (A) Anterior view of the patellofemoral joint and associated key muscles and connective tissues, (B) anterior view of location of patella relative to the femur, (C) posterior view of the patella showing facets, (D) inferior view of the location of the patella relative to the femur.

is particularly important in the initial stages of knee flexion, before the patella becomes well seated and more stable at about 20° of flexion.

Patellofemoral Alignment and the Q Angle

The shape, height, mobility, and facing of the patella in the femoral groove, as well as its angular relationship to the tibia, are important for determining stability and tracking of the patella. This angular relationship is termed the Q angle. The **Q angle** or **quadriceps angle** is a static measurement of the angle that the patellar tendon makes relative to the shaft of the femur as seen in figure 5.16. Since the patella is relatively free to move upon the femur when the knee is extended, when the quadriceps femoris muscle contracts it will try to establish a straight line between its proximal attachment onto the femur and pelvis and its distal attachment onto the tibial tuberosity. Thus, the Q angle provides an

indication of the lateral force (vector) applied to the patella, which tends to make the patella track laterally in order to establish a straight-line relationship between the proximal and distal attachments of the quadriceps femoris muscle group. Females generally have larger Q angles than men, with a normal range considered to be 8° to 15° for males and 10° to 19° for females (Diduch, Scuderi, and Scott, 1997; Hamill and Knutzen, 1995; Palmer and Epler, 1990) when the knee is in extension and the quadriceps is relaxed. Although controversial, Q angles greater than 15° (Insall, Bullough, and Burstein, 1979; Quirk, 1987), 17° (Hamill and Knutzen, 1995), or 20° (Caillet, 1996; Smith, Weiss, and Lehmkuhl, 1996) are considered abnormal and a risk factor for patellofemoral problems.

Patellofemoral Mechanics

Underlying positioning, movement, and the forces associated with patellofemoral function are two

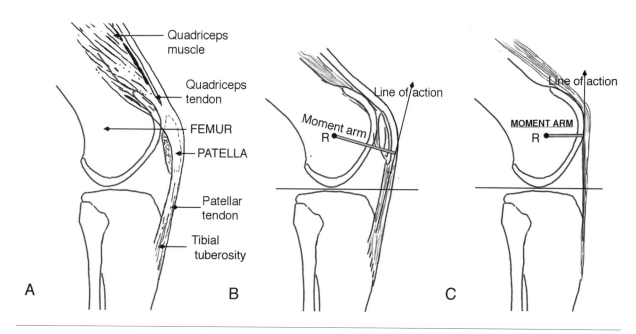

FIGURE 5.15   Function of patella to increase moment arm and torque of the quadriceps femoris (right knee). (A) Lateral view of the patellofemoral joint, (B) increase in moment arm due to the presence of the patella, (C) decrease in moment arm if the patella is absent.

important principles. These principles are the law of valgus and patellofemoral compression forces.

Law of Valgus

Because the femur normally runs slightly obliquely inward, the previously described Q angle is formed with its concomitant tendency to pull the patella laterally as seen in figure 5.17. This predisposition for lateral motion of the patella is referred to as the **law of valgus.** This underlying tendency in the normal knee can be further exaggerated in the abnormal knee by many structural and functional factors, including femoral anteversion, genu valgum, tibial torsion, a laterally placed tibial tuberosity, a patella that sits high (patella alta), an excessively mobile patella (hypermobile), tightness of the lateral stabilizers of the patella, and generalized quadriceps weakness. Lateral tracking causes the patella to abut against the lateral portion of the femoral groove. The resultant excessive shear forces can damage the cartilage lining the underside of the patella and cause patellofemoral dysfunction and pain.

It is important to realize that although many of the factors that tend to increase lateral tracking are structural and not readily changed, quadriceps strength can be easily improved and the vastus medialis is in a perfect position to counter this tendency for lateral tracking of the patella. Hence, adequate and balanced strength of the quadriceps is an essential

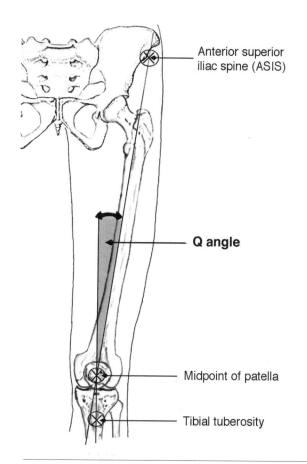

FIGURE 5.16   The Q angle (right knee, anterior view).

Patellofemoral Alignment: The Q Angle and Patellar Tracking

Perform the following procedures to measure your Q angle, and note the movements of the patella and presence of lateral patellar tracking.

1. Sit with your legs extended to the front and your quadriceps relaxed. Grasp the sides of your patella between your thumb and index finger, and move the patella from side to side. Note how mobile it is with the quadriceps relaxed. Passive movement of the patella up to half of its width medially and up to half of its width laterally is considered normal (Magee, 1997). Now, draw an "x" in ink on your tibial tuberosity and another "x" on the midpoint of your patella as shown in A. Then, draw one line connecting the tibial tuberosity and the midpoint of the patella and extending about 3 inches (7.6 centimeters) past the patella. Draw a second line from the midpoint of the patella upward, in line with the anterior superior iliac spine of the pelvis. The angle that is described with its apex at the midpoint of the patella is the Q angle. Use a protractor or goniometer to measure it and note if it is above "normal" values for your gender.

2. Now slowly tighten your quadriceps, focusing on "pulling" the kneecap up toward your waist without letting the knee move backward into hyperextension. While keeping the quadriceps contracted, draw another "x" on the midpoint of the patella, and note any lateral excursion of the patella ("lateral patellar tracking") that has occurred as shown in B. Also, with the quadriceps firmly contracted, grasp the sides of the patella between your thumb and index finger and carefully attempt to move the patella from side to side. Note how limited passive movement of the patella is when the quadriceps is contracted and how important the quadriceps is for stabilizing and directing movement of the patella.

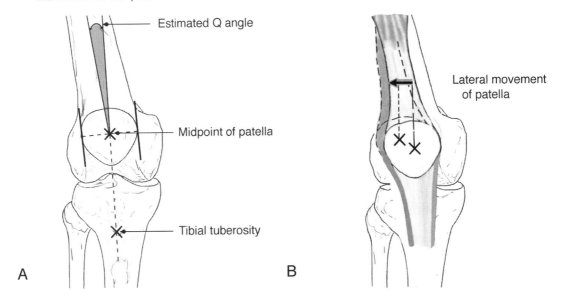

Estimated Q angle

Midpoint of patella

Tibial tuberosity

A

Lateral movement of patella

B

measure for promoting sound patellar mechanics and preventing patellofemoral injuries.

Patellofemoral Compression Forces

Another important consideration in patellar mechanics is patellofemoral compression forces. **Patello-** **femoral compression force** is the force pressing the kneecap back against the underlying femur. This force can become quite large, and an understanding of its genesis is important for preventing and alleviating patellofemoral problems.

The two most important determinants of patellofemoral compression forces are the magnitude

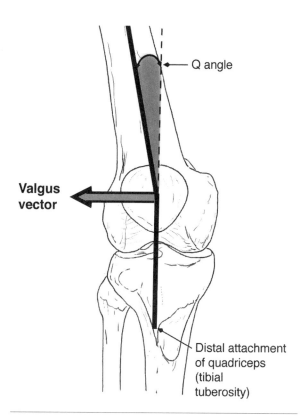

FIGURE 5.17 Law of valgus. Orientation of quadriceps in the frontal plane, Q angle, and consequent valgus vector (right knee, anterior view).

of quadriceps contraction and the angle of knee flexion. That is, the harder the quadriceps contracts the greater the compression force, and the farther the knee bends the greater the compression force. However, often these two factors are linked together. For example, when one bends the knee from a standing position such as in a grand plié, the center of gravity of the body falls increasingly posterior to the axis of rotation of the knee joint as the plié proceeds. This increases the effect that gravity has to make the knees bend further (increased moment arm of the resistance), requiring greater quadriceps force to counter this effect of gravity and a resultant higher compression force.

At the same time, as the knee bends, the effect of the changing angle between the quadriceps tendon and patellar tendon also contributes to the rising compression force. When the knee is in full extension or very slight flexion, the patella is being pulled upward almost parallel to the femur, and the quadriceps tendon and patellar tendon are almost in line. Hence, this force is acting primarily in a vertical direction, and there is little or no patellofemoral compressive force (C 1) irrespective of the magnitude of quadriceps tension (Fm 1) as seen in figure 5.18A. However, as knee flexion proceeds, the angle between the quad-

riceps tendon and patellar tendon changes; now the force does not just act vertically, but rather there is a larger component of the quadriceps force that acts in a direction to create compression of the patella against the underlying femur (C 2) as seen in figure 5.18B. Thus, with increasing knee flexion, an increasing quadriceps force (Fm 3) and an increase in the percentage of this force that is being directed toward the patellofemoral joint act together to increase compression forces (C 3) as seen in figure 5.18C.

Drawing from activities of daily living, as the angle of knee flexion and magnitude of quadriceps contraction increase from walking to stair climbing to deep knee bends, associated compression forces have been calculated to rise from approximately .5 to 1.2 times body weight to 3.3 times body weight to 7.6 times body weight (Reilly and Martens, 1972). For a dancer weighing 120 pounds (54 kilograms) these activities would be associated with approximately 60 to 144 pounds (27-65 kilograms), 396 pounds (180 kilograms), and 912 pounds (414 kilograms) of compression force, respectively. Examples of movements from dance that would have high patellofemoral compression forces include the grand plié, fondu, lunge, movements used to get up from and down to the floor, and the jump. Large jumps have been estimated to be associated with forces of about 20 times body weight (Dowson and Wright, 1981), that is, about 2,400 pounds (1,089 kilograms) of compression force for a 120-pound dancer.

Muscular Analysis of Fundamental Knee Movements

As previously described, the knee is primarily capable of flexion and extension, with some transverse rotation. The knee joint functions to help support the weight of the body as well as to change the length of the lower limb in accordance with movement requirements. For example, in walking, through appropriate timing of flexion and extension of the knee, vertical movement of the whole body's center of gravity is minimized and energy economy maximized. A summary of the key muscles capable of producing the fundamental movements of the knee is provided in table 5.2.

Knee Flexion

Remember that knee flexion involves bringing the posterior surfaces of the upper leg and lower leg

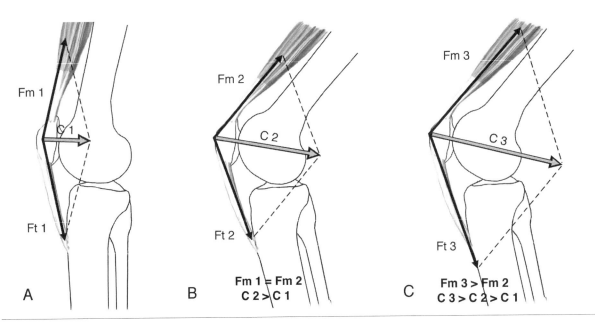

FIGURE 5.18   Increasing patellofemoral compression force. (A) Knee almost straight, (B) greater knee flexion, (C) greater magnitude of quadriceps contraction.

closer together. The hamstrings and other flexors of the knee (table 5.2) are used concentrically when flexion is occurring against gravity or resistance as in prone knee curls (table 5.3E, p. 276) or standing knee curls (table 5.3F, p. 277). The knee flexors are also used concentrically to flex the knee as the lower limb swings backward during walking and running gait. In dance, the knee flexors can also be used to shorten the length of the limb to facilitate turning, as in fouetté turns, and to effect a desired shape such as in a passé, attitude, or the back leg of the stylized stag leap seen in figure 5.19.

However, during standing with the weight of the body supported by the foot, the situation is differ-

ent. Once the knee is "unlocked" and begins to flex, gravity becomes the primary force and tends to create further flexion of the knee. Under these circumstances the knee flexors are not working to create knee flexion; rather the knee extensors are working to either maintain that angle of knee flexion (isometrically) as seen in figure 5.20 or control further flexion (eccentrically) as when the body is being lowered to the floor. So, the knee extensors (quadriceps femoris) act in this postural or "antigravity" role very frequently in dance on the support leg or legs. In impact movements such as jumping, this eccentric knee flexion is vital for shock absorption and deceleration of the falling body.

TABLE 5.2   Knee Movements and the Muscles That Can Produce Them

Knee joint movement	Primary muscles	Secondary muscles
Flexion	Hamstrings	Popliteus* Gracilis Sartorius Gastrocnemius
Extension	Quadriceps femoris	Tensor fasciae latae
External rotation	Biceps femoris	Tensor fasciae latae
Internal rotation	Semitendinosus Semimembranosus Popliteus (when foot free)	Gracilis Sartorius

*Unlocks the knee at beginning of knee flexion.

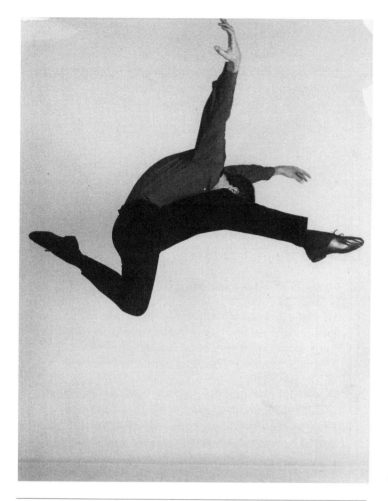

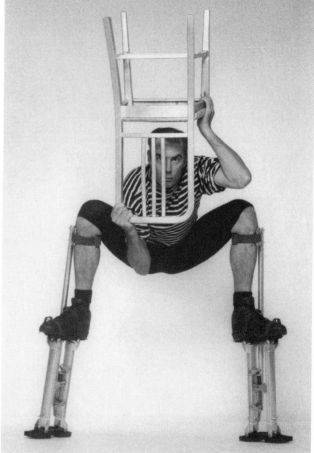

FIGURE 5.19   Sample dance movement showing knee flexion and associated prime movers.

Photo: Roy Blakey. Dancer: Douglas Nielsen in Viola Farber's "Last Call."

FIGURE 5.20   Knee extensors working isometrically to prevent gravity from producing further knee flexion.

Photo: Roy Blakey. Dancer: Douglas Nielsen.

Knee Extension

Remember that knee extension involves "straightening" the knee or decreasing the angle of knee flexion. The four quadriceps muscles are the extensors of the knee and are used concentrically to extend the knee both when the foot is free and when it is weight bearing. When the foot is free (open kinematic chain), the quadriceps are used to produce knee extension isometrically in exercises such as straight leg raises (table 5.3B, p. 275) and concentrically in exercises such as terminal knee extension (table 5.3C, p. 275) and sitting knee extension (table 5.3D, p. 276). In dance, the knee extensors can be used concentrically to produce a straight position of the knee in the gesture leg in the développé or isometrically to maintain a straight position of the knee of the gesture leg in the tendu, dégagés

(brushes), battements (kicks), and the movement shown in figure 5.21.

When the foot is weight bearing (closed kinematic chain), the quadriceps are used concentrically to extend the knee. This movement is used in walking up stairs or rising from sitting in a chair. Examples of strengthening exercises that include this form of knee extension are the wall squat (table 5.3G, p. 277) and plié/leg press (table 5.3H, p. 278) and lunge (table 5.3I, p. 278). In dance, this form of knee extension is used during rising from a plié or fondu. Concentric powerful use of the knee extensors is also operative in movements such as the takeoff in jumping to help effect the desired vertical rise of the center of gravity and propel the body through space as seen on the left leg in figure 5.21. Knee extension is also used isometrically in dance to maintain an extended knee on the support

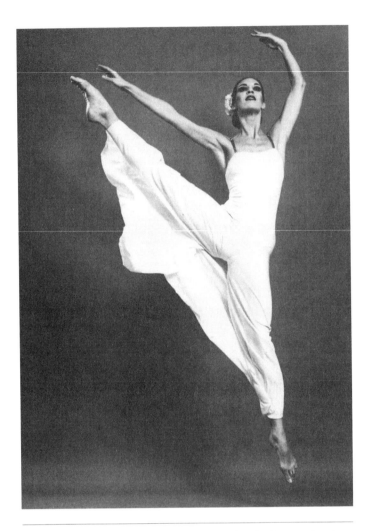

FIGURE 5.21   Sample dance movement showing knee extension.
© Martha Swope. Dancer: Susan McLain in "Diversion of Angels" with the Martha Graham Dance Company.

leg in many movements performed at the barre or center floor.

Knee Rotation

The internal rotators and external rotators of the knee listed in table 5.2 are key for controlling twisting or pivoting movements of the body when the foot is on the ground, as in association with changes in direction. In dance the subtle rotations of the tibia are also sometimes used when the foot is in the air to enhance the aesthetics of a movement. For example, in a back attitude, slight external rotation of the tibia and "winging" of the foot are sometimes encouraged in classical ballet to help effect the desired turned-out line of the lower extremity. Less frequently, rotations of the tibia are actually incorporated into the movement, as in performing a rond de jambe

en l'air that includes circling of the foot (en dehors and en dedans). With this movement dancers are classically instructed to keep the knee stationary as the foot describes a semicircle, oval, or tear shape (depending on the teacher's approach).

Key Considerations for the Knee in Whole Body Movement

When analyzing more complex movement that encompasses multiple joints, it is important to take into account the actions of multijoint muscles and specifically Lombard's paradox.

Actions of Two-Joint Muscles

Of the 12 muscles that act on the knee joint, all except the vasti muscles and popliteus cross the hip joint or the ankle joint in addition to the knee joint. When these muscles contract to produce movement at the knee, they also tend to move other joints. In some cases the multiple actions of a given muscle can be used together. For example, in a développé to the front, the actions of the rectus femoris (hip flexion and knee extension) are both utilized to effect the motion. However, this is actually a difficult situation for the muscle in that it is shortening across both joints and can easily reach such a shortened position that it has difficulty generating force (active insufficiency). And many dancers may experience discomfort or cramping in the rectus femoris when performing a développé to the front, especially when working on increasing the height of the leg, until adequate strength of other hip flexors, such as the iliopsoas, is developed.

However, more frequently, the multiple actions are not desired simultaneously, and the muscle remains the same length or is actually lengthened across one joint as it shortens across the other joint. An example of the former condition occurs with relevés in which the gastrocnemius remains the same length across the knee joint, as no change in joint angle occurs there, while it shortens across the ankle joint to effect ankle plantar flexion. An example of the second condition occurs when one extends the leg back from a passé position (such as with an arabesque) in which the rectus femoris is being lengthened across the hip joint (via hip hyper-extension) as it is shortening across the knee joint to produce knee extension. This latter condition allows a more favorable length of the muscle to be maintained such that greater force can be generated and active insufficiency delayed. Consciously using this principle when performing this movement—that is, concentrating on fully hyperextending the hip and feeling the rectus femoris stretch across the hip and the hip extensors (hamstrings) lift the knee up, before extending the knee—can often help you maintain a greater height of the leg as the knee is extended.

Lombard's Paradox

As discussed in chapter 2, in accordance with Lombard's paradox, when the hamstrings and rectus femoris simultaneously contract, extension of both the knee and hip will tend to predominate (Lombard and Abbott, 1907). This co-contraction of the quadriceps and hamstrings to produce knee and hip extension is frequently used during everyday as well as dance movements, as in standing up from a chair, the up-phase of pliés, and the takeoff phase of jumps.

Special Considerations for the Knee in Dance

When taking into account the mechanics of the tibiofemoral and patellofemoral joint, there are several issues in dance that warrant further discussion. These issues include use of the grand plié, twisting of the knee in turnout and other movements, knee hyperextension, and specific muscle use as they relate to achieving the desired aesthetic of common types of dance while keeping knee injury risk low.

The Grand Plié

There is much controversy about the use of a full squat or grand plié. Concerns cited are the large stresses applied to the menisci and posterior cruciate ligament (Escamilla, 2001) and the dislocating force due to the approximation of the calf and back of the thigh and the parallel component of the hamstring muscles (angle of muscle attachment—chapter 2), as well as very high associated patellofemoral compression forces. These concerns have led to the common recommendation of limiting active knee flexion (such as accompanies squats, pliés, and lunges) to about 90° or a position in which the thigh is parallel to the floor (parallel squat) for recreational athletes or deconditioned older individuals.

However, the application of these recommendations to competitive athletes, including well-conditioned dancers, is highly debatable. Critics of this conservative approach hold that a fuller range of motion is needed to develop adequate strength and explosive power necessary for high-level athletic performance. They also hold that such exercises, if performed with good technique and advanced appropriately, can actually have a protective effect through strengthening the knee structures and involved musculature, such that greater forces can be withstood during activity before injury occurs.

Looking at this issue as specifically related to dance, there are several additional factors that should be taken into account. First, potential risk to the knee is probably lessened by (1) the traditional use of music and counts to encourage a slow and controlled descent and rise from a plié; (2) the commonly used directive to "lift out of your knees," as well as to avoid hesitating, or "sitting," at the bottom of the plié and to instead keep movement continuous; (3) the use in some dance forms of a barre, which can aid with balance, as well as in some cases provide some unweighting of the knees; (4) the lack of external weights (such as barbells) so that only body weight is of concern; and (5) the common use of turned-out positions that may recruit other muscles such as the hip adductors and lessen the required magnitude of quadriceps contraction and resultant patellofemoral compression forces. Furthermore, performing pliés in different positions may represent slightly different benefits and risks. For example, third- and fourth-position grand pliés performed center floor not only require marked strength in the quadriceps but also high skill levels to maintain balance, turnout, and alignment and have been found to involve greater overall longitudinal rotation at the knee relative to second-position grand pliés (Barnes et al., 2000).

Lastly, potential functional strength benefits should be considered. Many female dancers have lower absolute quadriceps strength levels than some other types of athletes or than might be desired (Kirkendall et al., 1984; Koutedakis, Agrawal, and Sharp, 1998; Koutedakis et al., 1997; Mostardi et al., 1983), and grand pliés (as well as jumps and hinges) are among only a few exercises that include sufficient overload to effectively enhance strength. Not to provide adequate stimulus to improve quadriceps strength and not to allow practice of motor patterns including marked knee flexion in a slower, more controlled manner might actually be a disservice to dancers and increase their risk when choreography demands the use of full knee flexion, often at a faster tempo and in a more complex movement pattern later in the class or in rehearsal and performance (figure 5.22).

"Lift Out of Your Knees"

The instruction to "lift out of your knees" is sometimes used by teachers in an effort to reduce knee stress when dancers are performing demanding movements such as grand pliés or movements involving going down to the floor.

This cue of "lifting out of your knees" is often further explained as "don't let your weight drop into your knees." One could interpret these cues from an anatomical perspective in several ways. One interpretation is that they encourage the use of muscles to control motion at the knee, rather than allowing excessive momentum and reliance on passive constraints. For example, eccentric contraction of the quadriceps muscles (in conjunction with co-contraction of many other muscles) can be used to control the flexion of the knee as the body lowers toward the floor; and when full flexion is approached, this muscle contraction is maintained rather than the dancer's relaxing the quadriceps and "sitting in the plié," relying on passive tissues such as the ligaments of the knee to maintain the flexed position. Such an approach is advantageous in terms of creating more joint stability and less ligamental stress.

Another interpretation of this cue relates to contraction of muscles above the knee, particularly of the hip and torso. For example, using the hip extensors eccentrically and "pulling up" with the abdominal muscles and back extensors to help maintain desired positioning of the torso relative to the knee during knee flexion may reduce knee stress. The potential influence of muscle use on forces borne by the body was demonstrated in one study that included jump technique cueing, which resulted in greater use of the hamstrings and 22% reduction in peak impact forces (Hewett et al., 1999).

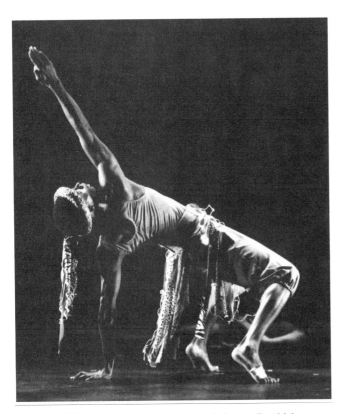

FIGURE 5.22 Sample dance movement demanding high levels of knee flexion, quadriceps strength, and neuromuscular coordination.

Photo courtesy of Keith Ian Polakoff. CSULB dancer Dwayne Worthington.

Considering all these factors, although the recommendations of limiting knee flexion to about 90° for beginning recreational athletes seem prudent, another approach is warranted in the dance arena. One recommended approach would be to use grand pliés judiciously in dancers with "healthy knees," with limited consecutive repetitions and close attention to technique and appropriate conditioning and skill level. Appropriate skill and strength should be present so that the descent and rise are controlled, the knees go as much to the side as hip turnout permits, and the pelvis stays vertical as shown in figure 5.23A—versus the common error of tilting the torso and pelvis anteriorly with resultant internal rotation of the femur and in-facing of the knees as shown in figure 5.23B. Keeping in mind the dislocating forces when in full flexion, dancers should be advised to maintain an active contraction of muscles with a quick reversal in direction at the bottom of pliés to enhance joint stability and avoid a position in which support is provided solely by passive constraints such as ligaments.

Due to the inherent greater strength and balance challenges, a more conservative approach can be employed when a barre is not used for first-, third-, fourth-, and fifth-position grand pliés, as is commonly done in modern and jazz dance. Such center floor movements should be used with more skilled dancers who do not experience knee discomfort; and when one is teaching these movements to more beginning dancers, a logical progression should be used. For example, skill can be developed (1) facing the barre

with two-hand support; (2) side to the barre with decreasing one-hand support; (3) center floor with range increasing in accordance with ability to maintain balance and body placement; and (4) center floor with choreographic-specific challenges such as adding off-center torso and arm movements.

The Hinge

Hinge movements take on various forms but generally involve keeping the torso in line with the knees as the knees flex and lower toward the floor on a diagonal. They represent an important element of dance vocabulary in jazz and some forms of modern dance, including Horton and Graham techniques, as seen in figure 5.24. The position of the torso makes this movement even more challenging than the grand plié in terms of quadriceps strength and neuromuscular coordination. Hence, a well-designed progression similar to that used with grand pliés is recommended for less-skilled or -conditioned dancers, or those new to this movement. An example of a progression would be (1) a series of wall squats (table 5.3G, p. 277) performed very slowly or with holds; (2) side to the barre with one-hand support while performing a hinge with gradually increasing

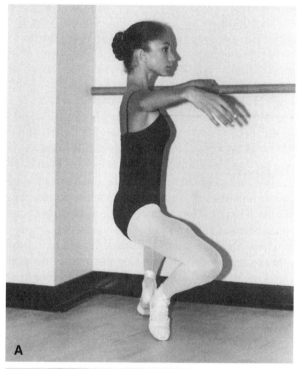
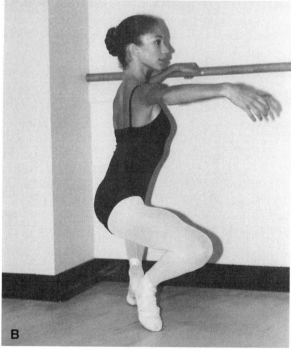

FIGURE 5.23 First-position grand plié with (A) desired body placement and (B) undesired body placement.

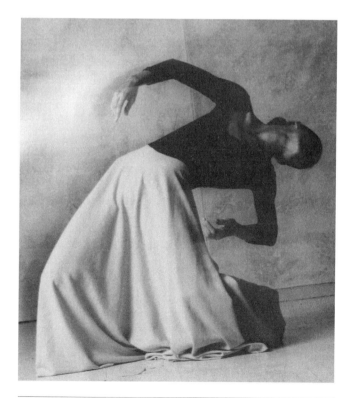

FIGURE 5.24 Example of a hinge (side tilt) as seen in the Graham technique.

Photo courtesy of Scott Peterson. Dancer: Susan McLain.

range while form is maintained; (3) center floor with range gradually increasing while form is maintained; and (4) gradual addition of choreographic-specific challenges such as adding torso or arm movements or classic pre- and post-linking movements. When adequate strength and skill are developed, the risks are dramatically lowered, and hinges offer both an important artistic element and an effective means of developing strength and skill for many demanding movements that require lowering the body weight to(ward) the floor or raising the body away from the floor.

Twisting of the Knee in Dance

Although the relative rotary motion between the tibia and femur expands functional movement capacities, excessive rotation can produce potentially injurious ligamental or patellofemoral stress. Thus, particular care must be taken to avoid excessive rotation with turnout or other dance movements.

Forcing Turnout

Some dancers use excessive rotation from the knee downward to achieve turnout, and this practice is termed "screwing the knee" or **forcing turnout.** To avoid forcing turnout during dynamic movement, it is important to recall that knee flexion allows more rotation of the tibia due to slackening of ligamental constraints, as well as external rotation of the femur associated with unlocking the knee. Thus, when the knee bends, such as at the base of a plié or during a weight shift, it is easy to shift the heel forward to obtain greater turnout of the feet. However, this practice should be avoided because when the knee straightens, the femur internally rotates and the ligaments become taut, and undesired torsional stress will occur at the knee if the foot is positioned excessively outward (figure 5.25). Conversely, when extending the knees it is easy to exaggerate the associated internal rotation of the femur if external rotation is not maintained at the hip joint. Again, the distal tibia is being held more externally rotated by the foot against the floor as the femur internally rotates, resulting in torsional stress at the knee. Both of these undesired practices also create a more laterally positioned tibial tuberosity relative to the midpoint of the patella, increasing the Q angle and increasing patellofemoral stress.

Unfortunately, how much rotation from the knee downward is "normal" versus potentially injurious is controversial. In reality, dancers training in dance forms where "perfect" turnout is emphasized derive significant portions of their turnout from the knee, the ankle-foot, or both; and in a study of elite ballet dancers only approximately 58% of active turnout came from the hip (Hamilton et al., 1992). While some individuals are critical of the use of full turnout of the feet, the issue is complex in that use of such positioning of the feet at an early age may facilitate the development of hip external rotation, and the incidence of knee injuries has not been shown to be higher in schools that emphasize greater turnout than schools that allow less lateral positioning of the feet. Furthermore, some rotation of the tibia is normal. For example, 7 to 14° of external rotation was found to occur during stair climbing (Hamill and Knutzen, 1995). In one study of dance, about 27° of knee external rotation was found to accompany a plié, and about 22° of knee external rotation occurred on the support leg during a penché (Worthen, Patten, and Hamill, 1998). So, further research is needed to clarify the relationship between tibial rotation and injury risk.

However, whatever the aesthetic demands of the school of dance, it is logical that the greater the proportion of turnout that can be achieved from the

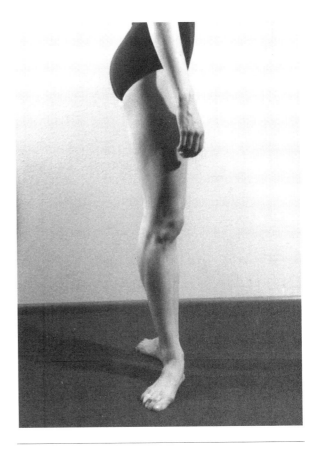

FIGURE 5.25   Dancer demonstrating extreme forced turnout while standing in first position.

DANCE CUES 5.2

"Bring the Heel Forward"

The instruction to "bring the heel forward" or "present the heel" is sometimes used by teachers in an effort to maximize turnout in open kinematic chain movements in which the foot is moving on the floor or coming off the floor, such as with a tendu or dégagé.

A desired anatomical interpretation is to think of the upper leg and lower leg as one continuous unit in which rotation that started at the proximal end (the hip joint) will result in rotation at the bottom end—such that the back of the heel will rotate from its original position of facing backward (when the leg is parallel) medially and forward. To reinforce this concept, the image is sometimes used of reaching the leg out and spiraling it around the axis running lengthwise through the middle of the limb. This movement can be thought of as like that of a screwdriver, where rotation of the proximal end by the hand results in rotation at the distal end. In contrast to this desired initiation, some dancers respond to this cue by bringing the heel forward from externally rotating the tibia relative to the femur at the knee joint. Hence it can be helpful to incorporate the hip into this cue, such as by cueing to start the rotation by bringing the trochanter back and continuing the rotation down the leg such that the heel rotates "in and forward."

hip, the less rotation will be required from the knee downward. The need to emphasize fully developing external rotation from the hip is given further support by findings that (1) ballet students exhibit increased active range of hip external rotation but not increased external rotation below the hip when compared to nondancing university students (Khan et al., 1997); (2) elite female ballet dancers with more total injuries had lower values of total turnout (Hamilton et al., 1992); and (3) in personal clinical experience, many dancers with patellofemoral pain syndrome experienced relief of symptoms by improving turnout technique.

To lessen knee stress, emphasize utilizing the hip external rotators to help direct the knee over the foot during movements such as pliés, and avoid shifting the heel forward when the knee is flexed. Furthermore, maintain as much external rotation as possible at the proximal end of the femur (hip joint), and avoid exaggerating the slight internal rotation of the femur relative to the tibia (associated with the locking mechanism of the knee) when extending the knees in movements such as rising from a plié. When the foot is free, such as in brushes, emphasis should be on rotating the hip and carrying the external rotation down the leg such that the "heel comes forward," rather than "bringing the heel forward" from excessive tibial rotation. In the author's experience, most dancers do not fully utilize or maintain the potential hip external rotation that their bodies possess.

Valgus Stress in Dance

Floor work in jazz and modern often includes positions that incorporate internally rotating the back leg, with the lower leg and foot facing back as seen in figure 5.26. Although performance of such positions is often not recommended for sedentary or recreational athletes, it is an important element of some dance forms; and many dancers have adequate hip range of motion to allow performance of such positions without undue knee stress. However, if inadequate hip or quadriceps flexibility is present (particularly in men with limited hip internal rotation), such positions might cause excessive valgus knee stress and knee discomfort.

If dancers do experience knee discomfort, they should perform supplemental stretching daily; and the position can be temporarily modified as shown in figure 5.26 as adequate hip flexibility is developed.

Valgus, varus, and rotational stresses also occur at the knee in dynamic movement as when the dancer changes direction, moves side to side, or moves on a diagonal. Studies looking at sidestepping and crossover cutting maneuvers suggest that such movements can place large stresses on the anterior cruciate and collateral ligaments of the knee that are of sufficient magnitude to cause ligament injury if the muscles of the knee do not provide adequate stability (Besier, Lloyd, Cochrane, and Ackland, 2001). These stresses are markedly higher in situations in which changes are unanticipated and the muscles do not

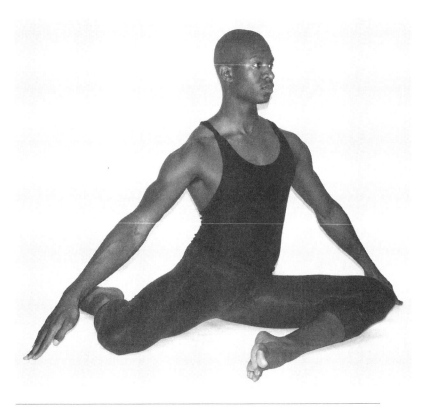

FIGURE 5.26   Potential valgus stress of can be reduced by allowing the right ischial tuberosity to lift slightly off the floor.

have adequate time to counter the increased loads placed on the knee (Besier, Lloyd, Ackland, and Cochrane, 2001). It is likely that dancers who train regularly will develop strategies for standard dance vocabulary that will help minimize the stress to the knee ligaments.

Hyperextended Knees in Dance

When the body is standing erect, the gravity line falls slightly in front of the knee joint axis, leading to a "locking" of the knee in extension by a small gravitational torque. This locking is also due to the terminal rotation associated with full knee extension previously discussed (e.g., the locking mechanism of the knee). Because this end position is passive and does not involve contraction of lower extremity muscles, dancers with genu recurvatum will not exhibit the same passive endpoints, and the knees will not stop at extension but rather will continue to a position of hyperextension (figure 5.27A). Hyperextended knees are very prevalent in dancers, and one study (Trepman et al., 1994) showed that all of the dancers studied exhibited knee hyperextension when standing in turned-out first position, but with significantly greater magnitude in ballet

than modern dancers (average of 13° vs. 5°). However, even dancers with extreme hyperextension can learn to control the extent of hyperextension allowed both in standing and in dance movements.

Two tactics for controlling knee hyperextension in dance include (1) limiting the degree of knee extension and (2) limiting the degree of femoral internal rotation. The first approach relies on the principle of stopping the knee earlier as it extends, when the center of mass of the whole body is just over the axis of the knee joint rather than anterior to the knee joint, so that passive knee hyperextension is avoided. Sometimes cueing to do just this, that is, to simply not straighten the knees so far or to "pull the knees straight up" versus "pushing the knees back," may be sufficient to prevent the problem. Similarly, thinking of "pulling up" just below the back of the knee at the same time that the front of the knee is being "pulled up" can encourage co-contraction of the hamstrings and quadriceps femoris. Since the hamstrings are flexors of the knee, if recruited early enough when the knee is still slightly bent, they can be used to prevent excessive knee extension. Alternatively, keeping the knees farther forward, in front of the ankle, as they are straightened can also prevent the center of mass of the body from moving anterior to the axis of the knee where it will tend to produce knee hyperextension.

The second approach relies on the linking of femoral internal rotation with hyperextension of the knee. Since the final ranges of knee extension naturally incorporate internal rotation of the femur due to the locking mechanism of the knee, focusing on using the external rotators at the hip to limit this internal rotation of the femur and keep the knees facing directly forward rather than twisting inward can prevent undesired knee hyperextension. Excessive internal femoral rotation can also be avoided by focusing on "pulling up" with the abdominal muscles while bringing the bottom of the pelvis forward to create a neutral pelvis, so that the femoral internal rotation associated with an anterior tilt of the pelvis is avoided.

However, with whichever method is used, since the hyperextended position will "feel straight" to a dancer who is used to hyperextending the knees, this new position will often feel as though the knees are bent. Often a mirror and visual correction must be used initially by the dancer until the internal sensation of "straight" is relearned.

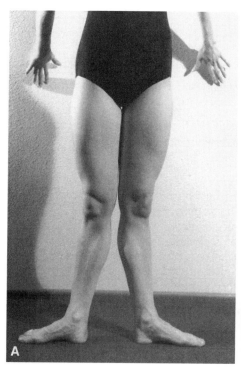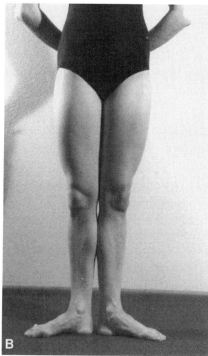

FIGURE 5.27 Knee hyperextension. (A) Standing with the heels separated and knees hyperextended; (B) correction of knee hyperextension, allowing the heels to be brought closer together.

Knee Hyperextension and Genu Varum

When genu varum is present, allowing the knees to hyperextend can increase the distance between the knees, giving the leg a more "bowed" look. In contrast, using the approaches just described to correct knee hyperextension—so that the knees are farther forward relative to the ankles and the knees face forward rather than inward as the inner thighs (hip adductors) are slightly contracted to pull the legs "together and up"—can help minimize the distorted appearance of genu varum. And over time, some dancers appear to be able to reduce apparent genu varum.

Overdevelopment of the Quadriceps

In some dance forms such as ballet, there is the desire to develop the body so that the legs appear "long"; and "short, thick, overdeveloped" thighs are avoided. Although genetics, body type, and limb length contribute to the appearance of the thighs, and dancers are encouraged to embrace the body type they have, training can also influence this development. While some hold that thigh development is simply related to the amount of quadriceps stress or

overload and resultant increase in size (hypertrophy), others conjecture that other factors such as the type of muscle contraction (higher emphasis on concentric vs. eccentric), speed of muscle contraction, or the range of motion utilized by the sport may also influence subtle differences in muscle development. In the dance arena, many dancers' bodies can change to develop a "longer," less "bulky" look after training at schools that emphasize this aesthetic. Further scientific investigation into this area is warranted, but two possible mechanisms for decreased thigh development are movement economy and altered muscle recruitment patterns.

In terms of movement economy, dancers with marked thigh development sometimes appear to be using excessive effort with movement, sometimes described by dance teachers as "gripping" or "working tensely." In contrast, dancers with the desired "long" muscle sometimes appear to be working more economically, without apparent wasted effort. Two examples of these extremes are shown in figure 5.28, where the execution of a second-position plié was associated with 25% versus 125% of a maximum isometric quadriceps contraction in a highly skilled ballet dancer noted for her "long lines" (figure 5.28A) versus a less skilled dancer noted for working with excessive "gripping" (figure 5.29B). Considering the marked difference in muscle effort associated with performance of the same movement, one could theorize that the second dancer would have greater hypertrophy of the quadriceps from dance training. This concept of greater economy being associated with skill level was given further support by another study that found significantly lower levels of activation of the rectus femoris and biceps femoris in key phases of a turned-out demi-plié in more experienced dancers (Ferland, Gardiner, and Lèbé-Neron, 1983).

In terms of altered muscle recruitment patterns, it may be that dancers with greater thigh development recruit the quadriceps femoris more in various dance movements. This might relate to alignment issues such as positioning of the torso or the amount of turnout used at the hip. For example, leaning

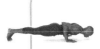

Controlling Hyperextended Knees
When the Foot Is Weight Bearing

Stand with your side to a mirror in a parallel first position and fully straighten your knees. Note if the knees appear slightly bent, straight (extended), or if they bow backward (hyperextension or genu recurvatum). If your knees are hyperextended, try the following exercises to help control this hyperextension.

· **Limiting the degree of knee extension.** While looking in the mirror, slowly bend and then straighten your knees. Identify the position visually and kinesthetically in which the knees are just straight and not overextended. Then, try to find this position kinesthetically and just use a visual check in the mirror to see if you were accurate. Focus on pressing down into the floor with the whole foot and keeping the ischial tuberosities ("sitz bones") facing down and forward over the ankles rather than facing back and over the heels as the knees straighten (A).

· **Limiting the degree of femoral internal rotation.** Now, bend your knees slightly and let your knees drop in. Then, use your hip external rotators (deep outward rotators) to bring the knees out relative to the foot as shown in B. Repeat this procedure several times; and when you have clear ability to activate the external rotators, concentrate on using these same deep outward rotators to keep your knee facing straight ahead as you slowly straighten your knees just to an extended, not a hyperextended, position. Also focus on using the abdominal–hamstring force couple to keep the "bottom of the pelvis under" so that the pelvis maintains a neutral position as the knees straighten. Notice when you relax the deep outward rotators and the abdominals whether the knees go "in and back" and the pelvis tilts anteriorly.

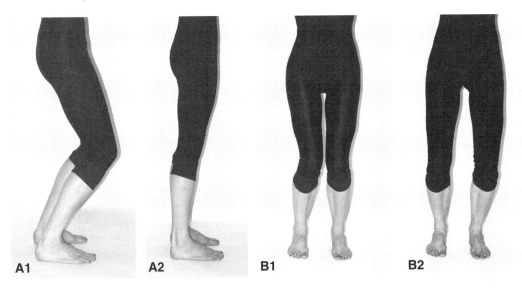

A1   **A2**   **B1**   **B2**

For the dancer with extreme genu recurvatum, these technique cues can be used to allow the heels to be brought closer together during standing in turned-out first position (figure 5.27B). Working with the feet separated and knees hyperextended tends to stretch out the posterior capsule and other restraints, increasing the degree of knee hyperextension over time and necessitating progressively greater separation of the heels. For dancers who are used to working with their heels separated more than an inch, it may be necessary to gradually bring the heels closer together over several months as skill for controlling hyperextension is developed and new balance strategies are learned.

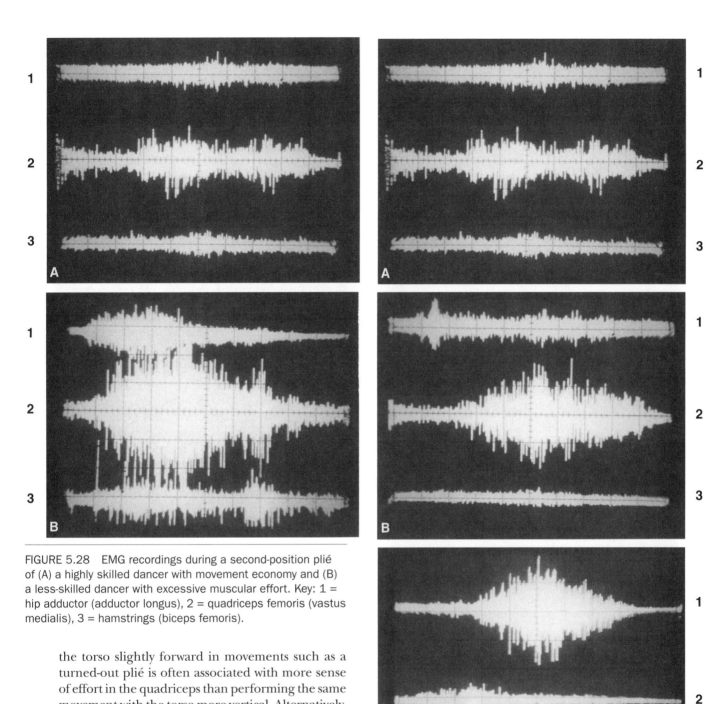

FIGURE 5.28   EMG recordings during a second-position plié of (A) a highly skilled dancer with movement economy and (B) a less-skilled dancer with excessive muscular effort. Key: 1 = hip adductor (adductor longus), 2 = quadriceps femoris (vastus medialis), 3 = hamstrings (biceps femoris).

the torso slightly forward in movements such as a turned-out plié is often associated with more sense of effort in the quadriceps than performing the same movement with the torso more vertical. Alternatively, degree of quadriceps activation may relate more to habit and preferential muscle recruitment strategies. The electromyography (EMG) tracings from the dancers shown in figures 5.28 and 5.29 exhibit a wide variety of recruitment patterns in terms of magnitude of quadriceps contraction and of relative contribution of the hamstrings and hip adductors. Teaching dancers to emphasize greater use of the hip extensors and hip adductors may allow less contribution of the knee extensors, which would be potentially advantageous in terms of reducing patellofemoral compression forces as well as meeting quadriceps

FIGURE 5.29   Example of muscle activation patterns for a skilled dancer performing a second-position grand plié with (A) routine performance, (B) cueing to "let the knees drop in," and (C) cueing to "reach the knees side." Key: 1 = hip adductor (adductor longus), 2 = quadriceps femoris (vastus medialis), 3 = hamstrings (biceps femoris).

development aesthetics. Such recruitment patterns could theoretically be encouraged by cues that direct students to use more of the inner thighs (hip adductors) and back of the leg (hamstrings). An example in which cueing designed to emphasize greater use of the hip muscles (e.g., reaching the knees as close to directly side as possible on the down-phase and then pulling the inner thighs up and together on the up-phase of a plié) changed muscle recruitment patterns such that greater activity in the adductor and hamstrings occurred, as shown in figure 5.29C. In contrast, cueing to promote the undesired technique of "letting the knees drop inward" resulted in greater activation of the quadriceps in this skilled dancer (figure 5.29B).

While excessive use of the quadriceps femoris should be discouraged in order to meet aesthetics in some dance forms, this does not mean that the quadriceps should not be used and that the quadriceps should not be strong. As previously discussed, the quadriceps are essential for controlling positioning of the knee. The issue is one of relative contribution of the quadriceps and magnitude of contraction, not of avoiding its use.

Conditioning Exercises for the Knee

Adequate strength and flexibility of the muscles crossing the knee are important for performance of demanding movements such as jumps, hinges, falls, floor work, and grand pliés. A balance of strength and flexibility is also important for preventing injury.

Selected Strength Exercises for the Knee

The most key muscle groups acting on the knee and patellofemoral joints are the quadriceps femoris (knee extensors) and hamstrings (knee flexors). For joint stability and proper mechanics it is essential that both of these muscle groups have both adequate and balanced strength. With the common use of the quadriceps as antigravity muscles, they can be three times stronger than their antagonists, the hamstrings (Hamill and Knutzen, 1995), and it is important that dancers not neglect strengthening the hamstrings. Sample exercises for these muscles are provided in table 5.3, and a brief description of their importance follows. Since the hamstrings and one component of the quadriceps femoris (rectus femoris) act on the hip as well as the knee, some strengthening exercises for these muscles were described in chapter 4. Exercises for other members

of the pes anserinus group and tensor fasciae latae were also described in this previous chapter on the hip, while exercises for the gastrocnemius are described in chapter 6.

Knee Extensor (Quadriceps Femoris) Strengthening

The knee extensors are very important antigravity muscles that act to control the lowering of the body, propel the body through space, or maintain an extended position of the knee. Furthermore, adequate quadriceps strength plays an important role in knee joint stability, the prevention or progression of knee osteoarthritis (Suter and Herzog, 2000), and proper tracking of the patella. While some female dancers are concerned about developing excessive bulk in the quadriceps femoris muscles, adequate strength is essential for injury prevention; and the exercises in table 5.3 can generally be used to develop strength without excessive bulk because the amount of weight (resistance) and volume (number of sets and reps) are generally too low to stimulate a large increase in muscle size (hypertrophy).

The knee extension can be strengthened isometrically by pulling the kneecap upward (quad sets) or isotonically by resisting knee extension. For dancers who have a history of kneecap problems or who experience knee discomfort with grand pliés, it is advisable to begin with exercises such as the quad set (table 5.3A) and straight leg raise (table 5.3B) in which the knee is isometrically maintained in a position of extension so that patellofemoral compression forces are low. Exercises incorporating only the final 20° to 30° of extension, such as the terminal knee extension (table 5.3C) exercise, can also be useful for providing greater overload to the quadriceps while patellofemoral compression forces still remain relatively low. However, for males without patellar problems and females who have developed adequate patellar stability and are pain free, performing knee extension exercises utilizing a larger range of motion (table 5.3D) is valuable to develop the strength needed for demanding dance movements utilizing greater degrees of knee flexion.

When one performs any of these extension exercises, proper technique is important. Due to the prevalence of knee hyperextension in dancers, it is important to take care that the knee is brought only to a straight position and not beyond straight to a position of hyperextension. The persistent use of hyperextension in these exercises can actually decrease knee stability and irritate tissues rather than provide the desired increase in joint stability and muscle strength.

(Text continues on p. 279.)

TABLE 5.3 Selected Strength Exercises for the Knee

Exercise name (Resistance)	Description (Technique cues)	Progression
Muscle group: Knee extensors **Muscles emphasized: Vastus medialis**		
Joint movement: Knee extension maintained		
A. Quad set 	Sit on the floor with the legs extended forward, and pull the kneecap up toward the hip by firmly contracting the quadriceps and holding the contraction for 5 seconds. Slowly release the muscle. (Focus on pulling the kneecap up without pushing the knee back to avoid hyperextension.) *Variation 1:* Perform with one leg extended and the other knee bent with the foot on the floor.	1. Increase reps from 8 to 12. 2. Increase sets from 1 to 2 and then 3.
Muscle groups: Knee extensors and hip flexors **Muscles emphasized: Quadriceps femoris, especially vastus medialis**		
Joint movement: Hip flexion with knee extension maintained		
B. Straight leg raise (Ankle weight) 	Sit with one knee bent with the foot on the floor while the other leg is extended to the front with a weight cuff on the ankle. Perform a quad set and then, while maintaining a firm contraction of the quadriceps, raise the extended leg, hold for 4 counts, and lower it to the starting position. (Use the quadriceps to maintain a straight but not hyperextended position of the knee, as the hip flexors are used to lift and lower the whole leg.)	1. Increase the weight from 2 pounds to 10 pounds gradually, in 1- to 2-pound increments.
Muscle group: Knee extensors **Muscles emphasized: Quadriceps femoris, especially vastus medialis**		
Joint movement: Knee extension		
C. Terminal knee extension (Ankle weight) 	Sit with one knee bent with the foot on the floor while the other leg is extended to the front with a foam support or a towel roll under the distal thigh and a weight cuff on the ankle. Slowly extend the knee to a straight position, hold 4 counts with the quads firmly contracted, and return to the starting position. (Avoid letting the knee hyperextend.) *Variation 1:* Perform sitting in a chair with the outstretched knee bent about 30°. *Variation 2:* Perform on a knee extension machine, only utilizing a range of the last 30° of extension.	1. Increase the weight from 5 pounds to 15 pounds gradually, in 1- to 3-pound increments.

(continued)

TABLE 5.3 **Selected Strength Exercises for the Knee** *(continued)*

Exercise name (Resistance)	Description (Technique cues)	Progression
Muscle group: Knee extensors **Muscles emphasized: Quadriceps femoris, especially vastus medialis**		
Joint movement: Knee extension with hip flexion maintained		
D. Sitting knee extension (Reformer) 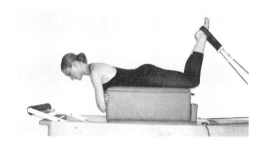 *Variation 1*	Sit on a Reformer, using the arms to support one thigh and the strap over the foot of that leg. Then slowly extend the knee to a straight position, pause, and return to the starting position. (Keep the thigh stationary while the foot pulls the strap as the knee extends to a straight but not hyperextended position.) *Variation 1:* Perform in the same position, only sitting on the floor with a looped band anchored under the support foot and around the instep or ankle of the gesture leg.	1. Increase the resistance from one spring gradually in small increments. 2. Bring torso more vertical with lumbar spine neutral.
Muscle group: Knee flexors **Muscles emphasized: Hamstrings**		
Joint movement: Knee flexion		
E. Prone knee curl (Reformer)	Lie prone on the box with the knees slightly bent and the straps on the feet. Then slowly bring the heels toward the buttocks, pause, and slowly lower the leg to the starting position. (Firmly contract the abdominals to maintain a neutral pelvis and avoid an anterior pelvic tilt.) *Variation 1:* Perform with one leg at a time. *Variation 2:* Perform on a knee-curl weight apparatus. *Variation 3:* Perform one leg at a time with an elastic band looped around the feet to provide resistance.	1. Gradually increase springs. 2. Increase range of knee flexion. 3. Lift knees half an inch off the box (slight hip hyperextension), and maintain this position throughout the exercise without letting the pelvis tilt anteriorly.

Exercise name (Resistance)	Description (Technique cues)	Progression

Muscle group: Knee flexors
Muscles emphasized: Hamstrings

Joint movement: Knee flexion

F. Standing knee curl (Ankle weight) 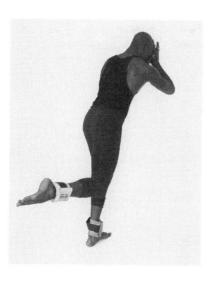	Stand with body weight supported on one leg, with the foot about 2 feet away from a wall and the forearms resting on the wall. Begin with the top of the other foot about 1 foot behind the support leg, and slowly bring the heel toward the buttocks with a weight around the ankle, pause, and slowly return to the starting position. (Keep the knee in place as it flexes, and avoid letting it move forward.) *Variation 1:* After flexing the knee about 30°, lift the whole leg back and up toward the ceiling (hip extension). *Variation 2:* Perform with a band tied in a loop under the arch of the support foot and around the gesture leg providing resistance.	1. Increase the weight from 5 pounds to 12 pounds gradually, in 1- to 2-pound increments.

Muscle groups: Knee extensors and hip extensors
Muscles emphasized: Quadriceps femoris

Joint movement: Knee extension with hip extension

G. Wall squat 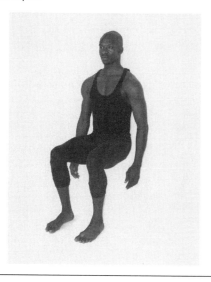	Stand with the back against a wall with the feet parallel, hip width apart, and about 1 1/2 to 2 feet from the wall. Slowly bend the knees until the thighs are parallel to the floor with the knees above the ankles, hold for 4 counts, and slowly straighten the knees to return to the starting position. (Maintain a firm contraction of the abdominals so that the pelvis is in a neutral position with the back of the sacrum and midthoracic spine staying in contact with the wall throughout the exercise.)	1. Gradually increase the hold from 4 counts to 5 seconds. 2. Add dumbbells in each hand.

(continued)

TABLE 5.3 Selected Strength Exercises for the Knee *(continued)*

Exercise name (Resistance)	Description (Technique cues)	Progression
Muscle groups: Knee extensors and hip extensors **Muscles emphasized: Hamstrings/abdominal–hamstring force couple**		
Joint movement: Knee extension with hip extension		
H. Plié/leg press (Reformer) (Weight apparatus)	Start supine on a Reformer, with feet parallel in line with hip joints on the foot plate, and knees bent. Slowly extend the knees until they are just straight, pause, and slowly bend the knees to return to the starting position. (Avoid hyperextending the knees; guide knees over second toe; maintain a stable torso and neutral pelvis.) *Variation 1:* Increase range by allowing the feet to come off the plate until the knees bend to about 90°, and add a relevé after the knees straighten. *Variation 2:* Perform in turned-out positions. (Turn out in accordance with hip external rotation with the knees straight.) *Variation 3:* Perform on a leg-press machine in parallel position, keeping the heels in contact throughout the exercise.	1. Gradually increase the resistance from three springs. 2. Perform with one leg with lower resistance.
Muscle groups: Knee extensors and hip extensors **Muscles emphasized: Hamstrings and quadriceps femoris**		
Joint movement: Knee extension with hip extension		
I. Lunge	Stand with feet parallel and about hip width apart and arms down by each side holding a dumbbell. Step far forward with one foot and then slowly lower the body until the front knee is bent to about 90°. Then slowly straighten the knee, and push off with the front foot to return to the starting position. (Guide knee over front foot and keep torso vertical rather than lean forward or backward.)	1. Gradually increase weight.

Exercise name (Resistance)	Description (Technique cues)	Progression
Muscle groups: Knee extensors and hip extensors **Muscles emphasized: Hamstrings and quadriceps femoris**		
Joint movement: Knee extension with hip extension		
J. Forward lunge (Pilates chair)	Stand facing the combo chair. Bring the pedal down with one foot, and place the other foot on the top platform of the chair. Then slowly raise the body up over the top foot, pause, lower the body and pedal down until the top knee is bent about 90°, and raise up again. (Guide front knee over foot; avoid excessive forward lean of the torso, and maintain an almost vertical position; focus on pressing the top foot firmly down and engaging the hip extensors as the body is lifted over the top foot; work only in a range where good form can be maintained and no knee discomfort is experienced.)	1. Gradually decrease springs.

Knee Flexor Strengthening

The flexors of the knees, including the hamstrings, are important for achieving and maintaining bent positions of the gesture leg such as used with a passé or attitude. With the tremendous demands for hamstring flexibility in dance, it is advisable to follow the knee flexion exercises described next with hamstring stretching exercises so that the hamstrings do not become tighter, or to utilize exercises emphasizing hip extension to strengthen the hamstrings.

Prone and standing knee curls emphasize resisted knee flexion. The prone knee curl (table 5.3E) can be performed with springs or an elastic band resisting knee flexion. The standing knee curl (table 5.3F) can also be performed with elastic resistance, but also afford a relationship to gravity that will allow an ankle weight to effectively resist knee flexion. The back leg raise shown in chapter 4 (table 4.5D, p. 214) offers a variation that emphasizes the hip extension function of the hamstrings.

Closed Kinematic Chain Strength Exercises

As discussed in chapter 1, closed kinematic chain exercises for the lower extremity involve movement at multiple joints (hip, knee, and ankle) while the foot remains fixed or encounters considerable resistance. This is in contrast to an open kinematic chain exercise in which the distal segment of the extremity (e.g., the foot) is free to move. Strength exercises previously described for the knee such as terminal knee extension and prone knee curl are examples of open kinematic chain exercises. Examples of closed kinematic chain exercises described in table 5.3, G through J, include the wall squat, plié/leg press, lunge, and forward lunge.

The wall squat (table 5.3G) provides an effective way of particularly strengthening the quadriceps while working on maintaining trunk stabilization and avoiding the common error of leaning the torso forward in pliés. The plié/leg press (table 5.3H) offers resistance to develop strength in the knee

CONCEPT DEMONSTRATION 5.3

Controlling Hyperextended Knees When the Foot Is Not Weight Bearing

Sit with one leg outstretched in front of you and the other knee bent with the foot on the floor. Practice maintaining a straight but not hyperextended knee in the following exercises.

- **Quad set** (table 5.3A, variation 1). Place two fingertips about 1 1/2 inches (3.8 centimeters) above the patella and about 1/2 inch (1.3 centimeters) medial to the inner border of the patella. Focus on pulling the kneecap up toward your hip without pushing the knee back into hyperextension. A firm contraction should be felt in the muscle under your fingertips (vastus medialis). If you have difficulty avoiding pushing your knee back, place the fingertips of your other hand behind your outstretched knee to help prevent your knee from hyperextending. Co-contraction of the quadriceps and gastrocnemius (knee flexor) may be necessary to establish a straight but not hyperextended position. For most dancers (depending on the size of the calf muscle), the heel of the outstretched leg should stay on the floor, and lifting of the heel off the floor indicates that the knee is being hyperextended.

- **Straight leg raise** (table 5.3B). Perform a quad set and then raise the leg off the ground, hold for four counts, and then lower the leg back to the starting position. Use your fingertips to check that the vastus medialis is staying contracted, and make sure the knee stays straight and not hyperextended throughout the movement. Avoid the common error of hamstring substitution. When the knee hyperextends, the line of pull of the hamstrings can switch from behind to in front of the axis of the knee joint, and thus the hamstrings can produce extension rather than its normal function of flexion of the knee. When raising the leg off the floor, some dancers will hyperextend the knee and then use the hamstrings (vs. the quadriceps) to maintain the hyperextension, while other hip flexors such as the iliopsoas are used to lift the leg. With this substitution, the vastus medialis will not be felt firmly contracting under the fingertips. This undesired substitution will not produce the desired strengthening of the quadriceps or develop a desired muscle activation pattern.

in a manner similar to that used with pliés and the preparation for turns and jumps. It can be performed with traditional weight apparatus (leg press machine) or on a reformer with a large number of springs offering resistance. The lunge (table 5.3I) and particularly the forward lunge (table 5.3J) are used to develop lower body strength but can produce injury if performed improperly, with too much overload, or with underlying biomechanical problems. Thus, such exercises should be reserved for adequately skilled and conditioned dancers without a history of knee problems and performed only with qualified supervision.

With any of these closed kinematic chain exercises, proper technique is particularly important. In addition to stabilization and focus on proper positioning of the torso, care must be taken to guide the knee over the second toe, avoid letting the knee fall inward, and lower only to a point at which correct form can be maintained and no knee pain is experienced.

Closed kinematic chain exercises have gained great popularity in the fitness and rehabilitation arenas in recent years because they better replicate functional movements in terms of the loads placed upon the joints and the complex muscle contraction involved in coordinating multiple joints. It has also been proposed that they place less stress on the anterior cruciate ligament and are associated with less patellofemoral compression force in the angles of 0° to 53° of knee flexion (Hungerford and Barry, 1979). However, some of their theoretical advantages have been questioned by recent research findings (Irrgang and Neri, 2000); for example, it appears that both open and closed kinematic chain exercises can be effective in improving joint proprioception (Perrin and Shultz, 2000). Furthermore, open kinematic chain exercises may offer advantages in terms of producing effective overload with less resistance, helping to correct muscle imbalances, and replicating dance demands of the gesture leg. So, one recommended approach is to include a combination of open and closed kinematic chain strengthening exercises in supplemental conditioning programs for dancers (Clippinger, 2002). In terms of rehabilitation, medical professionals will select appropriate exercises in accordance with the specific injury and relative advantages and disadvantages of these two types of exercises.

Selected Stretches for the Knee

Table 5.4 provides the normal range of motion for general populations (non-dance) as well as the structures that primarily limit further ranges of motion for knee flexion and extension. And sample stretches to improve range in these movements are described shortly and shown in table 5.5.

In addition, adequate flexibility of some of the multijoint muscles that cross the knee is important for optimal knee mechanics. For example, tightness in the iliotibial band can exert lateral forces on the patella and increase knee injury risk (Jenkinson and Bolin, 2001; Reid et al., 1987). Similarly, adequate flexibility in the hip adductors is important for correct placement of the knees over the feet in positions such as turned-out second (Clippinger, 2005). Distally, tightness of the calf muscles limits the depth of the plié and can contribute to compensatory foot pronation and resultant suboptimal knee mechanics. Stretches for the hip abductors and adductors were described in chapter 4, and calf stretches are described in chapter 6.

Knee Extensor (Quadriceps) Stretches

Despite having markedly increased flexibility in many other areas, dancers are frequently low in flexibility in the knee extensors or quadriceps femoris muscle group. This tendency for tightness appears to be more prevalent (at least in ballet dancers) in dancers with many years of training and almost universal in male ballet dancers; 75% of female and 100% of male elite ballet dancers tested exhibited quadriceps tightness (Clippinger-Robertson, 1991). Another study of preprofessional ballet dancers showed that 95% of these dancers had at least minimal tightness of the rectus femoris (Molnar and Esterson, 1997). A quick screening test is shown in Tests and Measurements 5.4 that can be easily used to check quadriceps flexibility. Stretches for this muscle group are often neglected in the dancer's regular stretching routine. Tight quadriceps muscles may increase the risk for patellofemoral problems, so it is important that adequate flexibility be achieved and maintained.

To effectively stretch the vasti components of the quadriceps, the knee must be brought into full flexion, and the position of the pelvis is irrelevant since these muscles do not cross the hip. In contrast, due to the proximal attachment of the rectus femoris on the anterior pelvis, care must be taken that the pelvis is in a neutral or tucked position, since an anterior pelvic tilt will slacken the rectus femoris and decrease stretch effectiveness. Because the rectus femoris is a hip flexor, bringing the hip into hyperextension prior to bringing the knee toward the buttocks will also increase the stretch to the rectus femoris.

The quadriceps are commonly stretched by using the hand to bring the heel toward the buttocks while standing, sitting on a chair (chair quadriceps stretch, table 5.5B), lying on one side, or lying prone (heel-to-buttocks stretch, table 5.5A). For whichever variation is being used, it is important to realize that due to knee joint structure, when the knee fully flexes the distal tibia should angle medially relative to the shaft of the femur. Hence, this normal motion should be allowed and twisting of the tibia should be avoided. The chair quadriceps stretch (table 5.5B) allows the quadriceps to be stretched in a position in which the torso is vertical and maintaining a neutral pelvis can be more readily achieved. The low lunge quadriceps stretch provides a challenging position for the more flexible dancer with adequate hip flexor flexibility in that the weight is on the thigh and above the

TABLE 5.4 Normal Range of Motion and Constraints for Primary Movements of the Knee

Knee joint movement	Normal range of motion*	Normal passive limiting factors
Flexion	0-135°	Soft tissue apposition: posterior aspects of thigh and calf or heel and buttocks Muscles: quadriceps femoris
Extension	0-10°	Capsule: posterior portion Ligaments: cruciates, medial collateral, lateral collateral, and oblique posterior (a ligament located posteriorly) Muscles: hamstrings (when hip in marked flexion)

*From American Academy of Orthopaedic Surgeons (1965).

TABLE 5.5 Selected Stretches for the Knee

Exercise name (Method of stretch)	Description (Technique cues)	Progression
Muscle group: Knee extensors **Muscles emphasized: Quadriceps femoris**		
Joint position: Knee flexion with hip extension		
A. Heel-to-buttocks stretch (Static) 	Stand on one leg with a slight posterior pelvic tilt. Bend the gesture leg and, with one hand grasping the foot, gently bring the knee back until the thigh is approximately vertical. Then bring the heel toward the buttocks until a moderate stretch is felt across the front of the thigh while a neutral position of the pelvis is maintained. (Maintain a firm contraction of the abdominals to prevent the pelvis from tilting anteriorly and avoid twisting the knee.) *Variation 1:* Perform lying on the floor on one side, using the upper arm to pull the heel of the upper leg toward the buttocks. *Variation 2:* Perform lying prone on the floor.	1. Bring the heel closer to the buttocks. 2. Bring the knee further back before bringing the heel to the buttocks to increase the stretch applied to the rectus femoris.
B. Chair quadriceps stretch (Static) 	Sit sideways to the back of a chair with one foot on the ground and the other knee hanging over the front edge of the chair, approximately perpendicular to the floor. Use the hand on the same side to bring the heel of the hanging knee toward the buttocks until a moderate stretch is felt along the front of the thigh. (Maintain a firm contraction of the abdominals to prevent an anterior pelvic tilt; reach the hanging knee directly down toward the floor, and avoid twisting the knee.)	1. Same as exercise A.

Exercise name (Method of stretch)	Description (Technique cues)	Progression
Muscle group: Knee flexors **Muscles emphasized: Hamstrings**		
Joint position: Knee extension with hip flexion		
C. Standing hamstring stretch (Static)	Stand on one leg with the other leg lifted to the front while the ankle is supported on a barre, chair, or box. While maintaining a straight knee, lean the torso over the outstretched leg until a moderate stretch is felt along the back of the knee or back of the thigh. (Tighten quadriceps if necessary to maintain the knee in a fully straight but not hyperextended position; lean the torso forward by flexing at the hip while keeping the upper back extended versus rounded forward.)	1. Gradually increase the height of the object that supports the outstretched leg. 2. Bring the torso closer to the front leg.

patella on the back leg (figure 5.30A). However, this stretch is often inappropriate for more beginning-level or tight dancers, in whom inadequate flexibility necessitates an uncomfortable position in which the weight is borne on the patella (figure 5.30B). In such instances, alternatives such as performing the lunge stretch without bringing the heel to the buttocks (with the lower leg on or off the floor; figure 5.30C) or substituting a prone, side-lying, or standing position (figure 5.30D) are advised.

Knee Flexor Stretches

When the hip is flexed as in a front développé, lack of adequate hamstring flexibility can limit the ability to fully straighten the knee. Because the hamstrings also cross the hip, stretches for these muscles were described in connection with the hip in chapter 4. However, there are other times when the hip is not flexed that some dancers may not be able to fully straighten their knees. This may be due to structural factors such as the angle between the tibia and femur, as well as soft tissue restraints such as the ligaments and capsule listed in table 5.4, and the prudence of

stretching such structures is controversial. Hence, it is important that such dancers see an orthopedist to determine their restraints and whether it is advisable for them to stretch the knee. However, if not contraindicated, very careful, gentle, and consistent stretching of the knee such as using the standing hamstring stretch (table 5.5C) can often result in gradual improvement (often taking months or a year to achieve a "straight" look). Because the structures being stretched are not primarily muscular, stretches should be done with particular care when the body is adequately warmed, avoiding excessive force or pain that can result in injury.

Knee Injuries in Dancers

The fact that the knee joint is located between the longest bones of the body and that, although broad, it is a very shallow articulation, leaves it very vulnerable to valgus and varus stresses with resultant potential injuries to the ligaments and menisci. This potential vulnerability is further heightened by the rotation allowed at the knee when it is in a flexed

Screening Test for Quadriceps Femoris Flexibility

While the dancer is lying prone, the examiner applies light pressure on the ankle to bring one heel toward the buttocks as shown in the figure. Stop if any pain is experienced. The dancer should focus on using the abdominal muscles to prevent the pelvis from anteriorly tilting throughout the test. The goal is to be able to easily bring the heel to the buttocks with the foot relaxed, but if they cannot be easily approximated, the examiner uses a ruler to measure the distance between the heel and the buttocks while maintaining light pressure. Holding the ankle at a right angle makes the test more challenging, but some dancers will be stopped by approximation of the posterior thigh and calf muscles versus quadriceps tightness with this test variation.

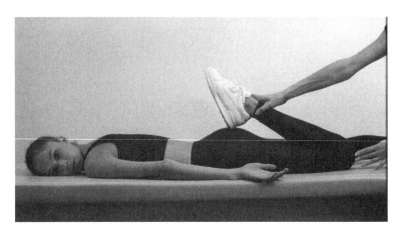

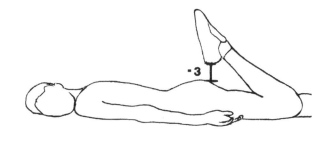

position. Anteriorly, the quadriceps, patella, and patellar tendon (collectively termed the extensor mechanism) serve key antigravity, deceleration, acceleration, and stability functions and also can be readily involved in both acute and chronic injuries.

With this general injury vulnerability and the large demands placed on the knee with jumping, floor work, and repetitive flexion, it is not surprising that knee injuries are common in dancers. The percentage of total injuries involving the knee has been reported as 16.1% to 17.3% for ballet dancers (Garrick, 1999; Quirk, 1987) and 14.5% to 18% for dancers at performing arts schools (Rovere et al., 1983; Wiesler et al., 1996). A survey of modern dancers revealed the knee was the most commonly reported site of injury with 20.1% of dancers reporting injury to this area (Solomon and Micheli, 1986), while a survey of Broadway dancers found 15% of dancers reported sustaining an injury to the knee during their production (Evans, Evans, and Carvajal, 1996).

Prevention of Knee Injuries

Given that the absolute strength of the quadriceps in some dancers may be lower than desirable and that low thigh power production tends to be linked with greater severity of lower extremity injuries (Koutedakis et al., 1997), many dancers would benefit from including supplemental quadriceps and hamstring strengthening (the latter for balance) in their regular training regimes. In addition to isolation exercises, this training would also ideally include exercises aimed at developing functional strength, such as jumping drills, in which proprioception and neuromuscular skills could be developed in movements commonly associated with injury. One study showed that a program utilizing bounding drills (plyometric training) reduced ACL injury to almost one-third of that seen in untrained athletes (Hewett et al., 1999).

Adequate flexibility of the quadriceps and paying close attention to technique may also help reduce

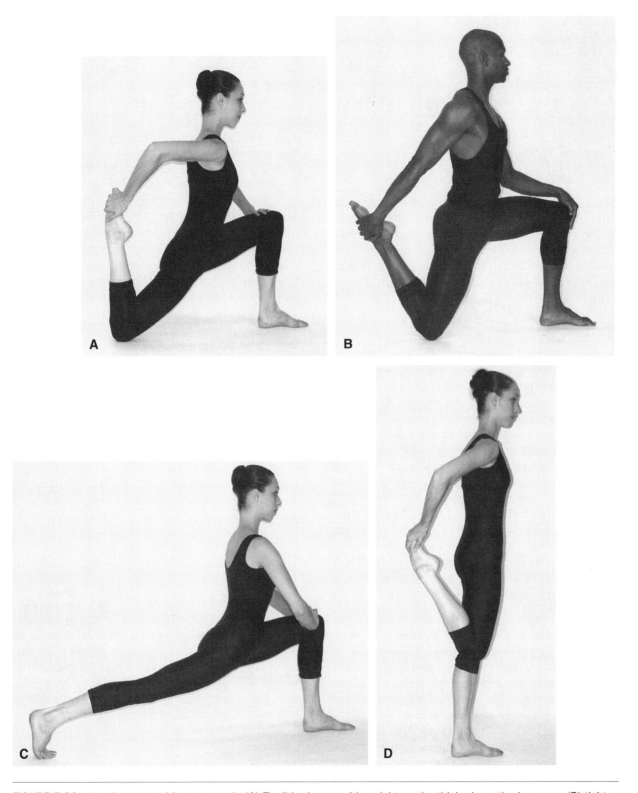

FIGURE 5.30 Low lunge quadriceps stretch. (A) Flexible dancer with weight on the thigh above the kneecap, (B) tighter dancer with weight on the kneecap, (C) alternate hip flexor stretch, (D) alternate quadriceps stretch.

injury risk. In terms of technique, excessive twisting of the tibia relative to the femur, inadequate stabilization of turnout from the hip, letting the knees "fall in" relative to the feet, overuse of the quadriceps, or excessive foot pronation can put undue stress on the knee and may increase the risk for certain types of knee injuries.

Common Types of Knee Injuries in Dancers

Many different types of injuries can occur around the knee. A discussion of a few of these injuries that more commonly occur in dancers follows, and interested dancers are referred to the publications written by James Garrick (1989, 1999), Ronald Quirk (1987), and other authors cited in this section for a more detailed presentation of knee injuries.

Knee Ligamental Injuries

Serious ligamental injuries to the knee are very common in skiing and contact sports. Although they are less common in dance, when they do occur they can severely affect the dancer's ability to dance, and prompt medical treatment is essential. With youth, particular care must be taken that adequate medical treatment be obtained, since the ligaments of the knee are generally stronger than the growth plates and injury to a ligament may also involve epiphyseal injury.

The ligaments are key to the stability of the knee, so when a ligament is torn, knee stability is temporarily jeopardized. The two most commonly involved ligaments in dancers are the medial collateral ligament and the ACL. Dancers with extreme generalized joint mobility (hypermobility) are probably more vulnerable to such ligamental injury.

Medial Collateral Ligament Injury   The most commonly occurring ligamental injury in sport involves the medial collateral ligament (Caillet, 1996). Such injuries often result from a medially directed force against the lateral side of the knee (valgus-deforming force) that tends to open up the inside of the knee as seen in figure 5.31. In dance, this type of force can occur when a dancer falls on another, as may happen, for example, in contact improvisation. Noncontact injuries of the medial collateral ligament may also result from deceleration, pivoting, or forcing turnout and pushing the knee forward relative to the foot, such as in fifth-position turned-out pliés (Quirk, 1988). It appears that the medial collateral ligament is particularly vulnerable to twisting of the tibia externally (Hall, 1999).

Symptoms of this injury include pain on the inside of the knee where the medial collateral ligament is located. When the ligament is palpated, tenderness and swelling are commonly present. Tests performed by the physician that are designed to stress this ligament (see Tests and Measurements 5.1 on p. 242) will also generally be positive.

Treatment will vary greatly depending on the severity of the ligamental sprain and the approach of the attending physician. More serious sprains may involve initial bracing or immobilization and use of crutches or a cane for locomotion (Diduch, Scuderi, and Scott, 1997; Mercier, 1995), while less serious sprains may require only temporary limitation of specific dance movements such as fifth position. Quadriceps strengthening, and later strengthening of the other muscles that cross the knee, are instituted, with care taken to use positions and ranges of motion that are pain free and that avoid undue valgus stress. With its location outside of the joint (extra-articular), this ligament has good healing capacity (Scioscia, Giffin, and Fu, 2001). Hence, recovery from tears of the medial collateral ligament with conservative treatment tends to be excellent, with a very good prognosis for future full return to dance.

Anterior Cruciate Ligamental Injury   One of the most dreaded injuries for the dancer is rupture of the ACL as seen in figure 5.32. Anterior cruciate injury occurs most frequently in sports that involve deceleration, twisting, pivoting, and jumping—all motions that occur in dance. Females appear to

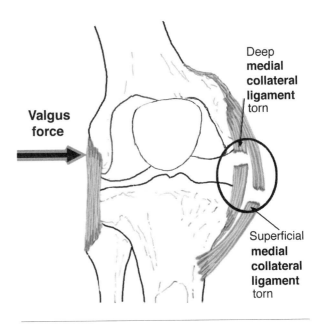

FIGURE 5.31   Injury to the medial collateral ligament (right knee, anterior view).

have a markedly greater incidence of anterior cruciate tears than males in competitive sport; different sources estimate two to seven times greater risk in females (Diduch, Scuderi, and Scott, 1997; Ireland, 2000; Scioscia, Giffin, and Fu, 2001). This increased incidence in females has been attributed to the shape and size of the femoral notch, less muscular development, greater ligamental laxity, less developed proprioception, greater hamstring flexibility that may lessen the hamstrings' potential protective effect on the ligament, and anatomical alignment tending to create a greater Q angle (Boden, Griffin, and Garrett, 2000; Scioscia, Giffin, and Fu, 2001).

A common mechanism for injury to this ligament in contact sports is a blow to the lateral knee that includes external rotation. In noncontact ACL injury, a common position on landing involves the body's falling such that the hip is adducting and internally rotating, with the knee collapsing into valgus while the tibia translates forward from an externally rotated position. This position is termed "the position of no return" and is shown in figure 5.32B. The most prevalent mechanism of injury in modern, ballet, and jazz dance appears to be landing in hyperextension from a jump on one leg as shown in figure 5.32C (Liederbach and Dilgen, 1998).

Classically the dancer feels a "pop" and is unable to continue dancing at the time of ligamental injury. The knee generally feels unsteady, with significant pain and ensuing rapid swelling. However, because ligaments themselves do not generally contain pain receptors, the degree of pain is not necessarily a

good indicator of the degree of injury, and dancers should seek medical evaluation if instability is present, even if pain is limited. Tests performed by the physician that are designed to test integrity of this ligament, including the anterior drawer test (Tests and Measurements 5.1C on p. 242), will generally be positive, and some orthopedists will utilize equipment to measure the exact anterior displacement of the tibia allowed on the injured side in comparison to the uninjured side.

Recommended treatment for minor anterior cruciate injuries may involve initial immobilization in a compression dressing with ice and elevation followed by hamstrings and quadriceps strengthening (Mercier, 1995). However, if the rupture is complete, this is one injury for which early surgical repair is often recommended for active individuals. Dancers with anterior cruciate deficient knees will often describe their knee as separating or "going out" (e.g., tibia sliding forward and then coming back) with movements such as walking down stairs. Repeated episodes of instability may cause further instability, injury to the menisci, and joint surface degeneration (Evans, Chew, and Stanish, 2001; Suter and Herzog, 2000). Hence, surgery to improve stability and joint function is often recommended, and Weiker (1988) holds that surgical repair of an ACL tear offers an 85% to 95% chance of being able to continue a professional dance career in contrast to only a 25% to 30% chance without surgery.

The ACL tends to heal poorly because it is located within the joint (intra-articular), where joint fluid

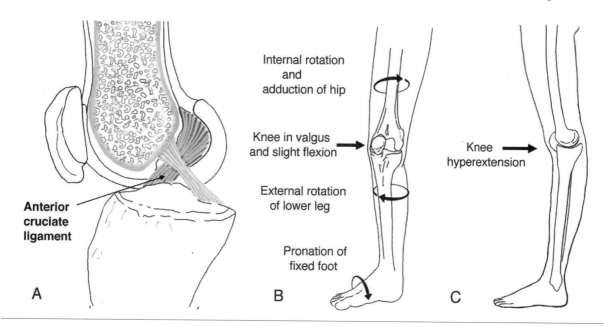

FIGURE 5.32   Injury to the anterior cruciate ligament (right knee, medial view). (A) Abnormal anterior movement of the tibia, (B) position of no return, and (C) classic mechanism in dance.

interferes with fibrin clot formation essential for the healing process (Scioscia, Giffin, and Fu, 2001). So, reconstruction rather than repair of the torn ligament is often the treatment of choice with dancers. One commonly used method utilizes a graft taken from the central one-third of the patellar tendon of the injured dancer (including a bony block from the tibial tuberosity and another from the patella), which is then fixed to the tibia and femur. Another method utilizes a graft taken from the injured dancer's medial hamstrings.

Whether a surgical or conservative approach is taken, the dancer should seek rehabilitative treatment from a qualified physical therapist who is working closely with the attending physician. Open kinematic chain knee extension exercises such as terminal extension can place large stresses on the ACL that may cause damage to an injured or reconstructed ligament. Hence, there are specific recommendations regarding the appropriate range of motion, appropriate use of open and closed kinematic chain exercises, and loading of the joint in different phases of rehabilitation that must be closely followed. Also, unlike what occurs with many other injuries, hamstring strength is particularly emphasized, as the hamstrings can pull the tibia posteriorly, aiding the anterior cruciate in its function. Long-term rehabilitation goals for anterior cruciate as well as other knee injuries are to maximize dynamic stability of the knee and prepare it to function with the diverse loading presented with dance training (Boden, Griffin, and Garrett, 2000; Brown and Clippinger, 1996; Irrgang, 1993; Loosli and Herold, 1992).

Meniscal Injury

The meniscus is designed to move with the tibia on the femur in a well-coordinated manner. However, if this coordinated movement becomes disrupted, the meniscus can become trapped between the opposing articular surfaces of the tibia and femur with resultant injury from compression, torque, or traction. The meniscus can be split, broken into pieces, or loosened by tearing of its ligamentous attachments. The medial meniscus has been reported to be torn 10 (Mercier, 1995) to 20 times (Caillet, 1996) more frequently than the lateral in general populations. One study of dancers also showed a predominance of medial meniscus tears, with 13 of the 15 meniscal tears examined arthroscopically involving the medial meniscus (Silver and Campbell, 1985). This increased vulnerability of the medial meniscus is probably related to its reduced mobility due to its attachment to the medial collateral ligament and joint capsule.

One of the most common mechanisms of injury of the meniscus is extension from a flexed, abducted position of the knee (valgus stress) while the leg is externally rotated with the foot fixed. In contact sports, such as football, this mechanism is often sudden and traumatic. However, in dance, it is believed that this mechanism may be operative chronically, that is, that repetitive forced turnout may result in long-term wearing and splitting of the meniscus (Quirk, 1987; Scioscia, Giffin, and Fu, 2001; Silver and Campbell, 1985). Dancers have also reported meniscal injury associated with losing balance or twisting when in a position of deep knee flexion such as that associated with floor work in modern or jazz, or center floor first or fifth grand pliés. In full flexion the menisci are pinched between the articulating bones; and if there is a twist in this vulnerable position, injury can readily occur. To lessen injury risk, full weighted knee flexion should be used cautiously, with appropriate progressions for beginners, and with an emphasis on good form.

In some cases of acute meniscal injury, a "popping" or "tearing" sensation is experienced, followed by severe pain (Mercier, 1995). More frequently, symptoms include moderate pain that gradually subsides (Diduch, Scuderi, and Scott, 1997). It is common to have localized tenderness on the joint line over the meniscus. Swelling is generally slow, often not reaching a maximum until the day after the initial injury, and may recur on multiple occasions (Scioscia, Giffin, and Fu, 2001). Grand pliés may be painful, and range of knee motion may be limited. There is often an apprehension about assuming the position of a full squat. In the days or even weeks following the initial injury, painful locking, catching, or giving way, especially with flexion and twisting movements, often occurs. Quadriceps femoris atrophy generally proceeds rapidly.

Initial recommended treatment for meniscal injury often involves limiting activity, ice, compression, elevation, and anti-inflammatory medications, followed by quadriceps strengthening (Diduch, Scuderi, and Scott, 1997; Mercier, 1995). Many small meniscal tears, especially small ones located in the outer third of the meniscus where the blood supply is adequate (figure 5.33B), can heal spontaneously. However, if the knee does not respond adequately to conservative therapy or there are repeating episodes of catching, locking, or giving way, surgery is often recommended. These episodes can relate to encroachment of the torn portion of the meniscus into the joint, where it can be caught between the condyles, as shown in figure 5.33, C and D. If allowed to continue, this mechanical impingement

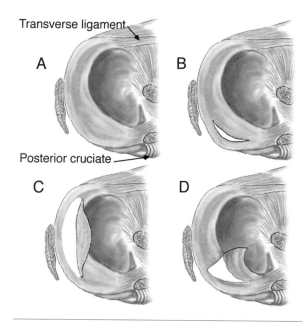

Transverse ligament

A   B

Posterior cruciate

C   D

FIGURE 5.33   Meniscal injury (right knee, superior view). (A) Normal meniscus, (B) small circumferential tear, (C) partial tear encroaching into the joint ("bucket handle" tear), (D) tear of posterior area encroaching into the joint ("posterior horn" tear).

is believed to cause damage and arthritic changes to the articular surface of the knee.

However, even if surgery is indicated, if the type of injury allows, surgery is often performed through a small scope (arthroscopic surgery) with an attempt to preserve or repair whatever part of the meniscus is viable or has sufficient blood supply to allow healing (Quirk, 1987; Scioscia, Giffin, and Fu, 2001). Such an approach allows for a shorter recovery period and less risk of future degenerative arthritis than open surgery involving full removal of the meniscus. The stress to the loaded tibiofemoral joint has been estimated to be three times higher when the meniscus is removed (Hall, 1999).

Recovery from meniscal injury, even when surgery is required, is generally excellent. Over the long term, this type of injury holds a very good prognosis for full return to dance.

The Terrible Triad

With some injuries, multiple structures can be involved. When a rotational component is added to the medially directed force on the knee, the ACL and medial meniscus, as well as the medial collateral ligament, can be injured simultaneously. This combination injury is termed the **"terrible triad"** (G. *trias*, three). It is a serious injury that requires prompt medical diagnosis and treatment.

Extensor Mechanism Injury

Any component of the extensor mechanism—including the quadriceps muscle itself, the tendons of the quadriceps, and the patella—can be injured, but the latter two are particularly commonly involved. A description of several injuries involving these latter two structures follows.

Patellofemoral Pain Syndrome   **Patellofemoral pain syndrome** refers to anterior knee pain that relates to the patella and associated retinacular support as seen in figure 5.34A. In cases in which there is documented damage to the thick cartilage that lines the backside of the patella, patellofemoral pain can be more specifically classified as **chondromalacia patella,** which literally means soft ("malacia") cartilage ("chondro"). Patellofemoral pain is the most prevalent type of knee pain in adolescents and young adults, and one of the most common complaints bringing athletes to sports medicine clinics (Caillet, 1996; Garrick, 1989; Mercier, 1995; Weiker, 1988). Patellofemoral pain is commonly seen in activities involving high-impact or repetitive knee flexion. Since dance contains both of these elements, it is not surprising to find patellofemoral pain syndrome prevalent in the dance population. In a survey of 362 pre-professional and professional modern and ballet dancers, 38% reported having three or more classic symptoms of patellofemoral pain syndrome associated with dance at some time during their dance training (Clippinger-Robertson et al., 1986).

In addition to the high and repetitive compression forces associated with dance, there are other underlying anatomical and biomechanical factors that tend to increase risk for patellofemoral pain. For example, factors that tend to produce decreased stability of the patella such as genu recurvatum and weakness of the vastus medialis—as well as factors that tend to produce patellar malalignment such as genu valgum, excessive femoral anteversion, an increased Q angle, or a tight iliotibial band—can all increase risk for patellofemoral pain syndrome (Grabiner, Koh, and Draganich, 1994; Reider, Marshall, and Warren, 1981; Sheehan and Drace, 1999; Winslow and Yoder, 1995). Some of these latter malalignments are commonly seen grouped together, and the composite is termed the miserable malalignment syndrome as seen in figure 5.34B. In general, patellofemoral pain syndrome occurs more frequently in females than in males. This is believed to be due to the greater Q angle and valgus vector associated with the wider pelvis, the tendency for greater genu recurvatum, or greater quadriceps weakness found in females versus males. In essence, patellar instability

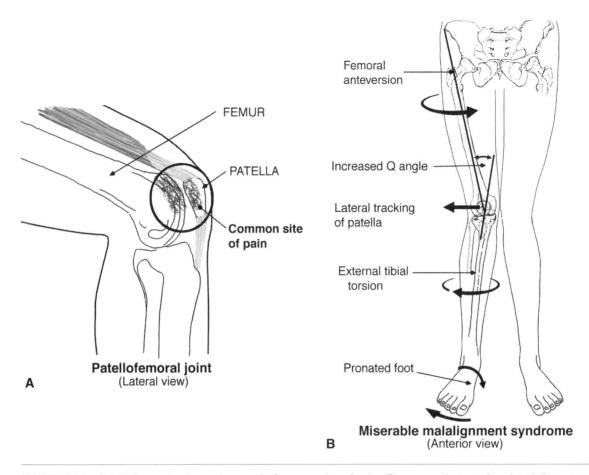

FIGURE 5.34   Patellofemoral pain syndrome. (A) Common site of pain, (B) commonly associated malalignments.

and malalignment factors are believed to allow abnormal lateral excursion of the patella against the lateral lip of the femoral groove, causing excessive patellar shear stress.

Classic symptoms of patellofemoral pain syndrome include (1) generalized (nonspecific) pain behind or around the patella, and particularly medial to the patella; (2) pain with knee flexion such as in grand pliés; (3) pain with extended sitting; (4) pain going down stairs; and (5) weakness, swelling, and pain during or after activity. One of the symptoms that most clearly distinguishes patellofemoral pain syndrome from other knee injuries is pain with extended sitting, such as in a theater, a car, or a plane. While other injuries often are pain free with rest, the quadriceps are slightly stretched by the bent knee position accompanying sitting, producing a small amount of patellofemoral compression and thus pain. A medical evaluation will classically reveal pain when applying pressure to the backside of the patella, and swelling and crepitus may be present (Mercier, 1995). Relative atrophy of the vastus medialis is also usually apparent, and other malalign-

ment or instability factors previously discussed are commonly present.

Initial recommended treatment often involves ice after activity, modified activity, and anti-inflammatory medication (Garrick, 1989; Roy and Irvin, 1983). Dance movements associated with high compression forces or pain, such as pliés, lunges, jumps, and floor work, should be temporarily avoided or modified to utilize a pain-free range (table 5.6).

However, the most important aspect of successful long-term rehabilitation is the development of quadriceps strength to counter the valgus tendency and restore optimal patellar tracking. Unfortunately, quadriceps atrophy appears to occur rapidly, and reflex inhibition can reduce the ability of the quadriceps to produce desired force within hours (Kennedy, Alexander, and Hayes, 1982; Urbach et al., 1999). Many classic exercises used to strengthen the quadriceps muscles will tend to aggravate the condition. Hence, a closely supervised physical therapy program initially using isometric (e.g., quad set and straight leg raise, table 5.3, A and B) and small arc exercises (terminal knee extension, table 5.3C)

TABLE 5.6 Dance Movements That Were Frequently Reported to Aggravate Knees of Ballet and Modern Dancers With Patellofemoral Complaints

Dance movement	Ballet	Modern	Both
Plié	60% (27)	69% (41)	65% (68)
Jumps	27% (12)	22% (13)	24% (25)
Flexion to extension	18% (8)	22% (13)	20% (21)
Turnout	20% (9)	10% (6)	14% (15)
Kneeling/floor work	0% (0)	20% (12)	12% (12)
Number of respondents	45	59	104

Dancers who reported three or more classic symptoms of chondromalacia patella
From Clippinger-Robertson et al. (1986).

in which compression forces are low, and with careful attention to activating appropriate muscles and avoiding knee hyperextension, is usually very effective. When quadriceps atrophy or apparent inhibition is marked, electrical stimulation of the quadriceps femoris muscle while the dancer superimposes conscious contraction may also be prescribed.

Attention to and correction of any underlying abnormalities or technical errors that can be improved, such as a tight iliotibial band, genu recurvatum, or forced turnout, can also be helpful. In the author's experience, working with dancers to maintain turnout at the hip and emphasize use of the hip adductors, while de-emphasizing use of the quadriceps during movements such as turned-out pliés, can also often provide symptom relief (Clippinger-Robertson et al., 1986). In some cases, taping techniques (McConnell taping) or a brace (patellar stabilization brace) may have a subtle positive influence on joint mechanics (Jenkinson and Bolin, 2001; Powers et al., 1999) while adequate quadriceps strength is being developed.

Although in a vast majority of cases conservative treatment emphasizing quadriceps strengthening will be successful in relieving symptoms, in a small number of nonresponsive cases, surgery may be recommended (Weiker, 1988). One common surgical approach is to resurface the posterior side of the patella and try to encourage cartilage healing. Another surgical approach utilizes various procedures to improve the alignment of the extensor mechanism.

Jumper's Knee **Jumper's knee** refers to injury to the patellar tendon right at its junction with the inferior pole of the patella as seen in figure 5.35. Some authors have also included injury to the quadriceps tendon at its junction with the superior patella

within this terminology (Bergfeld, 1982; Blazina et al., 1973; Cook et al., 2000). Jumper's knee is believed to involve an initial acute tear of the quadriceps tendon during a movement involving an explosive contraction of the quadriceps muscle. Then, before this site has time to heal, additional trauma aggravates the injury and it becomes chronic, often with a small area of granulation tissue at the site of the original tear (Quirk, 1987).

As its name implies, this injury is particularly common in athletes participating in sports involving jumping, such as volleyball or basketball players. It can also be found in sports that repetitively stress the quadriceps such as running, kicking, or climbing. Considering that dance contains both jumping and many repetitive movements that stress the quadriceps, it is not surprising that jumper's knee occurs readily in dancers. Factors that have been theorized to further increase the risk for this injury in dancers include participation in very athletic roles involving a lot of jumping (Quirk, 1987), excessive increase in dance workload, abrupt change in dance style, performing on hard floors, inadequate quadriceps strength, growth spurts, and calf tightness leading to a limited plié that requires large forces to be absorbed in a short period of time (Khan et al., 1995; Poggini, Losasso, and Iannone, 1999; Quirk, 1987).

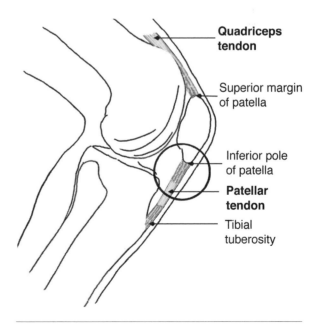

FIGURE 5.35 Jumper's knee and associated site(s) of pain (right knee, lateral view).

Pain is classically of insidious onset and is centered in the tendon just superior or just inferior to the patella (Blazina et al., 1973). This pain is generally "aching" in nature and usually goes away after a period of rest. In milder forms of tendinitis, the pain will often appear at the beginning of activity, disappear or decrease significantly after "warming up," and then reappear after completion of activity. In more advanced stages, the pain becomes more persistent and will tend to be present before, during, and after activity. In general, this pain is aggravated by performing jumps and can be reproduced by extending the knee against resistance. In some cases, the pain is accompanied by a sensation of "weakness" or "giving way."

Commonly recommended treatment for milder forms of jumper's knee involves heat or extra warm-up prior to activity (or both), ice after activity, anti-inflammatory medication, and in some cases physical therapy modalities (Bergfeld, 1982). Jumping and other high-load flexed movements of the knee are temporarily avoided as quadriceps strengthening and stretching are initiated (Diduch, Scuderi, and Scott, 1997). Although quadriceps strengthening is essential, full arc or plyometric types of exercises often aggravate the condition and should be avoided. Instead, initial treatment often involves terminal knee extension exercises (table 5.3C, p. 275) performed in a pain-free range of motion, as well as straight leg raises (table 5.3B, p. 275) with the knee in a position that is pain free (often requiring a very slightly flexed vs. fully extended position). Later stages of therapy may include eccentric quadriceps strengthening. In addition, technique factors such as poor landing mechanics with jumping should be corrected if indicated. In most cases, conservative treatment will lead to successful rehabilitation. However, if it should fail, some physicians recommend that the small area of granulation tissue within the quadriceps tendon be surgically excised (Quirk, 1983, 1987).

Osgood-Schlatter Disease

Osgood-Schlatter disease also involves the quadriceps tendon; but in contrast to jumper's knee, it involves the inferior attachment of the patellar tendon where it joins to the tibial tuberosity as seen in figure 5.36. This condition is not really a disease but rather involves an injury to the growth center of the tibial tuberosity (apophysis) due to traction produced by the quadriceps via the patellar tendon (Micheli, 1987). This injury usually becomes evident between 8 and 15 years of age, and especially during the peak of the adolescent growth spurt (Mercier, 1995; Stanitski, 1993). Although in the general population it is more prevalent in males

than females, in adolescent dancers it is common in both genders. Osgood-Schlatter disease is common in athletics involving rigorous or repetitive quadriceps contraction such as with running, jumping, and grand pliés. Factors discussed in the context of patellofemoral pain syndrome that tend to produce patellar malalignment will also increase the stress to the quadriceps tendon and may increase the risk for Osgood-Schlatter disease as well.

Osgood-Schlatter disease is characterized by pain and swelling over the tibial tuberosity. The tibial tuberosity is generally exquisitely tender to the touch or when pressure is applied, such as with kneeling, and it sometimes becomes enlarged.

Recommended treatment often includes ice after activity and anti-inflammatory medications (Stanitski, 1993). Dance should be modified to reduce movements that produce tendon stress and pain such as the grand plié, deep fondu, and jump. Knee pads with a felt or foam horseshoe fashioned to take the direct pressure off the tibial tuberosity can be worn if dance choreography requires floor work, and braces are sometimes prescribed (Micheli, 1987). Quadriceps strengthening, quadriceps stretching, and correction of any related technique factors can also sometimes provide relief. Luckily, this condition is almost always self-limiting and goes away when the tuberosity unites with the main part of the tibia (Diduch, Scuderi, and Scott, 1997; Quirk, 1987). However, if pain persists into adulthood, it is impor-

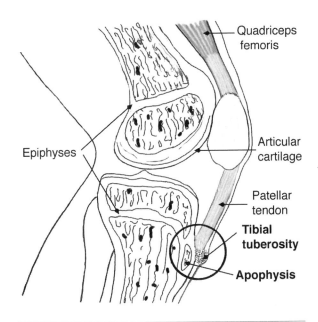

FIGURE 5.36   Osgood-Schlatter disease involves injury to the growth center associated with the tibial tuberosity (left knee, sagittal section).

tant for the person to get rechecked by a physician, as in some cases a fragment of the tibial tuberosity may actually fully detach.

Rehabilitation of Knee Injuries

Although treatment approaches will vary in accordance with the type of injury and other factors, one common rehabilitation concern is effective restoration of quadriceps strength and function. The quadriceps femoris muscles, and particularly the vastus medialis, appear to be quite prone to muscle inhibition following surgery, injury, or even relatively minor trauma or swelling (Hopkins et al., 2001). **Muscle inhibition** is the inability to fully activate the motor units in a given muscle with a voluntary contraction. This inhibition tends to produce muscle weakness, atrophy, and decreased neuromuscular control. Researchers have found 20% deficits in quadriceps strength to be common, with more severe deficits ranging from 30% to 45% occurring in some instances (Hurley, Jones, and Newham, 1994; Suter and Herzog, 2000).

The inhibition and related strength deficits can also be very persistent, evident months and even years after the original injury. For example, an average of 20% knee extensor inhibition was found in patients 22 months after ACL reconstructive surgery. Such decreases in quadriceps strength potentially interfere with restoration of normal knee function, increase the risk of reinjury, and may predispose the knee joint to degenerative diseases such as osteoarthritis. This extensor inhibition has been shown to occur commonly with both acute and chronic injuries and may involve the uninjured as well as the injured limb, making it inadvisable to use the noninjured side as "normal" when one is performing strength tests (Urbach et al., 1999). Hence, effective rehabilitation is recommended for even relatively minor knee injuries so that more serious or recurrent knee injuries can be avoided.

Summary

The knee joint proper is formed between the respective medial and lateral condyles of the femur and tibia and is called the tibiofemoral joint. The tibiofemoral joint is a modified hinge joint that primarily allows flexion and extension, but also some transverse rotation. Although the articular contact area is very broad, the shallowness of the joint makes it inherently unstable. Additional necessary stability is provided through a combination of ligaments, the joint capsule, the menisci, and strong muscles.

The cruciate ligaments are key stabilizers to limit anterior-posterior movement and rotation, as well as guiding the sliding of the femur relative to the tibia during knee flexion. The collateral ligaments are key stabilizers in the frontal plane to limit medial-lateral movement and valgus-varus stress. The iliotibial band provides additional lateral support to the knee. Overlying the ligaments and capsule are 12 muscles and their tendons, which provide additional support as well as movement. The action of the quadriceps femoris is knee extension, while the hamstrings and remaining muscles produce knee flexion, slight rotation, or both. In a weight-bearing position, once the knee begins to flex, gravity will tend to make it flex further. Hence, the knee extensors play a critical role not only to produce concentric knee extension, but also to isometrically maintain a bent position of the knee or eccentrically control additional flexion of the knee.

Tibiofemoral design favors both stability and mobility, partly achieved through static structural elements, such as the broadness of the joint (favoring stability) and the shallowness (favoring mobility). These contrasting demands are also met through the tibiofemoral joint's ability to change its characteristics with position. When the knee is straight, broad articular surfaces provide support, major ligaments are taut, rotation is limited, and stability is favored. However, when the knee bends, the collateral ligaments become slack, forces that would tend to dislocate the joint increase, rotation increases, and mobility is favored. This mobility is desirable to allow pivoting-type movements when the foot is weight bearing and positioning of the foot in space when the foot is free. However, this increased instability also can leave the joint at greater risk for injury. Common alignment deviations such as genu varum, genu valgum, and genu recurvatum can also influence injury predisposition. To foster optimal knee mechanics and prevent injury it is important that dancers develop adequate and balanced strength and flexibility in the key musculature; emphasize optimal mechanics; and avoid positions or movements that produce excessive valgus, varus, or rotation of the knee.

The patellofemoral joint is formed between the posterior surface of the patella and the underlying femoral groove. In contrast to what occurs with the tibiofemoral joint, the stability of the patella is low when the knee is in a position of extension but increases as flexion of the knee proceeds. However, because it is a sesamoid bone and there is not a true "joint" between the patella and the underlying femur, stability and excursion of the patella are markedly influenced by anatomical and biomechanical factors such as the law of valgus. The law of valgus and related Q angle give rise to a tendency for lateral tracking of the patella that can be exaggerated by alignment abnormalities, inadequate quadriceps strength, or twisting of the tibia, such as occurs with forced turnout. To encourage optimal patellofemoral mechanics and lessen the risk of injury, it is important that dancers develop adequate quadriceps strength and balanced muscle activation patterns and that they focus on correct alignment between the hip, knee, and foot.

Study Questions and Applications

1. Locate the following bony landmarks on a human skeleton: (a) medial femoral condyle and epicondyle, (b) lateral femoral condyle and epicondyle, (c) tibial plateau, (d) tibial tuberosity, and (e) patella.

2. Draw the following muscles on a skeletal chart, and use an arrow to indicate the line of pull of each muscle. Then, next to each muscle, list its actions: (a) rectus femoris, (b) vastus lateralis, (c) vastus intermedius, (d) vastus medialis, (e) biceps femoris, (f) semitendinosus, (g) semimembranosus, and (h) popliteus.

3. Locate the following muscles on your partner, and have your partner perform actions that these muscles produce while you palpate their contraction: (a) quadriceps femoris, (b) biceps femoris, (c) semitendinosus, and (d) semimembranosus.

4. Sitting in a chair, resist knee flexion by putting your left foot behind your right foot while pulling back with the right leg (resisted isometric knee flexion). Place your right hand under the right side of the back of the thigh and your left hand under the left side of the back of the thigh. Palpate the hamstrings as you pull back with (1) the tibia and foot externally rotated, (2) parallel, and (3) internally rotated relative to the femur. Explain the differences you feel in muscle contraction during these conditions.

5. Demonstrate two exercises for strengthening and two exercises for stretching the following muscles: (a) quadriceps femoris, (b) hamstrings.

6. Delineate differences in exercise design required in order to focus on the rectus femoris versus the vasti muscles for both strengthening and stretching exercises.

7. Mark the midpoint of your patella and tibial tuberosity with a pen or adhesive dot. Then perform a standing first-position demi-plié, and note the change in relationship between the dots on the patella and tibial tuberosity when the knee extends on the up-phase of the movement. Explain how this relates to the locking mechanism of the knee.

8. Use a marking pen to draw the Q angle on your knee (or your lab partner's knee) according to the directions provided earlier in this chapter. Then, sitting with both legs extended forward, note any lateral motion of the patella as you perform a quad set. Compare your Q angle with that of three other dancers. Describe how the law of valgus relates to this lateral tracking of the patella, and list two other alignment deviations that will tend to enhance this tendency for lateral tracking.

9. Place one hand on the front of the thigh about 6 inches (15 centimeters) above the patella and the other behind and above the knee on the hamstring muscles. Palpate these muscles while performing a demi-plié in first position (parallel), and note that contraction is present in both muscle groups. Explain how this can be occurring even though they have antagonistic functions at the hip and knee.

10. Perform an analysis of a back attitude, accounting for the joint movements, muscles groups, and sample muscles of the hip and knee of the gesture leg. Then, describe how active and passive insufficiency could be operative.

(continued)

Study Questions and Applications   *(continued)*

11. A dancer's teacher has noted that his knees are "hyperextending" at takeoff and "falling in" when landing in plié.

   a. Describe what joint motions could be occurring at the spine, hip, and knee that could contribute to these technique errors.

   b. Describe how the "locking mechanism" of the knee could contribute to these technique errors and how its negative effect could be minimized.

   c. Identify appropriate strength and flexibility exercises that could be utilized to maximize jump height and help prevent the undesired motions of the knee.

   d. Provide three cues that could be utilized to try to implement the desired technique adjustments.

CHAPTER SIX

The Ankle and Foot

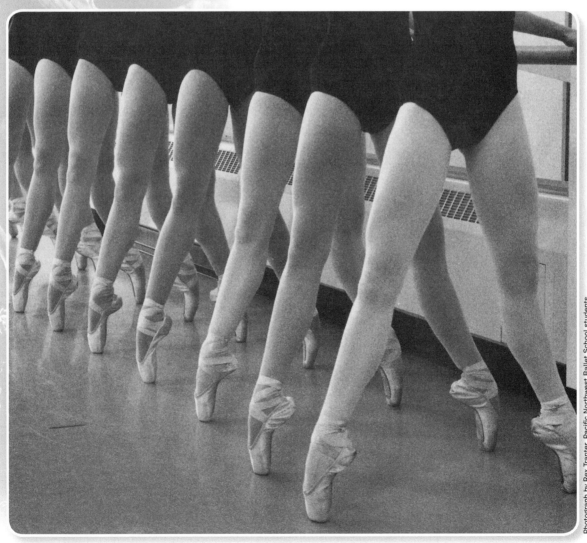

Photograph by Rex Tranter. Pacific Northwest Ballet School students.

With this chapter we turn to the ankle and the foot. The ankle serves as the connection between the foot and leg, vital for translation of forces and motion of the foot relative to the leg and of the leg relative to the foot. The foot is a complex structure that has evolved from a flexible grasping organ to a relatively rigid structure, which allows it to meet the demands associated with weight bearing and locomotion. The presence of various arches and the relative positioning of various joints allow the foot to play the dual role of a rigid lever for propulsion and a flexible accommodating structure for shock absorbency. One of the hallmarks of dancers is the marked development of fine strength, fine articulation, and range of motion of the feet in plantar flexion as demonstrated in the photo on page 297 and as exemplified by pointe work. However, with the large forces being generated at and absorbed by the ankle-foot complex, it is not surprising that this is the most common site of injury in dance.

This chapter will present basic anatomy and mechanics of the ankle and foot that influence optimal performance and the vulnerability of these joints to injury. Topics covered will include the following:

- Bones and bony landmarks of the ankle and foot
- Joint structure and movements of the ankle and foot
- Description and functions of individual muscles of the ankle and foot
- Alignment and common deviations of the ankle and foot
- Mechanics of the ankle and foot
- Muscular analysis of fundamental movements of the ankle and foot
- Key considerations for the ankle and foot in whole body movement
- Special considerations for the ankle and foot in dance
- Conditioning exercises for the ankle and foot
- Ankle and foot injuries in dancers

Bones and Bony Landmarks of the Ankle and Foot

The tibia, fibula, and 26 bones of the feet all take part in the various joints of the ankle and foot. The bones of the feet are composed of 7 tarsals (G. *tarsos*, sole of the foot), 5 metatarsals (G. *meta*, after), and 14 phalanges (L. *phalanx*, bone between two joints

of the toes or fingers) as seen in figure 6.1, which help form arches that run across (transverse arch) the foot and the length (longitudinal arches) of the foot. In regard to specific bones, the tibia can be easily palpated under the skin along the anterior lower leg and hence is often casually termed the "shinbone." This bone is the larger, stronger, and more medially located of the two lower leg bones. It ends distally with a concave surface and a medial projection that extends further inferiorly termed the **medial malleolus** (L. *malleus*, hammer). The projection of the medial malleolus can be easily palpated on the medial side of the ankle (see figure 6.5, p. 303). The thinner, more laterally located fibula also ends distally with a projection, termed the **lateral malleolus** (figure 6.2B), that can readily be palpated on the lateral side of the ankle. These inferior structures of the tibia and fibula come in

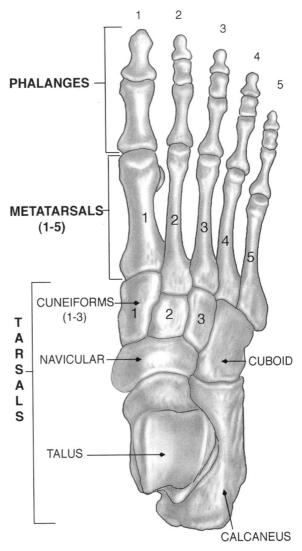

FIGURE 6.1 Bones of the foot (right foot, superior view).

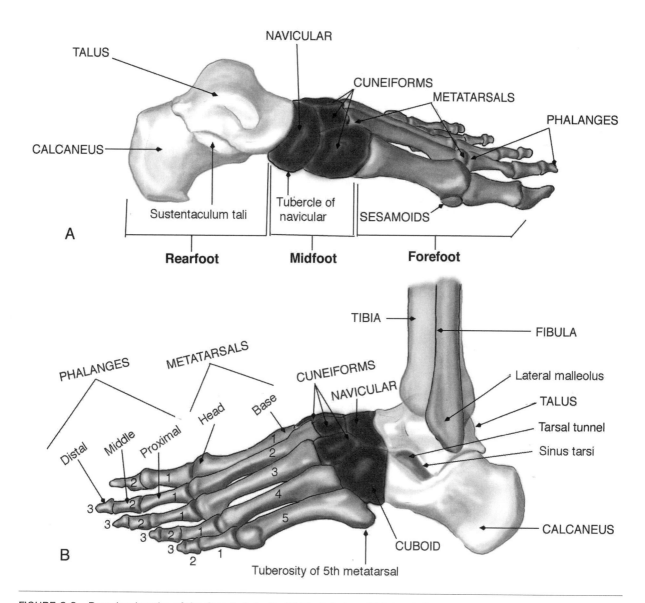

FIGURE 6.2   Bony landmarks of the foot (left foot). (A) Medial view, (B) lateral view.

contact with the upper surface of the large tarsal bone called the **talus** (L. ankle, ankle bone, figure 6.2A) to form the ankle joint.

The talus is often termed the cornerstone of the foot because forces coming down from the lower leg are translated forward and back on the foot through the talus. The talus sits on the largest tarsal bone, the **calcaneus** (L. *calcaneum,* heel). The calcaneus projects backward to form the "heel" and can be easily palpated in the heel area. There is a small space formed between a portion of the talus (its narrower neck) and the underlying calcaneus that is termed the **tarsal tunnel** or canal. This bony tunnel opens up laterally as a small bony depression filled with soft tissues called the **sinus tarsi** (L. *sinus,* cavity + G. *tarsus,* sole of the foot) (figure 6.2B). This landmark

is important for locating the lateral ligaments of the ankle and is often a site of swelling with lateral ankle sprains.

Anteriorly, the calcaneus articulates with the tarsal bone called the **cuboid** (G. *kybos,* cube + *eidos,* resemblance) as seen in figure 6.2B, and the talus articulates with the tarsal bone called the **navicular** (L. boat shaped) as seen in figure 6.2A. The navicular contains a small projection termed the **tubercle of the navicular** (L. *tuberculum,* a swelling). This projection can be palpated about 1 to 1 1/2 inches (2.5-3.8 centimeters) anterior to and about a finger breadth below the medial malleolus. This landmark can be used for evaluation of the arches of the feet.

The remaining three tarsal bones, termed the **cuneiforms** (L. *cuneus,* wedge), are located in a row in front of the navicular and are called the first, second, and third cuneiform going from medial to lateral. These cuneiforms are each in line with the three medial metatarsals, while the two lateral metatarsals are in line with the cuboid. Each **metatarsal** consists of a **base** (proximally), a **body,** and a **head** (distally). While the bases of the metatarsals articulate with the cuboid and cuneiforms, the heads articulate with their respective phalanges. The heads of the metatarsals can be easily palpated on the underside of the foot (plantar surface) at the base of the toes when the toes are repetitively flexed and extended. The metatarsals and toes are numbered 1 through 5, from medial to lateral. There are three phalanges in each of the toes except the great toe. These are termed the **proximal, middle,** and **distal phalanges** for toes 2 through 5 (the lesser toes). The first toe is termed the **hallux** (L. *hallux,* great toe), and it contains only two phalanges, the proximal and distal phalanges. Located directly below the head of the first metatarsal are two small sesamoid bones called the **medial** and **lateral sesamoid** (figure 6.2A).

Due to the large number of bones in the foot and the complexity of the joints, it is customary to refer to segments of the foot rather than individual bones for some descriptions of motion or mechanics. The segments of the foot are the rearfoot, midfoot, and forefoot (figure 6.2A). The **rearfoot,** or hindfoot, is composed of the talus and calcaneus. The **midfoot** is composed of the navicular, cuboid, and cuneiforms. The **forefoot** is composed of the metatarsals and phalanges.

Joint Structure and Movements of the Ankle and Foot

There are 34 joints in the ankle-foot complex (Smith, Weiss, and Lehmkuhl, 1996). The ankle, subtalar, and transverse tarsal joints are particularly key for desired functioning of this region, and their movements are intimately linked. Other more distal joints are important for subtle adjustments of the foot and movements of the toes. A summary of the primary joints of the ankle and foot is provided in table 6.1. Most of these joints are named according to the bones that compose the joints (e.g., tarsometatarsal), making learning the names easier and logical. Many joint capsules and approximately 100 ligaments provide stability for these joints and provide constraints for movements of the ankle-foot complex. For purposes of simplicity, this text will cover only selected primary ligaments of the rearfoot.

Ankle Joint Classification and Movements

Because the "ankle joint" is formed between the bones of the lower leg and the upper portion of the talus, its technical name is the **talocrural** (L. *crus,* leg) joint. The ankle joint is classified as a hinge joint and is more specifically formed by the articulation of the superior dome of the talus with the distal tibia and fibula (figure 6.3). The tibia is the primary weight-bearing bone of the lower leg, and it translates most of the weight between the femur and the talus, while the medial malleolus extends to provide medial support for the ankle. The fibula serves as a lateral strut, providing additional stability by helping to form a slot or mortise into which the talus can fit. The fibula has also been estimated to transmit about 6% to 7% of the load when the ankle is in a neutral position, but up to one-sixth of the load of the leg when the ankle-foot is in a position of dorsiflexion and eversion (DiFiori, 1999; Sammarco, 1980).

The distal tibia and fibula form a fibrous joint (distal tibiofibular joint), and the very strong interosseous membrane and adjacent ligaments (including the anterior and posterior tibiofibular ligaments) allow the tibia and fibula to function as a structural unit like a mortise. This mortise fits over the convex superior portion of the talus, gripping it tightly along its flattened sides to provide much-needed stability for this joint, while still allowing for small movements of the fibula relative to the tibia—necessary to accommodate the changes in contact area with the talus accompanying ankle joint movement. A cast of this mortise would closely replicate the shape of the talus, making it the most congruent joint found in the human body.

Due to this mortise architecture, with the medial and lateral malleolus extending downward, only small side-to-side movements and rotation are permitted at this joint; and consistent with its classification as a hinge joint, the fundamental motions allowed are flexion and extension. The specialized terms of ankle dorsiflexion and plantar flexion are used because there is lack of agreement as to which movement would be considered flexion and which extension: Functional and anatomical perspectives would suggest opposite answers. So as seen in figure 6.4, a neutral or anatomical position is when the foot forms a 90° angle with the tibia, and dorsiflexion refers to bringing the top of the foot (dorsum) and the shin closer together such as in "flexing the foot." Conversely, plantar flexion refers to the opposite motion of bringing the bottom or sole of the foot (plantar surface) and the shin away from each other such as in "pointing the foot." The

TABLE 6.1   Summary of Joints of the Ankle and Foot

Name	Type of joint	Movements
Ankle and foot		
Ankle (talocrural)	Hinge	Plantar flexion Dorsiflexion
Subtalar	Gliding	Inversion Eversion Abduction Adduction Slight plantar flexion Slight dorsiflexion

Transverse tarsal
  Talonavicular
  Calcaneocuboid
	Modified ball and socket
	Gliding
		Primarily inversion and eversion
		Slight abduction
		Slight adduction
		Slight plantar flexion
		Slight dorsiflexion

Other intertarsal	Gliding	Primarily slight dorsiflexion and some plantar flexion
Tarsometatarsal	Gliding	Primarily slight dorsiflexion and some plantar flexion
Toes		
Metatarsophalangeal	Condyloid	Flexion of the toes on the metatarsals Extension of the toes on the metatarsals Abduction of the toes on the metatarsals Adduction of the toes on the metatarsals
Interphalangeal	Hinge	Flexion of the digits (phalanges) of the toes Extension of the digits (phalanges) of the toes

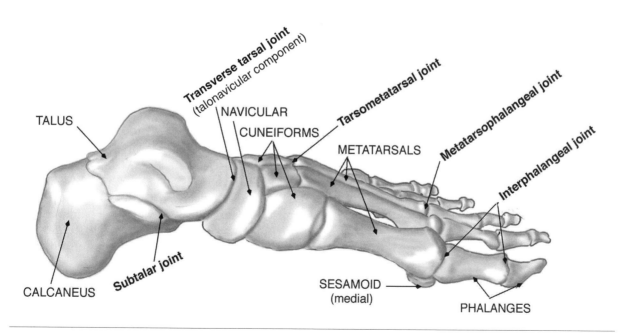

FIGURE 6.3   Key joints of the foot (left foot, medial view).

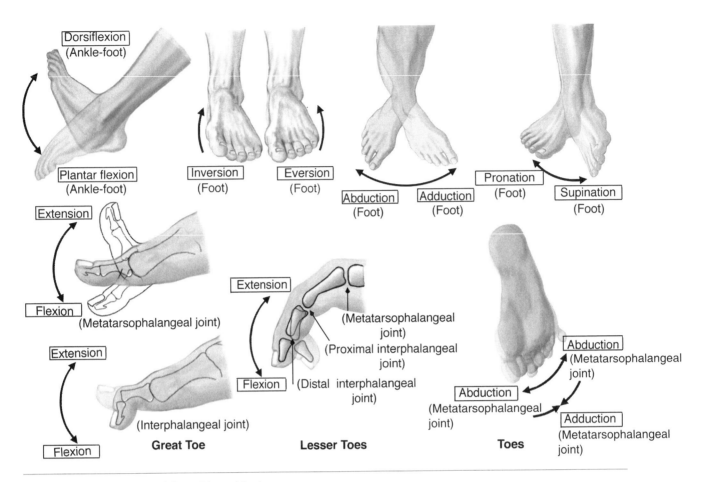

FIGURE 6.4   Movements of the ankle and foot.

axis for this movement is close to a frontal plane, but it deviates slightly posteriorly and inferiorly from the medial to lateral side, and it also does not stay fixed but rather shifts slightly with dorsiflexion and plantar flexion. You can obtain a rough estimate of the axis by putting your thumb and forefinger on the medial and lateral malleolus and imagining a line running through these points. However, there are very large individual differences, and divergent averages are given by different sources for the location of this axis. For example, Levangie and Norkin (2001) hold that on average the axis is rotated laterally 20° to 30° in the transverse plane and inclined 10° downward on the lateral side, while Kreighbaum and Barthels (1996) suggest much lower average values of 13° rotation and 7° inclination.

Subtalar Joint Classification and Movements

The subtalar joint (L. *sub*, under + *talar*, relating to talus) is formed between the inferior portion of the talus and the superior portion of the calcaneus

(figure 6.3). The articular surfaces of these bones fit well together, and additional stability is provided by a flattened area on the medial calcaneus termed the sustentaculum tali (L. *sustenataculum*, a prop or support + *tali*, relating to talus) that acts like a shelf to help support the medial talus. This joint is generally classified as a gliding synovial joint (Moore and Dalley, 1999), but it allows more movement than is often associated with a gliding joint.

The specialized terminology of *inversion-eversion, abduction-adduction,* and *plantar flexion-dorsiflexion* can be used to describe these movements (figure 6.4). *Inversion* involves lifting the *in*ner border of the foot so that the distal portion of the calcaneus and sole of the foot face medially or *in*ward. Eversion is the opposite movement, involving lifting the outer border of the foot so that the distal heel and sole of the foot face laterally. Abduction can be thought of as moving the forefoot away from the median plane or midline of the body, while adduction refers to the opposite movement of the forefoot toward the midline of the body. Note, however, that this specialized form of abduction-adduction of the foot occurs primarily in a transverse plane around a vertical axis, more akin to horizontal abduction-horizontal adduction of the shoulder or hip. The slight dorsiflexion and plantar flexion that occurs is in the same direction as described with the ankle but involves the talus upon the calcaneus rather than the talus relative to the mortise joint.

Ankle Joint Capsule and Rearfoot Ligaments

The ankle joint is surrounded by a thin fibrous capsule that is relatively weak, but it is reinforced on each side by strong ligaments, called the medial and lateral collateral ligaments. Other closely approximated ligaments hold the tibia and fibula together at the mortise joint (anterior and posterior tibiofibular ligaments), and still others provide key stability to the subtalar joint.

Medial Collateral Ligament

The medial collateral ligament (*collateral*, side by side)—also called the **deltoid ligament** (G. *deltoeides*, triangular)—is composed of four parts that fan out from their attachment on the medial malleolus to their respective attachments on the surrounding bones. As can be seen in figure 6.5, one division runs downward (tibiocalcaneal ligament) from the medial malleolus to attach onto the medial aspect of the calcaneus; two components run from the medial malleolus diagonally downward and forward to attach onto the talus and navicular (anterior tibiotalar ligament and tibionavicular ligament); and

the last component runs from the medial malleolus diagonally downward and backward to attach onto the talus (posterior tibiotalar). Together these ligaments prevent forward or backward displacement of the tibia or of the talus and are vital for providing medial stability to the ankle joint. Because one band attaches onto the calcaneus, the deltoid ligament also provides stability for the subtalar joint and helps limit eversion and abduction of the foot. These ligaments also help link movements between the tibia, ankle joint, and subtalar joints, particularly inversion of the foot and external rotation of the tibia (Hintermann, 1999). As with the knee, the integrity and function of the ligaments can be demonstrated by manual stress tests performed by a physician. If the medial side of the joint opens up and a gap is formed with eversion, injury to the deltoid ligament is suggested.

The deltoid ligament is very strong and extensive. This strength is important because the medial malleolus does not extend distally as far as the lateral, and so the lesser stability from bony architecture is in part compensated for by the greater massiveness of the medial ligaments. In fact the deltoid is so strong that when forces are large enough to cause injury, the medial malleolus may be avulsed and other bones fractured rather than the deltoid ligament's being ruptured.

Lateral Collateral Ligament

The lateral collateral ligament is composed of three discrete bands, shown in figure 6.6, that connect the lateral malleolus with adjacent bones of the foot. The **anterior talofibular ligament (ATFL)** runs almost

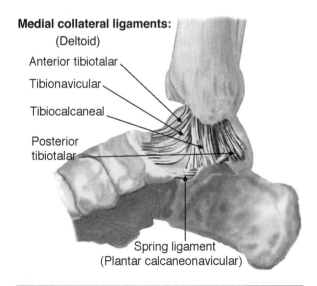

FIGURE 6.5 Key ligaments of the medial aspect of the ankle (right foot).

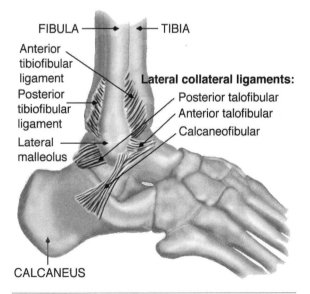

FIGURE 6.6 Key ligaments of the lateral aspect of the ankle (right foot).

horizontally anteriorly from the lateral (fibular) malleolus to the lateral talus and limits anterior movement of the talus relative to the fibula, or posterior movement of the fibula relative to the talus. It also can limit adduction and inversion of the foot, especially when the foot is plantar flexed. The **posterior talofibular ligament (PTFL)** is directed posteriorly from the posterior portion of the lateral malleolus to the talus and prevents excessive posterior slippage of the talus on the fibula or anterior slippage of the fibula on the talus. The **calcaneofibular ligament** runs downward and slightly backward from the distal end of the lateral malleolus to attach onto the lateral aspect of the calcaneus. It spans both the ankle joint and subtalar joint and is very important for preventing inversion and adduction of the foot when the foot is dorsiflexed (Hintermann, 1999).

As a whole, the lateral collateral ligaments are important in coupling movements between the tibia and foot, particularly eversion of the foot and internal rotation of the tibia. They are also very vital for lateral ankle stability and, more specifically, for preventing excessive inversion of the foot. Their relative contribution appears to shift with the position of the foot, such that the PTFL and calcaneofibular ligament are taut and provide primary stability in ankle-foot dorsiflexion, while the ATFL becomes taut and is particularly responsible for providing stability in plantar flexion. With the frequent use of plantar flexion in dance and the fact that this is the weakest of the lateral collateral ligaments, it is not surprising that the ATFL is commonly injured in dancers. These lateral ligaments are so essential for ankle stability that when they are seriously or repeatedly injured, the ankle often becomes chronically unstable (see Ankle Sprains on p. 360 for more information), and abnormal movement may be present when manual stress tests are performed by a physician (see Tests and Measurements 6.1) (Malone and Hardaker, 1990; Sammarco and Tablante, 1997).

Spring Ligament

The subtalar joint also has its own joint capsule and additional ligaments, including the spring ligament and interosseous talocalcaneal ligaments, that provide additional stability. The **spring ligament** (plantar calcaneonavicular ligament) shown in figure 6.5 is a broad ligament that spans between the sustentaculum tali of the calcaneus and the undersurface of the navicular. It forms a taut sling under the head of the talus, thereby helping to support the weight of the body received by the talus and to maintain the medial longitudinal arch. Permanent stretching of this liga-

ment is believed to contribute to a lowered medial longitudinal arch and a "flatfoot."

The tarsal tunnel, formed by a concave groove (sulcus) in the inferior talus and superior calcaneus, runs from the medial to the lateral sides of the ankle and is filled with short and strong bands called the **interosseous talocalcaneal ligaments** (L. *inter*, between + *os*, bone). These ligaments function to bind these bones together and contain abundant neural receptors that are believed to be important for the quick responses necessary for maintaining balance and helping to prevent injuries such as ankle sprains (Smith, Weiss, and Lehmkuhl, 1996).

Transverse Tarsal Joint Classification and Movements

The transverse tarsal joint lies just in front of the talus and calcaneus and forms a shallow "S" when viewed from above (figure 6.3). The **transverse tarsal joint** is actually a combination of the **talonavicular** (between the talus and navicular) and **calcaneocuboid** (between the calcaneus and cuboid) joints. The talonavicular is generally classified as a modified ball-and-socket joint, while the calcaneocuboid is classified as a gliding joint (Hamilton and Luttgens, 2002; Moore and Dalley, 1999) or saddle joint (Hall-Craggs, 1985; Magee, 1997). Although the shape of each joint by itself would tend to allow more free motion, the navicular and cuboid bones articulate with each other in a manner that allows very little motion between them and hence restricts overall motion and makes both joints act functionally as a single segment. Together, these joints allow inversion-eversion and lesser degrees of plantar flexion-dorsiflexion and abduction-adduction.

These movements at the transverse tarsal joint can be used to provide additional range to the same movements of the rearfoot or to move the forefoot in a direction opposite to that of the rearfoot. An example of the former occurs when plantar flexion of the transverse tarsal joint is added to that of the subtalar joint and ankle joint to allow the dancer to "point" the foot further. An example of the latter occurs with walking, where transverse tarsal inversion can be used to keep the lateral forefoot from rising off the ground when eversion of the subtalar joint and internal rotation of the tibia are occurring. However, this ability to counterrotate the forefoot is greater when the rearfoot everts and dramatically diminishes as the subtalar joint inverts. Hence, when extreme inversion of the foot occurs such as when one steps wrong off of a curb or lands wrong from a jump, the forefoot has limited ability to counter-

Selected Orthopedic Stress Tests for the Ankle

Two tests are shown that are commonly performed by physicians to test the stability of the ankle and evaluate lateral ligamental injury. Consider each test in terms of both the restraints offered by a normal intact ligament and the excessive motion allowed when injury occurs.

Anterior Drawer Test

When one hand is used to push backward on the lower tibia while the other hand is used to pull the calcaneus (and talus) forward, the ATFL resists this motion. When the ATFL is torn, the talus will slide anteriorly from under the tibia. This is termed a positive **anterior drawer sign** as shown in A.

Talar Tilt Test

When the foot is inverted, the calcaneofibular ligament resists this varus stress. When the calcaneofibular and anterior talofibular ligament are torn, excessive calcaneal varus is permitted, and the talus will gap and rock in the ankle mortise. This is termed a positive **talar tilt sign** as seen in B.

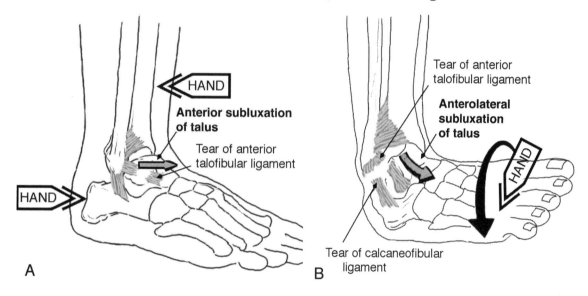

rotate, and an ankle sprain can readily occur unless muscles (the evertors of the foot) act quickly to counter this undesired extreme inversion.

Classification and Movements of Other Joints of the Midfoot and Forefoot

The remaining joints between the tarsal bones (intertarsal joints), as well as the joints between the tarsal bones and the proximal ends of metatarsals 2 through 5 (tarsometatarsal [TMT] joints), are gliding joints. These joints permit small motions that continue the function of the transverse tarsal joint, acting to continue or counter the motions of the hindfoot in accordance with the goal of the movement. The tarsometatarsal joints also contribute to

"cupping" or "flattening" of the foot when it is weight bearing, similar to that which occurs in the hand to facilitate grasping objects.

The joints between the heads of the metatarsal bones and the adjacent proximal phalanges—the **metatarsophalangeal joints (MTP)**—are condyloid joints. These joints allow a considerable amount of motion in flexion (30-45°) and extension (90°), with greater motion allowed in extension (Smith, Weiss, and Lehmkuhl, 1996). This extension motion (sometimes termed hyperextension) is important in weight-bearing functions such as in walking or rising onto the toes in demi-pointe, allowing the toes to maintain contact with the ground while the heel rises. The motion of abduction-adduction is more limited and is oriented relative to a line through the second toe. So, abduction of the toes would involve movement of the toes away from the second toe, while adduction would involve bringing the toes back toward the second toe.

Lastly, the joints between adjacent phalanges—the **interphalangeal (IP) joints**—are hinge joints. They allow flexion and extension of the toes. Flexion refers to bringing the plantar surfaces of the digits closer together such as when curling the toes under, while extension refers to decreasing the flexion of the digits, or straightening the toes.

The Composite Movements of Pronation and Supination

Due to the oblique orientation of the axes of the ankle, subtalar joint, and transverse tarsal joints and the close structural interrelationship of many of these joints, an isolated movement of an individual joint in a single plane is rare or even not possible, depending on the joint. In functional movement, many motions of the foot are composites, involving joints in the rearfoot, midfoot, and forefoot in multiple planes. Two particularly important examples of such movements are pronation and supination. When bearing weight, pronation can be described as a composite movement that involves dorsiflexion (primarily from the ankle), eversion (primarily of the rearfoot), and abduction (primarily of the forefoot), while supination involves the opposite motions of plantar flexion, inversion, and adduction (Hall, 1999). As will be discussed later in this chapter, these combination movements serve very important functions in weight-bearing activities such as walking, running, and dancing.

Special Structures of the Ankle and Foot

There are many specialized structures associated with the ankle and foot that enhance their function. A description of some of these structures that are particularly important follows.

Plantar Fascia

A special very strong and inelastic band of connective tissue called the **plantar fascia** (L. plantaris, relating to the sole of the foot + sheet of fibrous tissue) is located in the sole of the foot as shown in figure 6.7. It attaches from the heel (underside of the calcaneus) and runs forward, fanning out and dividing into slips that attach to the sheaths of the flexor tendons of the toes, underside of the proximal phalanges, and ligamentous structures near the heads of the metatarsals. The plantar fascia is covered only by fat and the skin, and can be readily palpated on the underside of the medial arch of the foot when the foot and toes are simultaneously dorsiflexed.

CONCEPT DEMONSTRATION 6.1

Foot Supination and Pronation

Stand in a parallel first position with your feet facing straight ahead and your knees slightly bent.

· **Identifying foot inversion and eversion.** Without changing the position of your knee or the facing of your forefoot, slightly lift the inner border of the heel and arch of one foot, thinking of rotating about the longitudinal axis of the foot running through the second toe. This motion is inversion of the foot. Now, slightly lift the outer border of the heel and foot. This motion is eversion of the foot. Notice that the amount of possible movement of the foot is small if the knee remains facing straight ahead and is not allowed to move inward or outward relative to the foot.

· **Identifying foot supination.** While still standing in first position, rock your body weight back onto your heels so that the front of your foot can move. Keeping your weight back, carefully and slowly lift the inner borders of your feet and notice how the front of your feet tend to point very slightly inward. The position you are in reflects all three elements of foot supination: plantar flexion (relative), inversion, and forefoot adduction.

· **Identifying foot pronation.** Returning to your original first position, bend your knees (plié) and allow your knees to fall inside your feet as you carefully lift the outer borders of your feet. Notice how the front of your feet point very slightly outward. The position you are in reflects all three elements of foot pronation: dorsiflexion, eversion, and forefoot abduction.

In addition to protecting and dividing the muscles of the plantar area of the foot into compartments, this fascial structure is very important for support of the medial longitudinal arch of the foot. It creates a trusslike structure (Frankel and Nordin, 1980), which is a rigid structure composed of elements that are fastened at their base to prevent movement between the individual elements and to maintain their shape (figure 6.8A). Thus, the rearfoot and forefoot are held together by the plantar fascia, and the flattening of the arch that would be expected during standing and bearing weight on the foot is prevented. Furthermore, due to its attachment onto the base of the phalanges, when the toes extend, such as before toe-off in walking, the band is tightened by being stretched across the metatarsophalangeal joints (windlass effect) as shown in figure 6.8B. This tightening of the band tends to raise the medial longitudinal arch and supinate the foot, which in turn locks the midtarsal joints and makes the foot more stable for toe-off in walking and running (Levangie and Norkin, 2001). This support of the arch and stabilization of the foot via the windlass mechanism are also operative whenever dancers go on demi-pointe (figure 6.8C).

Deep Fascia and Intermuscular Septa of the Lower Leg

Strong sheets of fascia divide muscles of the lower leg and foot into three primary **compartments**—anterior, posterior, and lateral. The posterior compartment

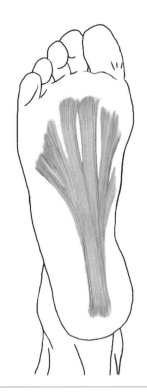

FIGURE 6.7 The plantar fascia (right foot, inferior view).

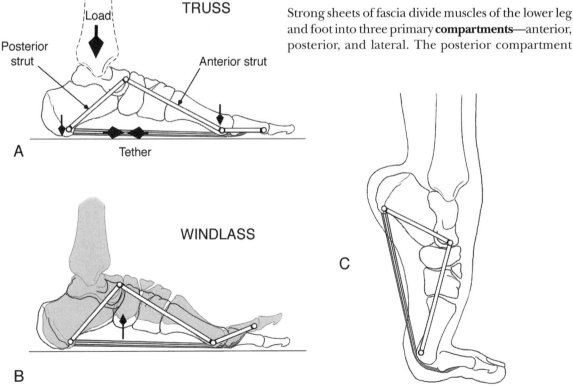

FIGURE 6.8 The function of the plantar fascia (right foot, medial view). (A) Tether of a truss in standing, (B) windlass effect with metatarsophalangeal extension, (C) windlass effect with demi-pointe.

can be further subdivided into the superficial posterior compartment and the deep posterior compartment as seen in figure 6.9. These compartments provide a functional division of muscles in that all of the muscles in a given compartment share at least one common action at the ankle-foot complex. The bone and strong fascia forming boundaries for each compartment limit the compartment's ability to expand, which in select individuals can lead to undesired increases in compartment pressures.

Retinaculum

Thickened bands of connective tissue called retinaculum (L. band, halter) are located around the ankle and foot that help hold tendons in place and keep them from bowing forward across the front of the ankle or sliding in front of the medial or lateral malleolus. For example, the **superior peroneal (fibular) retinaculum** extends from the lateral malleolus to the fascia of the back of the leg and lateral side of the calcaneus (figure 6.10). It functions to help hold the peroneal muscles in place behind the lateral malleolus.

Tendon Sheaths

Many of the tendons in the foot are encased by synovial tissue, forming tendon sheaths that protect the tendons from excessive friction. For example, on the dorsum of the foot, tendon sheaths surround the tendons of the tibialis anterior, extensor hallucis longus, and extensor digitorum longus muscles (figure 6.10).

Heel Pad

The **heel pad** is composed of fat cells located within chambers formed by fibrous tissue walls (septa) constructed in a manner to withstand strain and pressure. This pad has been found to be very important for shock absorption (Jorgensen, 1985), and loss of the shock absorbency of this fat pad has been shown to be associated with an increased shock wave amplitude at heel strike and increased soleus activity and load on the Achilles tendon. The effectiveness of the cushioning offered by the heel pad tends to decline with age, with noticeable decline in most individuals past 40 years of age (Levangie and Norkin, 2001).

Sesamoids

Two small sesamoid bones lie beneath the head of the first metatarsal, located within the tendon of the flexor hallucis brevis (figure 6.2A, p. 299). Their function is similar to that of the patella located in the quadriceps femoris at the knee. They increase the moment arm of the muscle within which they are located, increasing the muscle's ability to produce torque. They also help distribute the load and pressure beneath the metatarsal head during walking and running. Furthermore, they help protect the tendons of their associated muscle and the tendon of the flexor hallucis longus that runs between them—all of which without the sesamoids would be subjected to great compression forces with each step or when one goes on demi-pointe.

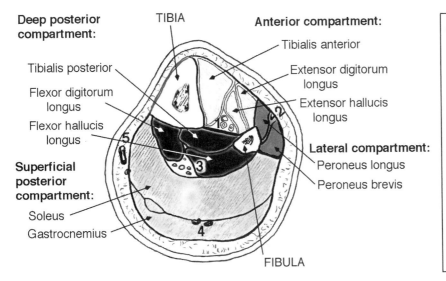

FIGURE 6.9   Compartments of the lower leg (right leg, transverse section).

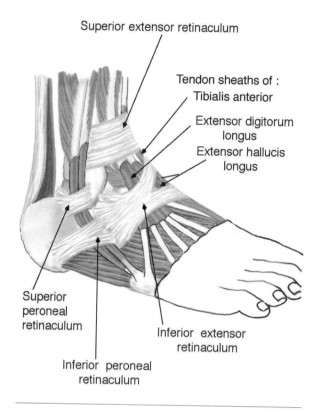

Superior extensor retinaculum

Tendon sheaths of :
Tibialis anterior

Extensor digitorum
longus

Extensor hallucis
longus

Superior
peroneal
retinaculum

Inferior extensor
retinaculum

Inferior peroneal
retinaculum

FIGURE 6.10 Examples of retinaculum and tendon sheaths (right foot, lateral view).

Bursae

There are many bursae in the region of the ankle and foot. Some of these bursae can become inflamed and painful in dancers. For example, the bursa located between the attachment of the Achilles tendon onto the heel and the overlying skin (**superficial calcaneal bursa**—figure 6.11) can easily become irritated by ill-fitting ballet or street shoes, while the deeper bursa is at greater risk for inflammation when there is a prominent upper angle of the calcaneus (Mercier, 1995). A heel lift, padding, use of a ballet shoe that ends lower on the heel, or modification of dance shoes to reduce pressure to the area can sometimes afford relief for the more superficial bursa.

Muscles

In addition to the many ligaments and joint capsules of the ankle-foot complex, many muscles act to provide stability as well as produce the complex movements of the many joints in this region. Some of these muscles play a vital role in shifting the body weight to the desired position relative to the foot, as well as absorbing the large forces associated with impact during weight-bearing movements such as walking, running, and jumping.

Description and Functions of Individual Muscles of the Ankle and Foot

There are 24 muscles of the ankle and foot. Twelve of these muscles are located entirely within the foot and are called **intrinsic muscles** (L. *intrinsecus*, on the inside). The remaining 12 muscles have distal tendon attachments on the foot but otherwise lie outside the foot. Hence, these muscles are called **extrinsic muscles** (L. *extrinsecus*, from without). The extrinsic muscles of the foot can be grouped by location into anterior, posterior, posteromedial, and lateral crural muscles. Each of these groups has at least one shared action at the ankle-foot, and each is located in the same osseofascial compartment of the leg (figure 6.9).

All of these extrinsic muscles cross at least two joints and so have actions at more than one joint. However, for purposes of simplicity, the actions at the ankle, subtalar, and midtarsal joints and other relevant joints are not differentiated here. Instead, dorsiflexion and plantar flexion are listed relative to the ankle-foot, while, since the ankle cannot contribute to other movements, inversion and eversion are listed only relative to the foot. Also, for purposes of simplicity and in keeping with many anatomy texts, the actions of foot abduction and adduction will not be included on charts. However, in general, the muscles with the action of foot inversion can also produce foot adduction, while the muscles with the action of foot eversion can also produce foot abduction. Many of the names of the muscles of the ankle and foot reflect the action that the given muscle performs, making it easier to learn these muscles. (See Individual Muscles of the Ankle and Foot, pp. 310-323.)

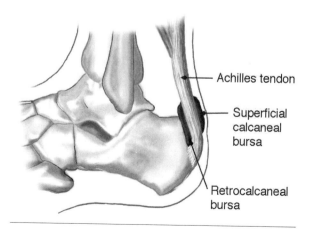

Achilles tendon

Superficial calcaneal bursa

Retrocalcaneal bursa

FIGURE 6.11 Bursae of the heel (left foot, lateral view).

Individual Muscles of the Ankle and Foot

Anterior Crural Muscles

The anterior crural muscles are located on the front of the lower leg. They are contained within the anterior compartment of the leg and include the tibialis anterior, extensor digitorum longus, extensor hallucis longus, and peroneus tertius. Because these muscles all pass anteriorly to the axis of the ankle joint, they have the common action of dorsiflexion. When the foot is free, this dorsiflexion can be used to raise the toes and front of the foot and to prevent their striking the ground in movements such as walking and running. Loss of the ankle dorsiflexors causes the foot to hang down, a condition termed "drop-foot" (Smith, Weiss, and Lehmkuhl, 1996) when swinging the leg forward in walking. Loss of the dorsiflexors also prohibits the desired smooth lowering of the foot to the ground during walking, and a distinctive slap or clop occurs (Moore and Agur, 1995).

Attachments and Primary Actions of Tibialis Anterior

Muscle	Proximal attachment(s)	Distal attachment(s)	Primary action(s)
Tibialis anterior (tib-ee-A-lis)	Upper two-thirds of lateral tibia and adjacent interosseous membrane	Medial and inferior surfaces of medial cuneiform and base of first metatarsal	A-F dorsiflexion Foot inversion

Tibialis Anterior

As its name implies, the **tibialis anterior** (*tibial,* tibia + *anterior,* toward the front) originates from the front of the shin (figure 6.12). It runs down the anterolateral portion of the shin and then crosses inward over the top of the ankle to insert onto the medial undersurface of the foot (first cuneiform and base of first metatarsal). The tibialis anterior is responsible for the roundness of the lower leg in this region, and its paralysis results in a flatness or even concavity in this area accompanied by an excessively prominent anterior tibia (Smith, Weiss, and Lehmkuhl, 1996). This muscle is a powerful dorsiflexor of the ankle-foot and is estimated to provide 80% of the dorsiflexion power of the foot (Frey and Shereff, 1988; Scheller, Kasser, and Quigley, 1980). During weight bearing, this dorsiflexion function can be used to bring the body weight forward over the foot to prevent the body from falling backward or to ready the body for an upcoming movement such as a quick rise onto the toes (Karpovich and Manfredi, 1973). Due to its medial progression to the undersurface of the foot, when the muscle contracts it is capable of producing slight inversion of the foot as well as dorsiflexion. During movement when the foot is weight bearing, this inversion function of the tibialis anterior helps support the medial longitudinal arch and prevent excessive pronation.

Palpation: The tendon of the tibialis anterior can be easily seen and palpated where it crosses the front of the ankle when the foot is actively dorsiflexed. The upper belly of the tibialis anterior can be palpated on the lateral side of the anterior margin of the tibia.

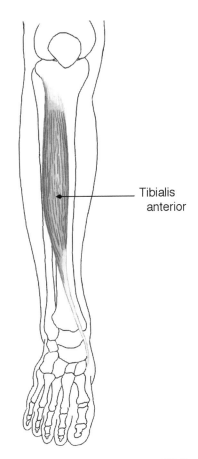

Tibialis anterior

FIGURE 6.12　The tibialis anterior (right foot, anterior view).

Attachments and Primary Actions of Extensor Hallucis and Digitorum Longus

Muscle	Proximal attachment(s)	Distal attachment(s)	Primary action(s)
Extensor hallucis longus (ek-STEN-sor HAL-u-sis LON-gus)	Anterior fibula and adjacent interosseus membrane at the middle half of leg	Upper surface of base of distal phalanx of great toe (hallux)	Great toe extension A-F dorsiflexion Foot inversion
Extensor digitorum longus (ek-STEN-sor di-ji-TOR-um LON-gus)	Lateral condyle of tibia Upper anterior fibula	Upper surface of lesser toes and their extensor expansions	Lesser toe extension A-F dorsiflexion Foot eversion

Extensor Hallucis Longus

The great toe or hallux has an extensor of its own, called the **extensor hallucis longus (EHL)** (figure 6.13). This is fitting, in that the great toe is very important in locomotion. The superior muscular portion of the extensor hallucis longus (*extensor,* extend + *hallux,* great toe + *longus,* long) is located deep to the tibialis anterior and peroneus tertius, but it rises to the surface to lie between these muscles in the distal third of the lower leg. Its tendon crosses the front of the ankle, just lateral to the tibialis anterior, and runs slightly medially to attach to the dorsal surface of the great toe. As its name implies, it has a primary action of extending the first MTP joint and the IP joint of the great toe. Due to its crossing anterior to the ankle joint axis and its medial line of pull, this muscle can also assist with ankle-foot dorsiflexion and foot inversion.

Palpation: The tendon of this muscle is located just lateral to the tibialis anterior at the front of the ankle. If you bring the big toe up toward the shin (hallux extension) the tendon will become more prominent and you can palpate the tendon from the top of the big toe and along the dorsum of the foot.

Extensor Digitorum Longus

The **extensor digitorum longus** (**EDL;** *extensor,* extend + *digit,* finger or toe + *longus,* long) and the associated peroneus tertius are the most laterally located muscles of the anterior crural muscles (figure 6.14). The extensor digitorum longus has a long tendon that begins about halfway down the lower leg; and when it crosses the front of the ankle joint, this tendon divides into four slips that attach distally to the dorsal surface of each of the lesser toes. As the name extensor digitorum longus implies, its primary action is to extend the toes (extension of the MTP and both proximal and distal IP joints of the four lesser toes). Crossing the front of the ankle with tendons running laterally, it also can produce ankle-foot dorsiflexion and foot eversion. The extensor digitorum longus can work together with the tibialis anterior as a helping synergist, neutralizing out the inversion of the tibialis anterior to allow the often-desired neutral dorsiflexion of the ankle-foot.

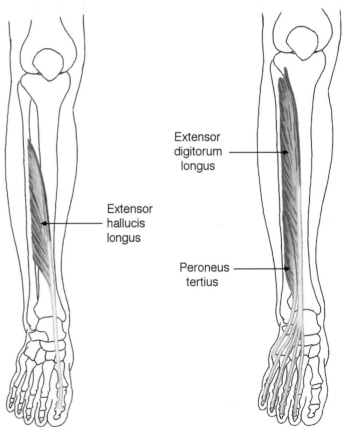

FIGURE 6.13   The extensor hallucis longus (right foot, anterior view).

FIGURE 6.14   The extensor digitorum longus and peroneus tertius (right foot, anterior view).

Palpation: The tendon of the extensor digitorum longus can be found just lateral to the tendon of the extensor hallucis longus at the level of the ankle. Extending toes 2 through 4 against resistance provided by your hand will make the tendons more prominent; and while the single tendon can be palpated near the ankle, distally the tendon divides into four parts, all of which can be palpated from below the ankle to their attachment on the top of the toes.

Attachments and Primary Actions of Peroneus Tertius

Muscle	Proximal attachment(s)	Distal attachment(s)	Primary action(s)
Peroneus tertius (per-o-NEE-us TER-shus)	Anterior fibula and adjacent interosseus membrane in lower third of leg	Upper surface of base of fifth metatarsal	A-F dorsiflexion Foot eversion

Peroneus Tertius

The **peroneus tertius** (*perone*, fibula + *tertius*, third) is considered misnamed by some because it is not contained in the lateral peroneal compartment and produces ankle-foot dorsiflexion versus the plantar flexion produced by the other peroneals. It is actually considered part of the extensor digitorum longus, and it is considered its fifth tendon. The peroneus tertius originates from the lower fibula and interosseus membrane and inserts onto the dorsal surface of the base of the fifth metatarsal (figure 6.14). Due to its lateral placement and the fact that it crosses in front of the ankle joint axis, its actions are ankle-foot dorsiflexion and eversion of the foot. The peroneus tertius has been observed only in humans and great apes, although it is not present in all humans.

Palpation: When it is present, you can palpate the tendon of the peroneus tertius just lateral to the extensor digitorum longus tendon going to the fifth toe while performing the same movement as for palpation of the extensor digitorum longus.

Posterior Crural Muscles

The posterior crural muscles are located on the back of the lower leg. These muscles are contained within the superficial posterior compartment of the leg and include the gastrocnemius, soleus, and plantaris muscles. The plantaris is considered a vestigial, rudimentary muscle that is absent in about 8% of humans (Rasch, 1989). In addition to being a weak assistant flexor of the knee, the plantaris contributes to plantar flexion. However, because its contribution is so minimal in terms of force production relative to the gastrocnemius and soleus (Levangie and Norkin, 2001), the plantaris will not be discussed further in this text. The posterior crural muscles all produce ankle-foot plantar flexion and are very important for propulsion.

Attachments and Primary Actions of Triceps Surae

Muscle	Proximal attachment(s)	Distal attachment(s)	Primary action(s)
Triceps surae			
Gastrocnemius (gas-truk-NEE-mee-us)	Posterior aspect of medial and lateral condyles of femur	Posterior calcaneus via Achilles tendon	A-F plantar flexion (Knee flexion)
Soleus (SO-lee-us)	Posterior aspect of upper tibia, fibula, and interosseus membrane	Posterior calcaneus via Achilles tendon	A-F plantar flexion Stabilizes lower leg on foot

Gastrocnemius

The gastrocnemius (*gaster*, belly + *kneme*, leg) is a double-bellied superficial muscle that attaches above the knee on the medial and lateral femoral condyles and is responsible for most of the rounded appearance or prominence of the "calf" of the leg (figure 6.15). It runs down the back of the lower leg as two separate bellies (medial and lateral) until about halfway down the back of the calf, where the heads join onto an aponeurosis that becomes the tendocalcaneus or **Achilles tendon.** This tendon continues down the lower leg to attach to the heel (calcaneus) and is the largest and strongest tendon in the body (Whiting and Zernicke, 1998). The gastrocnemius contains a preponderance of fast-twitch fibers (Smith, Weiss, and Lehmkuhl, 1996) and is a very powerful plantar flexor of the ankle, making it vital for the execution of forceful movements such as jumping.

Because the gastrocnemius crosses the knee, it can also assist with knee flexion. And, because it crosses the knee, position of the knee will also influence the ability of the gastrocnemius to be stretched or produce force. Creating a position of passive insufficiency by extending the knee and dorsiflexing the ankle-foot will favor effective stretching, while creating a position of active insufficiency by flexing the knee and plantar flexing the ankle-foot will reduce the ability of the gastrocnemius to produce force and require that the soleus play a greater role in producing necessary plantar flexion. One can capitalize on this differential use of these muscles by performing calf (plantar flexor) strengthening exercises with the knees bent and straight.

Palpation: The gastrocnemius can be seen contracting and can be easily palpated at the upper calf when you rise onto your toes (relevé; e.g., plantar flexion).

Soleus

The **soleus** (*soleus,* fish or sole) derives its name from its flat appearance, resembling the sole (a flat fish). This muscle lies deep to the gastrocnemius as seen in figure 6.16. It can be seen below the prominent double-bellied gastrocnemius and more medially in the lower posterior leg. Unlike the gastrocnemius, it does not cross the knee joint. Rather it originates from the posterior tibia and fibula and runs down the back of the lower leg to insert together with the gastrocnemius into the posterior calcaneus via the Achilles tendon. The soleus muscle is an important plantar flexor of the ankle and plays an important postural role to steady the leg upon the foot in standing. The soleus contains a high percentage of slow-twitch fibers, allowing it to perform sustained tonic activity (Smith, Weiss, and Lehmkuhl, 1996); and electromyographic data support the idea that it is the soleus that is active

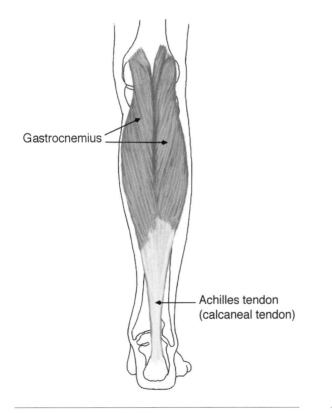

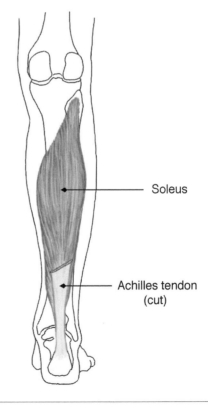

FIGURE 6.15   The gastrocnemius (right foot, posterior view).

FIGURE 6.16   The soleus (right foot, posterior view).

regularly during standing posture to keep the body from falling forward (Basmajian and DeLuca, 1985). Although some controversy still exists, there is some support for the concept that the medial half of the soleus may also act as an invertor of the calcaneus (Levangie and Norkin, 2001). The soleus and gastrocnemius together contain three muscle bellies and hence are termed the **triceps surae** (L. *tri,* three + *caput,* head + *sura,* calf of the leg).

Palpation: Although much of the soleus is covered by the more superficial gastrocnemius, the soleus protrudes on both sides of the gastrocnemius in the lower calf. You can feel the soleus contracting in the lower calf area when you go onto demi-pointe while sitting in a chair with the knee bent.

Posteromedial Crural Muscles

The posteromedial crural or deep posterior crural muscles are located in the deep posterior compartment of the leg. They include the popliteus, flexor hallucis longus, flexor digitorum longus, and tibialis posterior muscles. The primary function of the popliteus is at the knee, as was discussed in chapter 5. Although the remaining three muscles are located posteriorly, as they approach the ankle they course medially, running behind the medial malleolus to attach onto the foot. The resultant line of pull of these three muscles allows them to all function as inverters of the foot as well as plantar flexors.

Attachments and Primary Actions of Tibialis Posterior

Muscle	Proximal attachment(s)	Distal attachment(s)	Primary action(s)
Tibialis posterior (tib-ee-A-lis)	Posterior aspect of upper half of interosseous membrane and adjacent tibia and fibula	Plantar surface of navicular, with offshoots to adjacent bones	Foot inversion A-F plantar flexion Supports arch

Tibialis Posterior

The **tibialis posterior** *(tibial,* tibia + *posterior,* toward the back) lies deep to the triceps surae in the medial portion of the deep posterior compartment. It originates from the upper interosseous membrane and adjacent portions of the tibia and fibula. It runs medially down the back of the leg, passes under the medial malleolus, and then runs forward to attach onto the inferior surface of the navicular bone and (by means of fibrous expansions) into adjacent tarsal bones and into the bases of the metatarsals as seen in figure 6.17. Its line of pull makes it a powerful invertor of the foot whether the foot is plantar flexed or dorsiflexed. The tibialis posterior also assists with weight-bearing ankle-foot plantar flexion. The tibialis posterior is considered an important muscle for preventing undesired pronation; and with its fibrous expansions and sling-like support of the talus, it is in a desirable position to help maintain the medial longitudinal arch and lock the tarsal joints during movements. Due to these latter roles, the tibialis posterior is considered a key medial dynamic stabilizer of the foot (Frey and Shereff, 1988; Levangie and Norkin, 2001). The importance of the tibialis posterior in this function is evidenced by the eversion, loss of height of the medial longitudinal arch, and forefoot abduction that accompany rupture of the tibialis posterior tendon.

Palpation: The tendon of the tibialis posterior can be palpated just below the medial malleolus as it travels forward toward the navicular. Pointing the foot and bringing the big toe inward (ankle-foot plantar flexion and inversion of foot) will make the tendon become more prominent.

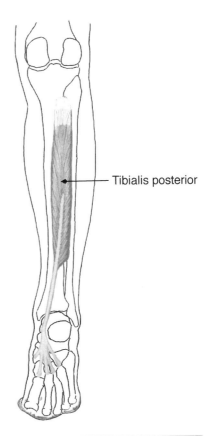

— Tibialis posterior

FIGURE 6.17   The tibialis posterior (right foot, posterior view).

Attachments and Primary Actions of Flexor Digitorum and Hallucis Longus

Muscle	Proximal attachment(s)	Distal attachment(s)	Primary action(s)
Flexor hallucis longus (FLEK-sor HAL-u-sis LON-gus)	Posterior aspect of lower two-thirds of fibula Lower interosseous membrane	Plantar surface of base of distal phalanx of great toe	Great toe flexion A-F plantar flexion Foot inversion
Flexor digitorum longus (FLEK-sor di-ji-TOR-um LON-gus)	Posterior surface of tibia and tibialis posterior fascia	Bases of distal phalanges of toes 2-4; each tendon passes through opening in corresponding tendon of flexor digitorum brevis	Flexion of lesser toes A-F plantar flexion Foot inversion

Flexor Hallucis Longus

The **flexor hallucis longus** (**FHL;** *flexor,* flex + *hallux,* great toe + *longus,* long) originates from the posterior aspect of the fibula, runs medially across the back of the leg to cross behind the medial malleolus, and then forward along the medial portion of the plantar aspect of the foot to attach to the undersurface of the great toe (figure 6.18). As its name implies, the primary action of this muscle is to flex the great toe at the MTP and IP joints. However, in movement, this action appears to be more important in establishing firm contact of the great toe on the ground in closed kinematic chain movements and producing a powerful push-off such as during walking, running, and jumping (Femino et al., 2000; Moore and Agur, 1995) rather than actually producing flexion that bends the big toe under. The flexor hallucis longus also assists with ankle-foot plantar flexion and inversion of the foot. Similar to what occurs with the tibialis posterior, this inversion can serve to raise the medial longitudinal arch, lock the transverse tarsal joint, and thereby stabilize the foot. The course of the flexor hallucis longus under the sustentaculum tali is particularly advantageous for supporting the talus and preventing excessive pronation. During standing on the toes, this muscle is also important for preventing excessive "rolling in," supporting the medial longitudinal arch, and helping to stabilize the hallux.

Palpation: You can palpate the distal portion of the flexor hallucis longus by placing two fingers under the proximal phalanx of the great toe while actively flexing the great toe.

Flexor Digitorum Longus

The **flexor digitorum longus** (**FDL;** *flexor,* flex + *digit,* finger or toe + *longus,* long) originates from the posterior aspect of the upper tibia and from the fascia covering the tibialis posterior, and runs down the posterior medial tibia (figure 6.19). As its name implies, the primary function of the flexor digitorum longus is to flex the digits of the toes. The distal tendon of the flexor digitorum longus divides into four separate tendons, each inserting into the base of the distal phalanges of toes 2 through 5, producing flexion of both the distal and proximal IP joints. This motion produces a pressing of the toes against the ground that is key to application of force to the ground during push-off in closed kinematic chain movements such as running or jumping, and can be used more subtly to help maintain stability. The flexor digitorum longus also assists with ankle-foot plantar flexion, foot inversion, and maintaining the longitudinal arch during dynamic weight bearing.

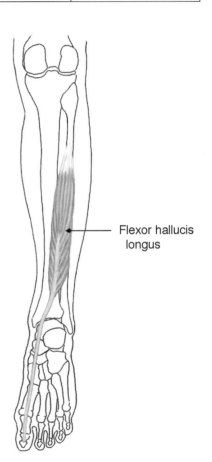

Flexor hallucis longus

FIGURE 6.18   The flexor hallucis longus (right foot, posterior view).

Palpation: You can palpate the distal portion of the flexor digitorum longus tendons by placing a finger under the middle phalanx of any of the lesser toes (toes 2 through 5) while actively flexing that toe. Proximally, the tibialis posterior, flexor digitorum longus, and flexor hallucis longus all cross behind the medial malleolus in close proximity. The mnemonic "*Tom, Dick, and Harry*" can be used to help remember the relative order of these muscles (figure 6.20). Their tendons are positioned from anterior to posterior in the following order: tibialis posterior (*Tom*), flexor *d*igitorum longus (*Dick*), and flexor *h*allucis longus (*Harry*). Hence, the tendon that can be seen and felt just posterior to the medial malleolus is that of the tibialis posterior, with the other two sequentially behind this tendon.

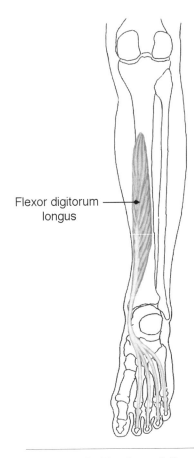

Flexor digitorum longus

FIGURE 6.19   The flexor digitorum longus (right foot, posterior view).

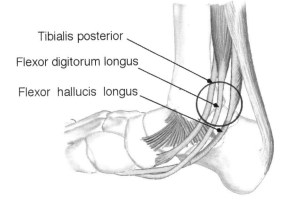

Tibialis posterior

Flexor digitorum longus

Flexor hallucis longus

FIGURE 6.20   Relative position of *t*ibialis posterior (Tom), flexor *d*igitorum longus (Dick), and flexor *h*allucis longus (Harry) (right foot, medial view).

DANCE CUES 6.1

"Use the Floor"

The directive to "use the floor" is commonly used by teachers in association with movements like tendus and dégagés. As just discussed, one of the important roles of the tibialis posterior and long flexors of the toes is to press the toes into the ground for "pushing off" in locomotor movements. So, one desired anatomical interpretation of this cue is to emphasize pressing down into the floor as the foot slides forward on the floor, rather than just shape the foot into plantar flexion with little or no contact with the floor as it moves forward. The former approach of emphasizing pressing into the floor is a useful way of strengthening these posteromedial crural muscles (and many of the intrinsic muscles of the feet), as well as rehearsing the skill of pushing down into the ground to generate the forces (ground reaction forces) that are responsible for propelling the body in the desired direction. If performed with the desired but often unrealized emphasis, the relatively simple movements of tendus and dégagés can provide significant benefits for dancers.

Lateral Crural Muscles

The lateral crural muscles are located on the lateral portion of the lower leg in the lateral compartment of the leg. The lateral crural muscles are composed of the peroneus longus and peroneus brevis. These muscles are closely associated in terms of origin and function and are sometimes jointly referred to as

Attachments and Primary Actions of Peroneal Muscles

Muscle	Proximal attachment(s)	Distal attachment(s)	Primary actions(s)
Peroneus longus (per-o-NEE-us LON-gus)	Lateral tibial condyle Lateral aspect of upper two-thirds of fibula	Lateral aspect of first cuneiform Proximal first metatarsal	Foot eversion A-F plantar flexion Depresses head of first metatarsal
Peroneus brevis (per-o-NEE-us BRE-vis)	Lateral aspect of lower two-thirds of fibula	Tuberosity at proximal end of fifth metatarsal	Foot eversion A-F plantar flexion

the peroneal muscles. These lateral crural muscles cross the lateral portion of the ankle behind the malleolus and both produce eversion of the foot and ankle-foot plantar flexion.

Peroneus Longus

The **peroneus longus** (*perone*, fibula + *longus*, long) originates from the lateral and upper portions of the tibia and fibula. It courses superficially along the lateral lower leg and then continues under the foot to insert onto the undersurface of the first cuneiform and first metatarsal (at the base of the great toe), as shown in figure 6.21. Because the peroneus longus passes behind the lateral malleolus to insert onto the plantar surface of the foot, its line of pull is such that it can assist with ankle-foot plantar flexion as well as perform its primary function of foot eversion. In addition, because the peroneus longus courses all the way under the foot to the inner aspect, it has the ability to pull the medial aspect of the foot down into the supporting surface and help control downward pressure of the first metatarsal head in closed kinematic chain movements. Thus, the peroneus longus is in a position to shift the body weight medially and help initiate pronation during walking, as well as help position the great toe appropriately for push-off. The peroneus longus is also in a position to offer support to various arches of the feet. First, the peroneus longus passes under the apex of the lateral longitudinal arch and thereby provides support for this arch. Second, its medial attachment allows it to support the transverse arch, functioning like a bowstring by pulling the medial border toward the lateral border and helping to limit the depression of the cuboid (Levangie and Norkin, 2001; Soderberg, 1986).

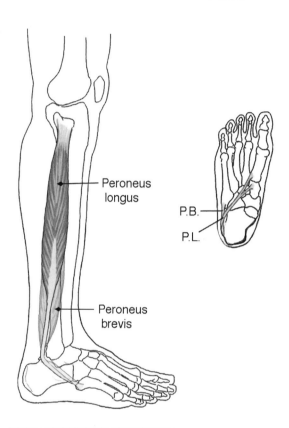

FIGURE 6.21 Peroneus longus and brevis (right foot, lateral and inferior views).

Peroneus Brevis

The **peroneus brevis** (*perone*, fibula + *brevis*, short) originates lower on the fibula than the longus and runs deep to the longus for much of its upper course. As its name suggests, the peroneus brevis is a shorter muscle than the peroneus longus, attaching distally onto the lateral foot (proximal fifth metatarsal) rather than coursing underneath the foot as seen in figure 6.21. It shares a similar proximal line of pull to the peroneus longus, and so it also assists with ankle-foot plantar flexion and is a prime mover for foot eversion. The peroneals' line of pull also enables them to produce abduction of the forefoot, a motion used by dancers to create a beveled foot, a commonly used position in many ballet and some modern schools of dance.

When weight bearing, both the peroneus longus and brevis are considered important dynamic stabilizers of the foot and the lower leg relative to the foot. These muscles provide an important counterbalance for the invertors of the foot such as the tibialis anterior, tibialis posterior, and flexor hallucis longus and are essential for preventing ankle inversion sprains.

Palpation: The tendons of the peroneals can be made more prominent by pointing and beveling the foot (plantar flexion and eversion). They can be palpated below and above the lateral malleolus. The peroneus brevis passes closest to the lateral malleolus, while the longus lies just posterior to the brevis. The peroneus brevis is more prominent with ankle-foot plantar flexion and eversion of the foot, and its course can be followed along the lateral foot to the base of the fifth metatarsal.

Summary of Extrinsic Ankle-Foot Muscle Attachments and Actions

A summary of the attachments of the extrinsic muscles of the ankle and foot is provided in table 6.2, and these muscles and some of their attachments are shown in figures 6.22, A and B, 6.23, A, B, and C, and 6.24, A and B. From these resources, deduce the line of pull and resultant possible actions of the primary extrinsic muscles of the ankle and foot, and then check for accuracy by referring to figures 6.22C, 6.23D, and 6.24C.

TABLE 6.2   Summary of Attachments and Primary Actions of Extrinsic Muscles of the Ankle-Foot

Muscle	Proximal attachment(s)	Distal attachment(s)	Primary action(s)
Anterior muscles			
Tibialis anterior (tib-ee-A-lis)	Upper two-thirds of lateral tibia and adjacent interosseous membrane	Medial and inferior surfaces of medial cuneiform and base of first metatarsal	A-F dorsiflexion Foot inversion
Extensor hallucis longus (ek-STEN-sor HAL-u-sis LON-gus)	Anterior fibula and adjacent interosseus membrane at the middle half of leg	Upper surface of base of distal phalanx of great toe (hallux)	Great toe extension A-F dorsiflexion Foot inversion
Extensor digitorum longus (ek-STEN-sor di-ji-TOR-um LON-gus)	Lateral condyle of tibia Upper anterior fibula	Upper surface of lesser toes and their extensor expansions	Lesser toe extension A-F dorsiflexion Foot eversion
Peroneus tertius (per-o-NEE-us TER-shus)	Anterior fibula and adjacent interosseus membrane in lower third of leg	Upper surface of base of fifth metatarsal	A-F dorsiflexion Foot eversion
Posterior muscles			
Triceps surae			
Gastrocnemius (gas-truk-NEE-mee-us)	Posterior aspect of medial and lateral condyles of femur	Posterior calcaneus via Achilles tendon	A-F plantar flexion (Knee flexion)
Soleus (SO-lee-us)	Posterior aspect of upper tibia, fibula, and interosseus membrane	Posterior calcaneus via Achilles tendon	A-F plantar flexion Stabilizes lower leg on foot
Posteromedial muscles			
Tibialis posterior (tib-ee-A-lis)	Posterior aspect of upper half of interosseous membrane and adjacent tibia and fibula	Plantar surface of navicular, with offshoots to adjacent bones	Foot inversion A-F plantar flexion Supports arch
Flexor hallucis longus (FLEK-sor HAL-u-sis LON-gus)	Posterior aspect of lower two-thirds of fibula Lower interosseous membrane	Plantar surface of base of distal phalanx of great toe	Great toe flexion A-F plantar flexion Foot inversion

Muscle	Proximal attachment(s)	Distal attachment(s)	Primary action(s)
Posteromedial muscles (continued)			
Flexor digitorum longus (FLEK-sor di-ji-TOR-um LON-gus)	Posterior surface of tibia and tibialis posterior fascia	Bases of distal phalanges of toes 2-4; each tendon passes through opening in corresponding tendon of flexor digitorum brevis	Flexion of lesser toes A-F plantar flexion Foot inversion
Lateral muscles			
Peroneus longus (per-o-NEE-us LON-gus)	Lateral tibial condyle Lateral aspect of upper two-thirds of fibula	Lateral aspect of first cuneiform Proximal first metatarsal	Foot eversion A-F plantar flexion Depresses head of first metatarsal
Peroneus brevis (per-o-NEE-us BRE-vis)	Lateral aspect of lower two-thirds of fibula	Tuberosity at proximal end of fifth metatarsal	Foot eversion A-F plantar flexion

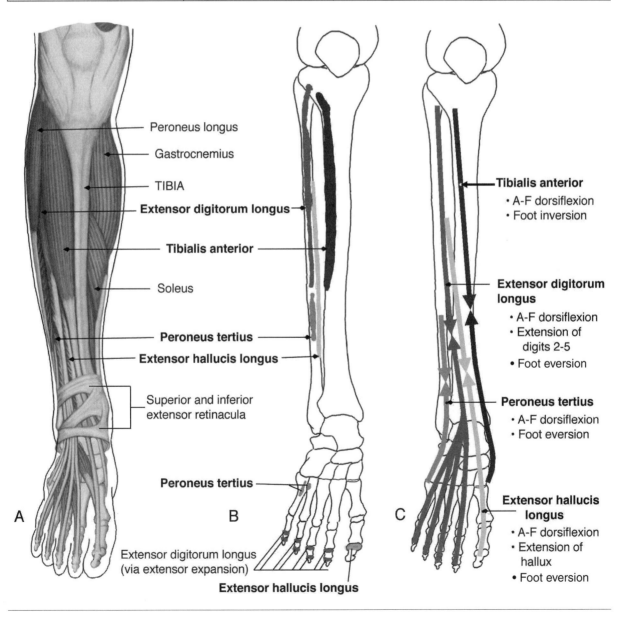

Peroneus longus
Gastrocnemius
TIBIA
Extensor digitorum longus
Tibialis anterior
Soleus
Peroneus tertius
Extensor hallucis longus
Superior and inferior extensor retinacula

Peroneus tertius
Extensor digitorum longus (via extensor expansion)
Extensor hallucis longus

A
B
C

Tibialis anterior
• A-F dorsiflexion
• Foot inversion

Extensor digitorum longus
• A-F dorsiflexion
• Extension of digits 2-5
• Foot eversion

Peroneus tertius
• A-F dorsiflexion
• Foot eversion

Extensor hallucis longus
• A-F dorsiflexion
• Extension of hallux
• Foot eversion

FIGURE 6.22   Anterior view of primary muscles acting on the ankle and foot (right foot). (A) Muscles, (B) attachments, (C) lines of pull and actions.

319

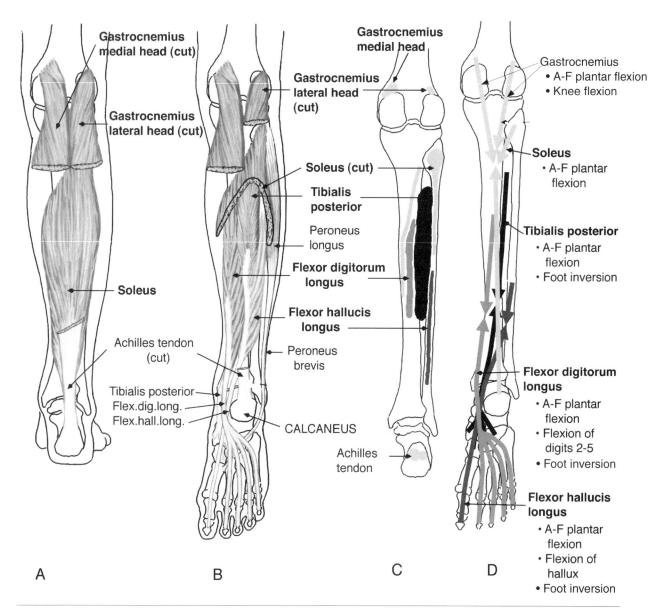

FIGURE 6.23   Posterior view of primary muscles acting on the ankle and foot (right foot). (A) More superficial view of muscles, (B) deeper view of muscles, (C) attachments, (D) lines of pull and actions.

Intrinsic Muscles of the Foot

Remember that by definition the intrinsic muscles have both their proximal and distal attachments within the foot, but some of these intrinsic muscles have similar functions to the extrinsic muscles. To help distinguish between extrinsic and intrinsic muscles with similar functions, the terms short (brevis) and long (longus) are sometimes used. For example, the extrinsic extensor of the great toe is called extensor hallucis longus while the intrinsic extensor is called extensor hallucis brevis. This short extensor of the hallux (extensor hallucis brevis), as well as the short extensors of the digits (extensor digitorum brevis), is located on the dorsum of the foot as seen in figure 6.25. The remaining 10 intrinsic muscles are called the plantar muscles and can be grouped into four layers as seen in figure 6.26. While the first three groups are located on the plantar aspect of the foot in progressively deeper layers, layer 4 is actually located between the metatarsals and phalanges.

The intrinsic muscles of the foot are responsible for abduction, adduction, flexion, and extension of the toes. Some of these muscles are also important for dynamic maintenance of the arches, propulsion, and fine adjustments of the feet. One of the important and often overlooked functions of the intrinsic muscles is to maintain the IP joints in extension to aid the flexor hallucis longus and flexor digitorum longus in producing a powerful push-off in locomotor movements. If the toes are not maintained in

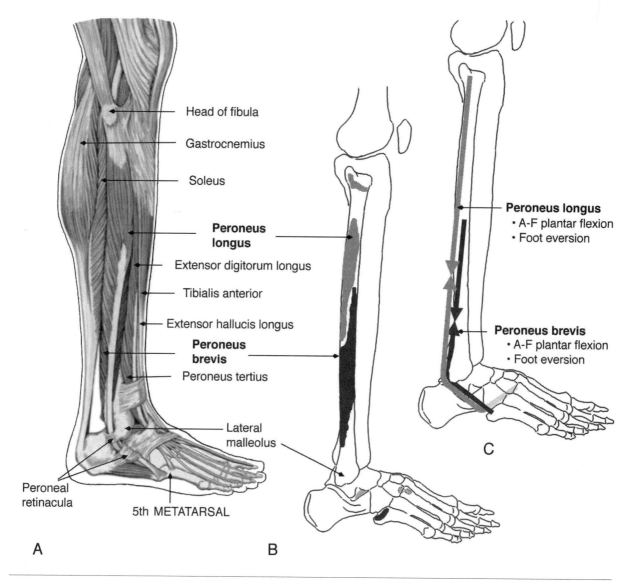

A

B

C

Peroneus longus
- A-F plantar flexion
- Foot eversion

Peroneus brevis
- A-F plantar flexion
- Foot eversion

Head of fibula

Gastrocnemius

Soleus

Peroneus longus

Extensor digitorum longus

Tibialis anterior

Extensor hallucis longus

Peroneus brevis

Peroneus tertius

Lateral malleolus

Peroneal retinacula

5th METATARSAL

FIGURE 6.24 Lateral view of primary muscles acting on the ankle and foot (right foot). (A) Muscles, (B) attachments, (C) lines of pull and actions.

extension they curl under, markedly decreasing the effectiveness of push-off. A detailed presentation of the intrinsic muscles of the feet is beyond the scope of this book. However, it is important for dancers to realize the extensiveness of these muscles and to remember that these muscles are very important in dancers due to the high-magnitude, precise, and intricate demands incurred by the feet. For interested readers, table 6.3 presents the names, locations, and functions of these muscles.

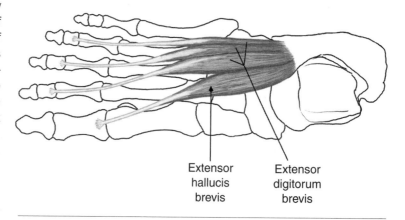

Extensor hallucis brevis

Extensor digitorum brevis

FIGURE 6.25 The dorsal intrinsic muscles of the foot (right foot, superior view).

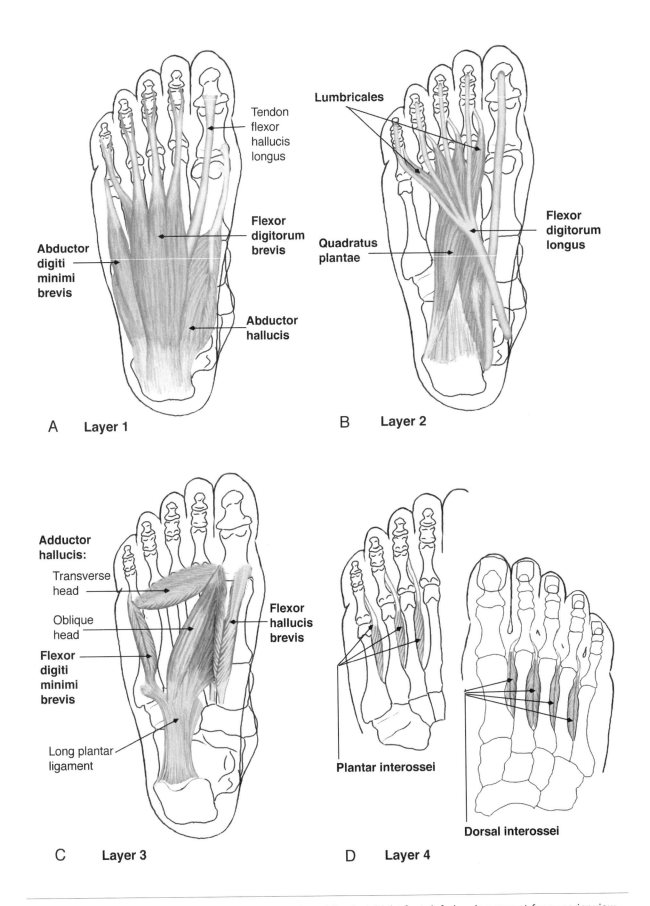

A Layer 1

Tendon flexor hallucis longus

Flexor digitorum brevis

Abductor digiti minimi brevis

Abductor hallucis

B Layer 2

Lumbricales

Flexor digitorum longus

Quadratus plantae

C Layer 3

Adductor hallucis:

Transverse head

Oblique head

Flexor digiti minimi brevis

Long plantar ligament

Flexor hallucis brevis

D Layer 4

Plantar interossei

Dorsal interossei

FIGURE 6.26 The layers of the plantar intrinsic muscles of the foot (right foot; inferior view except for superior view used for layer 4, dorsal interossei).

TABLE 6.3   Summary of Attachments and Primary Actions of Intrinsic Muscles of the Foot

Muscle	Proximal attachment(s)	Distal attachment(s)	Primary action(s)
Dorsal aspect			
Extensor hallucis brevis	Lateral portion of dorsal surface of calcaneus	Dorsal surface of base of distal phalanx of great toe	Extension of MTP joint of great toe
Extensor digitorum brevis	Lateral portion of dorsal surface of calcaneus	Tendons of extensor digitorum longus (toes 2-4)	Extension of MTP and IP joints of toes 2-4
Plantar aspect			
First layer			
Abductor hallucis	Tuberosity of calcaneus Plantar aponeurosis	Medial side of base of proximal phalanx of great toe	Abduction and flexion of MTP joint of great toe
Flexor digitorum brevis	Tuberosity of calcaneus Plantar aponeurosis	Both sides of middle phalanges of toes 2-5	Flexion of MTP and proximal IP joints of toes 2-5
Abductor digiti minimi brevis	Tuberosity of calcaneus Plantar aponeurosis	Lateral side of base of proximal phalanx of fifth toe	Abduction of MTP joint of toe 5 Flexion of proximal IP joint of toe 5
Second layer			
Quadratus plantae	Two heads: Medial surface Lateral margin of plantar surface of calcaneus	Tendons of flexor digitorum longus	Assists flexor digitorum longus with flexion of distal IP joints of toes 2-5
Lumbricals	Tendons of flexor digitorum longus	Medial aspect of expansion over toes 2-5	Flexion of MTP joints of toes 2-5 Extension of proximal and distal IP joints of toes 2-5
Third layer			
Flexor hallucis brevis	Plantar surfaces of cuboid and lateral cuneiform	Both sides of base of proximal phalanx of great toe	Flexion of MTP joint of great toe
Adductor hallucis	Oblique head: bases of metatarsals 2-4 Transverse head: plantar ligaments of metatarsophalangeal joints	Tendons of both heads attach to lateral side of base of proximal phalanx of great toe	Adduction of MTP joint of great toe Flexion of MTP joint of great toe Assists in support of transverse metatarsal arch of foot
Flexor digiti minimi brevis	Base of fifth metatarsal	Base of proximal phalanx of fifth toe	Flexion of MTP joint of toe 5
Fourth layer			
Plantar interossei (three muscles)	Bases and medial sides of metatarsals 3-5	Medial sides of proximal phalanges of toes 3-5 and tendons of extensor digitorum longus	Adduction of toes 3-5 Flexion of MTP joints of toes 3-5 Extension of distal IP joints of toes 3-5
Dorsal interossei (four muscles)	Adjacent sides of metatarsals 1-5	First: medial side of proximal phalanx of second toe Second to fourth: lateral sides of toes 2-4 and tendons of extensor digitorum longus	Abduction of MTP joints of toes 2-4 Flexion of MTP joints of toes 2-4 Extension of distal IP joints of toes 2-4

Alignment and Common Deviations of the Ankle and Foot

There are numerous alignment problems that can involve the ankle and foot, including abnormal positioning of the tibia, arches, rearfoot, and toes. Some of these problems are described in terms of the direction of the deviation of the bones; and similar to the situation with the knee, valgus refers to a lateral deviation of the distal segment while varus reflects a medial deviation of the distal segment. As with some other regions of the body, a thorough medical evaluation is necessary to distinguish between structural and functional alignment problems. Furthermore, it is important to realize that ankle and foot deviations are very common in both dancers and the general population, and that their significance for injury and the need for correction are highly controversial.

Tibial Torsion

As discussed in the previous chapter, the tibia generally exhibits external rotation along its length, termed external tibial torsion, such that in the average adult the ankle mortise faces about 15° laterally with the tip of the medial malleoli slightly anterior and superior relative to the lateral malleoli as seen in figure 6.27. However, individual variation can be great, with measures ranging from 4° of internal tibial torsion to 56° of external tibial torsion being reported (Smith, Weiss, and Lehmkuhl, 1996). Internal tibial torsion is associated with walking with the feet turned inward relative to the knee (toeing-in), while exaggerated external tibial torsion is associated with walking with the feet turned out relative to the knees (toeing-out). Theoretically, an increase in external tibial torsion might be advantageous for maximizing turnout of the feet. However, one study of professional ballet dancers did not show an increase in average external tibial rotation above that found in the general population (Hamilton et al., 1992).

Arches of the Feet

The bones of the feet are not arranged in a flat structure, but rather involve a series of longitudinal and transverse arches to form a structure similar to an elastic half-dome as seen in figure 6.28A. You can better visualize these arches by standing with your feet side by side and noting that while the lateral margins of both feet stay in contact with the ground, the inner soles of the feet form a shallow dome; the central portion forms an arch that is generally not in contact with the ground. This central concavity is due to the **medial longitudinal arch**—consisting of the three medial metatarsals, the cuneiforms, the navicular, and the calcaneus. The medial longitudinal arch is the higher of the longitudinal arches and is the arch that people are generally referring to when talking about the foot. It is designed to allow accommodation to uneven surfaces, change in direction, and easy shift of the body weight from one side of the foot to the other. In contrast, the **lateral longitudinal arch**—consisting of the two lateral metatarsals, the cuboid, and the calcaneus—is designed for stability and weight bearing and generally is in contact with the ground during standing.

While the longitudinal arches are responsible for the doming in a lengthwise direction, the **transverse arch** is key for the doming in a medial-lateral direction. The transverse arch consists of the tarsal bones in the midfoot (navicular, cuneiforms, and cuboid) and the metatarsals. This transverse arch can be further divided into the tarsal, posterior metatarsal, and anterior metatarsal arches (Magee, 1997). The height of the **tarsal transverse arch,** particularly influenced by the cuneiforms, varies markedly between individuals and is instrumental in creating the high instep valued in classical ballet. The **anterior metatarsal arch** is also very important for dancers, and a loss of this arch is often evidenced by callus formation under the head of the second metatarsal and by metatarsal pain.

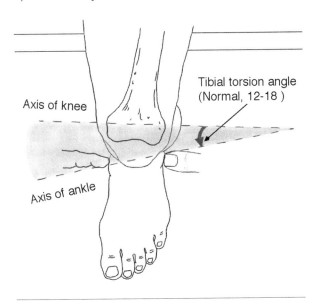

FIGURE 6.27 Tibial torsion (left foot, superior view).

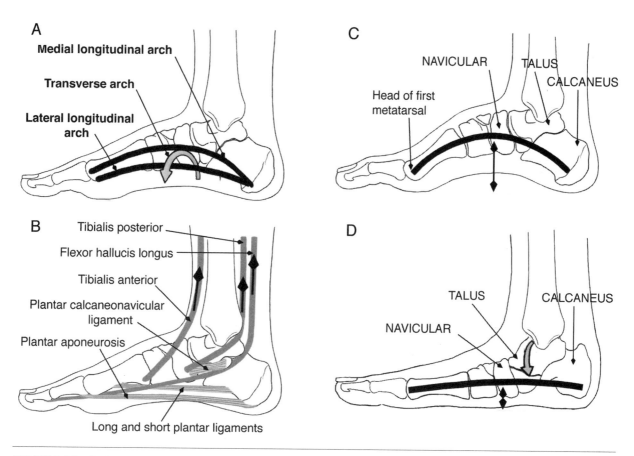

FIGURE 6.28 Arches of the foot. (A) Normal bony arches, (B) key ligaments and muscles that can help support the medial longitudinal arch, (C) pes cavus, (D) pes planus.

In relaxed standing (static stability), these arches are supported by the shapes of the bones, the plantar fascia, and the ligaments that help hold these bones together, without assistance from the muscles of the feet (Basmajian and DeLuca, 1985; Smith, Weiss, and Lehmkuhl, 1996). However, during movement (dynamic stability), various extrinsic and intrinsic muscles add active support and serve as a second line of stability for the arches of the feet, called into play as demands increase (figure 6.28B).

Presence of these arches allows the feet to withstand greater forces while still maintaining their integrity, to better absorb shock, and to have greater mobility and stability. When bearing weight, the foot tends to spread slightly, which helps to absorb the impact of the force; but the strong arches with their springlike quality from associated ligaments and fascia resist excessive spreading and provide an elastic recoil that assists in locomotion (Hamill and Knutzen, 1995).

Pes Planus (Flatfoot)

When the foot demonstrates a decrease or loss of the medial longitudinal arch, it is called a flatfoot, or **pes planus** (L. *pes*, foot + *planus*, flat). A footprint of this type will show much greater area of contact than a normal foot (figure 6.29B). A flatfoot can be further classified as a flexible flatfoot or a rigid flatfoot or pes planus. With a rigid pes planus, there is a decreased arch both when bearing weight and not. This type of flatfoot is often secondary to structural or pathological factors and is relatively rare. In contrast, with a flexible or functional pes planus, an arch is present when not bearing weight or when on demipointe, but when the dancer stands, the medial longitudinal arch flattens; the head of the talus moves inferomedially and causes the foot to pronate (figure 6.28D). This movement of the talus also brings the adjacent navicular with it, a landmark readily used for evaluation of the arches. It has been postulated that congenital ligamentous laxity or excessive pronation over time may cause stretching of the soft tissues, such as the spring ligament and tibialis posterior tendon, with resultant loss of height in the medial longitudinal arch of the foot during weight bearing (Hamilton and Luttgens, 2002; Smith, Weiss, and Lehmkuhl, 1996; Soderberg, 1986). The flexible flatfoot has been reported to occur in about 15% of the general population (Omey and Micheli, 1999) and is common in dancers.

Individuals with flatfeet have been shown to have more firing of muscles during standing, probably to try to prevent further flattening of the arches and offer stability to the intertarsal joints. There is some evidence that pes planus and its associated excessive pronation increase the risk for certain types of injuries such as shin splints, plantar fasciitis, and metatarsal stress fractures. However, the general proposed association of flexible pes planus with increased injury risk is controversial and complex, perhaps because the additional undesired stress to the structures working to support the medial arch may at least in part be counterbalanced by the beneficial shock absorbency offered by this foot type.

Pes Cavus (High-Arched Foot)

The condition opposite to pes planus is **pes cavus.** Pes cavus (L. *pes*, foot + *cavus*, hollow) involves an abnormally high arch (figure 6.28C), and a footprint would show less area of contact than for a normal foot or flatfoot (figure 6.29, A and C). How much of pes cavus is congenital and how much it can be developed is controversial, but in the author's experience, dancers can increase their arch to some degree with supplemental conditioning and dance training. Although the aesthetic of this cavus foot type is valued in most forms of dance, this foot type is generally a more rigid foot type, allowing limited pronation for shock absorbency. Hence, it may increase the risk for certain types of injuries such as stress fractures, tarsal sprains from going over the foot on pointe, plantar fasciitis, and metatarsal

problems (Conti and Wong, 2001; Hamilton, 1982; McCrory et al., 1999; Yakut et al., 1997).

Rearfoot Valgus and Varus

Another important consideration for foot alignment is the position of the calcaneus. Because the calcaneus is part of the medial longitudinal arch, the subtalar joint, and one of the transverse tarsal joints, its position will influence the position of the rearfoot, midfoot, and forefoot.

Rearfoot position can be estimated by the intersection at the subtalar joint of a line running down the back of the lower third of the tibia and a line bisecting the back of the calcaneus as seen in figure 6.30 (Kreighbaum and Barthels, 1996). A line that bisects the calcaneus would ideally be approximately perpendicular to the floor during standing and when the dancer is viewed from behind (Kreighbaum and Barthels, 1996). This would be considered a neutral position of the rearfoot (figure 6.30A). If the line that bisects the calcaneus deviates outward distally more than 2° (Levangie and Norkin, 2001), creating an everted foot, this condition is termed **rearfoot valgus** (L. turned outward) (figure 6.30B). This condition is commonly associated with excessive pronation during gait and requires midtarsal inversion to bring the lateral toes down to the ground in the same plane with the hallux during standing. A dancer with rearfoot valgus will find it easy to "roll in," or place too much of the body weight on the inside of the foot and tend to lift the outside toes off the floor.

If the line that bisects the calcaneus deviates inward versus outward distally, this malalignment

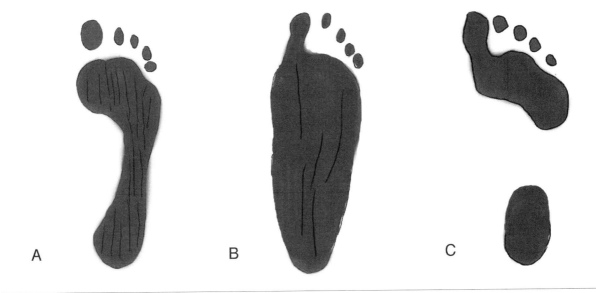

FIGURE 6.29   Footprint associated with (A) normal foot, (B) pes planus, (C) pes cavus.

Pes Planus

Perform the following observations to identify the presence of flexible or rigid pes planus.

1. While sitting down (non-weight bearing), mark the following landmarks on one foot:

    a. Inferolateral aspect of the head of the first metatarsal

    b. Tubercle of the navicular

    c. Distal point of the medial malleolus

    Note the relationship of these three points. If the tubercle of the navicular falls on the line between the head of the first metatarsal and the medial malleolus, this is considered a normal arch. In contrast, if the tubercle of the navicular drops markedly below this line, this is considered rigid flatfoot, or rigid pes planus.

2. Now stand up, placing weight on the foot that has the markers, and note if the relationship of the points changes. If the three points still stay in line, this would still be considered a normal arch. However, if the navicular was in line when non-weight bearing but drops below the line when weight bearing, this is considered a flexible flatfoot, or flexible pes planus. The degree to which the navicular drops is reflective of the severity of the pes planus.

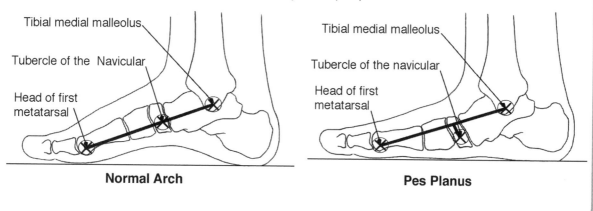

Normal Arch   Pes Planus

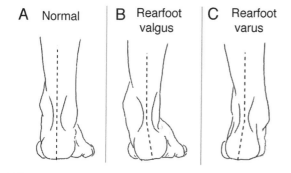

FIGURE 6.30   Rearfoot position (right foot, posterior view). (A) Neutral, (B) rearfoot valgus, (C) rearfoot varus.

is called **rearfoot varus** (L. bent inward) (figure 6.30C). Rearfoot varus is commonly associated with excessive supination during gait and increased risk for ankle sprains, and it requires midtarsal eversion to bring the medial toes down to the ground in the same plane with the lateral toes during standing. A dancer with rearfoot varus will find it easy to "roll out," with too much of the body weight placed on the outside of the foot and inadequate weight borne by the hallux.

Position of the Toes

The arches and position of the rearfoot, as well as genetic factors, can also influence the position of the toes. Prevalent problems involving the toes include claw toes, hammertoes, and hallux valgus.

Claw Toes and Hammertoes

Claw toes and hammertoes represent conditions in which the lesser toes, usually particularly the second toe, remain excessively flexed. With **claw toes** the

MTP joint is generally in fixed hyperextension and both IP joints are in fixed flexion as seen in figure 6.31. With **hammertoes,** the MTP joint is generally in fixed hyperextension, the proximal IP joint is in fixed flexion, and the distal IP joint is in hyperextension such that the tip of the toe becomes depressed downward (Levangie and Norkin, 2001; Mercier, 1995). These conditions are commonly associated with pes cavus in which the exaggerated arch involves a lowering of the heads of the metatarsals relative to the rearfoot. These conditions tend to place excessive stress on the metatarsal heads, can interfere with balance and placement on demi-pointe and pointe, and leave the flexed joints vulnerable for blisters and corns.

It is important for dancers and teachers to realize that these conditions are generally due to shortened toe flexors or intrinsic muscle imbalance, and relaxing the toes will not produce the desired correction. However, aggressive daily stretching by using one hand to bring the toes (appropriate IP joints) into extension while holding the MTP joint in a neutral position can sometimes offer gradual but noticeable improvement. In addition, using the intrinsic interossei and lumbrical muscles to stabilize the MTP joint in a neutral versus hyperextended position can also decrease clawing during standing flat versus on demi-pointe or pointe (Levangie and Norkin, 2001). These muscles can create the desired flexion of the MTP joint without producing undesired further IP flexion of the toes. Furthermore, the extrinsic and intrinsic toe extensors can be used to actively extend the toes as much as the flexion contractures

will allow. Strength and use of these muscles can be improved with doming exercises performed sitting (table 6.6J, p. 349), followed by repetition of the exercise standing, focusing on very slightly lifting the metatarsal heads up (vs. letting them drop) as the toes reach forward (IP extension). Mild deformities can also sometimes be improved or relieved with over-and-under taping to adjacent toes, selection of dance and street shoes that are not too short, use of various pads or toe caps to avoid pressure sores and corns from the associated abnormal friction from shoes, and making sure that the dancer is standing with his or her body weight appropriately positioned (vs. too far back) so that the toe flexors are not having to be used excessively to maintain stability. Although in the general population, surgery may be recommended for resistant forms of these deformities, this type of surgery is generally not recommended for the dancer.

Hallux Valgus and Bunions

Hallux valgus (L. great toe + turned outward) is a lateral deviation of the distal end of the great toe (hallux) at the MTP joint, often also involving a deviation of the first metatarsal toward the midline of the body (metatarsus primus varus) as seen in figure 6.32. This bony deviation changes the line of pull of the muscles that cross the MTP joint, such that many of these muscles will tend to have a bowstring effect that further increases the valgus deformity, and in more advanced cases causes the sesamoids to displace to the lateral side of the head of the first metatarsal. This valgus deviation of the hallux also tends to make the medial aspect of the first metatarsal head become more prominent, and the resultant friction and trauma from overlying footwear can readily lead to a bony outgrowth (exostosis), an inflamed bursa between the exostosis and skin, and a callus on the overlying skin. This bony and soft tissue enlargement on the inside of the head of the first metatarsal is termed a bunion.

Hallux valgus has been reported to affect as many as 22% to 36% of adolescents; a greater prevalence is in active females, and particularly female ballet dancers (Kravitz et al., 1986; Omey and Micheli, 1999). The etiology is still controversial, but it likely involves both familial factors and other factors that tend to increase lateral deviation forces on the hallux such as tight shoes, pointe work, metatarsus primus varus, pes planus, excessive pronation, forcing turnout, and joint hyperlaxity. In early stages, use of shoes with a wider toe box, a felt pad, a toe separator, hallux valgus taping, control of pronation, and strengthening the arch muscles and the abductor of the hallux may give some relief. However, in later stages, loss of

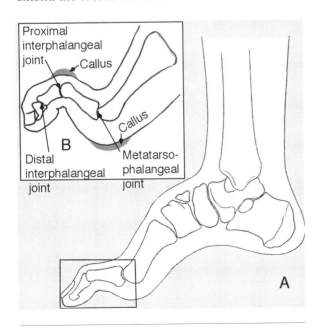

FIGURE 6.31   Claw toes associated with pes cavus (right foot, medial view). (A) Hallux, (B) second toe.

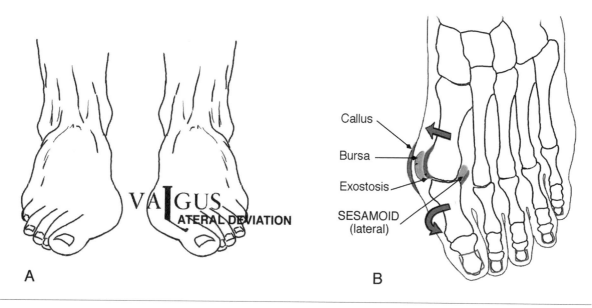

FIGURE 6.32   (A) Hallux valgus (anterior view) with (B) bunion formation (left foot, superior view).

range of motion, pain, and the degree of deviation often prohibit optimal mechanics and make these approaches ineffective. Although surgery is often recommended in this later stage for other populations, its use with performing dancers is controversial; and some orthopedists recommended against it due to the tendency to lose hallux extension that is necessary for dance (Baxter, 1994; Dyal and Thompson, 1997; Howse, 1983).

Foot Type

The foot as a whole can be classified into different types based on its shape and the relative length of the toes. One classification divides feet into three types: (1) the squared foot, in which the first and second toes are the same length; (2) the Egyptian foot, in which the first toe is longer than the second; and (3) the Morton's or Greek foot, in which the second toe is longer than the first. It is generally held that a relatively short, broad, square foot type is less prone to injury, and there is some support for this conjecture in dancers (Ende and Wickstrom, 1982; Hamilton et al., 1997).

The foot type and relative lengths of the metatarsals and toes will also influence what bones of the foot remain in contact during rising onto the ball of the foot. The axis at which the foot bends (e.g., where toes extend at the MTP joints), called the **metatarsal break,** is not perpendicular but rather makes an oblique angle from about 50° to 70° to the long axis of the foot (Sammarco, 1980). Thus, on demi-pointe, the lateral two or three metatarsals will generally

not remain in contact with the floor, and contact of the lateral toes will depend on the angle of this metatarsal break and the length of the toes. Hence, the directive sometimes given by dance teachers to keep all the metatarsals and toes in contact with the floor when on demi-pointe is not appropriate for most dancers. Probably a better cue is to focus on keeping the body weight centered over the first and second metatarsal heads with the middle of the back of the calcaneus in line with the middle of the back of the lower tibia (i.e., neutral rearfoot position without undue inversion or eversion of the rearfoot or midfoot). However, this neutral positioning will have to be modified slightly for schools of dance that desire the beveled line on demi-pointe or pointe. With pointe, the foot type, pointe shoe design, and aesthetic concerns (neutral vs. beveled) will influence toe contact and weight placement. One study that involved performing relevés with pointe shoes showed that the greatest pressures were over the hallux, and the pressures over the second toe varied with the length of the toe, such that greater pressures were present with a long second toe or with capping of the second toe (Teitz, Harrington, and Wiley, 1985).

Mechanics
of the Ankle and Foot

The design of the ankle-foot complex is such that certain positions offer greater stability and certain positions offer more mobility, important for meeting the many functions this structure must serve.

While weight is distributed in a manner to avoid excessive stress to any one structure with standing, in movement the use of dorsiflexion, plantar flexion, pronation, and supination alter foot characteristics and stability.

Weight Distribution on the Foot During Standing

During ideal standing, approximately 50% of the body weight should be borne by the heel and the remaining 50% transmitted across the metatarsal heads (Sammarco, 1980). When weight bearing, the anterior transverse metatarsal arch tends to flatten so that all five metatarsal heads come in contact with the ground. However, the load is not generally borne evenly by these metatarsals. Instead, the load on the metatarsal head of the great toe should be about twice that of each of the metatarsal heads of the lesser toes (figure 6.33). This is a helpful guideline to keep in mind, as many dancers stand with excessive weight on their heels or on the medial or lateral metatarsal heads. Wearing high heels can also alter this weight

distribution and tends to increase loads borne by the metatarsal heads associated with the lesser toes while decreasing the load borne by the metatarsal head of the hallux (Rasch, 1989).

Influence of Ankle Dorsiflexion and Plantar Flexion on Stability

The integrity offered by the mortise architecture of the ankle is not uniform in all positions. Although there are large individual variations in shape, the talus is generally slightly wedge-shaped with the anterior articulating surface being broader than the posterior (figure 6.34A). This structure produces a snug and stable fit when the ankle is in dorsiflexion or a neutral position with the foot at a 90° angle to the tibia, such as when standing (figures 6.34, B and D). However, when the ankle goes into plantar flexion, such as when wearing shoes with high heels, raising up on the toes, or jumping, the narrower por-

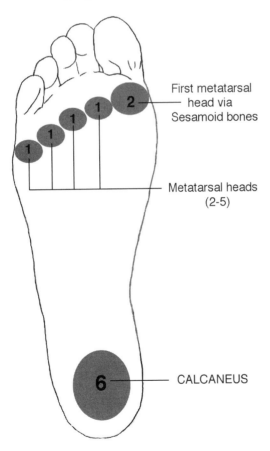

FIGURE 6.33   Ideal weight distribution on the foot during standing (right foot, inferior view).

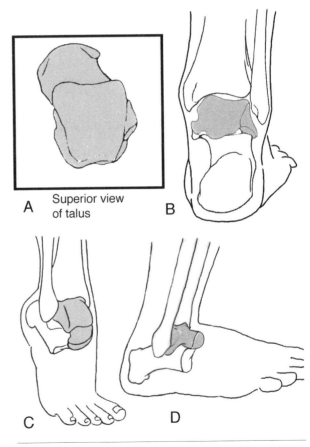

FIGURE 6.34   Change in ankle stability with position. (A) Talus with wider anterior articular surface, (B) talus sitting in mortise formed by malleoli and reinforced by ligaments, (C) decreased stability in plantar flexion with narrower portion of talus in mortise, (D) increased stability in dorsiflexion with wider portion of talus in mortise.

tion of the talus lies within the malleoli, allowing for more joint play and less stability (figure 6.34C). This position of plantar flexion relies more on ligaments and muscles for stability and is commonly involved in the mechanism of ankle sprains.

Influence of Pronation and Supination on Foot Mechanics

In movement, transfer of the body weight and relative positioning of the bones of the feet can function to make the foot more or less stable (Levangie and Norkin, 2001). The position of supination places the weight of the body on the lateral longitudinal arch, which is designed for stability; and due to ligament design and axes of the transverse tarsal joint the foot is "locked" and stable. This stable position of the foot is desirable for transfer of weight to the foot and for providing a stable segment about which the rest of the body may move, as well as for use of the foot as a rigid lever for propulsion in movements such as walking, running, or jumping. However, the foot also has the need to be able to accommodate to uneven surfaces and absorb shock. These qualities are met by pronation, in which the foot "unlocks" and becomes the flexible structure necessary to allow for small movements between the tarsals and movement of the forefoot relative to the rearfoot. This pronation also shifts the weight of the body toward the medial longitudinal arch of the foot, which is designed for mobility. Thus, the arrangement of the various arches and joints allows the foot to act as a rigid lever for propulsion and an adaptive structure for force absorption and accommodation, initiated by use of the positions of supination and pronation.

Muscular Analysis of Fundamental Movements of the Ankle and Foot

Movements are simplified in this discussion to ankle-foot dorsiflexion, ankle-foot plantar flexion, foot inversion, and foot eversion without differentiation regarding the contribution of the various joints of the rearfoot and midfoot. Also for purposes of simplification, movements of the toes are not discussed in the text but merely included in table 6.4. When thinking about the movements of the toes, it is important to keep in mind that one of the key functions of the toes is to press down against the ground to propel the body in space. A summary of the key muscles capable of producing the fundamental movements of the ankle and foot is provided in table 6.4.

Plantar Flexion

Ankle-foot plantar flexion involves bringing the anterior surface of the shin and the dorsum of the foot away from each other. For example, the triceps surae and other plantar flexors of the foot (table 6.4) are used concentrically to point the foot as in tendus, dégagés, or the sitting point (table 6.6B, p. 344) when the foot is not weight bearing. When the foot is weight bearing, the same muscles are used to rise onto the toes, such as in pointe work (figure 6.35) and the calf raise (table 6.6A, p. 343) or to propel the body into space, as in jumps (table 6.6C, p. 345). Although many muscles are capable of producing plantar flexion, due to their size and location (effective leverage due to large distance of Achilles tendon from the axis of the ankle joint), the gastrocnemius and soleus are the primary muscles, while other muscles can make only a small contribution. Their primary importance is demonstrated by the inability of an individual to rise onto the toes when paralysis of the triceps surae is present (Smith, Weiss, and Lehmkuhl, 1996).

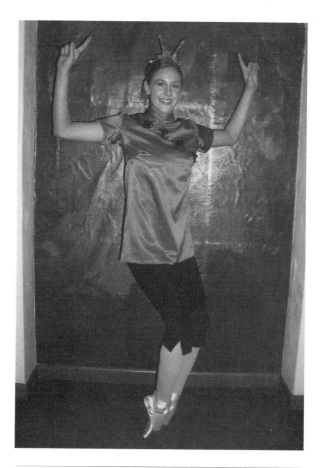

FIGURE 6.35   Sample dance movement showing ankle-foot plantar flexion.

Photo by Richard Newman. Dancer: Lauren Newman with Inland Ballet Theatre.

TABLE 6.4 Ankle-Foot Movements and the Extrinsic Muscles That Can Produce Them

Joint movement	Primary muscles	Secondary muscles
Ankle-foot		
Plantar flexion	Triceps surae: Gastrocnemius Soleus	Tibialis posterior Flexor hallucis longus Flexor digitorum longus Peroneus longus Peroneus brevis
Dorsiflexion	Tibialis anterior Extensor digitorum longus	Extensor hallucis longus Peroneus tertius
Foot		
Inversion	Tibialis posterior Tibialis anterior	Flexor hallucis longus Flexor digitorum longus Extensor hallucis longus
Eversion	Peroneus longus Peroneus brevis	Extensor digitorum longus Peroneus tertius
Toes		
Flexion		
Great toe	Flexor hallucis longus	*
Toes 2-5	Flexor digitorum longus	*
Extension		
Great toe	Extensor hallucis longus	*
Toes 2-5	Extensor digitorum longus	*

*Although there are no other extrinsic muscles, there are many intrinsic muscles listed in table 6.3 that can assist in producing these movements.

Dorsiflexion

Ankle-foot dorsiflexion involves bringing the anterior surface of the shin and the dorsum of the foot toward each other. The tibialis anterior and other dorsiflexors of the ankle-foot (table 6.4) are used concentrically to flex the unweighted foot, for example in the swing phase of walking; when the foot is actively flexed as a gesture in modern dance; in sitting dorsiflexion with weights (table 6.6D, p. 345); or before or after striking the floor in fla-

menco or tap dance (figure 6.36). Although all of the anterior crural muscles can produce dorsiflexion, the tibialis is the most powerful dorsiflexor.

When the foot is on the ground and weight bearing, the dorsiflexors can be used to very slightly pull the lower leg toward the foot, to help shift the weight of the body forward such as before a relevé or in preparation for moving forward in space. However, in most cases when the foot is weight bearing, gravity is the primary force and tends to create dorsiflexion of the foot. Hence, under these circumstances the dorsiflexors of the foot are not working concentrically to create dorsiflexion; rather the plantar flexors of the foot are used either to maintain the angle of dorsiflexion (isometrically), such as with standing in one place, or to control further dorsiflexion (eccentrically), such as during landing from a jump.

Inversion

Inversion of the foot involves lifting the inner border of the foot. When the foot is unweighted, inversion

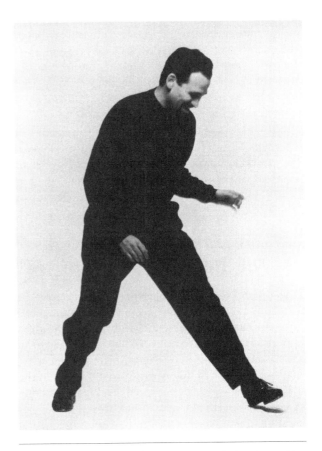

FIGURE 6.36 Sample dance movement showing ankle-foot dorsiflexion and associated prime movers.

Photo courtesy of Steve Zee and Jazz Tap Ensemble. Dancer: Steve Zee.

of the foot tends to be linked with forefoot adduction such as in the strength exercises sitting big toe up and away (table 6.6F, p. 347) and side-lying big toe up (table 6.6G, p. 347). However, this position is not commonly used in dance and is considered undesirable aesthetically in some dance forms such as ballet (sickling the foot). The flexor hallucis longus has been shown to be capable of producing inversion and forefoot adduction (Femino et al., 2000).

The functional significance of inversion is more operative when the foot is weight bearing. Here, the tibialis anterior, tibialis posterior, flexor hallucis longus, and other inverters of the foot (table 6.4) can be used to shift the weight very slightly laterally to create a locked and stable position of the foot, or to limit pronation, or both. This former slight lateral shift can be used in certain jumps (as seen in figure 6.37) to allow a stable base desirable for the generation of large forces that propel the body in space, as well as to create the desired direction of force (ground reaction force) so that the body will travel in the desired direction and the limb will be appropriately positioned relative to the rest of the body. Often, after the push-off phase is completed, the foot will be adjusted to a neutral or beveled position, in line with the choreographic aesthetic. In contrast, the latter function of limiting pronation is very important for keeping the center of gravity in the desired position over the foot so that balance can be more easily maintained. Appropriate control of pronation is also important for prevention of injuries such as shin splints.

Eversion

Eversion of the foot involves lifting the outer border of the foot. When the foot is unweighted, eversion is usually combined with forefoot abduction. This combination of movements is considered a desired aesthetic in some dance forms such as ballet, and is often referred to as "winging" or "beveling the foot" and often encouraged when the foot is pointed in movements such as an arabesque (figure 4.25, p. 189) or in strengthening exercises such as sitting little toe up and away (table 6.6H, p. 348). The peroneus longus appears to be particularly important in creating this combined movement of forefoot abduction, slight eversion, and plantar flexion (Femino et al., 2000).

This movement of eversion is also very important when the foot is weight bearing. Here, the everters (table 6.4) can be used to shift the weight very slightly medially to create an absorbent position of the foot such as in walking, or to create the beveled

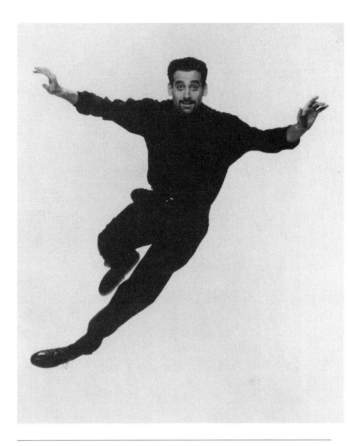

FIGURE 6.37 Sample dance movement showing foot inversion.
Photo courtesy of Steve Zee and Jazz Tap Ensemble. Dancer: Steve Zee.

line desired by many ballet schools when on demi-pointe or pointe as seen in figure 6.38. To achieve this latter aesthetic, the everters can be used to shift the body weight and position the forefoot and midfoot relative to the rearfoot while co-contraction of the plantar flexors and inverters is used to help maintain balance. The everters perform the important function of limiting supination of the foot. This latter function is very important for maintaining balance, preventing "falling out" of turns, and preventing ankle sprains.

Key Considerations for the Ankle and Foot in Whole Body Movement

When considering more complex full movements of the body it is helpful to look again at the role of foot pronation and supination, as these movements are not only important for the foot but also serve important functions during weight bearing for the body as a whole. The importance of pronation and supination

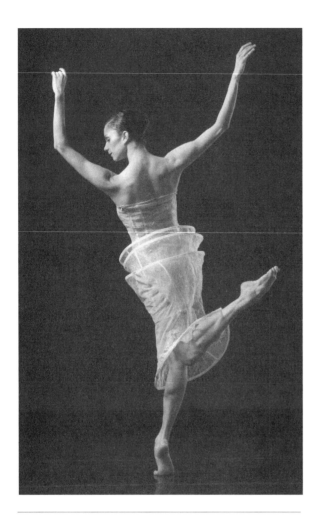

FIGURE 6.38   Sample dance movement showing foot eversion.

Photo courtesy of Marty Sohl. Alonzo King's Lines Ballet dancer Maurya Kerr.

will be further addressed through an examination of their role in walking, the negative implications of excessive pronation, and the coupling of the lower leg and foot with these movements.

Foot Pronation and Supination in Walking

The interplay of pronation and supination can be easily illustrated with walking gait. Walking is classically divided into two phases—the stance phase, or support phase, and the swing phase. During the **stance phase** the foot is in contact with the ground, while during the **swing phase** the foot is being swung forward in space to reach an appropriate position for the next step. The stance phase is the phase that places the weight-bearing demands on the ankle and foot and will be the focus of this discussion. The stance phase can be further subdivided into three periods—the contact period, midstance period, and

propulsive period. The foot initially contacts the ground (heel strike, or contact, period) on the lateral heel with the foot in a position of slight supination (Taunton, Clement, and Webber, 1981). This puts the foot in a stable position for transfer of weight onto the foot. Then as the body weight begins to shift over the foot, the tibia quickly begins to internally rotate on this fixed foot, producing pronation and a shift of the body weight medially. This foot pronation allows the foot to adapt to the surface and aids with shock absorption. Then, as the body moves farther over the foot in midstance, the foot begins to resupinate and body weight is shifted slightly laterally toward the head of the second metatarsal (Sammarco, 1980). This resupination stabilizes the forefoot and allows the foot to serve as a rigid lever upon which the plantar flexors can act to help push the body forward (propulsive period).

Excessive Pronation

Although as just described, pronation is an essential element of normal foot mechanics, excessive pronation may increase the risk for some types of injuries (Hall, 1999). When pronation is of high velocity or is excessive in amount, it is believed to place undue stress on the medial foot and the ligaments, fascia, and muscles that help support the medial longitudinal arch. Furthermore, when pronation is prolonged and extends into the propulsive period of gait when the foot should be resupinating, the foot is unstable rather than stable when propulsive forces are applied, placing undue stresses on the foot and decreasing the effectiveness of the push. Over time, repetitive abnormal pronation is also believed to cause stretching of tissues that support the arch and to contribute to the production of pes planus.

Excessive pronation can come from many causes including malalignment, muscle imbalances, and technique. In regard to malalignment, rearfoot varus and tibial varum require more pronation before the inner portion of the foot can contact the ground (Taunton, Clement, and Webber, 1981). In terms of muscle imbalance, if the triceps surae is tight, compensatory pronation will occur to unlock the transverse tarsal joints in order to gain the necessary apparent dorsiflexion. Inadequate strength in the extrinsic inverters of the foot and the intrinsic muscles that help maintain the medial longitudinal arch may also be a factor in failing to adequately limit extent or duration of pronation. With regard to technique, failing to maintain adequate turnout at the hip, such that the knees "fall inside the feet" during movements like pliés, can cause relative

Foot Supination and Pronation in Walking

· **Identify normal foot mechanics in walking.** Walking very slowly, mark on your body the normal foot mechanics during the stance phase of walking that were just described in the text and that are shown in A.

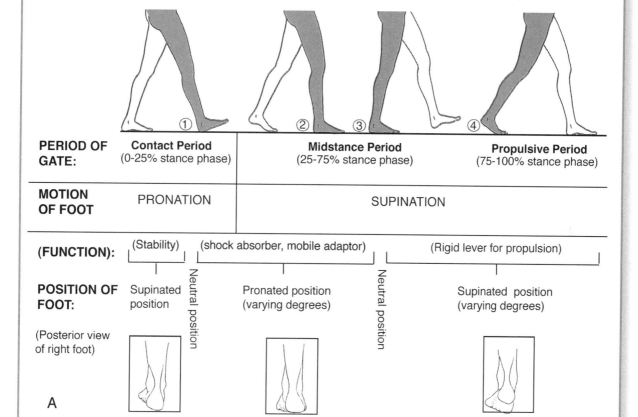

PERIOD OF GATE:	Contact Period (0-25% stance phase)	Midstance Period (25-75% stance phase)	Propulsive Period (75-100% stance phase)
MOTION OF FOOT	PRONATION	SUPINATION	
(FUNCTION):	(Stability)	(shock absorber, mobile adaptor)	(Rigid lever for propulsion)
POSITION OF FOOT: (Posterior view of right foot)	Supinated position · Neutral position	Pronated position (varying degrees) · Neutral position	Supinated position (varying degrees)

A

· **Observe three to five individuals walking.** Position yourself so that a dancer walks directly toward you and then directly away from you. Observe the mechanics listed in the text and notice if supination—pronation—supination occur and to what extent and with what timing. Notice differences between sides in the same individual and any malalignments in the knees, hip, and spine that might influence this gait.

· **Observe yourself walking.** Now observe yourself walking by walking toward a mirror or keying in to internal cues. Make the same observations as just described. Also note your shoe wear pattern. Look at the ideal pathway of the center of pressure on the foot shown in B, and consider what clues shoe wear can give regarding foot mechanics in walking.

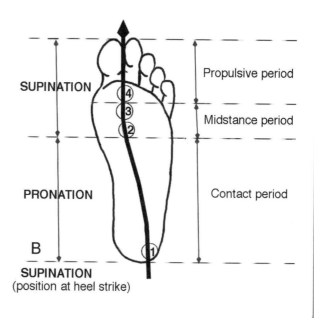

SUPINATION

Propulsive period

Midstance period

PRONATION

Contact period

B

SUPINATION
(position at heel strike)

internal rotation of the lower legs and compensatory pronation of the feet.

Coupling of the Leg and Foot

Due to the oblique axis of the subtalar joint, the shapes of various bones, and soft tissue interaction, there is a coupling of movements between the leg and foot when the foot is fixed and weight bearing as shown in figure 6.39 (Hintermann, 1999). Since the ankle joint is a hinge joint that does not allow much rotation, rotation of the lower leg is translated to the foot; and conversely, rotation (abduction and adduction) of the foot is translated to rotation of the lower leg. This coupling is such that supination is accompanied by external rotation of the leg, and external rotation of the leg is accompanied by mandatory supination (Soderberg, 1986). Conversely, pronation is accompanied by internal rotation of the leg, and internal rotation of the leg produces pronation of the foot.

During walking, this coupling is important for absorbing the rotations of the lower leg as the tibia internally and externally rotates at the beginning

and end of stance, respectively (Hamill and Knutzen, 1995). If this mechanism were not available, these rotations of the lower leg would tend to spin the foot on the ground or disrupt the integrity of the ankle joint by causing the talus to rotate within the mortise (Levangie and Norkin, 2001). This coupling is also important for the dancer to keep in mind in regard to technique, as rotation of the leg can be used to place body weight appropriately over the axis of the foot, such that excessive pronation or supination can be avoided. On the other hand, the common tendency of allowing the foot to pronate during standing will produce internal rotation of the tibia with resultant loss of turnout if the whole limb is allowed to follow, or knee stress if turnout of the femur is maintained at the hip while the tibia rotates internally.

Special Considerations for the Ankle and Foot in Dance

When one is trying to apply the mechanics of the ankle and foot to dance, there are several technique areas that deserve more discussion. One of these is the issue of achieving the desired aesthetics and placement in demi-pointe and pointe positions. Another issue is achieving desired foot placement when the knee bends, such as in pliés. In ballet, still another important concern is the introduction of pointe work.

Demi-Pointe, Pointe, and the Stirrup Muscles

The repetitive use of demi-pointe and pointe in dance places great demands on the foot and requires specialized strength, flexibility, and technique development. In terms of flexibility, extreme ankle-foot plantar flexion is required to achieve the desired aesthetic of these positions and allow the dancer to get high enough to allow the body weight to be appropriately placed over the ball of the foot (demi-pointe) or toes (pointe). For proper mechanics and aesthetics on pointe, it is recommended the dancer have 90° to 100° of ankle plantar flexion (Hamilton et al., 1992). About 90° of extension of the hallux at the MTP joint (figure 6.40) is also necessary for a desired high demi-pointe position (Sammarco, 1980).

In terms of plantar flexion strength and range, the ankle-foot plantar flexors have to contract forcefully to achieve and maintain this position of the foot, and ballet dancers have been reported to have very high

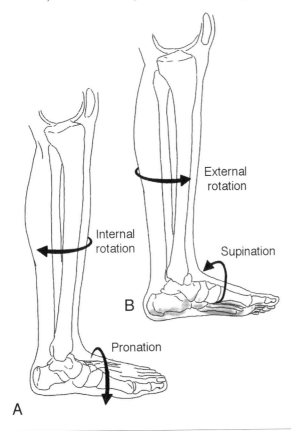

FIGURE 6.39   Coupling of the leg and foot (left foot, lateral view). (A) Internal rotation of leg and foot pronation, (B) external rotation of leg and foot supination.

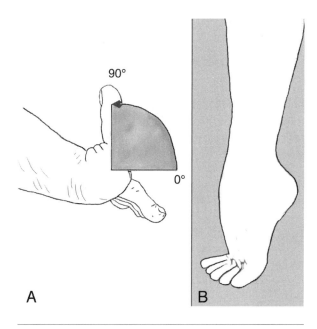

FIGURE 6.40   (A) Hallux range of motion and demi-pointe. About 90° of extension of the metatarsopha-langeal joint is necessary for (B) optimal positioning in demi-pointe.

levels of plantar flexor strength. Although the triceps surae muscles produce a large percentage of the plantar flexor torque, other plantar flexors can help slightly reduce the demands on the triceps surae and help achieve the desired aesthetic. Two such plantar flexors are the flexor hallucis longus and flexor digitorum longus. The flexor hallucis longus and flexor digitorum longus have been shown to have a shortening effect on the foot in a front-to-back direction (Smith, Weiss, and Lehmkuhl, 1996), and so can help achieve the desired "high-arch" look in pointe. Three other plantar flexors—the tibialis posterior, tibialis anterior, and peroneus longus—function together to lift the arch and help maintain balance on demi-pointe and pointe. These three muscles can be termed the **stirrup muscles** because they run behind the medial and lateral malleoli to converge to attach onto the undersurface of the medial longitudinal arch in a stirrup-like arrangement. All three muscles have attachments onto the plantar surface of the cuneiforms, with the tibialis anterior and peroneals also both attaching onto the base of the first metatarsal, while the tibialis posterior has additional attachments on the navicular and other metatarsal bases. Their attachments put them in a perfect position to lift the midfoot higher up in plantar flexion, irrespective of the position of the toes.

In terms of stability, the stirrup muscles can be used to keep the body weight appropriately positioned in a medial-lateral direction over the axis of the foot. Their co-contraction (in combination with other muscles) can be used to allow the weight to rise to the toes and lower from the toes without undesired inversion or eversion, and to make subtle adjustments of the body weight to enhance balance and dance aesthetics. For example, contraction, or pulling up, with the lateral stirrup muscles will shift the body weight medially on the foot (eversion) and prevent excessive rolling out (inversion) on the foot, such as is commonly seen in "falling out" of multiple pirouettes. Conversely, contraction, or pulling up, with the medial stirrup muscles will shift the body weight laterally on the foot (inversion) and prevent excessive rolling in (eversion) on the foot. In terms of these medial stirrup muscles, theoretically, the tibialis posterior should be emphasized more than the tibialis anterior when on demi-pointe or pointe due to its additional desired action of ankle-foot plantar flexion.

Pointing the Foot in Open Kinematic Chain Movements

This same balanced use of the stirrup muscles can be utilized during plantar flexion of the foot without weight bearing, such as in a tendu. The peroneals and tibialis posterior are used synergistically and in accordance with the aesthetic of the given dance form to create a neutral position or slightly "beveled" position of the foot and to get a more fully pointed position, with the desired "stretch" across the instep. Due to their more distal attachment, these stirrup muscles can be used to add slight plantar flexion at the intertarsal joints and tarsometatarsal joints, while the gastrocnemius and soleus, which attach proximally onto the calcaneus, would primarily effect plantar flexion at the ankle joint proper.

The flexor hallucis longus and flexor digitorum longus can also be used to achieve this more fully pointed look, and tension on the flexor hallucis longus has been shown to increase the height of the medial longitudinal arch (Femino et al., 2000). These muscles can also increase the point of the foot by bringing the MTP joint into flexion. However, to prevent the undesired curling under of the toes (IP flexion) accompanying use of these flexors, the intrinsic toe extensors (lumbricals and interossei) must be used synergistically to maintain the IP joints in extension. Lastly, other intrinsic muscles can be used to "lift the arch" and increase the point. Thinking of pulling the base of the toes and the underside of the arch back with strings running behind each side of the malleoli, while stretching across the

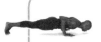

Stirrup Muscle Function in Relevé

· **Use the stirrup muscles to adjust your body weight placement.** Rise onto the ball of your foot using your hand on a wall or barre to help balance. Purposely shift your body weight outward so that your foot rolls out (inversion) and excess weight is borne by the fourth and fifth toes as seen in C. Then pull up with the outer stirrup muscles by thinking of lifting the underside of the outer border of the foot up toward the ceiling to bring your body weight back over the long axis of the foot. Now, shift your body weight inward so that your foot rolls in (eversion) with excess weight on the big toe as seen in D. Then pull up the inner stirrup muscles by thinking of lifting the underside of your medial arch toward the ceiling to bring your body weight back so it is centered between your first and second toe. Lastly, keeping your weight over the axis of the foot, contract both sides of the stirrup muscles together to keep your body weight appropriately positioned and to raise your arch slightly higher to help reach full height in a demi-pointe position as seen in A and B.

KEY   1 = Tibialis anterior   2 = Peroneus longus and brevis   3 = Tibialis posterior

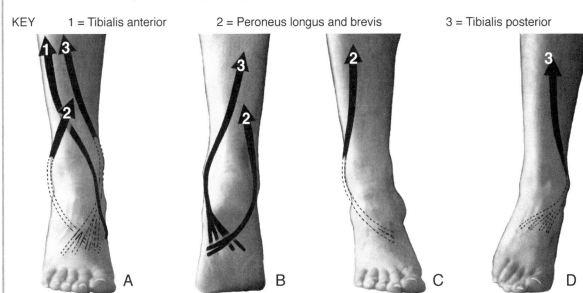

· **Perform a normal relevé.** Perform several relevés as you normally would and without thinking about the stirrup muscles. Note the placement of your body weight. Then, make any necessary correction with the stirrup muscles, and repeat a relevé trying to maintain correct positioning. Which muscle(s) do you need to focus on using more? What cue could you utilize to help make this correction quickly, such as when in class?

---

instep and reaching the toes out, can sometimes help achieve the desired muscle activation.

Knee-Foot Alignment

Due to the coupling of the leg and foot discussed previously, positioning of the knee relative to the foot is important for correct foot mechanics. Using the cue to keep the knee over the foot (a plumb line dropped from the center of the patella being

in line with the second toe) in standing movements involving bending one or both knees, such as pliés or weight shifts, can help encourage proper foot mechanics in many dancers and help prevent the common tendency of not maintaining adequate hip external rotation, letting the knees excessively fall in and the feet pronate. However, it is important to realize that the specific relationship of the knee to the foot that will yield the desired neutral subtalar and midtarsal foot position will vary greatly between

"Point From the Top of the Foot"

The instruction to "point from the top of the foot," often in conjunction with "and don't use your Achilles," is sometimes used by teachers in an effort to achieve a greater point of the foot without causing discomfort under the Achilles (posterior impingement). However, from an anatomical perspective, this cue can be confusing in that the muscles on top of the foot do not point the foot (they are dorsiflexors), and the Achilles and associated gastrocnemius and soleus are prime movers for plantar flexion. A more anatomically sound cue could focus on creating a stretch across the top of the foot by reaching the foot "out and down," focusing on articulating each of the joints that can contribute to plantar flexion/flexion (talocrural, subtalar, intertarsal, tarsometatarsal, and MTP joints) rather than just the ankle joint. In addition, focusing on using the stirrup muscles and the intrinsic muscles of the feet to pull the bottom of the metatarsals back toward the heel can increase the point of the foot with less tendency for impingement.

dancers, based on many factors including femoral torsion, tibial torsion, and forefoot abduction. Thus, although this cue is often helpful in a class setting, the individual dancer may need to adjust it slightly for his or her body. Furthermore, in dance forms that require the feet to face almost directly to the side, dancers should realize that this will tend to produce pronation of the foot and internal rotation of the tibia if hip external rotation is not sufficient. Focusing on using the external rotators of the hip and knee to maximize turnout at the hip and prohibit internal rotation of the tibia can help reduce the tendency toward or degree of foot pronation.

Beginning Pointe

Beginning pointe is a major and often highly anticipated step in the training of a female classical ballet dancer. With rising technical demands in professional dance, teachers and parents frequently have questions regarding the appropriate timing to begin pointe. The goal is to avoid injury in dancers who are still maturing while still allowing them to develop the proficiency on pointe that is necessary to be competitive in the ballet world. Unfortunately, the answer to this question is not simple; it encompasses many individual factors such as skeletal maturity, mental maturity, technical proficiency, and years of training. Considering all of these factors, several orthopedists who are noted for their expertise with dancers have recommended that dancers begin pointe at a minimum of 11 years of age if they have undergone three to four years of disciplined ballet training and exhibit sufficient strength, technical proficiency, and skeletal

and mental maturity (Hamilton, 1988; Sammarco, 1982; Weiker, 1988).

However, these age guidelines were in part based on the concern for injury of structures still in the growth process. And the limited number of injuries reported that appear to be related to premature pointe has led to some less conservative recommendations and a greater emphasis on functional readiness. In terms of age, two dance medicine groups suggest that if other criteria are met, with select individuals a minimum of 10 years of age may be appropriate (Solomon, Micheli, and Ireland, 1993), at least to begin pointe work at the barre (Ryan and Stephens, 1987). In terms of functional concerns, there is an increasing awareness of the varied age at which dancers reach adequate strength, flexibility, and technical proficiency. Hence, a greater emphasis on individual readiness may be appropriate. Suggested functional tests include the ability to plantar flex the foot in a line parallel to the line of the tibia (Solomon, Micheli, and Ireland, 1993) when measured with a goniometer or as evidenced in a tendu and relevé. Another commonly used test is the ability to maintain balance in retiré on demi-pointe with good alignment of the ankle, a straight knee, maintenance of turnout at the hip, and good pelvic and spinal alignment (Khan et al., 1995). The author also recommends use of a pirouette, noting the alignment just described with the retiré, with particular attention paid to the ability to prevent excessive rolling out on the foot. The ability to go on pointe without knuckling or sickling is another commonly held criterion.

While in general agreement with these suggestions, from a kinesiological perspective the author

CONCEPT DEMONSTRATION 6.4

Influence of Knee Position on Foot Mechanics

· **Knee position in a parallel plié.** Perform a demi-plié in parallel first position. As the knees bend, purposely guide the midpoint of the kneecap well inside the feet and notice how the feet tend to pronate. Now guide the knees over the feet, and find the path of the knee where the foot stays neutral without rolling in or out and with desired weight distribution on the foot. Lastly, purposely guide the midpoint of the kneecap well outside the feet, and notice how the foot inverts. Perform a parallel plié the way you normally would and see if you need to make any correction in knee placement so that a neutral position of the foot is maintained.

· **Knee position in a turned-out plié.** Repeat the procedures just described while performing a second-position demi-plié in turnout. Do you notice any difference with the addition of turnout? Adjust the facing of your feet slightly out and in from how you normally stand, and notice the effect on your feet. How do changes in foot position influence foot mechanics? How does maintaining turnout at the hip influence foot mechanics? How do these factors relate to coupling of the leg and foot?

would emphasize that there are unique challenges related to pointe work that will not be developed with demi-pointe. These demands include (1) greater challenge to the flexor hallucis longus due to the necessity of producing force at a shorter length (because it is not lengthened across the MTP joint as with demi-pointe) and its key role in pushing down into the ground to facilitate going from demi-pointe to pointe (MTP flexion); (2) greater strength and coordinated contraction required in other flexors and extensors of toes (particularly the great toe) to stabilize the toes in extension and prevent toe flexion (knuckling) when actually on pointe (figure 6.41); and (3) greater forces borne by the first two toes and balance challenges associated with decreasing the base of support from the ball of the foot to the small toe box of the pointe shoe.

Hence, in addition to the prior suggestions, the author would also encourage the use of supplemental conditioning exercises and an initial progressive use of pointe within the technique class to assist with the transition into pointe work. Some pointe-specific exercises are shown in figure 6.42, and other relevant exercises that will be described in the next section are included in the sample pointe preparation routine given in table 6.5. These exercises should be added three to six months prior to beginning pointe and performed only if no pain is experienced and there are no medical contraindications. The last two exercises are more advanced exercises and should be added only after the other exercises have been performed for about six weeks. If time is limited, the exercises with an asterisk are most specific to pointe

and can be prioritized, with additional exercises selected in accordance with the specific dancer's technique needs.

In terms of introduction of pointe work into technique class, the approach used by some ballet schools of starting with simple exercises at the barre for the last 15 to 30 minutes of technique class, which gradually progress in difficulty and duration, is very sound from a physiological perspective. Initial presentation of pointe work that is too difficult or too long in duration for current strength and coordination levels can result in the development of undesired compensations or injury. In contrast, a well-designed program that is initially performed two to three times per week and gradually progresses in duration and difficulty should allow the necessary development of strength and skill for more advanced work with sound technique.

Conditioning Exercises for the Ankle and Foot

The ankle-foot is a common site of injury in dance, and adequate strength and flexibility are necessary for lowering injury risk, as well as enhancing performance.

Strength Exercises for the Ankle-Foot

Sample strength exercises for the ankle-foot are provided in table 6.6, and a brief description of their importance follows. When strengthening exercises for

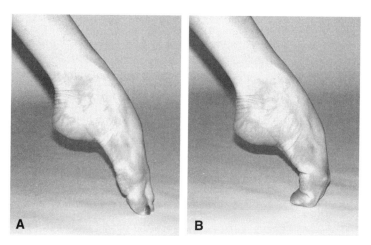

FIGURE 6.41   (A) Coordinated toe flexor and extensor co-contraction necessary for correct positioning when pointing the foot or going on pointe to avoid (B) undesired curling under of the toes (excessive IP flexion).

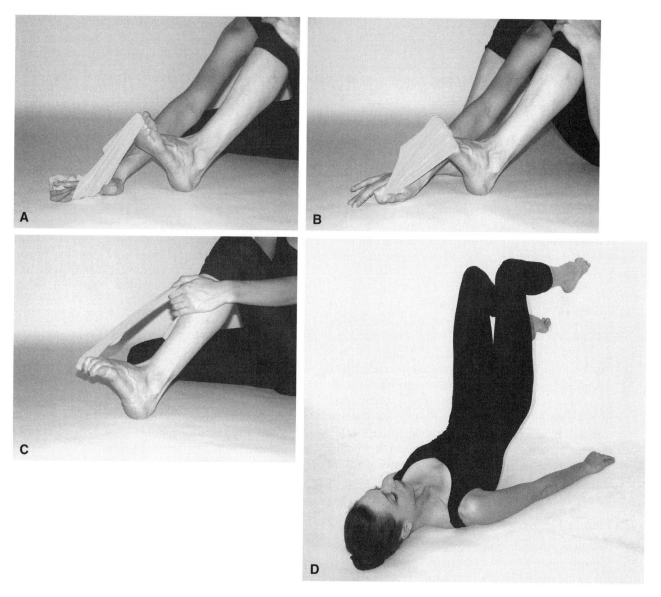

FIGURE 6.42   Sample exercises for beginning or improving pointe work. (A) Big toe extension, (B) toe extension, (C) big toe flexion, and (D) toe wall climbs.

TABLE 6.5   Sample Pointe Preparation Routine

Exercise	Repetitions	Purpose
*Demi to pointe (band) (table 6.6B, variation 2)	6 times (all toes)	Strength to help rise from demi to pointe
Big toe flexion (figure 6.42C)	6 times (great toe only)	Strength to help rise from demi to pointe
*Toe extensions (band) (figure 6.42A) (figure 6.42B)	6 times (great toe only) 6 times (all toes)	Stability on pointe and to prevent knuckling under
Sitting big toes up and away (band) (table 6.6F)	8-12 times	Prevent rolling in
Sitting little toes up and away (band) (table 6.6H)	8-12 times	Prevent rolling out
*Doming (table 6.6J)	8-12 times	MTP joint stability and strength to keep toes extended instead of curled (flexed)
Sitting dorsiflexion (band) (table 6.6E, variation 1)	8-12 times	Muscle balance
*Sitting pointe stretch (table 6.8F)	3 times with 20-second hold	ROM to allow ideal positioning of body over toes
Toe wall climbs (figure 6.42D)	1-4 times up and down	Strength to help rise from demi to pointe
Fondu forced arch (table 6.6A, variation 2)	6-12 times	Stirrup muscles and positioning of instep over toes

this region are performed, particular care must be taken with respect to developing balanced strength between antagonist muscles. For example, movements performed in class such as relevés and jumps tend to develop the ankle-foot plantar flexors, and an emphasis on supplemental strengthening of the dorsiflexors is recommended for many dancers to maintain a healthy ratio between these antagonists. Similarly, many dancers exhibit weakness in the foot everters relative to the foot invertors. When a known imbalance is present, one approach is to repeat the exercise in a second set of repetitions on the weaker side (after 2-3 minutes of recovery) for a limited time until a better balance in strength is achieved. For some key movements, exercises are included that use bands and weights. Bands offer a great advantage in terms of convenience and can be easily carried in a dance bag, and exercises can be performed during a break. However, for dancers who find that they have marked weakness in certain areas, weights may better allow them to develop greater strength throughout a wider range of motion and to easily monitor progress.

Plantar Flexor Strengthening

Adequate strength in the plantar flexors is important for work on demi-pointe and pointe, and for a powerful push-off such as used for turns and jumps. The ankle plantar flexors have also been found to play a vital role in absorbing energy when landing from a jump (Devita and Skelly, 1992). Ballet dancers have been shown to have plantar flexor strength markedly greater than that of many other athletes (Hamilton et al., 1992), reinforcing the importance of strength in this area for dancers. Adequate strength in the plantar flexors is also believed to be important for prevention of Achilles tendinitis; a study of runners showed lower strength levels of the plantar flexors in runners with Achilles tendinitis when compared to runners without tendinitis (McCrory et al., 1999).

Calf raises (table 6.6A) provide a functional way to work on building this strength and technique, while sitting point (table 6.6B) is a convenient exercise that can easily be performed with a band. Dancers can also strengthen these muscles functionally by performing repetitive jumps, starting with two feet and progressing to single-leg jumps (table 6.6C). The dancer must be thoroughly warmed up before performing jumps and should perform them on a resilient floor. Performing jumps on a Pilates Reformer also offers an opportunity to work on technique with increasing springs, height of jumps, or quickness and complexity of jumps for progression. Jumps are particularly useful for developing the explosive power of the gastrocnemius needed for both high and quick jumps used in dance choreography. In contrast, performing ankle-foot plantar flexion with the knees bent, as described in table 6.6A (variation 3), will emphasize greater use of the soleus.

(Text continues on p. 352.)

TABLE 6.6 Selected Strength Exercises for the Ankle-Foot

Exercise name (Resistance)	Description (Technique cues)	Progression
Muscle group: A-F plantar flexors **Muscles emphasized: Triceps surae and stirrup muscles**		
Joint movement: A-F plantar flexion		
A. Calf raise (Dumbbells) *Variation 2*	Stand on one foot with the other foot against the ankle of the support leg. Slowly rise onto the ball of the foot, pause, and slowly lower to the starting position. (Keep the body weight centered between the first and second toes, and avoid rolling in or rolling out; rise up high onto the ball of the foot, focusing on using the stirrup muscles to give a slightly greater lift to the arch of the foot.) *Variation 1:* Perform calf raises supine on Pilates Reformer. *Variation 2:* Fondu forced arch— Bend the support knee (fondu) and rise as high as possible onto the ball of the foot with a bent knee. Then straighten the knee (trying to keep the heel as high as possible), pause, and lower to starting position with a straight knee while standing on the floor or lying supine on the Reformer, with the foot on the jump board. *Variation 3:* Perform calf raises while sitting in a chair with the knees bent to 90°, leaning forward and using your hands on your thighs or a weight plate on top of the lower thighs for resistance.	1. Gradually increase the height of relevé. 2. Gradually increase from 5-pound to 10-pound dumbbells. 3. Add a brief hold at the top.

(continued)

TABLE 6.6 **Selected Strength Exercises for the Ankle-Foot** (continued)

Exercise name (Resistance)	Description (Technique cues)	Progression
Muscle group: A-F plantar flexors and MTP flexors **Muscles emphasized: Stirrup muscles and MTP flexors**		
Joint movement: A-F plantar flexion with MTP flexion		
B. Sitting point (Elastic band) *Variation 2*	Sit with one leg outstretched to the front with the band under the ball of the foot and the hands pulling the band taut. Slowly point the foot, leading with the ball of the foot and only adding the toes at the end of the movement. Pause, and slowly return to the starting position. (Focus on using the stirrup muscles to keep the foot in a neutral position throughout the movement and avoid inverting or everting the foot.) *Variation 1:* Perform with the knee slightly bent and the heel resting on the ground. *Variation 2:* Maintain the plantar-flexed position throughout the exercise, and start with the toes back (metatarsophalangeal extension) as if on demi-pointe. Then reach the toes out to be in line with the metatarsals (metatarsophalangeal flexion), pause, and slowly allow the toes to come back to the starting demi-pointe position.	1. Pull the band tauter for the starting position. 2. Use a heavier band.

Exercise name (Resistance)	Description (Technique cues)	Progression
Muscle group: A-F plantar flexors **Muscles emphasized: Gastrocnemius**		
Joint movement: A-F plantar flexion		
C. Single-leg jumps (Body weight) 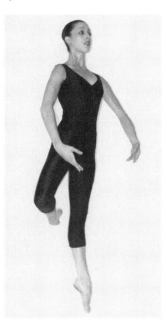	After adequate warm-up including jumps from two feet, perform repetitive jumps taking off from and landing on the same leg. Stand facing a barre with the fingertips on the barre if needed. (Focus on maintaining correct mechanics of the foot, and avoid excessive pronation or double heel strikes when landing.) *Variation 1:* Perform supine on the Pilates Reformer with a jump board.	1. Increase height while maintaining good technique. 2. Increase speed and height while maintaining good technique.
Muscle group: A-F dorsiflexors **Muscles emphasized: Tibialis anterior and extensor digitorum longus**		
Joint movement: A-F dorsiflexion		
D. Sitting dorsiflexion (Weight) 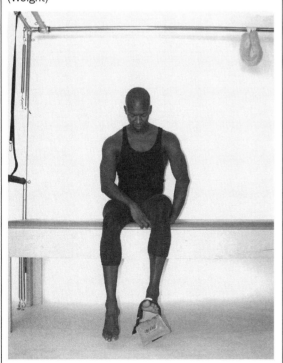	Sit with legs bent over the edge of a table, the Pilates Cadillac, or a counter with a weight hanging from the top of one foot with the ankle-foot in slight plantar flexion. Slowly raise the foot up toward the shin, pause, and slowly return to the starting position. (Keep the foot in a neutral position, guiding the space between the first and second toe toward the middle of the shin.) *Variation 1:* Focus on leading with the great toe and inverting the foot instead of keeping it in neutral to emphasize the tibialis anterior. *Variation 2:* Focus on leading with the fifth toe and everting the foot instead of keeping it neutral to emphasize the extensor digitorum longus and peroneus tertius.	1. Gradually increase how high the toes are lifted. 2. Gradually increase from 5 pounds to 15 pounds.

(continued)

TABLE 6.6 **Selected Strength Exercises for the Ankle-Foot** *(continued)*

Exercise name (Resistance)	Description (Technique cues)	Progression
Muscle groups: A-F dorsiflexors and foot inverters **Muscles emphasized: Tibialis anterior**		
Joint movement: A-F dorsiflexion with inversion		
E. Sitting big toe up and in (Elastic band) *Variation 2*	Sit with one leg outstretched and the other leg bent and supported by the arms. Loop the band under the arch of the outstretched leg and over the toes of the bent leg. Bend the knee enough to make the band taut. Then flex the foot (leading with the great toe), pause, and slowly return to the starting position. (Focus on bringing the great toe both up and in so that inversion is combined with dorsiflexion of the foot.) *Variation 1:* Sitting dorsiflexion—Dorsiflex the foot in a neutral position rather than leading with the big toe to emphasize general strengthening of the dorsiflexors. *Variation 2:* Sitting little toe up and in—Dorsiflex the foot, leading with the little toe to emphasize the extensor digitorum longus and peroneus tertius. *Variation 3:* Perform any of these exercises facing the end of the Pilates Cadillac with one foot in the strap that has a spring attached at the low end of the Cadillac.	1. Bring the heel of the bent leg closer to the buttocks so that the band is tauter. 2. Use a heavier band.

Exercise name (Resistance)	Description (Technique cues)	Progression
Muscle group: Foot inverters **Muscles emphasized: Tibialis posterior**		
Joint movements: Foot inversion and forefoot adduction with A-F plantar flexion		
F. Sitting big toe up and away (Elastic band) 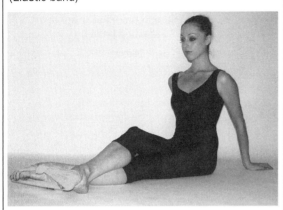 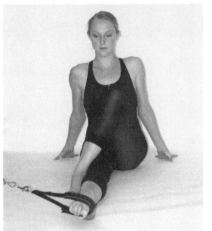 *Variation 2*	Sit with the lower legs crossed to the front and a band looped around the ends of the feet with the heels separated so that the band is taut. With feet pointed, move the front of the feet (leading with the great toes) up and away from each other, pause, and slowly return to the starting position. (Keep both feet pointed throughout the exercise, and isolate the movement to the feet, avoiding movement of the knees.) *Variation 1:* Secure the loop under or around something sturdy. Place only one foot in the loop, and move the foot up and away (leading with the great toe). *Variation 2:* Perform the same movement, sitting with the side to the end of the Pilates Cadillac and one foot in a strap that has a spring attached low to the end of the Cadillac.	1. Pull band tauter by moving the feet further away at the start. 2. Use a heavier band.
G. Side-lying big toe up (Weight) 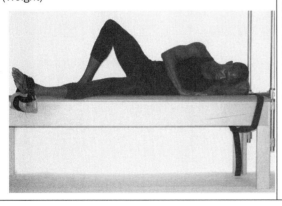	Lie on your side with a weight hanging from the end of your bottom foot. With the foot pointed, bring the forefoot up toward the ceiling, leading with the great toe. Pause, and slowly control lowering to the starting position. (Keep the foot pointed throughout the movement.)	1. Gradually lift the great toe higher. 2. Gradually increase the weight from 5 pounds to 15 pounds.

(continued)

TABLE 6.6 Selected Strength Exercises for the Ankle-Foot *(continued)*

Exercise name (Resistance)	Description (Technique cues)	Progression
Muscle group: Foot everters **Muscles emphasized: Peroneals**		
Joint movements: Foot eversion and forefoot abduction with A-F plantar flexion		
H. Sitting little toe up and away (Elastic band) *Variation 2*	Sit with legs outstretched to the front and a band looped around the ends of the feet with the feet separated so that the band is taut. With the feet pointed, bring the front of the feet away and up, leading with the little toes. Pause, and slowly control the return to the starting position. (Keep the feet pointed throughout the movement; isolate the movement to the feet, and concentrate on keeping the knees facing straight up to avoid including movement of the hip.) *Variation 1:* Secure the loop under or around something sturdy. Place only one foot in the loop, and bring the forefoot up and away (leading with little toes). *Variation 2:* Perform the same movement, sitting with the side facing the end of the Pilates Cadillac and one foot in a strap that has a spring attached low to the end of the Cadillac.	1. Move little toes further away. 2. Spread the feet farther apart for the starting position. 3. Use a heavier band.
I. Side-lying little toe up (Weight)	Lie on your side with a weight hanging from the end of your top foot. With the foot pointed, bring the forefoot up toward the ceiling, leading with the little toe. Pause, and smoothly lower the foot to the starting position. (Keep the foot pointed throughout the movement.)	1. Gradually lift the little toe higher. 2. Gradually increase the weight from 5 pounds to 15 pounds.

Exercise name (Resistance)	Description (Technique cues)	Progression

Muscle group: MTP flexors
Muscles emphasized: Intrinsic foot muscles (lumbricals and interossei)

Joint movement: MTP flexion with IP extension

Exercise name (Resistance)	Description (Technique cues)	Progression
J. Doming (Hand) 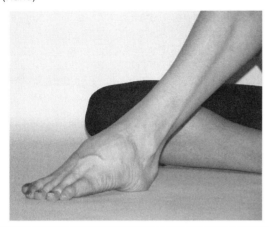	While sitting, press the toes firmly down and back into the floor as you raise the metatarsal arch of the foot. Hold for 5 seconds. (Keep the toes extended as you press them down and avoid letting them curl under.)	1. Add the use of one hand to resist the raising of the arch.

Muscle groups: MTP flexors and toe flexors
Muscles emphasized: Intrinsic foot muscles

Joint movements: MTP flexion and toe flexion

Exercise name (Resistance)	Description (Technique cues)	Progression
K. Towel curl (Weights) 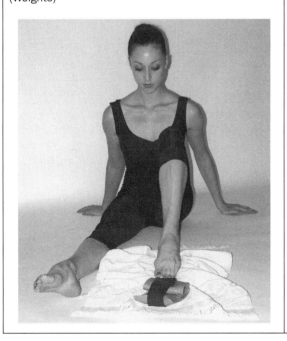	Sit with one knee bent and the heel on the floor with a 2-pound weight on a small towel in front of the foot. Push the close end of the towel slightly away so that wrinkles form in the towel. Grab a wrinkle in the towel with your toes, and then pull the towel toward you. (Focus on fully flexing the toes to grab the towel and then raise the metatarsal and medial longitudinal arches as you pull the towel.)	1. Gradually increase weight from 2 pounds to 10 pounds.

(continued)

TABLE 6.6 Selected Strength Exercises for the Ankle-Foot *(continued)*

Exercise name (Resistance)	Description (Technique cues)	Progression
Muscle groups: Foot everters and inverters **Muscles emphasized: Peroneals and tibialis anterior/A-F proprioception**		
Joint movements: Foot eversion and inversion with A-F dorsiflexion		
L. Side-to-side (Half foam roller) 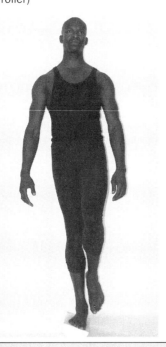	Stand with body weight on one foot placed on the flat side of a half foam roller while the other leg is slightly bent with the foot touching the ankle of the support leg. Slowly shift the body weight outward and then quickly evert the foot to return to center. Next, slowly shift the body weight inward and then quickly invert the foot to return to center. Place the fingertips on a wall or barre to aid with balance if needed. (Focus on making the adjustments from the ankle and foot rather than the hip.) *Variation 1:* Perform repetitively in the same direction (e.g., rolling out to center eight times and then rolling in to center eight times). *Variation 2:* Perform turned out. *Variation 3:* Perform on an ankle disk or balance board.	1. Use a slightly larger range of motion but in a safe territory so that an ankle sprain is avoided. 2. Perform with hands clasped behind the head. 3. Perform with eyes closed. 4. Perform on demi-pointe with very small movements, positioned so that the hand can be used to aid with balance when needed.
Muscle groups: A-F plantar flexors and dorsiflexors, and foot everters and inverters **Muscles emphasized: Foot everters and inverters/A-F proprioception**		
Joint movements: A-F plantar flexion, foot eversion, A-F dorsiflexion, and foot inversion combined to produce a circular motion		
M. Ankle disk circles (Ankle disk) 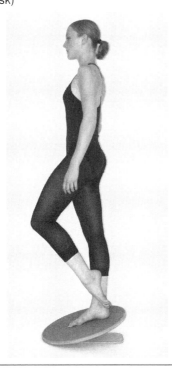	Stand with your weight on one foot and the foot positioned toward the center of the disk. Slowly shift your body weight, and use your feet so that you make a counterclockwise circle with the edge of the disk, contacting the ground sequentially. Place the fingertips on a wall or barre to aid with balance if needed. After six times, reverse the direction of the circle (clockwise). (Work to make the circle as smooth and symmetrical as possible, and emphasize using the ankle-foot muscles.)	1. Perform with minimal or no use of the hand for balance. 2. Use a disk with a larger half sphere attached to the bottom.

Exercise name (Resistance)	Description (Technique cues)	Progression

Muscle group: A-F plantar flexors
Muscles emphasized: Stirrup muscles/A-F proprioception

Joint movement: A-F plantar flexion

N. Ankle disk relevé (Ankle disk) 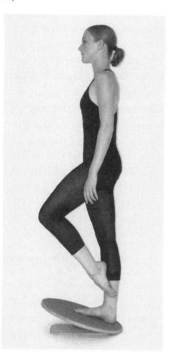 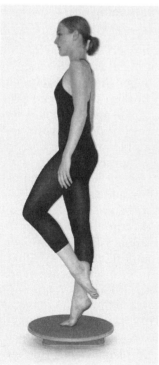	Stand with both feet on the disk and the ball of the foot positioned toward the middle of the disk so that on relevé the disk is balanced with no edge touching the ground. Start with the heels dropped and the back edge of the disk touching the ground. Slowly rise on the ball of the foot, and hold this position for 4 counts. Then smoothly lower to the starting position. Use one hand on a barre or wall to aid with balance if needed. (Keep the body weight centered between the first and second toes, and focus on using the stirrup muscles to help raise to a full demi-pointe position.)	1. Perform with minimal or no use of the hand for balance. 2. Perform with eyes closed. 3. Perform on one leg at a time.

DANCE CUES 6.3

"Lift From Under the Pelvis as You Rise to Relevé"

The cue to "lift from under the pelvis as you rise to relevé" is sometimes used by teachers to encourage maintaining vertical alignment of the pelvis and torso as the body rises. As discussed in chapter 3, with ideal standing alignment the center of mass of the body falls just in front of the ankle joint. So, to rise to demi-pointe or pointe, the center of mass of the body must move forward several inches so that it is placed over the new base of support. There are many tactics for facilitating this shift. One anatomical interpretation of this cue is to progressively shift the pelvis and torso forward as a unit (maintaining desired vertical alignment), by focusing on using the hip extensors to position the bottom of the pelvis over the moving base of support as the plantar flexors are used to raise the body and the abdominal muscles and back extensors are used to help keep the torso positioned over the pelvis. In turned-out positions, a focus on use of the lower deep outward rotators is added to the use of the abdominal–hamstring force couple, and for some dancers this has the feeling of lifting "up and forward" from under the pelvis. In contrast, one undesired approach to shifting the center of mass forward is to make the shift primarily from leaning the torso forward (hip flexion), distorting the desired body alignment and reinforcing undesired motor programs for maintaining balance.

Dorsiflexor Strengthening

Inadequate strength in the dorsiflexors may increase the risk for some injuries such as shin splints. There have been conflicting results, but at least some dancers tend to be low in dorsiflexor strength both in terms of balance with their plantar flexors and in relation to other athletes (Hamilton et al., 1992; Liederbach and Hiebert, 1997). This tendency does appear to be specific to dance form, with flamenco (Wilmerding et al., 1998) and tap dancers (Mayers, Judelson, and Bronner, 2003) not necessarily exhibiting this ratio imbalance or weakness that is seen in ballet dancers. Table 6.6 provides an exercise for strengthening these muscles with a weight (table 6.6D) or elastic band (table 6.6E, variation 1) for resistance. All of the muscles that produce ankle-foot dorsiflexion also produce either inversion or eversion of the foot, and so can also be strengthened with exercises that incorporate these motions with dorsiflexion.

Foot Inverter Strengthening

Adequate strength in the inverters of the foot is important for preventing excessive rolling in and the injuries associated with excessive pronation. Sitting big toe up and away (table 6.6F) and side-lying big toe up (table 6.6G) will strengthen the inverters in plantar flexion and are particularly helpful for preventing rolling in while on or going through demi-pointe or pointe. Sitting big toe up and in (table

6.6E) will strengthen the inverters in dorsiflexion and is particularly helpful for preventing rolling in while on flat or in plié.

Foot Everter Strengthening

When rising onto the toes, most beginning-level dancers and many trained dancers tend to invert the foot, and taken together the inverters of the foot tend to be stronger than the everters of the foot (Levangie and Norkin, 2001). Hence, development of adequate strength and use of the everters is important for achieving the desired dance aesthetic of rising up right over the axis of the foot. In addition, the peroneus longus can be seen as a direct continuation of the biceps femoris in terms of its location (Smith, Weiss, and Lehmkuhl, 1996), and appropriate use of these two muscles can aid with maintaining desired turnout throughout the segments of the lower extremity. Furthermore, adequate everter strength is important for preventing ankle sprains or their recurrence, and persistent peroneal weakness is common in dancers following injury (Ende and Wickstrom, 1982). Sitting little toes up and away (table 6.6H) and side-lying little toe up (table 6.6I) will strengthen these everters. Both exercises are done in plantar flexion because this is the position in which ankle sprains tend to occur and in which the foot is less stable. However, dancers who have problems with rolling out when standing flat may benefit from adding another set performed with the foot neutral versus plantar flexed.

Intrinsic Muscle Strengthening

Many exercises can be performed for the intrinsic muscles of the foot. Two that are particularly helpful for dancers are doming (table 6.6J) and towel curls (table 6.6K). Both of these exercises focus on strengthening muscles important for helping maintain the arches of the foot.

Ankle-Foot Proprioceptive Exercises

Proprioceptive exercises are exercises designed to challenge reflexes related to balance and movement coordination. They often incorporate tools such as balance boards, wobble boards, foam rollers, ankle disks, or the biomechanical ankle platform system (BAPS) board. Use of such exercises has been shown to be important for developing better balance, quick corrections of movements such as falling out of a turn, and prevention of injuries such as ankle sprains. Proprioceptive exercises are often advanced from single-plane to multiplane movement, from two feet to one foot, from eyes open to eyes closed, and from using a flat foot position to incorporating a relevé. Three examples of exercises with a proprioceptive emphasis are provided in table 6.6, L-N.

Stretches for the Ankle-Foot

Adequate flexibility in plantar flexion and dorsiflexion of the ankle-foot is particularly important for dancers. Table 6.7 provides average range of motion for these movements in the general population as well as the primary constraints to these movements. As previously described, adequate range of the great toe (MTP joint extension) is also important to allow correct positioning on demi-pointe.

Plantar Flexor (Calf) Stretches

Adequate flexibility in the plantar flexors and especially the gastrocnemius and soleus is essential for allowing the ankle-foot dorsiflexion needed in movements such as pliés and lunges. When the knee is bent, such as in a plié, the gastrocnemius is slackened across the knee joint, and the soleus is generally the primary constraint. When the knee is straight, the gastrocnemius is stretched as well as the soleus. Having adequate and symmetrical flexibility in the calf muscles is vital to give the dancer adequate time to absorb the large forces associated with landing from movements such as jumps. Furthermore, when the triceps surae is tight, the foot is often allowed to excessively pronate in order to unlock the midtarsal joint and allow greater apparent dorsiflexion. This excessive pronation can increase injury risk at the knee and foot.

Unfortunately, at least elite ballet dancers tend to have lower ranges of motion in ankle-foot dorsiflexion than even sedentary controls (Clippinger-Robertson, 1991; Hamilton et al., 1992; Liederbach and Hiebert, 1997). One study of elite ballet students showed that 67% lacked the 10° of dorsiflexion required for just normal walking gait (Molnar and Esterson, 1997). Another study showed a 50% reduction in dorsiflexion when compared to general norms (Hamilton et al., 1992). In this latter study, female ballet dancers with higher total injuries were also associated with lower bilateral plié and decreased ankle-foot dorsiflexion. In a study that followed both ballet and modern dance students for one year, those who reported previous leg injuries correlated significantly with lower dorsiflexion values and with more new injuries (Wiesler et al., 1996).

This research supports the strong need to incorporate regular calf stretching into the dancer's routine to counter the effect of training and decrease injury risk. Hamilton (1988) claims that just putting stretching boxes (incline boards) in the studios and encouraging regular stretching of the triceps surae markedly reduced the incidence of Achilles tendinitis

TABLE 6.7   Normal Range of Motion and Constraints for Plantar Flexion and Dorsiflexion of the Ankle-Foot

Ankle-foot joint movement	Normal range of motion*	Normal passive limiting factors
Plantar flexion	0-50°	Capsule: anterior portion Ligaments: anterior talofibular, anterior portion of deltoid Muscles: dorsiflexors of foot Bony opposition: posterior talus and posterior tibia
Dorsiflexion	0-20°	Capsule: posterior portion Ligaments: posterior talofibular, calcaneofibular, and deltoid Muscles: plantar flexors of foot Bony opposition: anterior talus and anterior tibia

*From American Academy of Orthopaedic Surgeons (1965).

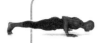

Influence of Foot Pronation on Dorsiflexion Range of Motion

Bring the right leg back to perform a standing lunge calf stretch with your side to a mirror.

· **Dorsiflexion range with a parallel foot.** Check the back foot so that it is parallel, facing straight ahead, and in line with the tibia. This position will tend to throw the body weight slightly outward on the foot and create a locked position of the midtarsal joints (slight foot inversion). Now bend the front knee, and lean the body forward until a stretch is felt in the back of the calf. Note the angle of dorsiflexion that can be reached on the back ankle-foot.

· **Dorsiflexion range with the foot toed out.** Now shift your weight forward onto your front foot, and adjust your back foot so that it is facing slightly outward relative to your tibia. Again, bend the front knee further, and lean the body forward until a stretch is felt in the back of the calf. Note that the foot unlocks and pronates, allowing a much greater angle of apparent dorsiflexion than could be reached before.

· **Relationship to technique.** Consider how this undesired use of pronation would influence the structures being stretched and would relate to dancers with shallow pliés or asymmetrical pliés (with less dorsiflexion on one side).

in professional ballet dancers. Table 6.8 provides two stretches with a straight knee to emphasize the gastrocnemius (table 6.8, A and B, p. 356) and two stretches with a bent knee to emphasize the soleus (table 6.8, C and D, p. 357). In all of these exercises, particular care must be taken that the foot is parallel (in line with the tibia) and that the foot remains neutral or slightly inverted versus pronated. It is also important that the stretch be experienced in the calf. If pain and limitation is experienced in the front of the ankle, the dancer should stretch only in a pain-free range and seek an evaluation from a sports medicine professional to rule out impingement or other medical conditions that could be worsened by forcing this stretch.

Stretches to Improve Pointing of the Foot

Adequate flexibility of the ankle-foot dorsiflexors is necessary to achieve the high ranges of plantar flexion used in movements such as pointing the foot and relevés. In contrast to the range for dorsiflexion, range of ankle-foot plantar flexion in dancers tends to be much greater than found in the general population. One study of elite professional ballet dancers showed the mean for female dancers to be 113° (Hamilton et al., 1992), and in another study of elite advanced and professional ballet dancers it was 97° (Clippinger-Robertson, 1991). These numbers reflect an extreme deviation from the American Academy of Orthopaedic Surgeons norm of 50°. In

ballet, at least 90° of plantar flexion is recommended to meet biomechanical and aesthetic demands for pointe work. Although other dance forms such as modern and jazz do not require as extreme measurements, high ankle-foot plantar flexion range is still important for aesthetics during pointing and for proper placement on demi-pointe. Hence, stretching the feet to gain adequate plantar flexion is important for meeting dance demands.

This plantar flexion range is not just from the ankle joint, but rather comes from a combination of the talocrural, subtalar, midtarsal, and metatarsophalangeal joints. The contribution of these other joints is often underestimated; and even with the general population, 10% to 40% of the range of plantar flexion comes from joints distal to the talocrural joint (Levangie and Norkin, 2001). However, as seen from table 6.7, although increasing this range includes stretching the dorsiflexors of the foot (particularly the tibialis anterior, extensor hallucis longus, and extensor digitorum longus), it also probably includes stretching joint ligaments and capsules. Hence such stretches should be done when the feet are fully warmed, and with very slow and careful application of stretch in a pain-free range.

Table 6.8 provides two stretches for improving range in plantar flexion—one performed standing and one sitting. The standing pointe stretch (table 6.8E, p. 358) offers a stretch that can easily be done either in class prior to moving across the floor or

TESTS AND MEASUREMENTS 6.3

Screening Test for Range of Motion for Ankle-Foot Plantar Flexion

Two tests are shown for measuring passive range of motion of the ankle-foot in plantar flexion. For many dancers this range will be influenced by the bony structure of the arches, joint capsules, and ligaments, as well as the constraints offered by the ankle-foot dorsiflexors. While the dancer is sitting with the legs extended to the front and one foot pointed, the examiner places one hand on the top of the instep of the pointed foot and gently presses down to bring the foot into further plantar flexion. For the first test (A) the axis of the goniometer is placed just below and slightly in front of the lateral malleolus, the stationary arm along the fibula, and the moving arm parallel to the bottom of the foot. It is considered "0" when the foot is at a right angle to the lower leg, and the amount the foot can point (plantar flexion) from this position is measured as positive degrees. While 50° is considered normal range in general populations, the average value for elite female ballet dancers in one study was found to be 97° (Clippinger-Robertson, 1991), and achieving a value of at least 90° is considered desirable for optimal body placement for demi-pointe and pointe.

If a goniometer is not available, one can place a ruler with its upper portion in line with the middle of the lateral portion of the tibia and middle of the medial malleolus as shown in B. Note whether the head of the first metatarsal is above, on, or below the line made by the top of the ruler. For pointe work, the goal is to have this landmark approximately on or below the line of the ruler.

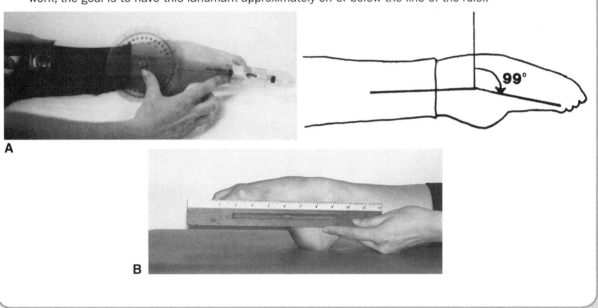

A

B

immediately following class. The sitting pointe stretch (table 6.8F, p. 358) offers the advantage of more easily being able to control the magnitude and location of the stretch. Quick application of high forces, such as associated with sticking the feet under a couch and lying back, can create ligament sprains and other injuries to the feet and should be avoided. Also, if pain and limitation is felt at the back of the ankle when the dancer is trying to perform these stretches, he or she should use one hand to hold the heel in place (attempting to prevent posterior impingement) while placing the other hand

about halfway down the foot and applying a smaller stretch as shown in table 6.8F. If pain is still present, the dancer should seek a medical evaluation to rule out medical conditions that could be aggravated by stretching too far or hard.

Great Toe Flexor Stretches

As previously described, about 90° of MTP joint extension of the great toe is needed to allow the dancer to go high onto demi-pointe, and to keep the weight over the axis of the foot rather than roll in or out in an attempt to get more range.

TABLE 6.8   Selected Stretches for the Ankle-Foot

Exercise name (Method of stretch)	Description (Technique cues)	Progression
Muscle group: A-F plantar flexors **Muscles emphasized: Gastrocnemius**		
Joint position: A-F dorsiflexion with knee extension		
A. Standing lunge calf stretch (Static) 	Stand in a lunge position with the front leg bent and the back leg straight. Shift your hips and pelvis forward until a stretch is felt in the calf of the back leg. (Keep both feet parallel and facing forward instead of letting the forefoot toe-out and the foot pronate; keep the heel of the back foot in contact with the ground.) *Variation 1:* PNF—From the above position, contract the calf muscle of the back leg by pressing the ball of the foot into the ground as if to plantar flex the foot. Relax, and shift the bottom of the pelvis slightly farther forward to increase the stretch of the back calf.	1. Move the back foot farther back, and shift the hips and torso farther forward.
B. Half foam roller calf stretch (Static) 	Stand facing a wall with the hands on the wall and one foot about 12 inches behind the other foot and the ball of the back foot resting on the flat surface of a half foam roller. Allow the front knee to bend as the back heel slowly presses back and down toward the floor, rocking the roller backward, until a stretch is felt in the calf of the leg that is back. (Keep the back foot facing forward and avoid toeing-out or pronation. Maintain good body placement such that a straight line could be drawn between the sides of the ankle, knee, pelvis, and shoulder.)	1. Bring the heel further down. 2. Shift the hips and torso further forward. 3. Use a larger-diameter roller.

Exercise name (Method of stretch)	Description (Technique cues)	Progression
Muscle group: A-F plantar flexors **Muscles emphasized: Soleus**		
Joint position: A-F dorsiflexion with knee flexion		
C. Standing lunge bent-knee calf stretch (Static) 	From the position used in exercise A, bring the back foot in about 8 inches (20 centimeters). Bend the back knee until a stretch is felt low in the calf of the back leg. (Keep both feet facing forward and avoid toeing-out or pronation.) *Variation 1:* PNF—From the above position, contract the calf muscle of the back leg by pressing the ball of the foot into the ground as if to plantar flex the foot. Relax, and slightly deepen the bend of the back knee to apply a greater stretch.	1. Bend the back knee further and shift body weight further forward over the back foot.
D. Half foam roller bent-knee calf stretch (Static) 	Perform the stretch as described in exercise B but with the back knee bent throughout the exercise and the trunk more vertical.	

(continued)

TABLE 6.8 Selected Stretches for the Ankle-Foot *(continued)*

Exercise name (Method of stretch)	Description (Technique cues)	Progression
Muscle groups: A-F dorsiflexors and toe extensors **Muscles emphasized: Extensor digitorum longus**		
Joint position: A-F plantar flexion with MTP and IP flexion		
E. Standing pointe stretch (Static)	Stand on the left foot, with the other leg slightly bent and the top of the distal right foot in contact with the floor. Gently press the right heel forward until a stretch is felt across the upper instep. If necessary, slightly bend the support knee and bend the right knee further to emphasize the stretch in the upper versus lower foot. Repeat on the other side.	1. Shift the body weight slightly further toward the foot being stretched.
F. Sitting pointe stretch (Static)	Sit with the right foot on the ground and the left knee bent, with the ankle resting on the right thigh. With the left hand grasping the heel and holding it in place, use the right hand to gently pull the foot into further plantar flexion until a stretch is felt across the front of the upper instep. Repeat on the other side. (Focus on using the right thumb to press the arch upward as the other fingers pull the forefoot slightly "out and then down.")	1. Pull the forefoot slightly further downward (i.e., greater A-F plantar flexion).

Exercise name (Method of stretch)	Description (Technique cues)	Progression
Muscle group: Flexors of great toe **Muscles emphasized: Flexor hallucis longus and brevis**		
Joint position: Extension of the great toe at the MTP joint		
G. Big toe stretch (Static)	While sitting, use the hand to pull the great toe slightly out and then gently back toward the top of the foot until a stretch is felt along the plantar aspect of the great toe. (Keep the great toe in line with the first metatarsal and the subtalar joint in a neutral position as you apply the stretch.)	1. Pull the great toe slightly farther back in a pain-free range but only to a maximum of 90°.

If the big toe cannot be brought back sufficiently to create a right angle, the big toe stretch (table 6.8G) should be carefully added to the dancer's regular stretching routine. This exercise involves stretching not only the flexors of the great toe but also often the joint capsule and ligaments. Hence, it should be performed slowly and gently. If pain and limitation is experienced, the dancer should stretch only in a pain-free range and seek a medical evaluation to rule out arthritis or other conditions that could be worsened by overzealous stretching.

Ankle and Foot Injuries in Dancers

Very large forces are generated and absorbed in the ankle-foot complex in dance. For example, ankle joint compression forces have been calculated to reach 5 times body weight during walking and 9 to 13 times body weight during running (Hamill and Knutzen, 1995). Considering these high forces and the complex structure and demands of the foot, it is not surprising that the ankle-foot complex is the site most frequently injured in dance. In three extensive

studies of ballet dancers, 38% (Garrick and Requa, 1988), 42.4% (Quirk, 1983), and 48.5% (Garrick, 1999) of all injuries involved the ankle-foot complex. Studies involving modern dancers showed that 26.6% (Solomon and Micheli, 1986), 36% (Schafle, Requa, and Garrick, 1990), and 38% (Hardaker and Moorman, 1986) of injuries were in the ankle and foot. Studies of flamenco dancers indicated incidences of injury to the ankle-foot complex of 45% and 40% (Salter-Pedersen and Wilmerding, 1998), and a study of tap dancers showed that 36% of all injuries occurred in the ankle and foot (Mayers, Judelson, and Bronner, 2003). So, despite differing demands of varied dance forms, all of the dance forms studied showed a high incidence of injury to the ankle and foot, although at least in ballet, with a higher incidence in female versus male dancers (Liederbach, 2000).

Prevention of Ankle and Foot Injuries

Considering the high incidence of injury involving the ankle and foot, prevention of injuries to this region should be a priority for dancers. Preventive conditioning measures include trying to avoid abrupt increases in dance training by maintaining condition during layoffs or breaks, performing supplemental strengthening exercises for the ankle-foot two to three times per week, and performing daily stretching to maintain adequate ankle-foot dorsiflexion to foster shock absorption and help avoid excessive foot pronation. Preventive technique considerations include utilizing appropriate placement of the body weight over the axis of the foot to avoid excessive inversion or eversion, utilizing the stirrup muscles to facilitate balance and a high demi-pointe or pointe position with less Achilles stress, maintaining turnout at the hip to prevent compensatory foot pronation, and "going through the foot" (emphasizing a toe-heel contact pattern) and using adequate plié depth to help lessen impact when landing from jumps (Devita and Skelly, 1992; Dufek and Bates, 1990). In terms of equipment considerations, careful selection of well-fitting shoes and use of floors with good resiliency and friction characteristics (Fiolkowski and Bauer, 1997) whenever possible can also help prevent injuries to the ankle and foot.

Rehabilitation of Ankle and Foot Injuries

As with injuries to other regions of the body, initial recommended treatment usually utilizes ice and anti-inflammatory medications to control pain and swelling. For dancers, many physicians recommend using nonsteroidal anti-inflammatory medications for many injuries such as tendinitis or plantar fasciitis, reserving corticosteroids for select conditions with unresponsive pain, as the repetitive use of steroids has been implicated in tissue weakening and rupture (Hardaker, 1989; Weiker, 1988)—particularly if activity is not adequately controlled immediately following injection (Roberts, 1999). Various other physical therapy modalities such as contrast baths, massage, ultrasound, electrical stimulation, or phonophoresis (ultrasound used to deliver hydrocortisone cream) are often used to reduce pain, increase range of motion, and promote healing.

As soon as symptoms allow, stretching and range of motion exercises are added in a pain-free range to help restore normal range of motion. Again, as symptoms allow, strengthening exercises are added, often progressing from isolation exercises to functional exercises and proprioceptive exercises as permitted by healing. Due to the fact that weight bearing can often aggravate more severe ankle and foot injuries, functional exercises are frequently initially performed where loading can be reduced, such as in a swimming pool or on a Pilates-based Reformer (Brown and Clippinger, 1996; Hender-

son et al., 1993), and then gradually progressed to normal weight bearing on land.

Proprioceptive exercises are also key in the rehabilitation process, as many injuries have been shown to impair reflex responses and subtle aspects of movement coordination that can interfere with full return to dance and increase the risk of injury recurrence. Last, as symptoms allow, specific dance movements that originally aggravated the condition, such as jumps or turns, are gradually reintroduced in a progressive manner, with particular care taken to correct any technique problems that could contribute to reinjury.

Because altered foot mechanics play an important role in many injuries of the ankle and foot, particular care should be paid to correcting any underlying technique problems. In some cases, assistive devices such as tape, arch supports, heel cups, and shock-absorbing inserts may be incorporated into the rehabilitation process. Potential mechanisms by which these supports work are still controversial and may relate to very slight changes in skeletal movement, shock absorption, or minimizing muscle work (Marshall, 1988; Nigg, Nursae, and Stefanyshyn, 1999; Scranton, Pedegana, and Whitesel, 1982; Yakut et al., 1997).

Common Ankle and Foot Injuries in Dancers

Given the large number of joints and ligaments composing the ankle-foot complex, it is not surprising that a vast number of different types of injuries can occur in this region. A discussion of selected key injuries follows, and interested dancers are referred to the writings of Hamilton (1988), Malone and Hardaker (1990), Norris (1990), Spilken (1990), and other authors cited in this section for a more detailed presentation of injuries to the ankle and foot.

Ankle Sprains

The ankle sprain is one of the most common acute (traumatic) injuries seen in dancers. Although termed an **ankle sprain,** technically this injury involves injury to ligaments of both the ankle joint and the subtalar joint. About 85% of ankle sprains involve inversion (Whiting and Zernicke, 1998) and tend to occur when the ankle is in a less stable position of relative plantar flexion, during loading or unloading of the foot such as in landing poorly from a jump, falling out of a turn, or miscalculating a step.

Ankle sprains are classically put into three grades based on the degree of damage. Hamilton (1988) describes Grade I as a mild sprain involving partial tear of the ATFL and occasionally the anterior tibiofibular ligament with little or no resultant instability. Grade II sprains are moderate sprains generally involving complete tears of the ATFL with minimal damage to the calcaneofibular ligament. A moderately positive anterior drawer sign is present, but a normal or minimally abnormal talar tilt is seen on stress X-ray films (Tests and Measurements 6.1, p. 305). Hamilton holds that this is the type of sprain most commonly seen in dancers. In the demi-pointe or pointe position, the ATFL is almost vertical and so is easily torn when an adduction-inversion force is applied, while the calcaneofibular ligament is in a position almost parallel to the floor where it will likely avoid large disruptive forces (figure 6.43A). Grade III injuries are severe ankle sprains and are rare. Grade III injuries involve a complete rupture of the lateral ligament complex and result in gross instability, with grossly positive drawer sign and stress films (figure 6.43B).

When the ankle is sprained, dancers will often hear a pop or experience a tearing sensation with immediate pain. However, it is important to realize that the extent of pain is not necessarily a good indicator of the seriousness of the injury. Swelling occurs quickly around the ligaments (lateral malleolus); and if the sprain is sufficiently serious, the dancer feels that the ankle is unstable and is unable to continue dancing or to walk normally. Depending on the severity, after several hours, swelling progresses, range of motion becomes limited, and discoloration may appear. On examination, both passive inversion of

the foot and ankle-foot plantar flexion will tend to produce discomfort.

In terms of treatment, many dance medicine physicians recommend surgical repair for Grade III sprains in professional dancers to achieve adequate ankle-foot stability and avoid early joint degeneration that can be associated with instability (Hamilton, 1988; Hardaker, 1989; Safran, Benedetti, et al., 1999). However, for Grade I and Grade II ankle sprains, a conservative treatment approach is generally recommended. Because this is a traumatic versus an overuse injury, initial treatment is aimed at limiting damage; and this is one injury for which RICE (Rest [relative], Ice, Compression [elastic ankle wrap], Elevation) is particularly relevant. Early protection such as taping, strapping, an air cast, functional walking orthosis, or a walking plaster cast may also be utilized in accordance with the injury severity.

As symptoms allow, a comprehensive rehabilitation program should be followed that includes stretches to help restore normal motion, strengthening exercises with a particular emphasis on the peroneals, functional exercises such as relevés while holding dumbbells, and proprioceptive exercises such as side-to-side or fondu développés performed on balance boards and foam rollers. Proprioceptive exercises are key for reestablishment of reflexes necessary for regaining a sense of the joint's feeling stable and prevention of reinjury (Eils and Rosenbaum, 2001). Impaired reflex response of the peroneals and increased postural sway have been shown to persist for weeks or even months after the

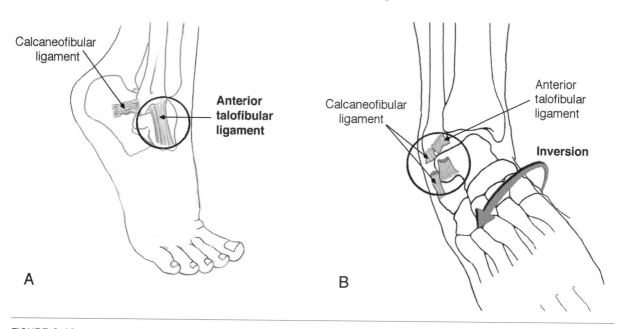

A

B

FIGURE 6.43   In plantar flexion (right foot), (A) the anterior talofibular ligament (ATFL) is almost vertical and can be readily sprained when (B) inversion-adduction force is applied.

initial injury (Nawoczenski et al., 1985), and in some populations the likelihood of lateral ankle sprain recurrence is as high as 70% to 80% (Hertel et al., 1999). However, one study of soccer players showed only a 5% recurrence of ankle sprains in athletes performing regular proprioceptive exercises versus 25% seen in controls (Tropp, Askling, and Gillquist, 1985). Hence dancers with ankle sprains are encouraged to undergo comprehensive rehabilitation (Sammarco and Tablante, 1997), consider the use of dance-specific ankle taping or braces (Rovere et al., 1988) with the initial return to dance, and continue select peroneal and proprioceptive exercises well after full return to dance.

Plantar Fasciitis

Plantar fasciitis is an inflammation of the plantar fascia, often involving microtears in the fascia that, if persistent, can lead to degeneration of collagen in the fascia (Shea and Fields, 2002). Because of the key role the plantar fascia plays in supporting the longitudinal arch, jumping is commonly implicated with this injury. Anatomical and biomechanical factors that can heighten injury risk include pes planus or pes cavus foot types, a tight triceps surae, and excessive foot pronation (Hall, 1999; Hamill and Knutzen, 1995; Kreighbaum and Barthels, 1996). In some cases a bone spur develops in conjunction with the plantar fasciitis, and on occasion the plantar fascia can rupture, often in association with impact loading after it has already been weakened from chronic inflammation, repeated cortisone injections, or both (Howse and Hancock, 1988; Roberts, 1999).

Plantar fasciitis is characterized by pain and tenderness on the underside of the calcaneus at the medial or central area (figure 6.44) where the plantar fascia attaches onto the calcaneus. Surprisingly, only a relatively small percentage of individuals complain of pain extending distally along the plantar fascia itself, and this may occur more in dancers with chronic cases. Generally, pain can be accentuated through passively extending the MTP joints, which in effect stretches the plantar fascia. A hallmark of this condition is morning stiffness. Some dancers complain that while taking the first few steps in the morning, it feels as though their feet are as stiff as boards.

In addition to ice, friction massage, and other physical therapy modalities, recommended rehabilitation focuses on heel raises done on a step to strengthen the triceps surae and eccentrically load the Achilles tendon (Shea and Fields, 2002), as well as strengthening the intrinsic muscles and extrinsic muscles that help support the longitudinal arch. Because of associated risk from pronation, efforts

to control pronation including orthotics, arch supports, and taping, as well as technique modification and triceps surae stretching (when indicated), can be helpful. Adding viscoelastic inserts or a heel cup to reduce shock can also sometimes offer relief (Marshall, 1988; Warren, 1983).

Ankle-Foot Tendinitis

Tendinitis (tendon + G. *itis*, inflammation) is an inflammation of a tendon or its covering/sheath (or both) due to microscopic tearing of collagen fibers secondary to overload (Fernández-Palazzi, Rivas, and Mujica, 1990). Although tendons have a tensile strength that is about twice that of muscle (Frey and Shereff, 1988), their collagen fibers have poor elasticity and so can be injured when forces are applied rapidly, obliquely, or during high-level eccentric contractions of their associated muscles.

When a tendon becomes injured, the surface becomes roughened and it will no longer move smoothly, but instead will tend to bind as it moves in its sheath or covering, causing further pain, swelling, tenderness, and sometimes crepitus. Furthermore, the new collagen that the body tries to lay down for

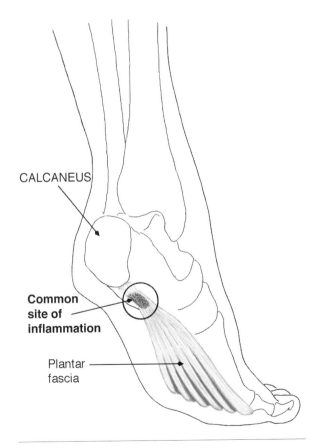

FIGURE 6.44   Common site of pain with plantar fasciitis (left foot, posterolateral view).

"healing" the tendon can be damaged by enzymes associated with inflammation, and so the inflammatory response must be limited through such modes as ice, anti-inflammatory medication (Frey and Shereff, 1988), and adequate relative rest. Additionally, it appears that these new collagen fibers orient in accordance with the forces applied to the tendon, suggesting that the high forces associated with eccentric contractions may help the fibers align in the desired longitudinal direction. However, one must take care when performing eccentric contractions that the movement is very slow and controlled, or injuries can sometimes be aggravated.

Tendinitis can occur in any of the tendons that cross the ankle. However, the Achilles tendon and tendon of the flexor hallucis longus are most commonly involved in ballet dancers.

Achilles Tendinitis

The Achilles tendon is not surrounded by the typical synovial tendon sheath, but rather by a sheath composed of fascia that is termed a paratendon. Inflammation and injury can occur to the paratendon, the tendon itself, or both. It is not surprising that this tendon is commonly injured when one considers that the triceps surae is responsible for generating a majority of the force used in plantar flexion and that this tendon has been estimated to bear forces 4 to 10 times body weight in running and jumping (Hamilton, 1988; Whiting and Zernicke, 1998).

Factors that have been theorized to increase risk of injury include a tight triceps surae, congenitally small or thin Achilles tendons, excessive pronation, rolling in or out when on demi-pointe or relevé, limited range in ankle-foot plantar flexion or presence of an os trigonum such that the triceps surae has to contract very hard in an effort to achieve adequate height in relevé/pointe, inadequate triceps surae strength and endurance, cavus foot type, and prominence of the posterior superior portion of the calcaneus (Ende and Wickstrom, 1982; Frey and Shereff, 1988; Hall, 1999; Hamilton, 1988; Hardaker, 1989; Howse and Hancock, 1988; Norris, 1990). Further research will be necessary to show which of these factors actually are predictive of Achilles tendinitis and to what degree. A study with runners showed that runners with Achilles tendinitis had more of a cavus foot type, greater maximum pronation magnitude and velocity, and lower plantar flexion strength and that they performed less stretching (McCrory et al., 1999). Floors also appear to be an important factor. In one study, 45% of cases of Achilles tendinitis occurred when dancing was on cement, while only 4% of cases started when dancing was on wood surfaces (Fernández-Palazzi, Rivas, and Mujica, 1990).

Achilles tendinitis is characterized by pain, tenderness, and swelling, most commonly about 0.8 to 2.4 inches (2-6 centimeters) above its attachment onto the heel (figure 6.45). This is an area where the tendon is narrower and where blood supply is poor (Frey and Shereff, 1988; McCrory et al., 1999). Dancers will also often complain of a feeling of tightness and stiffness, particularly when awakening in the morning, and decreased range of motion in pliés and other movements involving ankle-foot dorsiflexion. Sometimes a feeling of weakness is present. There may also be crepitus associated with active motion. Pain is generally reproduced or increased with resisted ankle-foot plantar flexion such as in relevés or jumps. Pain also tends to occur when the triceps surae is working eccentrically or the tendon is stretched, as in landing from jumps or the bottom of a plié.

Treatment is particularly challenging because healing and remodeling of the tendon are slow due to its relative avascularity, and it is often difficult for the dancer to stop long enough for it to heal. However, if the dancer continues dancing with Achilles tendinitis, it can lead to scar formation, areas of tissue death (necrosis) within the tendon itself, and sometimes rupture (Weiker, 1988). Hence, it is very important for the dancer to heed tendinitis in its early acute stages while tendon damage is minimal and to follow a well-supervised, comprehensive rehabilitation program that can appropriately progress exercises so that further tendon damage is avoided. Earlier stages of rehabilitation generally focus on the use of medications and modalities to limit the inflammatory response and reduce symptoms. Wearing 1/2-inch (1.3-centimeter) heel lifts or shoes with slight heels, viscoelastic heel inserts, Achilles taping,

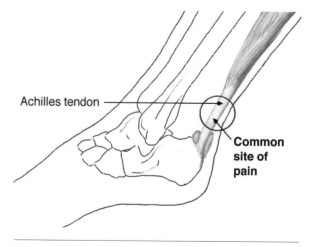

FIGURE 6.45   Common site of pain and thickening with Achilles tendinitis (left foot, lateral view).

control of excessive pronation (where indicated), and correction of related technique errors can also sometimes help reduce symptoms. Later stages of rehabilitation generally focus on restoring adequate and symmetrical flexibility and strength of the triceps surae. The desired inclusion of eccentric contractions can be achieved by performing calf raises while holding weights on a step or platform, where the lowering phase is emphasized by performing it more slowly.

When Achilles tendinitis does not respond to conservative treatment or an actual rupture of the Achilles tendon occurs, surgery may be recommended. Rupture usually occurs in male dancers over the age of 30 (Hamilton, 1988). The rupture commonly occurs in rigorous movements such as jumping or a quick change in direction, and the dancer classically feels as if he has been "shot" or "kicked in the back of the leg" (Teitz, 1986). Surgical repair of the tendon is often recommended for professional dancers because it has been shown to better restore plantar flexion strength (Scheller, Kasser, and Quigley, 1980).

Flexor Hallucis Longus Tendinitis   **Flexor hallucis longus tendinitis** has a uniquely high prevalence in ballet dancers (Hardaker, 1989). Its high occurrence in dancers is thought to relate to its important functions of stabilizing the foot and preventing excessive eversion in demi-pointe and pointe, as well as pressing the big toe down against the ground to help go from demi-pointe to a full pointe position, and helping to stabilize the big toe in full pointe when it is in a very shortened position. This muscle may also be particularly prone to tendinitis for anatomical reasons. The flexor hallucis longus tendon passes through a fibro-osseous tunnel at the back of the ankle just behind the medial malleolus (figure 6.46); and when strained or thickened, it will tend to bind rather than move smoothly. Because it crosses the ankle joint and toe joints, an excursion of 2 to 3 inches (5-7.6 centimeters) (Conti and Wong, 2001) of the tendon may be required when going from a plié to pointe, giving ample opportunity for irritation if it is not sliding smoothly in its fibro-osseous tunnel.

Flexor hallucis longus tendinitis is characterized by pain on the posterior medial aspect of the ankle, deeper than experienced with Achilles tendinitis (Fond, 1983). Tenderness, mild swelling, and in some cases crepitus may be present that are generally aggravated by flexion and extension of the great toe. Weakness of flexion of the great toe may be present with manual testing, and dancers may complain of a sense of weakness in the big toe on pointe. In more advanced cases, fusiform thickening of the tendon (nodules) can occur that can get stuck within the tendon sheath or canal and cause pain, popping, and impaired ability to move the big toe ("triggering of the big toe") as seen in figure 6.46. Affected dancers may complain of having the big toe get stuck in flexion or extension, and the release of the hallux is generally accompanied by a pop or snap on the posterior medial aspect of the ankle (Sammarco and Miller, 1979).

Recommended treatment for flexor hallucis longus tendinitis includes anti-inflammatory medications, deep friction massage, ice massage, and other modalities, as well as stretching and strengthening the flexor hallucis longus and related muscles in pain-free ranges as inflammation subsides (Fond, 1983; Norris, 1990). Temporary avoidance of relevé or pointe work is often recommended. Correction of any relevant technique errors such as excessive pronation or having the body weight too far medial or back (such that the toes tend to "grab" the floor) can also often be beneficial.

Nonsurgical treatment is usually successful in alleviating symptoms. When conservative treatment fails, surgery may be recommended in accordance with the particular case to remove dead areas of the tendon, reinforce the tendon, free the tendon from adhesions, open the tendon sheath or flexor retinaculum, remove a bony block, or do a combination of these (Hamilton, Geppert, and Thompson, 1996).

Shin Splints and Tibial Stress Syndrome

This text will use the term **shin splints,** also termed tibial stress syndrome, to refer to activity-related pain and generalized tenderness on the anterior or medial

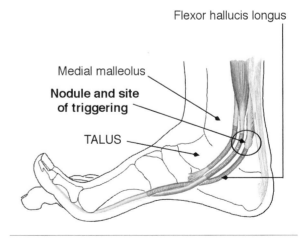

FIGURE 6.46 Chronic flexor hallucis longus tendinitis with a nodule near the entrance of the fibro-osseous canal (right foot, medial view).

shin (figure 6.47), from traction of muscles on their attachments onto the tibia that results in injury to and inflammation of the membrane covering the bone (periosteum), fascial inflammation, a stress reaction of the bone, or a combination of these. While the anterior shin pain was originally believed to involve the tibialis anterior and tibialis posterior muscles, there is evidence that the soleus (Hutchinson, Cahoon, and Atkins, 1998; Michael and Holder, 1985) and flexor hallucis (Kortebein et al., 2000) may also be responsible in some cases.

Shin splints often relate to too fast an increase or change in overload such as beginning to dance after a long layoff, participating in intensive workshops, working with a choreographer with an unaccustomed style, or changing to less resilient or raked floors as can happen on tour. Shin splints also have been postulated to be related to abnormal pronation since the muscles commonly involved in shin splints are all inverters that work eccentrically to control pronation. Theoretically, abnormal pronation could put excessive stress on these inverters and their proximal attachments onto the tibia (Brukner, 2000). Various studies, primarily involving runners, have shown an association of increased pronation with increased risk for shin splints (Kortebein et al., 2000; Soderberg, 1986; Sommer and Vallentyne, 1995). In the dance world, one study also found that dancers with shin splints tended to demonstrate more double heel strikes during jumps (Gans, 1985). A double heel strike occurs when a dancer places the heel on the floor upon landing, lifts it off the floor unintention-

ally, and then replaces the heel to push off for the next jump.

Shin splints are evidenced by regular aching or long-lasting shin pain that is associated with repetitive exercise such as dance. At first, pain tends to lessen or disappear after warm-up and return only with rigorous movements such as repetitive jumping, or with fatigue such as toward the end of class or rehearsal. However, if not heeded, over time the pain often increases in severity, does not disappear so readily with warm-up, and is brought on by less intense activity. This shin pain is usually accompanied by generalized tenderness along the lateral border and crest of the tibia (figure 6.47A) or the posteromedial border of the lower tibia (figure 6.47B).

Recommended treatment for shin splints often includes ice after activity and sufficient decrease in activity to allow a pain-free status. In dance, this often means removing movements like jumps and sometimes also limiting the duration of dance. When symptoms allow, strengthening of the involved muscles and developing a balance of strength between the dorsiflexors and plantar flexors of the foot are key, as low levels of dorsiflexor strength relative to plantar flexor strength may increase risk for shin splints (Gehlsen and Seger, 1980). Arch or shin taping, use of shock-absorbing insoles (Thacker et al., 2002), and use of arch supports or orthotics in street shoes to try to control excessive pronation (Michael and Holder, 1985) can also sometimes provide relief. For many dancers, technique modification involving maintaining turnout at the hips to limit pronation versus using the foot inverters to "hold up the arches" is essential for successful rehabilitation and prevention of shin splint recurrence. However, if despite conservative treatment pain persists or becomes severe, it is important that the dancer see a physician to rule out more serious conditions such as a stress fracture or compartment syndrome.

Exertional Compartment Syndromes of the Lower Leg

Compartment syndromes involve an activity-related marked increase in pressure within one or more of the compartments of the lower leg, producing pain and potentially interfering with the blood flow to the muscles so that they do not receive adequate oxygen (Blackman, 2000; Martens et al., 1984). While in the more common chronic or recurrent form (Geary and Kelly, 1997) the pressures drop rapidly when exercise stops, in rare instances and for reasons poorly understood, the condition progresses to an acute form in which pressures continue to increase and then stay elevated. If the rise is severe enough

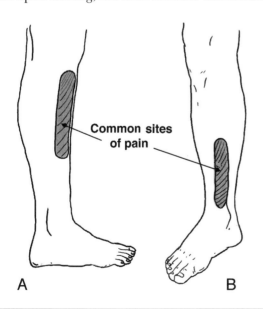

FIGURE 6.47 Pain associated with shin splints thought to reflect involvement of the (A) tibialis anterior and (B) tibialis posterior, flexor hallucis longus, or soleus.

and stays elevated long enough, it can lead to death of the involved muscle tissue and injury to the nerves unless the compartment is decompressed via surgical opening of the fascia (Mercier, 1995; Whiting and Zernicke, 1998). Although this condition occurs infrequently in dancers (Lokiec, Siev-Ner, and Pritsch, 1991), dancers should be aware of it because it can be a medical emergency with permanent dire consequences if medical treatment is not pursued quickly.

Recurrent compartment syndromes are classically associated with leg pain described as ill-defined deep cramping, aching, or burning that generally has a characteristic point of onset relative to exercise intensity or duration and that classically disappears shortly after activity is stopped. Some individuals, however, primarily experience ankle weakness, the inability to control the ankle when fatigued, and numbness of the foot. Shortly after exercise, a tenderness and tenseness over the muscle mass of the involved compartment may be present. For example, the anterior compartment is the compartment most commonly involved, and the condition may be evidenced by

weakness of ankle-foot dorsiflexion and toe extension; pain in the anterior compartment when the toes are extended; diminished sensation of the first dorsal web space; and tenseness, swelling, and tenderness in the anterior compartment (Geary and Kelly, 1997; Korkola and Amendola, 2001; Leach and Corbett, 1979) as shown in figure 6.48. When compartment syndromes are suspected, techniques can be used to allow pressures in the desired compartments to be measured during exercise.

Unfortunately at this time, there has been little success with conservative treatment (Martens et al., 1984); and common recommendations are to adjust training to a level below the level where pain and pressure become evident or to have surgery. Surgical approaches are directed at cutting the fascia in various ways so that pressures are prohibited from rising to dangerous levels, and these approaches have a reported high success rate.

Stress Fractures of the Lower Leg and Foot

The risk of lower leg and foot stress fractures can also be increased by factors that tend to heighten

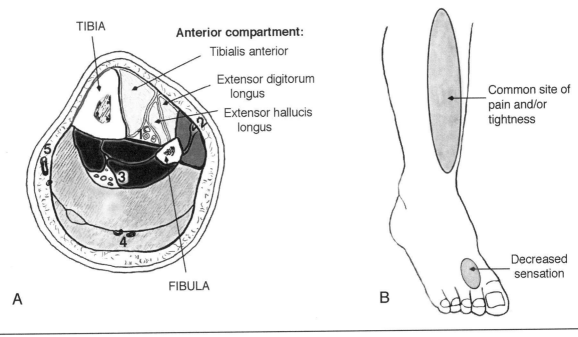

Associated nerves and blood vessels:

1 Anterior tibial artery,deep peroneal nerve

2 Superficial peroneal nerve

3 Posterior tibial artery

4 Small saphenous vein, sural nerve

5 Great saphenous vein, saphenous nerve

FIGURE 6.48   Exertional compartment syndrome of the lower leg involving the anterior compartment (right foot). (A) Transverse section of the lower leg showing the anterior compartment, and (B) common complaints.

the stress borne by these bones during activity, such as muscle fatigue or muscle weakness (Brukner, Bradshaw, and Bennell, 1998; Couture and Karlson, 2002; Hockenbury, 1999), a pes cavus foot type (Nigg, Nursae, and Stefanyshyn, 1999), and a pes planus foot type and other factors associated with excessive pronation (Hughes, 1985; Matheson et al., 1987; Taunton, Clement, and Webber, 1981). Studies of military recruits and runners suggest that factors related to excessive pronation are particularly important predisposing factors for stress fractures.

A **stress fracture** can occur in any of the bones of the lower leg or foot. In ballet dancers, the most common site is the metatarsals (Brukner et al., 1996), and the metatarsal most commonly affected is the second metatarsal, at its base (Harrington et al., 1993; O'Malley et al., 1996; Sammarco, 1982), as seen in figure 6.49. According to one study of elite ballet students, 45% of stress fractures occurred in the metatarsals, followed by 26% in the fibula, 13% in the tibia, and 3% in the cuboid (Lundon, Melcher, and Bray, 1999). Another study of professional ballet dancers showed 63% of stress fractures in the metatarsals and 22% in the tibia.

A stress fracture is generally associated with pain and tenderness, localized to the site of the fracture, that is aggravated by weight bearing or impact. The pain typically has a gradual onset and initially is often a low-grade aching associated with certain movements (such as jumps) or the duration of dance (e.g., the dancer hurts toward the end of class or rehearsal). However, if not heeded and dance is continued, the pain may progress such that it becomes more severe and more persistent and is more easily initiated. Abnormal changes often do not show up on an X ray for at least two weeks (Brukner, 2000), although other diagnostic techniques such as bone scans and magnetic resonance imaging can be helpful for establishing a definitive diagnosis at a much earlier stage (Hutchinson, Cahoon, and Atkins, 1998).

A cornerstone to successful treatment for a stress fracture is to temporarily unload and in some cases immobilize the bone sufficiently to allow completion of the remodeling process so that the bone is stronger and better able to handle loads (Hershman and Mailly, 1990). The limitation of activity necessary to achieve a pain-free situation will vary greatly by the site, severity, and length of injury. For example, a small stress fracture that is treated very early may require discontinuing only high-impact movements such as jumps and using viscoelastic inserts to reduce shock. In contrast, a more serious or long-standing stress fracture or a stress fracture in a site such as the tibia, noted for poor healing, may require not only total temporary stopping of dance but also immobilization with a brace, a wooden-soled shoe, crutches, or casting to even allow pain-free walking (Martire, 1994). Electrical stimulation may also have a positive effect on stimulating osteoblasts to lay down new bone (Brukner, 2000).

When healing is sufficient, a very gradual and progressive resumption of impact activity is initiated. There are many different approaches, but one approach is to have the athlete pain free 10 to 14 days before this gradual reintroduction begins (Matheson et al., 1987). Reintroduction of activity on an alternate-day basis may be beneficial, as rest days have been shown to reduce stress fracture incidence. Although the goal is to remain pain free, even well-designed progressions often have points at which bone pain recurs. If this should happen, an often effective approach is to rest one to two days until no pain occurs with walking and then resume activity at the pace below the level at which pain occurred (Brukner, 2000).

During rehabilitation, other stress fracture risk factors should also be addressed, including pain-free strengthening of associated muscles for better shock absorbency, correction of any underlying technique issues such as excessive pronation, stretching of the triceps surae if inadequate dorsiflexion is present, and addressing hormonal and dietary factors as discussed in chapter 1, if indicated. Adequate correction of risk factors is important not only to promote successful full return to dance but also to prevent recurrence. One study of stress fractures in

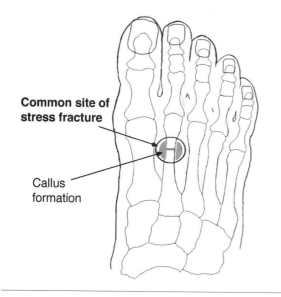

Common site of stress fracture

Callus formation

FIGURE 6.49 Common site of stress fractures in dancers (right foot, superior view).

professional dancers reported eight refractures out of the original 51 dancers studied (O'Malley et al., 1996). To have another stress fracture occur after prolonged rehabilitation not only is very discouraging for the dancer but also may jeopardize the dancer's career.

Impingement Syndromes of the Ankle

With pointing and flexing of the foot, the talus changes its position in the mortise. With the extreme range of motion utilized in dance, the talus can come into contact with the tibia either anteriorly or posteriorly; this contact is termed anterior or posterior impingement.

Anterior Ankle Impingement   When the ankle-foot is dorsiflexed as in walking, the front of the lower tibia normally is accommodated by a depression, called a sulcus, on the talar neck. However, with the extreme dorsiflexion used in dance, such as in demi-plié, some dancers can reach a point where the tibia actually comes directly in contact with the talus, and this contact between the bones is termed **impingement.** With repetitive impingement the bone itself can respond to the trauma by producing small outgrowths (osteophytes or bone spurs). These osteophytes then make impingement occur at an earlier degree of dorsiflexion, causing larger osteophytes and a vicious cycle (Hamilton, 1988). Anterior impingement tends to occur in sports involving jumping, and it is seen more commonly in male versus female dancers, perhaps due to the greater jumping demands that tend to be imposed on men.

Dancers with **anterior impingement syndrome** will often complain of dull, chronic aching anterior ankle pain that tends to be exacerbated with ankle-foot dorsiflexion. They will also commonly note that there is a decrease in the depth of their plié, and that they are stopping because of discomfort or the feeling of a block on the front of the ankle, well before they feel a stretch in their calf. Tenderness and swelling may also be present in this anterior aspect of the ankle (Hardaker and Moorman, 1986). Suspected anterior ankle impingement syndrome can be confirmed by the presence of exostoses where the front of the talus makes contact with the front of the tibia on X rays.

Recommended symptomatic treatment for this condition includes anti-inflammatory medications and a decrease in ankle-foot dorsiflexion through consciously making the plié shallower and using heel lifts (bilaterally) in street shoes (Malone and Hardaker, 1990), and if possible in dance shoes (e.g., jazz shoes). Unlike many other injury situations in which increasing strength and flexibility can

improve the condition, this is often not the case with impingement; and forced stretching of the calf to try to improve the plié depth will generally only aggravate the condition. While reduction in inflammation and technique modifications may sometimes offer some relief, if and when symptoms become severe enough to limit dance to an unacceptable degree, surgery is usually recommended to excise the exostoses. Although this is the only definitive treatment, in some cases exostoses recur, and repeat excision may be required, usually within three to four years (Hardaker, 1989).

Posterior Ankle Impingement and the Os Trigonum Syndrome   In contrast to anterior impingement syndrome, posterior impingement has a unique high occurrence in dance, probably due to the repetitive use of extreme ankle-foot plantar flexion. For the female ballet dancer, there is a particularly strong emphasis on maximizing plantar flexion to meet both aesthetic and biomechanical criteria in pointe work; and not surprisingly, posterior impingement occurs more frequently in female versus male ballet dancers. During extreme plantar flexion, the posterior portion of the talus is brought in approximation with the posterior aspect of the tibia. The posterior border of the talus has a lateral tubercle (termed the posterior process) that normally fuses with the body of the talus between 9 and 12 years of age (Kadel, Micheli, and Solomon, 2000). However, in some cases this process fails to fuse and remains a separate little bone, termed an **os trigonum.**

While some hold that the os trigonum actually represents a stress fracture of the posterior process (Howse and Hancock, 1988) and that failure to unite is due to repetitive trauma, this conjecture is still an area of controversy. If such an os trigonum is present, or if the posterior process is particularly long (Stieda's process), adjacent capsular and synovial tissues can be readily compressed or impinged against the posterior tibia as shown in figure 6.50. With repeated pinching and inflammation, these soft tissues can become thickened and fibrotic. In addition to posterior ankle impingement syndrome, this condition is called by other names including os trigonum syndrome.

With **posterior ankle impingement syndrome,** pain, tenderness, and sometimes swelling are generally experienced at the back of the ankle, behind the lateral malleolus and deep to the Achilles tendon. This pain tends to be reproduced when the ankle-foot is brought into full plantar flexion, such as in tendu, demi-pointe, and particularly pointe work. Passive plantar flexion may also reveal the feeling of a sudden hard stop or endpoint to the motion. A decreased passive range in plantar flexion and

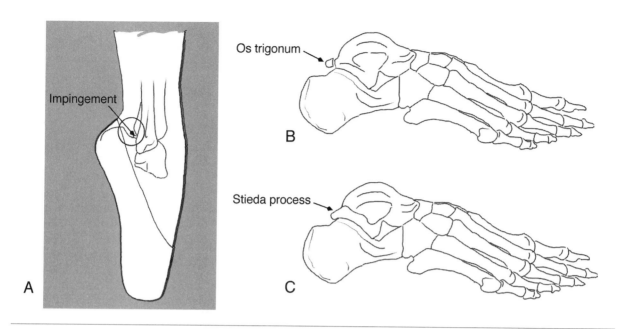

FIGURE 6.50   (A) Posterior ankle impingement risk increased by the presence of (B) an os trigonum or (C) a Stieda's process (right foot, lateral view).

decreased ability to point the foot (active range of plantar flexion) are often present. Weakness and numbness may also be present. The diagnosis is often confirmed by taking a lateral-view X ray with the ankle-foot in full plantar flexion, such as in standing on pointe or demi-pointe, and the use of other imaging techniques to ascertain soft tissue involvement (Hamilton, 1988; Marotta and Micheli, 1992).

Recommended initial treatment often includes nonsteroidal anti-inflammatories; limitation of ankle-foot plantar flexion in dance to pain-free limits; and physical therapy that includes an emphasis on restoring plantar flexion range of motion, strengthening ankle-foot plantar flexors, and correction in any technique errors such as insufficient use of the stirrup muscles on relevé, which could decrease stress to this area. If there is dual involvement of the flexor hallucis longus, which runs in the groove just medial to the posterior process, this condition must also be addressed. However, the great plantar flexion demands of dance training may preclude successful conservative treatment; and if conservative treatment fails, surgical excision of the os trigonum is often recommended for professional and other serious dancers and tends to allow the ability to return to full dance (Brodsky and Khalil, 1986; Marotta and Micheli, 1992; Weiker, 1988).

Sesamoiditis

Sesamoiditis is an inflammation of the sesamoid bones that lie within the flexor hallucis brevis.

Because of their location under the base of the big toe, these sesamoids bear large forces during movements such as going on demi-pointe or pushing off or landing in jumps. Hard floors, a cavus foot type (Spilken, 1990), and bunions have also been conjectured to increase the risk for sesamoiditis. In the case of inflamed bunions, the tendency to shift the body weight more medially or laterally to reduce pain puts undue stress on the sesamoid on that side, while with more advanced bunions, the angulation of the first metatarsal can displace the sesamoids from their normal positioning and produce excessive stress.

Sesamoiditis is characterized by pain and tenderness over one or both sesamoids (figure 6.51). One can readily locate the sesamoids by passively hyperextending the great toe (MTP extension) with one hand and palpating them over the head of the first metatarsal with the opposite hand. Pain is also often reproduced or exaggerated with demi-pointe.

In addition to the normal ice, anti-inflammatory medications, and physical therapy modalities, treatment is aimed at reducing the load borne by the sesamoids through various padding techniques. However, sesamoiditis often is difficult to treat in dancers because the hallux extension accompanying movements such as demi-pointe and the push-off in locomotor movements tends to aggravate the condition. Restriction of demi-pointe in and out of dance class and use of a felt pad in relatively rigid athletic shoes, or taping to limit hallux hyperextension (Dyal and Thompson, 1997), can sometimes be temporarily used to control symptoms. However if pain persists, other potential causes of pain including stress fractures or fractures of the sesamoids need to be evaluated. Detecting a fracture or stress fracture is not always as straightforward as one would expect, as approximately 6% to 30% of feet have sesamoids that are in two or more parts from birth (bipartite or multipartite sesamoids) and are asymptomatic (Van Hal et al., 1982). Sequential X rays or a bone scan, or both, are often used to help make the specific diagnosis. In some persistent cases, surgical treatment is required (Conti and Wong, 2001).

Morton's Neuroma

Morton's neuroma involves fibrous tissue growth that is fusiform in shape (small benign tumor) and forms around a sensory nerve in the foot as shown in figure 6.52. This nerve runs between each pair of metatarsals and divides near the end of the metatarsals to go to the adjacent side of the two adjacent toes. Due to their placement between the metatarsals and the ligaments that run between the metatarsals, these sensory nerves are vulnerable to being compressed, and it is this repeated compression that is believed to cause the outgrowth of the lining of the nerve and neuroma (Dyal and Thompson, 1997). This neuroma occurs most commonly in the third interspace (space between the third and fourth metatarsals), followed in frequency by the second interspace (between the second and third metatarsals).

Morton's neuroma is associated with a sharp, electrical or burning pain in the region of the third (or second) interspace that may radiate down into the adjacent toes. Numbness or tingling may also be evident in the adjacent toes. This pain can generally be reproduced or aggravated by gently squeezing the forefoot together or pressing between the appropriate metatarsals. The pain is also often aggravated by the wearing of narrow shoes, particularly narrow high-heeled shoes, and relieved by removal of the shoes.

Treatment involves anti-inflammatories and wearing wider dance and street shoes. Use of a felt metatarsal pad behind the metatarsal heads (Ryan and Stephens, 1987) and correction of any technique problems that could aggravate the condition, such as shifting the weight too far laterally, can sometimes alleviate compression. Interestingly, this condition often tends to clear after several years even when no treatment is performed (Weiker, 1988), but pain can often be limiting and surgery is often curative (Brown, 2002, personal correspondence).

Summary

The ankle joint proper is a hinge joint that primarily allows dorsiflexion and plantar flexion. This joint has a very strong bony structure that is enhanced by strong medial and lateral collateral ligaments. Below and in front of the ankle joint, the subtalar joint and transverse tarsal joints can contribute slightly more

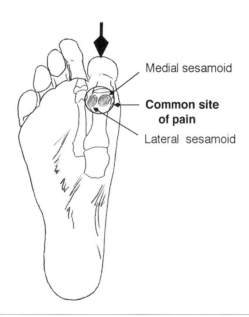

FIGURE 6.51   Common site of pain and tenderness with injury to the sesamoids (right foot, inferior view).

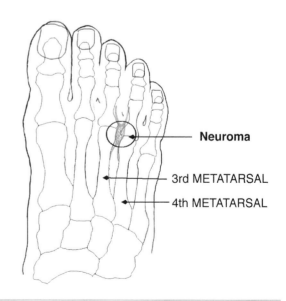

FIGURE 6.52   Morton's neuroma (right foot, superior view).

plantar flexion and dorsiflexion to that of the ankle, and also provide inversion, eversion, abduction, and adduction of the foot. Together, these joints give rise to the combined motions of pronation and supination. The MTP joints are condyloid joints that allow for flexion, extension, slight abduction, and slight adduction of the toes on the metatarsals. The IP joints are hinge joints that allow for flexion and extension of the digits themselves. These additional joints have capsules and ligaments that provide additional stability to the ankle-foot complex. Twelve extrinsic and 12 intrinsic muscles function to move the ankle and foot. The extrinsic muscles have a logical arrangement in which the anterior muscles cause dorsiflexion, the lateral muscles eversion, the posterior muscles plantar flexion, and the medial muscles inversion of the ankle or foot. Many of these muscles also have additional actions, important for movement, placement of body weight, and support of the arches of the foot.

The arrangement of the arches in the foot is important for meeting the diverse challenges of stability and mobility. When the foot is supinated, the foot becomes stable with a formed medial lon-gitudinal arch, allowing effective initial contact of the foot with the ground or propulsion of the body. In contrast, pronation unlocks the foot, making it more flexible and allowing it to function to accommodate uneven surfaces and absorb the large forces associated with movement. Individual differences in arch formation will influence the ability of the foot to meet these opposite demands, with the rigid pes cavus foot type being stable but less able to absorb shock, and the flexible pes planus foot type being able to easily accommodate but less stable.

While pronation and supination are normal foot movements, excessive amounts of either can easily lead to foot problems. Learning to use optimal placement of the foot when standing, desired knee-foot alignment, and coordinated use of the stirrup muscles can aid with the development of desired dance skill. Similarly, strengthening of the stirrup and other key muscles and stretching to achieve both adequate dorsiflexion and plantar flexion can help enhance ankle and foot function and prevent injuries. If an injury does occur, effective treatment and aggressive rehabilitation are vital to prevent recurrence or instability and to allow successful return to dance.

Study Questions and Applications

1. Locate the following bones and bony landmarks on a skeleton or drawing of a skeleton and then on your own body: (a) tibia and medial malleolus, (b) fibula and lateral malleolus, (c) talus, (d) calcaneus, (e) cuboid, (f) navicular and tubercle of the navicular, (g) cuneiforms, (h) metatarsals and their base and head, (i) phalanges (proximal, middle, and distal), (j) sesamoids.

2. Draw the following muscles on a skeletal chart, and use an arrow to indicate the line of pull of each muscle. Then, next to each muscle, list its actions: (a) gastrocnemius, (b) soleus, (c) tibialis anterior, (d) tibialis posterior, (e) peroneus longus, (f) peroneus brevis.

3. Locate the following muscles on your partner or your own body, perform or have your partner perform actions that these muscles produce, and palpate their contraction during these movements: (a) gastrocnemius, (b) soleus, (c) tibialis anterior, (d) extensor hallucis longus, (e) extensor digitorum longus, (f) tibialis posterior, (g) flexor hallucis longus, (h) flexor digitorum longus, (i) peroneus longus, (j) peroneus brevis.

4. Observe a partner while standing from behind, and note the position of his or her rearfoot. How would the presence of rearfoot valgus or varus tend to influence foot pronation?

5. Explore the concept of coupling of the leg and the foot. Note what happens to the lower leg when the foot inverts and when it everts. Now, note what happens to the foot when the lower leg internally rotates and when it externally rotates. How could this coupling relate to turnout and pronation in dance?

(continued)

Study Questions and Applications   (continued)

6. Working with a partner, demonstrate the fundamental movements of the ankle and foot (plantar flexion, dorsiflexion, inversion, and eversion) including both of the following:

    a. When the foot remains in contact with the ground (closed kinematic chain)

    b. When the foot is free to move (open kinematic chain)

    Then, provide a movement from dance that exemplifies each of these variations on the fundamental ankle-foot movements, and describe the primary muscle group and sample muscles used to effect these motions.

7. Demonstrate two exercises for stretching the gastrocnemius and soleus. How does the position of the knee influence which muscle is being emphasized?

8. Describe how one could attempt to correct a dancer who excessively pronates during a plié through making changes at the foot, the lower leg, and the hip. What approach do you think would be best over the long term and why?

9. Provide a strengthening exercise that would be the most important for preventing the following injuries, and identify the muscle group targeted by the exercise: (a) lateral ankle sprain, (b) shin splints.

10. A dancer has been having a difficult time performing multiple outside turns and keeps falling back out of her turns. Her teacher has noted that she is rolling out on her foot as the turn progresses. Describe how the stirrup muscles of the foot could relate to this technique error and how these muscles could be used to help correct the problem. Identify appropriate strength exercises that could be utilized to prevent the undesired motion of the foot and three cues that could be utilized to try to implement the desired technique adjustments.

CHAPTER SEVEN

The Upper Extremity

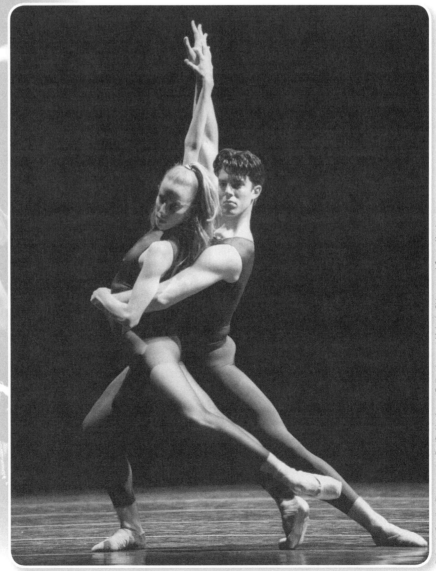

© Angela Sterling Photography. Pacific Northwest Ballet dancers Melanie Skinner and Casey Herd.

The upper extremities, which include the shoulder girdle, arms, and hands, are the focus of this chapter. The arms are intimately connected with movements of the shoulder girdle, and hence the shoulder girdle and shoulder joint should be viewed together as a functional unit. The shoulder girdle and shoulder joint are characterized by a design that maximizes mobility necessary for reaching, grasping, lifting, and throwing. Such mobility makes specific muscle strength development and activation important for correct technique and injury prevention. In dance, very specific and subtle use of the arms is often required to meet the aesthetics of the school of dance or a given choreographer. In some cases, stylized use of the arms is vital to portray the desired emotional quality of the dance movement. Furthermore, with partnering, the arms often come into play to help support a partner, as well as help express a relationship between the dancers as shown in the photo on the previous page.

The upper extremity will be covered all together in this chapter. While some sports such as throwing sports, swimming, weightlifting, and gymnastics place great stress on the upper extremity, dance tends to place greater stress on the lower extremity. Hence, the upper extremity is not covered in as much detail in this text as the lower extremity, and the emphasis is on the shoulder joint. Topics covered will include the following:

- Bones and bony landmarks of the shoulder complex
- Joint structure and movements of the shoulder girdle
- Joint structure and movements of the shoulder
- Description and functions of individual muscles of the shoulder complex
- Alignment and common deviations of the shoulder complex
- Shoulder mechanics
- Muscular analysis of fundamental shoulder movements
- Special considerations for the shoulder complex in dance
- Other joints of the upper extremity
- Description and functions of selected individual muscles of the elbow
- Structure and movements of the radioulnar joints
- Key considerations for the upper extremity in whole body movement

- Conditioning exercises for the upper extremity
- Upper extremity injuries in dancers

Bones and Bony Landmarks of the Shoulder Complex

The shoulder complex involves the clavicle (collarbone), scapula (shoulder blade), and humerus (upper arm bone) on each side of the body. When seen from above, the clavicle is shaped like a stretched-out "S" that is convex anteriorly in its medial portion and concave anteriorly in its lateral portion (figure 7.1). The medial end (sternal end) of the clavicle is slightly expanded, while the lateral end (acromial end) is markedly expanded and flattened; these shapes aid in articulation with the respective adjacent bones.

The scapula is a large, triangular-shaped flat bone that normally glides on the posterior rib cage. This bone has many muscles attached to it, and many different bony landmarks are used to clarify the sites of attachment of these muscles. As can be seen in figure 7.2, the scapula has three borders, the medial (vertebral), lateral (axillary), and superior borders, as well as three angles (the **superior, inferior,** and **lateral angles**). It also has two surfaces; the anterior surface, which lies close to the ribs, is termed the **costal surface,** while the posterior surface is termed the **dorsal surface.** The costal surface is slightly hollowed to form the **subscapular fossa.** The dorsal surface is divided by a large **spine,** into a smaller but deeper hollowed area above the spine called the **supraspinous fossa** and a larger but shallower **infraspinous fossa** below the spine. The spine of the scapula ends laterally in a large flattened process called the **acromion process** (G. *akron,* tip + *omos,* shoulder). This process articulates with the clavicle to form the acromioclavicular joint. The lateral

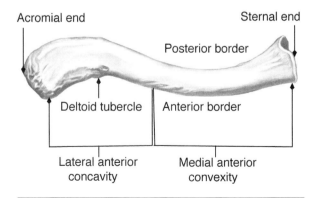

FIGURE 7.1   The clavicle (right clavicle, superior view).

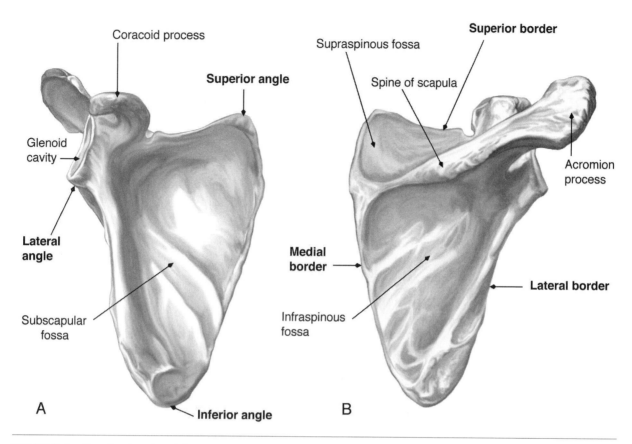

FIGURE 7.2   Bony landmarks of the scapula (right scapula). (A) Costal surface, (B) dorsal surface.

angle of the scapulae ends before it creates a true angle in an indented area termed the **glenoid fossa** (G. *glenoeides,* socket of joint) or **glenoid cavity.** Just medial to this glenoid cavity, a large, beaklike process projects forward from the scapulae termed the **coracoid process** (G. *korakodes,* like a crow's beak). This process is a site for attachments of key muscles and ligaments for the shoulder and shoulder girdle. With their positioning above the glenoid cavity, the acromion process and coracoid process also help protect the shoulder joint.

The humerus is a long bone with a cylindrical body that changes in form at both ends and is quite parallel in structure to the femur (figure 7.3). At the proximal end, the humerus expands to form the rounded head, the medial portion of which articulates with the glenoid cavity to form the shoulder joint. Slightly distal to this articular surface and on the anterior aspect of the humerus lie the more medially placed **lesser tubercle** and the more laterally placed **greater tubercle.** The greater tubercle can be palpated just below the acromion process when the arm is hanging by the side in an internally rotated position. The slight narrowing of the humerus between the articular surface of the head

of the humerus and the greater and lesser tubercles is termed the **anatomical neck** of the humerus, while the region where the head and tubercles join to the body of the humerus is termed the **surgical neck.** The lesser and greater tubercles are separated from each other by a groove called the **intertubercular sulcus** or **groove.** The tendon of the long head of the biceps brachii muscle lies within this groove. You can generally palpate this groove with two fingers below the acromion process when your arm is fully externally rotated with the elbow by your side. If you follow the intertubercular groove down the arm, its lateral portion leads to a roughened prominence about halfway down the humerus called the **deltoid tuberosity** (the site of attachment for the distal deltoid muscle). The landmarks of the distal end of the humerus will be described later with the elbow joint.

Joint Structure and Movements of the Shoulder Girdle

The shoulder girdle can be pictured as an incomplete ring formed by the two clavicles and two scapulae (figure 7.4). Anteriorly, the paired clavicles

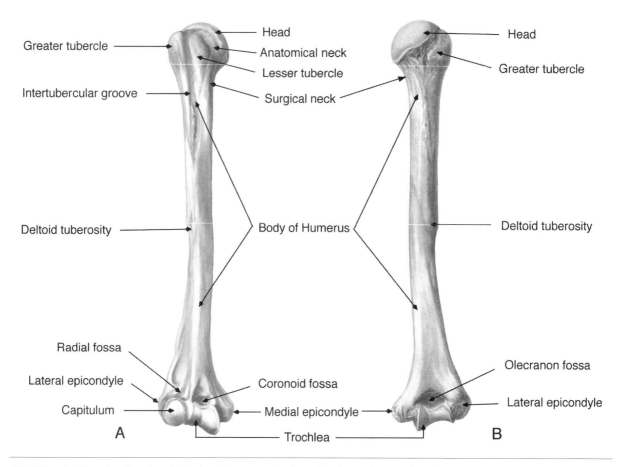

FIGURE 7.3   Bony landmarks of the right humerus. (A) Anterior view, (B) posterior view.

join onto the sternum and cartilage of the first rib (first costal cartilage) to form the **sternoclavicular joint** (figure 7.4B). The sternoclavicular joint can be classified as a saddle joint (Moore and Agur, 1995), and it contains a fibrocartilage articular disc that divides the joint cavity into two and serves as a shock absorber. This small joint serves as the only bony attachment of the entire upper extremity to the axial skeleton. However, the sternoclavicular joint is surrounded by a fibrous capsule that is reinforced by various strong ligaments, and it is a stable joint that is rarely dislocated.

Laterally, the paired clavicles join with the acromion processes of their respective scapulae at the **acromioclavicular joints** (figure 7.4A). This gliding joint (Moore and Agur, 1995) is surrounded by a capsule and reinforced by various strong ligaments. These ligaments limit the range of motion possible at this joint and prevent the clavicle and acromion process from being pulled apart (Kreighbaum and Barthels, 1996). However, they are not very effective at preventing the clavicle from riding over the top of the acromion when a lateral blow is applied to the shoulder, and two nearby strong ligaments (the

trapezoid and conoid coracoclavicular ligaments) further connect the clavicle to the scapula via the coracoid process and provide indirect support to help prevent such a dislocation.

Functionally, movements of the sternoclavicular joint, and to a lesser degree the acromioclavicular joint, contribute to movements of the shoulder girdle. It is less complex to describe the combined movements of these joints in terms of the resultant movements of the scapulae that they create. These movements of the scapulae on the thorax are sometimes referred to as occurring at the **scapulothoracic "joints,"** although these are not true joints. Possible movement pairs of the scapulae include scapular elevation-depression, abduction-adduction, and upward rotation-downward rotation (figure 7.5) (Smith, Weiss, and Lehmkuhl, 1996).

With **elevation,** the scapula as a whole moves upward toward the ear. This movement occurs when the shoulders are shrugged, such as in jazz isolations. **Depression** is the opposite movement to elevation and involves movement of the scapula as a whole downward. During standing, gravity will tend to depress the scapulae when the elevators of

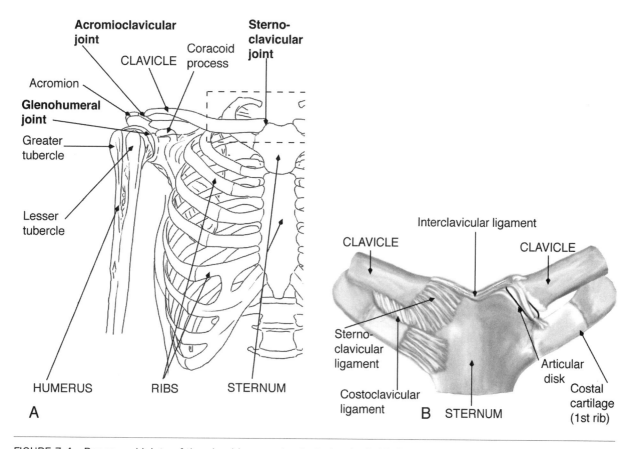

FIGURE 7.4   Bones and joints of the shoulder complex (anterior view). (A) Glenohumeral joint, acromioclavicular joint, and sternoclavicular joint, (B) more detailed view of sternoclavicular joint.

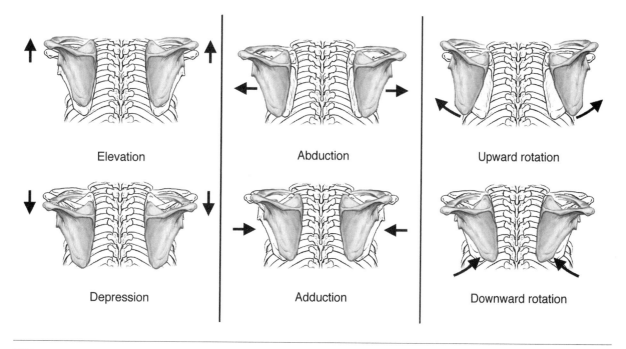

FIGURE 7.5   Movements of the scapulae.

the scapulae stop contracting. However, when the body weight is supported on the hands with the arms down by the sides, the scapular depressors must be contracted to hold the scapulae down to prevent undesired elevation and to stabilize the scapulae so the trunk can be elevated. **Abduction** or protraction of the scapulae involves movement of the scapulae away from the spinal column and each other, sometimes referred to in dance as "widening the shoulder blades." **Adduction** or retraction of the scapulae is the opposite motion to abduction, and it involves bringing the scapulae toward each other and toward the spinal column; in dance this is sometimes referred to as "pinching the shoulder blades." **Upward rotation** of the scapula involves turning the scapula about an axis through the spine of the scapula such that the glenoid cavity moves upward while the inferior angle moves laterally and anteriorly on the thorax. This motion is hard to produce in isolation but is an essential movement that accompanies overhead movements of the arm. The opposite motion, **downward rotation,** involves a downward rotation of the glenoid cavity. It can be exaggerated through bringing the hand behind the low back. Some authors also include tilts, not further described in this text.

Note that these movements do not have an exact counterpart in the lower extremity because the bones of the pelvis cannot move independently. However, the movements of the pelvic girdle as a whole relative to the spine at the lumbosacral joint serve a similar function of adjusting the relationship of the pelvis so that movements of the femur are fostered. However, one important difference is that due to the relatively rigid linking of the pelvis posteriorly with the sacrum (at the sacroiliac joints), movement of one side of the pelvis will have a direct effect on the opposite side. In contrast, due to the fact that the scapulae are only linked muscularly posteriorly, movement of one scapula and arm can occur independently with minimal effect on the position or function of the opposite arm.

Joint Structure and Movements of the Shoulder

While the movements of the scapula just described position the scapula to help facilitate movements of the arm, the movement of the arm actually occurs at the joint formed between the glenoid cavity of the scapula and the head of the humerus. This joint is called the shoulder joint or **glenohumeral joint** (see figure 7.4A). The glenohumeral joint is a triaxial,

ball-and-socket joint. Both the head of the humerus and glenoid cavity are covered with articular cartilage. This glenoid cavity is quite shallow, and only about one-fourth to one-third of the almost hemispherical head of the humerus makes contact with the glenoid cavity (Frankel and Nordin, 1980). Furthermore, the shape of the glenoid cavity is less curved and more elongated (pear shaped) while the head of the humerus is more spherical (Caillet, 1996), so that rather than simple rotation occurring about a fixed axis, the axis of rotation shifts as the shoulder joint moves and the humeral head moves linearly (translates) as well as rotates (Hall, 1999). So, the shoulder joint represents a very complex and much less stable ball-and-socket joint that is more prone to dislocation and recurrent subluxation than the hip joint.

As with other ball-and-socket joints, the shoulder joint has three degrees of motion: flexion-extension approximately in the sagittal plane (figure 7.6A), abduction-adduction approximately in the frontal plane, and external-internal rotation approximately in the transverse plane (figure 7.6B). The specialized terms of horizontal abduction and horizontal adduction (figure 7.6C) are given to movements of the arm occurring in a horizontal plane with the arm at shoulder height. Also, as with the hip joint, many movements that occur during dance do not occur in exact anatomical planes. Some texts give a specialized term, **scaption,** to one of these types of movement. Because the glenoid cavity faces slightly anterior to the frontal plane, some authors hold that a more natural movement is abduction in the plane of the scapula, or scaption, rather than pure abduction in the frontal plane. Another unique term used at the shoulder joint is elevation. The term elevation is generally used to describe movement of the humerus away from the side in any plane. Note that this is a movement of the arm, in contrast to the "elevation" used to describe movement of the scapula. Many of the movements at the glenohumeral joint can occur through a very large range of motion, and the shoulder joint is the most freely movable joint in the human body (Hall, 1999).

Shoulder Joint Capsule and Key Ligaments

The shoulder joint is surrounded by a sleevelike fibrous capsule lined with synovial membrane that is attached proximally to the perimeter of the glenoid cavity. Distally it is attached to the anatomical neck of the humerus, except medially, where it is attached slightly lower on the humerus. The capsule is loose; for example, when the arm is down by the side, there are hanging folds in the inferior portion of

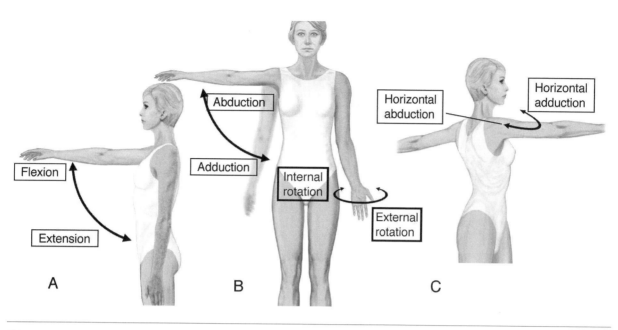

FIGURE 7.6   Movements of the shoulder joint. (A) Flexion-extension, (B) abduction-adduction and external rotation–internal rotation, (C) horizontal abduction–horizontal adduction.

the medial capsule that allow the arm to be raised to the side and overhead. This looseness of the capsule potentially allows 1 to 2 inches (2.5-5 centimeters) of separation between the humerus and scapula (Hamilton and Luttgens, 2002). However, despite its limitations, the capsule is still vital for joint stability (Warner et al., 1990).

The joint capsule is reinforced by various ligaments as seen in figure 7.7. Anteriorly, the capsule is strengthened by the **superior, middle,** and **inferior glenohumeral ligaments.** These ligaments help prevent excessive displacement or translation of the humerus, particularly in a forward direction. The inferior glenohumeral ligament has been shown to be a particularly key restraint for preventing anterior translation of the head of the humerus in higher ranges of shoulder abduction (Warner et al., 1990), while the middle and superior glenohumeral ligaments resist anterior translation in lesser degrees of abduction. The superior glenohumeral ligament is also vital for preventing inferior translation of the head of the humerus (Cavallo and Speer, 1998).

Superiorly, the capsule is reinforced by the **coracohumeral ligament** (not shown). This ligament runs from the base of the coracoid process into the capsule to attach to the greater tubercle and lesser tubercles of the humerus, helping to form a tunnel between these tubercles within which the tendon of the long head of the biceps brachii lies. A related ligament, the **coracoacromial ligament,** spans between the coracoid process and the acromion

process of the scapula to help form an arch above the head of the humerus. This arch, composed of the coracoid process, coracoacromial ligament, and acromion process, is termed the **coracoacromial arch** (Lyons and Orwin, 1998). The coracohumeral and coracoacromial ligaments help prevent superior dislocation of the humerus, and the latter can be implicated in shoulder impingement. Classically, **shoulder impingement syndrome** refers to a pinching of soft tissues, such as the supraspinatus tendon or subacromial bursa, between the head of the humerus and the overlying coracoacromial arch.

Specialized Structures of the Shoulder Joint

Various specialized structures are associated with the shoulder that provide additional joint stability and aid with shoulder function. These structures include the glenoid labrum and various bursae.

Glenoid Labrum

The **glenoid labrum** is a rim of fibrocartilage located at the perimeter of the glenoid cavity (figure 7.7B), functionally similar to the one found in the hip joint (acetabular labrum). The glenoid labrum is thicker around the circumference than centrally. It serves to increase the size and depth of the glenoid cavity, increasing the superior inferior diameter by 75% and anterior-posterior diameter by 50% (Richards, 1999). In addition, the labrum provides a site for attachments of the joint capsule, the glenohumeral ligaments, and various tendons including the long

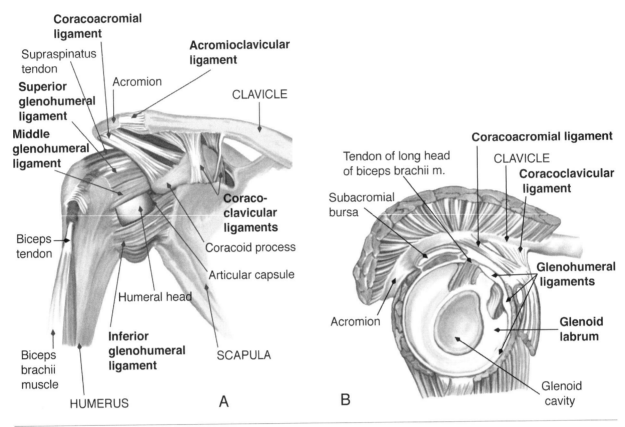

FIGURE 7.7 The shoulder joint (right shoulder). (A) Anterior view, (B) lateral view with head of the humerus removed.

head of the biceps brachii. The glenoid labrum has been found to be vital for joint stability, as well as increasing the surface area of contact of the head of the humerus (Levine and Flatlow, 2000) and serving to add a cushioning effect against the impact associated with forceful movements of the arms.

Bursae

There are various bursae located about the shoulder joint. Two bursae that lie deep to the deltoid muscle and separate and cushion the muscles of the rotator cuff from the overlying coracoacromial arch and sometimes become inflamed are the **subdeltoid** and **subcoracoid bursae**. These bursae are located close to each other, are sometimes connected, and hence are often jointly referred to as the **subacromial bursa** (see figure 7.7B) (Mercier, 1995).

Muscles

Limited stability is provided by the glenoid labrum and bony articulation, and the glenohumeral ligaments and capsule primarily provide restraints at the extremes of motion; hence, the muscles surrounding the joint are essential for providing stabilization

(particularly in midrange shoulder motion), as well as movement (Park, Blaine, and Levine, 2002). This stabilization role can be demonstrated by the fact that when these shoulder muscles are paralyzed, the shoulder joint will tend to sublux, with the weight of the hanging arm separating the head of the humerus from the glenoid cavity. This observation has led to the expression that the shoulder is a "muscle-dependent joint." Hence adequate strength, balanced strength, and coordinated activation of the muscles of this region are essential for optimal function and injury prevention.

Description and Functions of Individual Muscles of the Shoulder Complex

There are many ways in which the muscles of the shoulder complex can be organized and described. This text will use a functional approach, dividing the muscles into three groups—the scapular muscles, the rotator cuff, and other major glenohumeral muscles. (See Individual Muscles of the Shoulder Complex, pp. 381-394.)

Individual Muscles of the Shoulder Complex

Scapular Muscles

The **scapular muscles** are comprised of six muscles that connect the scapula with the axial skeleton (skull, spine, and rib cage). These muscles work both to hold the scapula in place (stabilization) and to generate the movements of the scapula previously described. The importance of these muscles is often underestimated, but they play a vital role in functional movements involving the arms. For example, the scapular elevators are essential for effective lifting movements, the scapular depressors for effectively pushing downward, the scapular abductors for forward pushing movements, the scapular adductors for pulling movements, the scapular upward rotators for elevating the arm overhead, and the scapular downward rotators for forceful adduction of the arm.

The scapular muscles can be subdivided into those located anteriorly and posteriorly. The anterior muscles are the subclavius, pectoralis minor, and serratus anterior. Due to its small size and negligible contribution to scapular motions, the subclavius will not be further discussed. However, the latter two muscles connect the scapula to the front of the rib cage and share the ability to pull the scapula anteriorly (scapular abduction). The posterior scapular muscles are the trapezius, rhomboids, and levator scapulae. These muscles serve to connect the scapula to the spine and are all capable of pulling the scapula posteriorly (scapular adduction). The individual scapular muscles also have other actions that are described next and summarized in table 7.1 on page 384.

Attachments and Primary Actions of Trapezius

Muscle	Proximal attachment(s)	Distal attachment(s)	Primary action(s)
Trapezius (trah-PEE-zee-us)	Base of skull Ligament of neck C7-T12 spinous processes	Outer third of clavicle Upper acromion Upper spine of scapula	Upper: Scapular elevation Scapular upward rotation Scapular adduction Middle: Scapular adduction Lower: Scapular depression Scapular upward rotation Scapular adduction

Trapezius

The **trapezius** (*trapezion,* irregular four-sided figure) is a superficial paired muscle located on the back of the neck and upper back on each side of the midline (figure 7.8). The paired relatively flat muscles derive their name from the fact that together they form a diamond shape, or trapezium. Due to its shape the trapezius is also sometimes called the "shawl" muscle (Smith, Weiss, and Lehmkuhl, 1996). Because of the different line of pull and innervation of different portions of the trapezius, it can be divided into three parts—the upper, middle, and lower trapezius. To visualize the actions, it is helpful to mentally construct the line of pull of these three portions. The upper portion courses downward and laterally; the middle portion is more horizontal; and the lower portion courses upward and outward. As a whole the trapezius tends to produce upward rotation and adduction of the scapula.

To understand how the trapezius could produce upward rotation, it is important to note that it attaches onto the upper

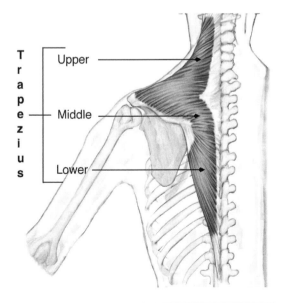

FIGURE 7.8 Superficial posterior scapular muscles: trapezius (left scapula).

scapula, forming a force couple (chapter 2) whereby the lower portion of the trapezius pulls down on the medial border of the scapula as the upper portion of the trapezius pulls up on the acromion. The combined action is to produce rotation in the same direction, that is, upward rotation of the scapula. Upward rotation of the scapula accompanies elevation of the arm, and so the trapezius works whenever the arm is raised to the side (shoulder abduction) and in higher ranges of raising the arm to the front (shoulder flexion). The lower portion of the trapezius also tends to depress the scapula, and this function is often emphasized in dance training. In contrast, the upper portion of the trapezius tends to elevate the scapula (as when you shrug your shoulders) and provides support for the distal end of the clavicle and acromion process of the scapula. This latter function comes into play when a heavy weight, such as a suitcase, is held in the hand (Hamilton and Luttgens, 2002). In such cases, tension and often fatigue or soreness are experienced in the upper trapezius. This latter lateral support function may also affect shoulder posture, in that weakness of the trapezius can result in a lower and forward position of the point of the affected shoulder consequent to the downward rotation of the scapula from the weight of the hanging arm and abduction of the scapula (Smith, Weiss, and Lehmkuhl, 1996). When the head is free to move, the upper trapezius can assist with extension, lateral flexion, and rotation (to the opposite side) of the cervical spine.

Palpation: Place the fingertips of your left hand just behind the outer third of the right clavicle with your right arm held overhead. You can feel the upper trapezius contracting when you bring your right shoulder up toward your ear (scapular elevation) in this position. On a partner, you can palpate the lower portion of the trapezius contracting medial to the inferior angle of the scapula when your partner actively pulls his or her shoulder blades together and down (scapular depression and adduction). You can see and feel the entire muscle contracting when your partner pulls the shoulder blades together with the elbows just above shoulder height (scapular adduction).

Attachments and Primary Actions of Levator Scapulae

Muscle	Proximal attachment(s)	Distal attachment(s)	Primary action(s)
Levator scapulae (le-VA-tor SKAP-u-le)	C1 to C4 or C5 transverse processes (from spine to superior border)	Medial border of scapulae	Scapular elevation Scapular downward rotation Assists with scapular adduction

Levator Scapulae

The **levator scapulae** (L. *levator,* a lifter) is a small muscle that lies beneath the upper trapezius and extends from the upper cervical vertebrae to the upper medial border of the scapula (figure 7.9). Hence, its line of pull is almost vertical, with a slight lateral progression as it runs inferiorly. Thus, its primary action is elevation of the scapula with the ability to contribute slightly to scapular adduction. During standing, due to the weight of the arm pulling downward on the glenoid cavity, contraction of the levator scapulae also tends to produce downward rotation of the scapula (Rasch and Burke, 1978; Smith, Weiss, and Lehmkuhl, 1996). Loss of the levator scapulae is associated with the shoulder's being depressed, especially when the trapezius is also not functioning adequately. Loss of both of these muscles is associated with a marked slope of the shoulders and a thin neck. When the head is free to move, the levator scapulae can produce lateral flexion and rotation (to the same side) of the cervical spine.

Palpation: Because the levator scapulae lies beneath the trapezius and commonly works in conjunction with the trapezius, it is difficult to palpate in isolation.

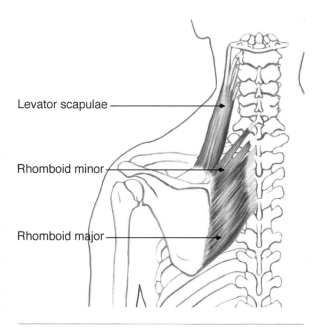

FIGURE 7.9   Deep posterior scapular muscles: levator scapulae and rhomboids (left scapula).

Attachments and Primary Actions of Rhomboids

Muscle	Proximal attachment(s)	Distal attachment(s)	Primary action(s)
Rhomboids (ROM-boidz)	C6 or C7 to T4 or T5 spinous processes	Medial border of scapula from spine to inferior angle	Scapular elevation Scapular adduction Scapular downward rotation

Rhomboids

The rhomboid (*rhomboid,* diamond shaped) muscles are paired muscles that lie beneath the trapezius muscle (figure 7.9). They derive their name from the fact that they are shaped like a rhombus (G. *rhombos*). They are often divided into the thinner and weaker upper portion called the **rhomboid minor** and the thicker and stronger lower portion called the **rhomboid major.** The rhomboids run down and outward from the spine to the medial border of the scapulae. Their line of pull is similar to that of the trapezius except that their attachment is onto the medial border of the scapula. Hence, when the rhomboids contract they produce downward rather than upward rotation of the scapula. They can also elevate and adduct the scapula. Since downward rotation of the scapula accompanies shoulder adduction or extension, the rhomboids are used when these motions are performed forcefully or against resistance.

Palpation: Have a partner stand with the back of his or her right hand against the low back, and place your fingers under the lower portion of the medial border of the right scapula. Then have your partner lift his or her right hand backward (away from the back), and you will feel the rhomboids contract to produce the necessary downward rotation of the scapula.

Attachments and Primary Actions of Serratus Anterior

Muscle	Proximal attachment(s)	Distal attachment(s)	Primary action(s)
Serratus anterior (ser-A-tus an-TEER-ee-or)	Lateral, outer aspect of lower 8 to 9 ribs	Inferior angle and medial border of scapula	Scapular abduction Scapular upward rotation Scapular depression (lower fibers)

Serratus Anterior

The **serratus anterior** (*serratus,* saw) is named for its serrated, or saw-toothed, anterior margin and can be seen on the anterolateral rib cage below the armpit. It actually runs from the lower eight or nine ribs under the scapula to attach onto the inferior angle and the entire length of the medial margin of the scapula (figure 7.10). Part of the anterior portion of this muscle is covered by the pectoralis major, and posteriorly it is covered by the scapula. The lowest four or five slips interdigitate with fibers of the external oblique abdominal muscles. The serratus anterior effectively attaches the medial scapula to the front of the thorax. The line of pull makes it an effective abductor of the scapula. The lower fibers of the serratus anterior and the trapezius also form a force couple for upward rotation of the scapula (figure 7.11), used when one lifts the arms to the side (shoulder abduction) and to the front (shoulder flexion). In addition, the lower fibers of the serratus anterior can assist with scapular depression.

Functionally, the serratus anterior has been shown to be active in pushing movements,

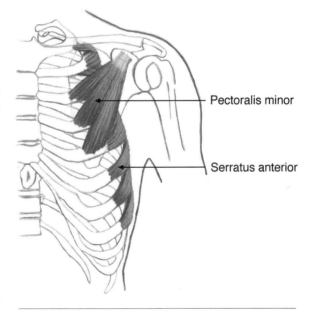

FIGURE 7.10   Anterior scapular muscles: serratus anterior and pectoralis minor (left shoulder, deep view).

"forward-reaching" movements, throwing, and bench pressing. In pushing movements, the serratus anterior is vital for stabilizing the scapula so that the pressure on the outstretched hand does not cause the scapula to move posteriorly. It has also been shown to be very active during swimming (Nuber et al., 1986). The importance of the serratus anterior for upward rotation is demonstrated by the difficulty of raising the arms above shoulder height (or even the inability to do so) when this muscle is paralyzed. Loss of this muscle is also associated with backward projection of the medial border of the scapula (termed "winging" of the scapula) and inadequate forward movement of the scapula on the thorax (scapular abduction), when the arm is reached forward (Smith, Weiss, and Lehmkuhl, 1996).

Palpation: Stand with the fingertips of the left hand placed on the anterolateral aspect of the ribs, just in front of the lower portion of the lateral border of the scapula. The serratus anterior can be felt contracting under the fingertips when the right arm is raised forward to an overhead position.

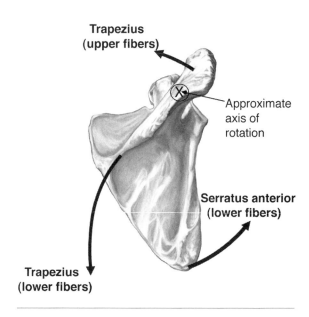

FIGURE 7.11   Force couple formed by the trapezius and serratus anterior for upward rotation of the scapula (right scapula, posterior view).

Attachments and Primary Actions of Pectoralis Minor

Muscle	Proximal attachment(s)	Distal attachment(s)	Primary action(s)
Pectoralis minor (pek-to-RA-lis MY-nor)	Outer surface of 2nd or 3rd to 5th ribs	Coracoid process of scapulae	Scapular abduction Scapular downward rotation Scapular depression

Pectoralis Minor

As its name implies, the **pectoralis minor** (*pectus,* chest, breast + *minor,* lesser) is a small muscle located in the upper area of the chest (deep to the pectoralis major) as seen in figure 7.10. The pectoralis minor runs from three upper ribs upward and outward to attach to the coracoid process of the scapula. Due to this line of pull it tends to produce abduction, depression, and downward rotation of the scapula. However, it probably acts more for fine motor control and to assist the previously described scapular

TABLE 7.1   Summary of Actions of the Scapular Muscles

	Scapular upward rotation	Scapular downward rotation	Scapular elevation	Scapular depression	Scapular abduction	Scapular adduction
Upper trapezius	x		x			x
Middle trapezius						x
Lower trapezius	x			x		x
Levator scapulae		x	x			x
Rhomboids		x	x			x
Serratus anterior	x			x (lower fibers)	x	
Pectoralis minor		x		x	x	

muscles rather than as a prime mover (Moseley et al., 1992). Posturally, it can pull the medial border and particularly the inferior angle of the scapula away from the rib cage (winged scapula). However, if the scapula is adequately stabilized, contraction of the pectoralis minor will instead act to elevate the upper ribs and contribute to a desired lifted posture of the chest (Hamilton and Luttgens, 2002), often used in dance as part of presentation.

Rotator Cuff

The **rotator cuff** is composed of the four muscles that span between the scapula and the proximal humerus—the supraspinatus, infraspinatus, teres minor, and subscapularis. These muscles form a hood or cuff about the head of the humerus, and their tendons actually merge into the capsule of the shoulder joint and provide a net compression force that helps stabilize the head of the humerus in the glenoid cavity. In addition to helping keep the humerus in contact with the glenoid cavity, these muscles produce rotation that is often used to position the head of the humerus or the arm to facilitate optimal mechanics. Some of these muscles also have other actions at the shoulder joint.

Attachments and Primary Actions of Supraspinatus

Muscle	Proximal attachment(s)	Distal attachment(s)	Primary action(s)
Supraspinatus (soo-prah-spi-NAH-tus)	Inner portion of supraspinous fossa of scapula	Top of greater tubercle of humerus	Shoulder abduction Stabilization of shoulder

Supraspinatus

The **supraspinatus** is a small but important muscle located under the upper portion of the trapezius. As its name implies, the supraspinatus (*supra,* above + *spin,* spine) originates above the spine of the scapula, in the supraspinous fossa, and runs laterally to attach to the top of the humerus (figure 7.12). Near the tip of the shoulder, the muscle fibers of the supraspinatus converge to form a short tendon that courses underneath the acromion and adheres to the capsule. This tendon is a common site of injury. The superior line of pull of this muscle allows the supraspinatus to be an effective abductor of the shoulder, and it appears to be particularly important for initiation of abduction when the arms are down by the sides (Hall-Craggs, 1985). Despite its relatively small size, the supraspinatus has been shown to be able to effect full abduction of the arm when the deltoid is not operative and is estimated to normally contribute about 50% of the torque for abduction when the deltoid is operative (Smith, Weiss, and Lehmkuhl, 1996). Its line of pull also allows this muscle to help pull the humerus into

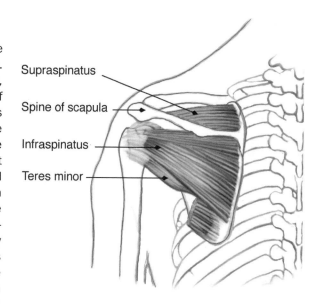

FIGURE 7.12   Posterior view of rotator cuff muscles: supraspinatus, infraspinatus, and teres minor (left shoulder, deep view).

the glenoid cavity and help prevent downward dislocation of the shoulder.

Palpation: Place the fingertips of your left hand just above the spine of the right scapula. The supraspinatus can be felt contracting under the trapezius when you quickly and repetitively raise your arm just about 8 inches (20 centimeters) to the side (shoulder abduction).

Attachments and Primary Actions of Infraspinatus and Teres Minor

Muscle	Proximal attachment(s)	Distal attachment(s)	Primary action(s)
Infraspinatus (in-frah-spi-NAH-tus)	Medial portion of infraspinous fossa of scapula	Middle of greater tubercle of humerus	Shoulder external rotation Stabilization of shoulder Shoulder horizontal abduction Component of SIT force couple
Teres minor (TE-reez MY-nor)	Dorsal aspect of lateral border of scapula	Lower greater tubercle and adjacent shaft of humerus	Same as infraspinatus

Infraspinatus and Teres Minor

The infraspinatus and teres minor are functionally aligned muscles located on the back of the scapula (figure 7.12). As its name implies, the **infraspinatus** (*infra,* below) runs from below the spine of the scapula (medial infraspinatus fossa) laterally and upward to attach onto the posterior aspect of the greater tubercle on the back of the humerus. The **teres minor** (*teres,* round + *minor,* lesser) runs from the inferolateral border of the scapula to attach just below the infraspinatus on the greater tubercle and on the adjacent shaft of the humerus. As with the supraspinatus, the tendons of these muscles are adherent with the shoulder capsule and are important for preventing dislocation of the shoulder. These muscles produce external rotation and horizontal abduction of the shoulder. They also participate in the SIT force couple, a force couple vital for proper shoulder mechanics that is discussed later in this chapter.

Palpation: While sitting in a chair, lean your torso forward about 30° and place the fingers of your left hand just to the outside of the lateral margin of the right scapula while your right arm is hanging straight down toward the floor. The infraspinatus and teres minor can be palpated when the arm is slowly externally rotated in this position. The infraspinatus can be felt contracting just below the lateral portion of the spine of the scapula. The teres minor can be felt contracting just below the infraspinatus.

Attachments and Primary Actions of Subscapularis

Muscle	Proximal attachment(s)	Distal attachment(s)	Primary action(s)
Subscapularis (sub-scap-u-LAR-is)	Costal surface of scapula (subscapular fossa)	Lesser tubercle of humerus	Shoulder internal rotation Stabilization of shoulder Component of SIT force couple

Subscapularis

As its name suggests, the **subscapularis** (*sub,* under + *scapular,* scapula) is located deep to the scapula (figure 7.13). The subscapularis courses from its attachment on the costal surface of the scapula laterally, upward, and slightly forward to attach onto the lesser tubercle of the humerus. This more anterior attachment on the humerus allows the subscapularis to function as an internal rotator of the humerus and to help prevent anterior subluxation or dislocation of the humerus. This muscle can also help prevent inferior dislocation of the shoulder. Due to the slope of the glenoid cavity, downward dislocation of the humerus requires lateral movement of the head of the humerus, which can be prevented by muscles with a horizontal line of pull including the subscapularis, infraspinatus, and teres minor (Hamilton and Luttgens, 2002). In addition, the subscapularis plays a part in the SIT force couple.

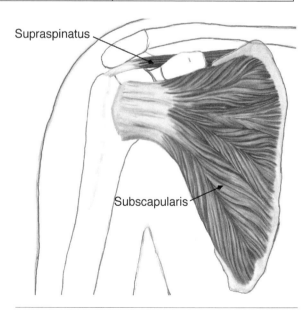

FIGURE 7.13 Anterior view of rotator cuff muscles: subscapularis and supraspinatus (right shoulder, deep view of costal surface of scapula).

Palpation: While sitting in a chair, lean your torso forward until it is about horizontal and gently place the fingers of your left hand in your right lower armpit against the costal surface of the scapula while your right arm is hanging straight down toward the floor. The subscapularis can be palpated contracting when the arm is slowly internally rotated in this position.

Other Major Glenohumeral Muscles

The remaining group of muscles generally spans greater distances and connects the humerus to the trunk (including the ribs, clavicle, sternum, scapula, spine, and pelvis). These muscles are important for generating the large movements of the arm. In addition to the muscles described in this section, the biceps brachii and the long head of the triceps brachii also cross the shoulder joint, but they will be discussed later in this chapter in connection with the elbow.

Attachments and Primary Actions of Pectoralis Major

Muscle	Proximal attachment(s)	Distal attachment(s)	Primary action(s)

Pectoralis major (pek-to-RA-lis MAY-jer)	Inner two-thirds of anterior aspect of clavicle
	Sternum
	Costal cartilage of ribs 1 or 2 to 6 or 7 near sternum
		Intertubercular groove of humerus extending down from tubercles about 3 inches (7.6 centimeters)	Clavicular:
			  Shoulder flexion
			  Shoulder abduction above 90°
			  Assists with shoulder adduction (lower ranges)
			Sternal:
			  Shoulder extension
			  Shoulder adduction
			Both:
			  Shoulder horizontal adduction
			  Shoulder internal rotation

Pectoralis Major

As its name suggests, the **pectoralis major** (*pect,* breast, chest + *major,* larger) is a large superficial muscle located on the chest, and its development can be readily observed in the area of the upper chest (figure 7.14). The lower border of the lateral pectoralis major forms a muscular fold (anterior axillary fold) and most of the front wall of the armpit. The pectoralis major runs from the inner clavicle, sternum, and costal cartilages of the upper six ribs laterally to attach via a flat tendon to the intertubercular groove of the humerus. Near the distal attachment, the muscle twists clockwise 180°, leaving it twisted when in anatomical position but untwisted when the arms are raised overhead. The muscle is fan shaped and is often divided into a clavicular or upper and a sternal or lower portion. The line of pull of the clavicular portion is such that it can produce shoulder flexion and aid with shoulder adduction. However, when the arm is above shoulder height, the line of pull moves above the axis of the shoulder joint and it can then produce the opposite action of shoulder abduction (chapter 2, figure 2.9, p. 44). In contrast, the proximal attachment of the sternal portion is low enough that it tends to consistently produce shoulder adduction (and shoulder extension if the arm is in a starting position where it is raised to the front). All portions of the pectoralis major tend to produce horizontal adduction and assist with shoulder internal rotation. The pectoralis major as a whole is particularly important in

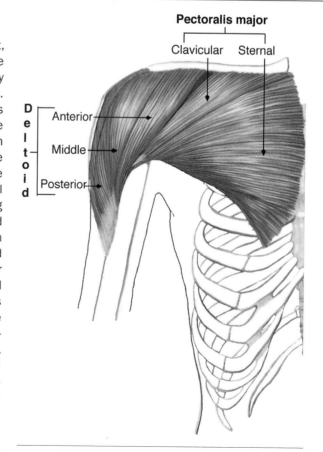

FIGURE 7.14   Anterior view of superficial shoulder muscles: pectoralis major and deltoid (right shoulder).

pushing, throwing, and punching movements (Hamilton and Luttgens, 2002). When the pectoralis major is missing, the arm can still be raised and lowered, but the power in shoulder flexion and extension is markedly diminished (Rasch and Burke, 1978).

Palpation: Use your left hand to pinch the fold of muscle that forms the front of the right armpit (axilla) while your right hand is placed on a stationary object such as a desk. You can feel the sternal head of the pectoralis major contracting under your fingers when you firmly press your right hand down onto the desk as if to extend the shoulder (isometric shoulder extension). To palpate the clavicular portion, move the fingers of your left hand just below the middle of the clavicle and your right hand under the desk. You can palpate the clavicular portion of the pectoralis major contracting when you firmly press your right hand upward against the desktop (isometric shoulder flexion).

CONCEPT DEMONSTRATION 7.1

Different Actions of Pectoralis Major

The differing functions of the clavicular and sternal portions of the pectoralis major can be demonstrated with the following exercise.

· **Shoulder flexion and extension.** Sit with your hands clasped at shoulder height with both elbows extended. Pull down with the right arm (shoulder extension) and up (shoulder flexion) with the left arm simultaneously, such that no net movement of the shoulders occurs. Note the lower sternal portion of the pectoralis major contracting on the right side of your chest and the upper clavicular portion of the pectoralis major contracting on the left side of your chest.

· **Shoulder horizontal adduction.** Press both hands and arms toward each other so that no net movement of the shoulder occurs (isometric horizontal adduction). Note the clavicular and sternal portions of the pectoralis major contracting on both the right and left sides of your chest.

Attachments and Primary Actions of Deltoid

Muscle	Proximal attachment(s)	Distal attachment(s)	Primary action(s)
Deltoid (DEL-toid)	Outer anterior aspect of clavicle Acromion of scapula Lower border of spine of scapula	Deltoid tuberosity of humerus	Anterior: Shoulder flexion Shoulder horizontal adduction Assists with shoulder internal rotation Middle: Shoulder abduction Shoulder horizontal abduction Posterior: Shoulder extension Shoulder horizontal abduction Assists with shoulder external rotation

Deltoid Muscle

The **deltoid** (*delta,* triangular) muscle is the superficial muscle that forms the round contour of the shoulder. As its name implies, it is triangular in shape (figure 7.15). The deltoid courses from the outer clavicle and acromion process and spine of the scapula downward and outward to attach onto the deltoid tuberosity located about halfway down on the lateral humerus. With its extensive proximal attachments, it crosses the joint in many ways and is best thought of functionally as three muscles—the anterior deltoid, middle deltoid, and posterior deltoid. The **anterior deltoid** traverses the front of the shoulder, and its lateral and downward course produces a line of pull allowing its primary actions of shoulder flexion and horizontal adduction (figure 7.14). It can also assist with abduction of the shoulder and probably internal rotation. The **middle deltoid** courses laterally over the top of the shoulder and then downward to attach onto the humerus, making it an important and powerful abductor of the shoulder (figure 7.15). Its activity increases progressively as the arm is raised and is greatest between 90° and 180° of shoulder abduction (Basmajian and DeLuca, 1985; Hamill and Knutzen, 1995), and the arm cannot be raised above shoulder height when this muscle is missing. The **posterior deltoid** crosses the back of the shoulder joint and can be thought of as having opposite actions to the anterior deltoid (figure 7.16). The posterior deltoid is an important shoulder extensor, and a loss of the ability to raise the arm backward above waist height tends to accompany loss of this muscle. The posterior deltoid also can

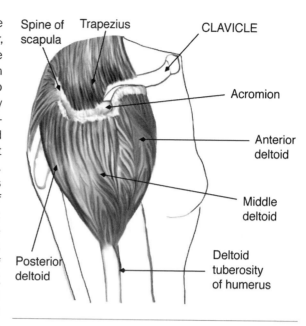

FIGURE 7.15   Lateral view of deltoid (right shoulder).

produce horizontal abduction, probably contributes slightly to shoulder external rotation, and helps prevent downward dislocation of the humerus.

Surprisingly, there is one movement in which the anterior and posterior deltoid can actually work together, and that is shoulder adduction. With shoulder adduction, their simultaneous synergistic contraction allows shoulder adduction while neutralizing out undesired other actions of shoulder flexion-extension, horizontal abduction-adduction, and external-internal rotation. In addition, the deltoid appears to function to help stabilize the shoulder joint, and often two or three parts of the deltoid tend to be active when the arm is moved, with greater activity in the portion of the muscle generating the desired movement (Rasch, 1989).

Palpation: The deltoid can easily be seen and palpated at the front, top, and back of the shoulder. Sit with the fingers of the left hand on the front of the right shoulder. You can feel the anterior deltoid contracting when you raise your right arm to the front slowly from low fifth (shoulder flexion). You can palpate the middle deltoid on the top of the shoulder just inferior to the tip of the acromion process when raising the right arm from low fifth to second position (involves shoulder abduction). The posterior deltoid can be felt contracting on the back of the shoulder when the right arm is raised backward (shoulder hyperextension).

Attachments and Primary Actions of Coracobrachialis

Muscle	Proximal attachment(s)	Distal attachment(s)	Primary action(s)
Coracobrachialis (kor-ah-ko-bra-kee-AL-is)	Coracoid process of scapula	Anteromedial aspect of middle of humerus	Shoulder flexion Shoulder adduction Shoulder horizontal adduction

Coracobrachialis

The **coracobrachialis** (*coraco,* coracoid + *brachi,* arm) is a small muscle located beneath the pectoralis major and anterior deltoid on the anteromedial aspect of the shoulder and arm. Its name describes its attachments, and it runs from the coracoid process of the scapula downward to attach to the anteromedial aspect of the humerus. It is pictured later in this chapter with the brachialis (see figure 7.42 on p. 417). The actions of the coracobrachialis include shoulder flexion and horizontal adduction, but due to its small size, its contribution is less significant than that of the pectoralis major or anterior deltoid. It can also work with other muscles to produce shoulder adduction.

Attachments and Primary Actions of Latissimus Dorsi

Muscle	Proximal attachment(s)	Distal attachment(s)	Primary action(s)
Latissimus dorsi (lah-TIS-i-mus DOR-see)	T6-L5 spinous processes Sacrum Crest of ilium Posterior aspect of lower 3 ribs	Lower intertubercular groove of humerus parallel to attachment of pectoralis major	Shoulder extension Shoulder adduction Shoulder horizontal abduction Shoulder internal rotation Depression of humerus

Latissimus Dorsi

The name of this muscle describes both its shape and location (*latissimus,* widest + *dorsi,* back), and it is the broadest muscle of the back and lateral thorax. The **latissimus dorsi** is located superficially, except where its upper portion is overlapped by the lower fibers of the trapezius, and laterally it helps form the back wall of the armpit (axilla). This very extensive muscle's proximal attachments include the lower spine, pelvis, and associated fascia (lumbodorsal fascia) as seen in figure 7.16. It runs upward and outward and then forward. Similarly to the pectoralis major, it twists 180° before attaching with a flat tendon to the anterior humerus, parallel to the attachment of the pectoralis major. Due to this anterior attachment it tends to produce shoulder internal rotation, as well as being a powerful extensor of the shoulder used in resisted "downward and backward pulling" motions of the arms, as in swimming, rowing, rope climbing, and pull-ups. When used in conjunction with the pectoralis major, the latissimus dorsi is also a powerful adductor of the arm (Hall-Craggs, 1985).

Due to its extensive bony and fascial attachments, the latissimus dorsi also serves an important function in stabilizing the trunk; and when the arms are fixed (closed kinematic chain movement), the distal attachment of the latissimus dorsi can aid with lifting the pelvis as in crutch walking, sitting push-ups, or dance floor work. Posturally, the latissimus dorsi can aid with depression of the humerus, and this function is sometimes emphasized in dance.

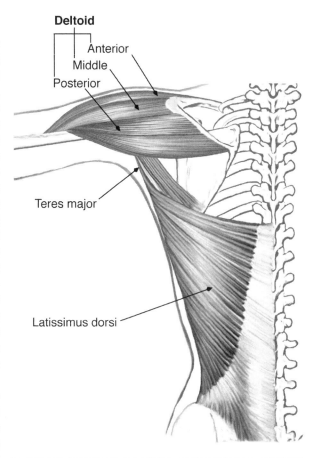

Deltoid
Anterior
Middle
Posterior
Teres major
Latissimus dorsi

FIGURE 7.16   Posterior view of superficial shoulder muscles: latissimus dorsi, teres major, and deltoid (left shoulder).

Loss of the latissimus dorsi is associated with forward displacement of the shoulder and loss of strength in downward movements of the arm against resistance.

Palpation: Place your left hand on a stationary object such as a desk, with the elbows slightly bent and the fingertips of your right hand about 8 inches (20 centimeters) below the back portion of your left armpit on your posterolateral rib cage. You can feel the latissimus dorsi contracting under your right hand when you press down firmly with your left hand (isometric shoulder extension).

Teres Major

The teres major (*teres,* round + *major,* larger) is similar in shape to the teres minor, only larger, hence its name teres "major." It runs from the lateral border of the lower scapula outward and upward to attach onto the anterior humerus (figure 7.16). When resistance must be overcome, the teres major comes into play and has the same actions as the latissimus major. Hence, it is sometimes called "the latissimus dorsi's little helper" (Rasch and Burke, 1978). When the arm is behind the back, the teres

Attachments and Primary Actions of Teres Major

Muscle	Proximal attachment(s)	Distal attachment(s)	Primary action(s)
Teres major (TE-reez MAY-jer)	Inferior angle of scapula	Medial lip of intertubercular groove	Shoulder extension Shoulder adduction Shoulder horizontal abduction Shoulder internal rotation (Depression of humerus)

major appears to assist with extension (hyperextension) and adduction, even when resistance is not present (Hamilton and Luttgens, 2002).

Palpation: Use the same movement as with the latissimus dorsi, only with the fingertips of your right hand placed just lateral to the inferior angle of the scapula. You can feel the teres major contracting under your right hand when you press down firmly with your left hand (shoulder extension).

Summary of Attachments and Actions of the Muscles of the Shoulder Complex

A summary of the proximal and distal attachments of the muscles of the shoulder complex—the scapular muscles, rotator cuff, and other glenohumeral muscles—is provided in table 7.2. Many of these muscles and their attachments are shown in figures 7.17, A and B, and 7.18, A and B. From these resources, deduce the line of pull and resultant possible actions of these muscles, and then check for accuracy by referring to figures 7.17C and 7.18C for the larger muscles responsible for the fundamental movements of the shoulder joint (e.g., "other glenohumeral muscles" category) and the primary action(s) column in table 7.2 for the scapular muscles and rotator cuff muscles. Note that figures 7.17 and 7.18 include the biceps brachii muscles and triceps brachii muscles to show their relationship to the glenohumeral joint. However, they are discussed later in this chapter with the elbow, and their attachments and actions are provided in table 7.6 (p. 420).

TABLE 7.2   Summary of Attachments and Primary Actions of the Muscles of the Shoulder Complex

Muscle	Proximal attachment(s)	Distal attachment(s)	Primary action(s)
Scapular muscles			

Trapezius (trah-PEE-zee-us)	Base of skull
	Ligament of neck
	C7-T12 spinous processes
		Outer third of clavicle
		Upper acromion
		Upper spine of scapula
			Upper: Scapular elevation
			   Scapular upward rotation
			   Scapular adduction
			Middle: Scapular adduction
			Lower: Scapular depression
			   Scapular upward rotation
			   Scapular adduction

Levator scapulae (le-VA-tor SKAP-u-le)	C1 to C4 or C5 transverse processes (from spine to superior border)	Medial border of scapula	Scapular elevation Scapular downward rotation Assists with scapular adduction
Rhomboids (ROM-boidz)	C6 or C7 to T4 or T5 spinous processes	Medial border of scapula from spine to inferior angle	Scapular elevation Scapular adduction Scapular downward rotation
Serratus anterior (ser-A-tus an-TEER-ee-or)	Lateral, outer aspect of lower 8 to 9 ribs	Inferior angle and medial border of scapula	Scapular abduction Scapular upward rotation Scapular depression (lower fibers)
Pectoralis minor (pek-to-RA-lis MY-nor)	Outer surface of 2nd or 3rd to 5th ribs	Coracoid process of scapulae	Scapular abduction Scapular downward rotation Scapular depression

(continued)

TABLE 7.2 Summary of Attachments and Primary Actions of the Muscles of the Shoulder Complex *(continued)*

Muscle	Proximal attachment(s)	Distal attachment(s)	Primary action(s)
Rotator cuff muscles			
Supraspinatus (soo-prah-spi-NAH-tus)	Inner portion of supra-spinous fossa of scapula	Top of greater tubercle of humerus	Shoulder abduction Stabilization of shoulder
Infraspinatus (in-frah-spi-NAH-tus)	Medial portion of infraspinous fossa of scapula	Middle of greater tubercle of humerus	Shoulder external rotation Stabilization of shoulder Shoulder horizontal abduction Component of SIT force couple
Teres minor (TE-reez MY-nor)	Dorsal aspect of lateral border of scapula	Lower greater tubercle and adjacent shaft of humerus	Same as infraspinatus
Subscapularis (sub-scap-u-LAR-is)	Costal surface of scapula (subscapular fossa)	Lesser tubercle of humerus	Shoulder internal rotation Stabilization of shoulder Component of SIT force couple
Other glenohumeral muscles			

Pectoralis major (pek-to-RA-lis MAY-jer)	Inner two-thirds of anterior aspect of clavicle
	Sternum
	Costal cartilage of ribs 1 or 2 to 6 or 7 near sternum
		Intertubercular groove of humerus extending down from tubercles about 3 inches (7.6 centimeters)	Clavicular:
			  Shoulder flexion
			  Shoulder abduction above 90°
			  Assists with shoulder adduction (lower ranges)
			Sternal:
			  Shoulder extension
			  Shoulder adduction
			Both:
			  Shoulder horizontal adduction
			  Shoulder internal rotation

Deltoid (DEL-toid)	Outer anterior aspect of clavicle
	Acromion of scapula
	Lower border of spine of scapula
		Deltoid tuberosity of humerus	Anterior:
			  Shoulder flexion
			  Shoulder horizontal adduction
			  Assists with shoulder internal rotation
			Middle:
			  Shoulder abduction
			  Shoulder horizontal abduction
			Posterior:
			  Shoulder extension
			  Shoulder horizontal abduction
			  Assists with shoulder external rotation

Coracobrachialis (kor-ah-ko-bra-kee-AL-is)	Coracoid process of scapula	Anteromedial aspect of middle of humerus	Shoulder flexion Shoulder adduction Shoulder horizontal adduction
Latissimus dorsi (lah-TIS-i-mus DOR-see)	T6-L5 spinous processes Sacrum Crest of ilium Posterior aspect of lower 3 ribs	Lower intertubercular groove of humerus parallel to attachment of pectoralis major	Shoulder extension Shoulder adduction Shoulder horizontal abduction Shoulder internal rotation Depression of humerus
Teres major (TE-reez MAY-jer)	Inferior angle of scapula	Medial lip of intertubercular groove	Shoulder extension Shoulder adduction Shoulder horizontal abduction Shoulder internal rotation (Depression of humerus)

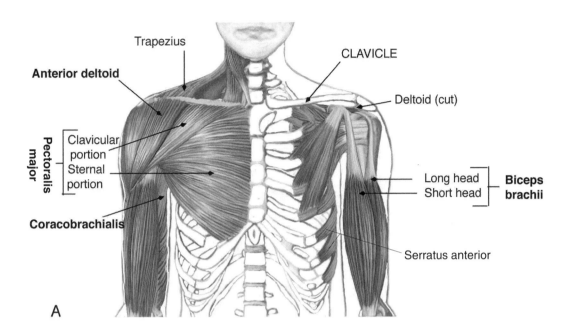

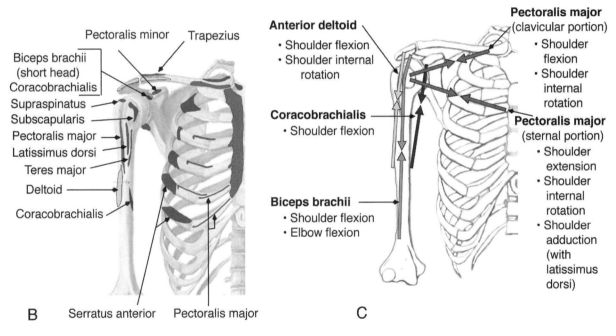

FIGURE 7.17 Anterior view of primary muscles acting on the shoulder complex. (A) Muscles, (B) attachments, (C) lines of pull and primary actions of selected glenohumeral muscles.

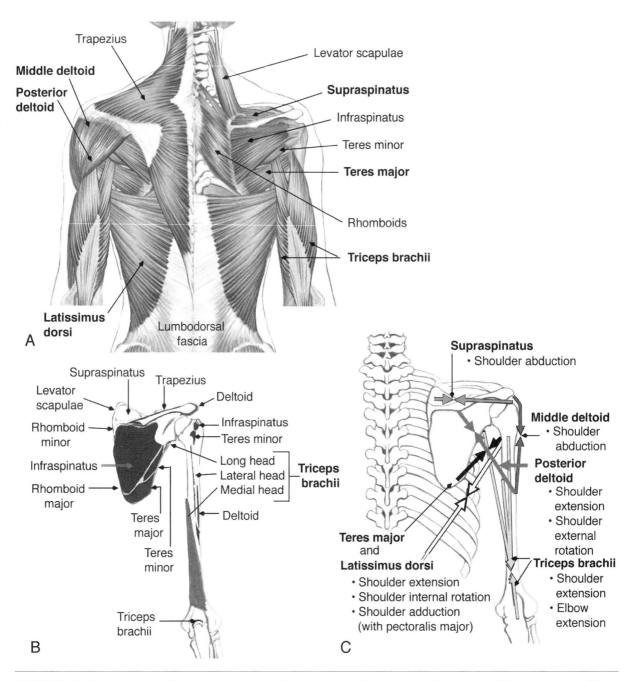

FIGURE 7.18   Posterior view of primary muscles acting on the shoulder complex. (A) Muscles, (B) attachments, (C) lines of pull and primary actions of selected glenohumeral muscles.

Alignment and Common Deviations of the Shoulder Complex

With normal alignment of the shoulder complex, the clavicles should be approximately horizontal, while the scapulae lie flat against the rib cage posteriorly and extend from approximately the second through the seventh rib (Rasch and Burke, 1978). Various deviations from this ideal alignment occur, including rolled shoulders and winged scapulae. Because these deviations are often associated with muscular imbalances, their occurrence is widespread, but they are generally more readily corrected than some of the deviations seen at other joints that involve more permanent structural elements.

Rolled Shoulders

Rolled shoulders involves a forward rounding of the shoulders that usually encompasses a position of excessive scapular abduction and often internal rotation of the humerus (figure 7.19). Correction requires strengthening of the scapular adductors (especially the trapezius and rhomboids) and in some cases stretching of the scapular abductors (particularly the pectoralis minor). When internal rotation of the humerus is also present, strengthen-

ing of the external rotators and stretching of the internal rotators (especially the pectoralis major and latissimus dorsi) can also be helpful. When rolled shoulders is a chronic posture, kyphosis is also frequently present, and strengthening of the upper back extensors (see chapter 3) is necessary. Several exercises for helping prevent and correct rolled shoulders are shown in figure 7.20 and described in tables 7.10 and 7.12. Double-shoulder external rotation (figure 7.20B and table 7.10I, progression 3, p. 439) offers a time-efficient exercise that combines shoulder external rotation, scapular adduction, and thoracic extension in a single exercise. The single-arm scarecrow (figure 7.20C and table 7.10H, variation 2, p. 439) provides an exercise for developing shoulder external rotation while maintaining torso stability when the arm is at shoulder height, a position commonly required in dance. Stretches to help improve rolled shoulders include the sitting arms overhead shoulder stretch (figure 7.20A and table 7.12C, variation 1, p. 450) and kneeling arms overhead shoulder stretch (described later in table 7.12B, p. 449), which emphasize stretching of the latissimus dorsi and lower fibers of the pectoralis major, as well as the wall shoulder stretch (described later in table 7.12D, p. 450), which emphasizes stretching of the anterior deltoid and the pectoralis major. In addition to exercises, cueing to bring the scapulae slightly down and together while one reaches the shoulders

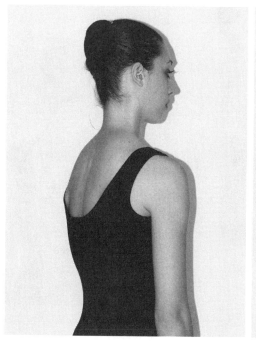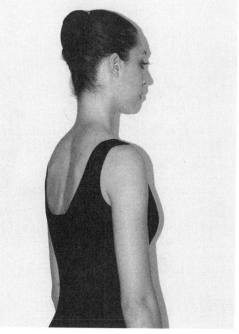

FIGURE 7.19   Shoulder alignment. (A) Rolled shoulders; (B) desired shoulder placement.

to the side can help correct rolled shoulders during static posture (figure 7.20D).

Winged Scapula

Since there is no bony attachment between the scapula and the back of the rib cage, the positioning of the scapula is greatly influenced by the relative strength, flexibility, and activation of the surrounding muscles, and particularly the muscles of scapular stabilization. In some cases, the medial border or the inferior angle of the scapula, or both, will project backward rather than lying flat against the rib cage in the desired manner (figures 7.21, A and B). This postural deviation, termed "winged scapula," can be caused by various muscular imbalances including a tight pectoralis minor or inadequate strength or activation of the serratus anterior or trapezius muscles. If the serratus anterior is not functioning synergistically with the trapezius, when the trapezius contracts to help upwardly rotate the scapulae during elevation of the arm, its unopposed action will tend to elevate the scapula, adduct the scapula, and produce a backward projection of the medial border

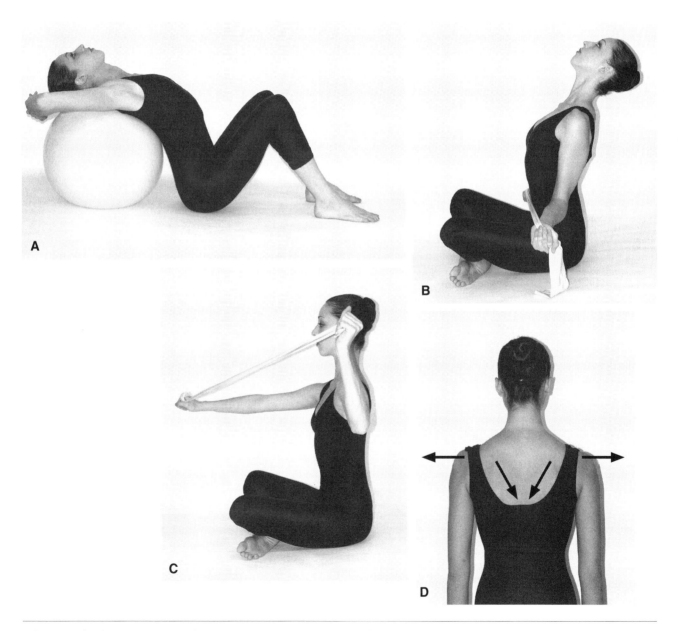

FIGURE 7.20   Sample exercises for improving rolled shoulders. (A) Sitting arms overhead shoulder stretch, (B) double-shoulder external rotation, (C) single-arm scarecrow, (D) technique cue to bring shoulder blades slightly down and together as the shoulders reach to the side.

DANCE CUES 7.1

"Pull Your Shoulders Back"

The directive to "pull your shoulders back" or "pull your shoulders back and lift your chest" is sometimes used by teachers in response to a student with rolled shoulders and functional kyphosis. One desired anatomical interpretation of this cue is to emphasize using the scapular adductors to help bring the shoulders to a desirable position and the thoracic spinal extensors to help correct the rounded upper back. However, some students respond to this directive by pinching the shoulder blades together (excessive scapular adduction) and "rib-leading" (excessive lumbar extension versus the desired upper thoracic extension). In such cases, cueing to "reach the shoulders to the side" as the upper back "lifts up toward the ceiling" or to bring the shoulder blades slightly down and together as the shoulders reach to the side may help achieve the desired placement.

of the scapula (figure 7.21C). The location of the serratus anterior (figure 7.21D) allows it to be a key abductor of the scapula, and hence this muscle can be recruited and strengthened by focusing on keeping the scapula "wide" (scapular abduction) versus allowing them to "pinch together" (scapular adduction) while performing a push-up (figure 7.21E) and by adding a little extra push at the top of the push-up, further abducting the scapulae (termed a "push-up plus," table 7.10A, variation 1, p. 434). In contrast, if the trapezius is not functioning properly, the unopposed action of the serratus anterior during elevation of the arm will tend to depress the scapula, abduct the scapula, and produce a backward projection of the inferior angle of the scapula (figure 7.21F). Since the trapezius' location allows it to function as a powerful adductor of the scapula (figure 7.21G), performing sitting rowing exercises with a band (figure 7.21H and table 7.10D, variation 2, p. 435) or prone rowing exercises with a weight while focusing on keeping the elbows at shoulder height as they are brought slightly behind the torso as the shoulder blades are pulled together (scapular adduction) can be used to recruit and strengthen this muscle. However, a winged scapula may also relate to other medical conditions including scoliosis or nerve injury, and if the winging is marked, evaluation by a physician is recommended.

Shoulder Mechanics

Coordinated movements between the shoulder girdle and arms are essential for optimal movement and preventing injuries. The scapulohumeral rhythm, combined external rotation with shoulder abduction, the SIT force couple, and synergies are utilized to foster this coordinated functioning of the shoulder complex.

Scapulohumeral Rhythm

Because the shallow glenoid cavity has contact with only about one-third of the surface area of the head of the humerus, the glenohumeral joint is rather susceptible to subluxation or dislocation. Hence, coordinated movements of the scapula are vital to position the glenoid cavity so that adequate contact with the head of the humerus can be maintained and the desired large range of movement of the humerus can be facilitated while the costal surface of the scapula is still kept in close contact with the thorax. This movement of the scapula also often works to help keep the prime movers at the shoulder joint at a favorable length to generate force and avoid active or passive insufficiency. This precisely coordinated, synchronous movement between the scapula and the humerus is termed the **scapulohumeral rhythm.**

This scapulohumeral rhythm involves characteristic scapular movements that supplement specific humeral movements. The most commonly discussed linking is the upward rotation of the scapula that accompanies shoulder abduction as shown in figure 7.22. After the initial movement of the arm that predominantly occurs at the glenohumeral joint, there is a linked relationship between upward rotation of the scapula and elevation of the arm such that after about 30° of abduction or 45° to 60° of flexion there is about 3° of glenohumeral motion for every 2° of scapular motion. So, with the total range of 180° flexion or abduction, the glenohumeral-to-scapula ratio is 2:1, that is, about 120° of glenohumeral motion and 60° of scapular motion as shown in figure

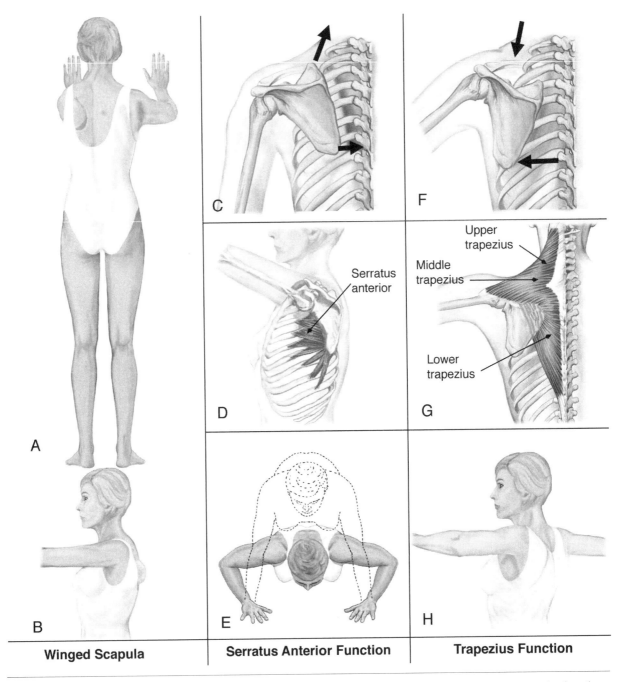

Winged Scapula   **Serratus Anterior Function**   **Trapezius Function**

FIGURE 7.21   Winged scapula. (A) Posterior view, (B) lateral view; due to (C)-(E) inadequate serratus anterior function or (F)-(H) inadequate trapezius function.

7.23 (Kreighbaum and Barthels, 1996; Levangie and Norkin, 2001). This upward rotation of the scapula not only allows the arm to reach a greater height but also moves the acromion process out of the way as the greater tubercle of the humerus approaches it with abduction (Kreighbaum and Barthels, 1996). This latter function is vital for preventing impingement.

Other commonly linked movements between the humerus and scapula in an upright position are listed in table 7.3. Note that there is a logical linking where opposite movements of a movement pair of the glenohumeral joint are linked with opposite movements of the scapula. For example, glenohumeral abduction is linked with scapular upward rotation, while glenohumeral adduction is linked with scapular downward rotation; glenohumeral flexion is linked with scapular abduction and upward rotation, while glenohumeral extension is linked

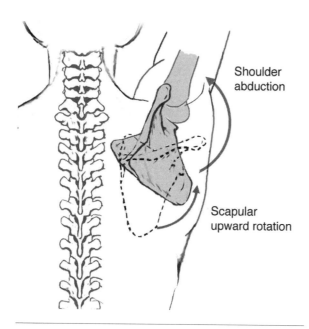

FIGURE 7.22 Upward rotation of the scapula accompanying elevation of the arm.

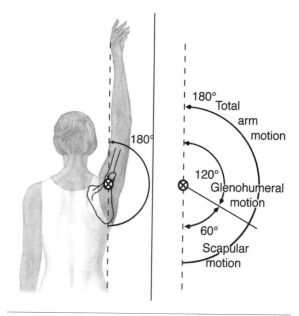

FIGURE 7.23 The scapulohumeral rhythm with shoulder abduction.

with scapular adduction and downward rotation; and glenohumeral external rotation is linked with scapular adduction, while glenohumeral internal rotation is linked with scapular abduction. Depending on the relationship to gravity and what types of external forces are present, these movements may be performed concentrically by the muscle(s) with the associated action (see table 7.4) or controlled eccentrically by the muscles that tend to produce the opposite motion. For example, when one is raising a weight to the side (shoulder abduction), the upward rotation occurs from synergistic concentric contraction of the upward rotators of the scapula. However, when the weight is lowered (shoulder adduction), the downward rotation of the scapula tends to be produced by gravity, and eccentric contraction of the upward rotators of the scapula works to control the downward rotation.

When the position changes from upright, things get more complex; and it is important to consider what effect gravity will have and which scapular muscles will have to work to stabilize the scapulae. For example, during a push-up, gravity tends to make the scapulae come together (scapular adduction), and the scapular abductors have to work to keep the scapulae in the desired position. In other cases, different types of external resistance such as the floor, a partner, or strength training apparatus influence necessary scapular muscle recruitment.

While some of these linked motions, such as upward rotation of the scapula, are necessary to allow high degrees of shoulder flexion or abduction,

other movements are less predictably linked and can be shaped by individual posture and movement patterns. In dance, these movements are sometimes consciously biased to meet a given aesthetic. For example, some schools of dance may prefer a more open position of the arms with slight scapular adduction, while others may prefer a "wider back" with a neutral position or even slight abduction of the scapula.

Influence of Shoulder Rotation on Abduction

In raising the arm to the side (shoulder abduction), range is also facilitated by using external rotation to position the humerus (Concept Demonstration 7.3). During the final 90° of abduction, this external

TABLE 7.3 Linked Movements of the Scapula That Accompany Movements of the Humerus at the Shoulder Joint

Movement of humerus	Movement of scapula
Flexion	Abduction and upward rotation
Extension	Adduction and downward rotation
Abduction	Upward rotation
Adduction	Downward rotation
Medial rotation	Abduction
Lateral rotation	Adduction
Hyperextension	Elevation

Influence of External Forces on Scapular Stabilization

Use the following exercise with a partner to demonstrate the influence of pushing and pulling on the muscles used to stabilize the scapula.

· **Pushing.** Face a partner with right palms in contact and arms at shoulder height with the elbows extended. Push against your partner, and note that if you relax the scapular muscles, the right scapula will tend to be pushed backward (scapular adduction). Now focus on keeping the scapula stationary as you push, and notice the serratus anterior, located near your armpit on the front of your chest, contracting to help stabilize the scapula with its function of scapular abduction.

· **Pulling.** Now face your partner with right hands grasped as if to shake hands. The next step is for both of you to slowly pull on each other's hand. Notice that if you relax the scapular muscles the right scapula will tend to be pulled forward (scapular abduction). Now focus on keeping the scapula stationary as you pull, and notice the contraction of the trapezius and other muscles between the shoulder blades to produce scapular adduction and prevent forward movement of the scapula.

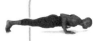

Influence of External Rotation on Overhead Arm Movements

Working with a partner, raise his or her left arm in abduction, as if to bring it overhead through second position to a high fifth position as directed in the following.

· **Internal rotation.** First, perform this motion slowly and gently while holding the arm in internal rotation. Note how the scapula elevates excessively, the shoulder "hikes," and it is difficult to bring the arm fully overhead.

· **External rotation.** Now, from this elevated position, slowly externally rotate the arm, and note how the scapula and shoulder "drop" and the arm can be easily brought overhead. Now slowly raise your partner's arm to the side from a low to high position, adding a gradual external rotation as the arm is raised, and note how this allows the desired dance aesthetic of keeping the shoulders down while bringing the arm overhead.

rotation of the humerus allows the greater tubercle of the humerus to pass behind the coracoacromial arch (Caillet, 1996; Magee, 1997), which permits an additional 30° of abduction of the humerus (Hamill and Knutzen, 1995). It is interesting to note the parallel situation at the hip, where external rotation of the femur and bringing the greater trochanter closer to the ischial tuberosities (sitz bones) allows much greater hip abduction range than when the femur is maintained in a parallel or internally rotated position. As with the hip, adequate strength and appro-

priate activation of the external rotators (particularly the infraspinatus and teres minor of the rotator cuff) are key for correct mechanics.

SIT Force Couple

When the arm is relaxed and hanging by the side, the head of the humerus tends to sit in the upper part of the glenoid cavity (Magee, 1997), and with contraction of the middle deltoid a large component of the muscle force will tend to pull the head

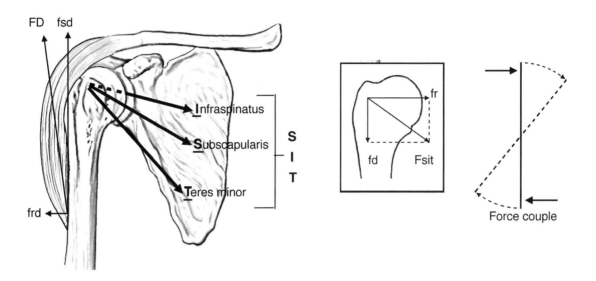

FIGURE 7.24 The SIT force couple. When the arm is down by the side and the middle deltoid contracts (FD) to produce shoulder abduction, a large component of this force (fsd, stabilizing component) tends to pull the head of the humerus upward while only a small component of this force (frd, rotary component) is capable of producing the desired joint movement. However, the SIT muscles provide a force (Fd, dislocating component) that acts to pull the humerus downward and a larger rotary component (fr) such that the resultant force of the SIT muscles (Fsit) acts as a force couple to counter the upward pull of the deltoid and facilitate the desired shoulder abduction.

of the humerus upward (stabilizing component) rather than produce the angular rotation needed for shoulder abduction. However, this natural positioning and upward pull of the deltoid are countered by members of the rotator cuff—the subscapularis, infraspinatus, and teres minor (figure 7.24). These muscles are collectively referred to as the **SIT force couple** (S for subscapularis, I for infraspinatus, and T for teres minor). The SIT force couple, perhaps aided by some additional muscles (Hamill and Knutzen, 1995), functions to depress the head of the humerus and counter the upward movement of the head of the humerus toward the acromion that could pinch the interposed soft tissues (shoulder impingement). The lower positioning of the humeral head into the wider portion of the glenoid cavity produced by the SIT force couple also facilitates the desired rotation of the shaft of the humerus (e.g., shoulder abduction).

Synergies

Many of the muscles of the shoulder complex have multiple actions, and sophisticated use of synergies is necessary to achieve the desired positions and movements of the arms, scapulae, and torso. For example, when the arms are raised forward from low fifth to high fifth, several synergies are operative. At the glenohumeral joint, the two primary shoulder

flexors used to raise the arm (anterior deltoid and pectoralis major) also tend to produce internal rotation of the shoulder. This undesired internal rotation can be neutralized by the synergistic action of external rotators such as the teres minor and infraspinatus. Meanwhile, another synergy is occurring to produce the desired upward rotation of the scapula (figure 7.25). In this case, the lower trapezius and lower fibers of the serratus anterior neutralize out the undesired action of scapular elevation produced by the upper portion of the trapezius. Similarly, the serratus anterior neutralizes out the undesired action of scapular adduction that would be produced by the trapezius if it were unopposed. These are examples of helping synergists (chapter 2), as they assist with the desired action of upward rotation of the scapula while neutralizing out potential undesired elevation or adduction of the scapula.

Muscular Analysis of Fundamental Shoulder Movements

As suggested by the previous discussion, analysis of shoulder movements is complicated by the use of muscles to stabilize the joint, prevent impingement, effect the linked movements of the scapula,

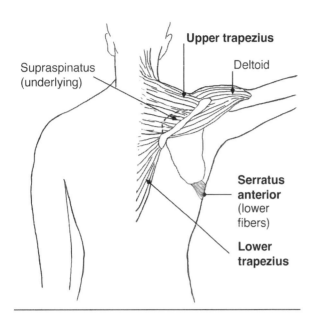

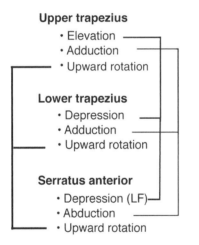

FIGURE 7.25   Example of scapular synergy ideally utilized during shoulder abduction.

and neutralize undesired secondary actions of the prime movers. In addition, due to the large range of motion possible at the shoulder, some muscles may change their relationship to the axis of motion at the shoulder joint, and hence their function, in different ranges of motion. For simplicity, this section will emphasize providing examples of the primary muscles capable of producing the desired shoulder movement and accompanying scapular movement(s). However, readers are encouraged to remember that this presentation represents a great simplification, that many other stabilizers and synergists would actually be operative, and that specific movement conditions such as speed and resistance would influence which muscles actually were recruited.

Shoulder Flexion

In open kinematic chain movement, shoulder flexion involves bringing the arm forward and upward relative to anatomical position in an approximate sagittal plane, such as when raising both arms forward from low fifth to high fifth positions or raising one arm forward from a low to an overhead position (right arm in figure 7.26). This same motion (concentric shoulder flexion) is used in strengthening exercises such as the front arm raise (table 7.10B, p. 434) and the kneeling biceps lift (table 7.10M, p. 442). The shoulder flexors are used concentrically in walking and running when the arms swing forward, in underhand throwing, in some underhand swings in racket sports, and in bowling. Concentric shoulder

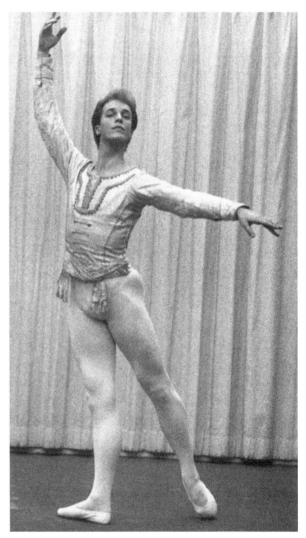

FIGURE 7.26   Sample dance movement showing shoulder flexion.

Photo courtesy of Myra Armstrong. Dancer: Lorin Johnson with American Ballet Theatre.

Shoulder Complex Movement and Muscles Used in a Push-Up

Observe a dancer performing a push-up (with the elbows staying in), focusing on the joint motion and muscles working at the shoulder complex.

· **Up-phase.** Note that in the up-phase of the push-up the motion at the shoulder is against gravity. Hence, the joint motion, shoulder flexion, would be produced via concentric contraction of the shoulder flexors. Examples of primary shoulder flexors are the anterior deltoid and pectoralis major (clavicular) muscles.

· **Down-phase.** Note that in contrast, during the down-phase, gravity would tend to produce the movement at the shoulder joint. Hence, although the joint motion is shoulder extension, the shoulder flexors would be working eccentrically to control the lowering of the body and prevent it from falling to the ground. So, the same shoulder flexors would be working on both the up- and down-phases of the movement—concentrically on the up-phase and eccentrically on the down-phase.

· **Scapular stabilization and movement.** Now examine the influence of gravity on the scapulae and note that the weight of the body will tend to make the scapulae come together or adduct, particularly on the down-phase of the movement. Use of the serratus anterior and other scapular abductors to keep the scapula "wide" throughout the push-up will help counter this tendency for adduction. Furthermore, the later stages of shoulder flexion (greater than 60°) tend to be linked with slight scapular abduction and upward rotation. Again, the serratus anterior, and to a lesser degree the trapezius, can be used to achieve the desired scapulohumeral rhythm.

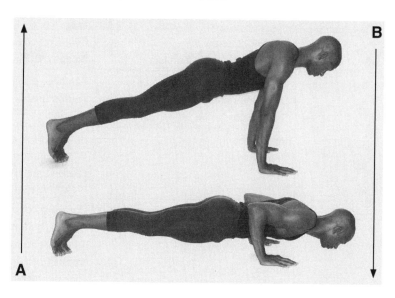

flexion also occurs in pushing motions when the hand is fixed (closed kinematic chain) and the elbow is by the side, such as in the up-phase of a push-up (table 7.10A, p. 432) or press-up (table 7.10C, p. 433). The shoulder flexors—primarily the anterior deltoid and the pectoralis major (clavicular portion, table 7.5)—would be used to effect these movements (table 7.4). Higher ranges of shoulder flexion tend to be accompanied by slight scapular abduction (serratus anterior) and upward rotation (trapezius and serratus anterior, table 7.4) of the scapula (table 7.3, p. 399). Because of the scapular abduction that naturally accompanies scapular upward rotation, the serratus anterior has been shown to play a more prominent role relative to the trapezius in shoulder flexion (Rasch, 1989).

TABLE 7.4 Scapular Movements and the Muscles That Can Produce Them

Scapular movement	Primary and secondary muscles
Elevation	Upper trapezius Levator scapulae Rhomboids
Depression	Lower trapezius Pectoralis minor Serratus anterior (lower fibers)
Abduction (protraction)	Serratus anterior Pectoralis minor
Adduction (retraction)	Trapezius Rhomboids Levator scapulae
Upward rotation	Serratus anterior Trapezius
Downward rotation	Rhomboids Pectoralis minor Levator scapulae

TABLE 7.5 Shoulder Movements and the Muscles That Can Produce Them

Shoulder movement	Primary muscles	Secondary muscles
Flexion	Anterior deltoid Pectoralis major (clavicular)	Coracobrachialis Biceps brachii
Extension	Pectoralis major (sternal) Latissimus dorsi Teres major	Posterior deltoid Triceps brachii
Abduction	Middle deltoid Supraspinatus	Anterior deltoid (>15°) Pectoralis major (clavicular, >90°) Biceps brachii (when shoulder externally rotated)
Adduction	Pectoralis major (especially sternal portion) with latissimus dorsi	Posterior deltoid Anterior deltoid Teres major Coracobrachialis Biceps brachii Triceps brachii
External rotation	Infraspinatus Teres minor	Posterior deltoid Coracobrachialis (from internal rotation to neutral)
Internal rotation	Subscapularis Teres major	Anterior deltoid Pectoralis major Latissimus dorsi Coracobrachialis (>90°)

Shoulder movement	Primary muscles	Secondary muscles
Horizontal abduction	Middle deltoid Posterior deltoid Infraspinatus Teres minor	Latissimus dorsi Teres major
Horizontal adduction	Anterior deltoid Pectoralis major	Biceps brachii (short head) Coracobrachialis

Shoulder Extension

In open kinematic chain movements, shoulder extension often involves moving the arm backward and downward from a position of flexion (such as from high fifth to low fifth) in approximately the sagittal plane. However, when the torso is upright, gravity will tend to produce this movement, and shoulder extension is primarily controlled with eccentric contraction of the shoulder flexors and scapular upward rotators. However, if the arm is brought beyond anatomical position (hyperextension), where the motion is now against gravity (as seen with the right arm in figure 7.27), or if the motion is opposed by another external resistance such as a wall pulley, elastic tubing, or springs (e.g., sitting row [table 7.10D, p. 435] or triceps kick back [table 7.10, E and O, pp. 436 and 444]), the shoulder extensors—including the posterior deltoid, latissimus dorsi, and teres major—would be used concentrically to produce the desired extension, accompanied by relative scapular adduction, and downward rotation (rhomboids, levator scapulae, and lower trapezius to neutralize undesired elevation). Similarly, with a pull-up (closed kinematic chain), extension would occur against gravity (e.g., lifting the body up against gravity), and the shoulder extensors (including the pectoralis major [sternal], latissimus dorsi, and teres major) would work concentrically on the up-phase to produce this shoulder extension. Here, this hanging position would tend to produce extreme elevation of the scapulae, and forceful and deliberate scapular depression (lower trapezius, serratus anterior) would ideally accompany shoulder extension.

Shoulder Abduction

When the hand is free to move (open kinematic chain), shoulder abduction refers to moving the arm sideways away from the midline of the body in approximately the frontal plane, as in raising the arms to the side from low fifth to high fifth, jumping jacks, or the side arm raise (table 7.10F,

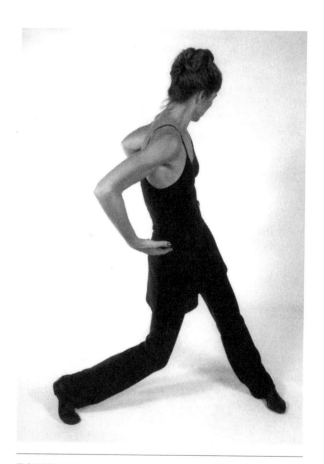

FIGURE 7.27   Sample dance movement showing shoulder extension.

Photo courtesy of Patrick Van Osta. CSULB dancer Jennifer Fitzgerald.

p. 437) performed with a weight. In dance, one or both arms are often held in a position of about 90° abduction to facilitate balance or achieve aesthetic goals (as seen with the left arm in figure 7.28). The shoulder abductors—particularly the supraspinatus and deltoid—would be used to effect these motions. When the shoulder is externally rotated, the biceps brachii can also aid with shoulder abduction (Smith, Weiss, and Lehmkuhl, 1996). When the arms are raised above shoulder height, the clavicular portion of the pectoralis major can also assist with abduction (table 7.4). Shoulder abduction (greater

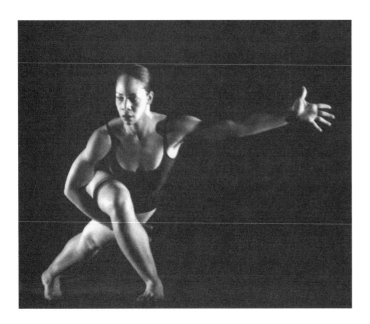

FIGURE 7.28   Sample dance movement showing shoulder abduction.
Photograph by Brooks Dierdorff. Dancer: Nicole Robinson.

than 30°) is accompanied by upward rotation of the scapula (serratus anterior and trapezius); and full abduction to an overhead position is not possible without this coordinated upward rotation of the scapula. The rotator cuff also contributes by helping depress the head of the humerus (SIT force couple: subscapularis, infraspinatus and teres minor) to prevent impingement in middle ranges of abduction and help counter potentially superiorly dislocating components of the force produced by the middle deltoid in higher ranges of abduction (Hall, 1999). In higher ranges of abduction, the rotator cuff also can produce slight external rotation (infraspinatus and teres minor) to help clear the greater tubercle relative to the acromion process and allow greater range of the arm.

Shoulder Adduction

In open kinematic chain movements, shoulder adduction involves moving the arm downward and inward toward the midline of the body from an abducted position in approximately the frontal plane, such as in bringing the arms from second to low fifth. However, when the torso is upright, gravity will tend to produce this movement, and shoulder adduction and its associated downward rotation are generally controlled by eccentric contraction of the shoulder abductors and scapular upward rotators. However, if the arms are brought beyond anatomical position in front of or behind the body where

the motion is now against gravity as shown in figure 7.29 (left shoulder "hyper"adduction combined with slight shoulder flexion), or if the motion is opposed by another external resistance such as a weight apparatus (e.g., lat pull-downs), elastic tubing, water (e.g., swimming the breaststroke), or another dancer, the shoulder adductors and scapular downward rotators (rhomboids, levator scapulae with lower trapezius or serratus anterior to neutralize elevation) come into play. Similarly, in closed kinematic chain movements such as the iron cross in gymnastics, the shoulder adductors would be used concentrically against gravity to raise the body. Unlike what occurs at the hip, where there is a specific muscle group that produces hip adduction, at the shoulder there are not specific muscles whose primary function is shoulder adduction. Instead, muscles located on the front and back of the shoulder are simultaneously contracted to produce shoulder adduction. For example, combined contraction of the pectoralis major and latissimus dorsi results in shoulder adduction, as would combined contraction of the anterior and posterior deltoid muscles.

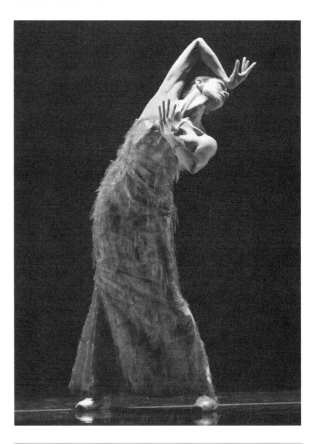

FIGURE 7.29   Sample dance movement showing shoulder adduction.
Photo by Edward Casati. Alonzo King's Lines Ballet dancer Maurya Kerr in "Baker Fix," dress by Colleen Quen Couture.

Shoulder External Rotation

When the hand is free to move, shoulder external rotation refers to rotating the humerus outward along its long axis in an approximately horizontal plane as when one rotates the arm outward from anatomical position so that the point of the elbow (olecranon process) faces into the side of the body. In strengthening exercises, this movement is often performed against external resistance with the elbows in a flexed position, as in the kneeling scarecrow (table 7.10H, p. 439) and double-shoulder external rotation (table 7.10I, p. 439). In dance, external rotation is often added to other movements of the arm such as shoulder flexion or abduction to create a desired aesthetic (right arm in figure 7.30). In sport, shoulder external rotation is incorporated into the backhand drive in racket sports and used in the underhand pitch. Mechanically, as previously described, the addition of external rotation to full shoulder abduction decreases shoulder stress and increases possible range without undesired scapular elevation. The shoulder external rotators—particularly the infraspinatus and teres minor of the rotator cuff (Warner et al., 1990)—would be used concentrically to effect this rotation. Shoulder external rotation tends to be linked with adduction of the scapula (trapezius, rhomboids).

Shoulder Internal Rotation

In open kinematic chain movements, shoulder internal rotation refers to rotating the humerus inward along its long axis in an approximately horizontal plane, as when one rotates the arm inward from anatomical position so that the point of the elbow (olecranon process) faces outward or forward. As with external rotation, strengthening exercises against external resistance often incorporate a position of elbow flexion, as in single-shoulder internal rotation (table 7.10J, p. 440). In dance, similarly to external rotation, internal rotation is often added to other movements of the arm such as shoulder flexion, extension, or abduction to create a desired aesthetic (left arm in figure 7.31). In sport, shoulder internal rotation is incorporated in overarm throwing; certain overhead and forehand strokes in racket sports; and the crawl, butterfly, and breaststroke in swimming. Internal rotation of the shoulder can be important for placement and force application of the hand. The shoulder internal rotators—including the subscapularis, teres major, latissimus dorsi, and pectoralis major—could be used concentrically to effect this rotation. The subscapularis (of the rotator

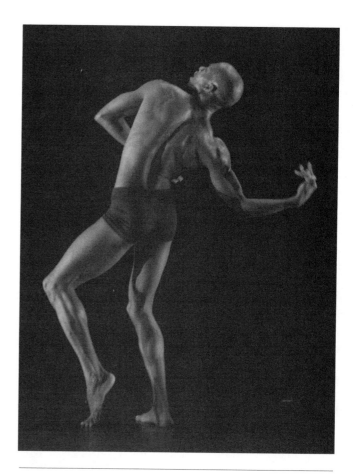

FIGURE 7.30   Sample dance movement showing shoulder external rotation.

Photo courtesy of Patrick Van Osta. CSULB dancer Dwayne Worthington.

cuff) is a particularly strong internal rotator that is capable of producing this motion in isolation. Many of the other muscles are called into play when more force is needed, in different joint ranges, or when a specific combination of movements is present. For example, the latissimus dorsi would tend to create shoulder extension with internal rotation, whereas the pectoralis major (clavicular portion) would tend to produce shoulder flexion and internal rotation. Shoulder internal rotation tends to be linked with abduction of the scapula (serratus anterior and pectoralis minor).

Shoulder Horizontal Adduction and Abduction

Although not among the fundamental movement pairs in the classic three planes associated with ball-and-socket joints, the specialized movements of horizontal adduction and horizontal abduction are included because of their common use in dance.

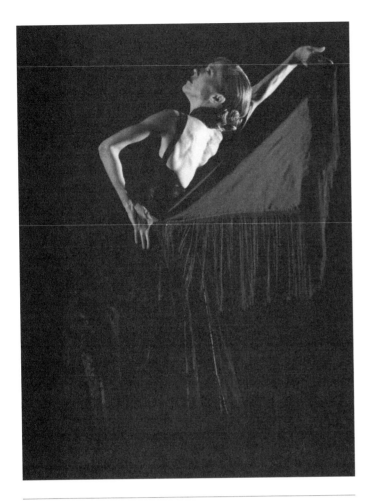

FIGURE 7.31   Sample dance movement showing shoulder internal rotation.

Photo courtesy of Keith Ian Polakoff. CSULB dancer Holly Clark.

Horizontal adduction refers to bringing the arms forward toward the midline from a horizontal position (90° abduction) and keeping the arms at shoulder height throughout this motion. An example from ballet is bringing the arms forward from second position to the front. When the torso is upright, the horizontal adductors—including the anterior deltoid, pectoralis major, and coracobrachialis—can produce this movement, while the shoulder abductors (supraspinatus and middle deltoid) are used to maintain the arms at shoulder height. If you wanted to strengthen these muscles with weights, lying supine would provide a more effective position for gravity to resist horizontal adduction (e.g., supine fly or bench press). Shoulder horizontal adduction tends to be linked with abduction of the scapula (serratus anterior and pectoralis minor).

Horizontal abduction refers to the opposite movement of bringing the horizontally placed arms back away from the front of the body while keeping them at shoulder height, similar to the movement of bringing the arms from middle fifth to second position or accompanying some spinal hyperextension movements commonly used in African dance or jazz dance. When the torso is upright, the horizontal abductors—including the infraspinatus, teres minor, middle deltoid, and posterior deltoid—can produce this movement, while the shoulder abductors are again used to maintain the arms at shoulder height. If you wanted to strengthen these muscles with weights, lying prone on a bench would allow a more effective position for gravity to resist horizontal abduction (e.g., prone fly or row with elbows out). Shoulder

DANCE CUES 7.2

"Hold Your Shoulder Blades Down"

The directive to "hold your shoulder blades down" is sometimes used by teachers in response to a student who excessively lifts the shoulders as the arms are raised overhead. As just discussed, one desired anatomical interpretation of this cue is to emphasize using the scapular depressors (particularly the lower trapezius and serratus anterior) to neutralize the undesired elevation (particularly of the upper trapezius). However, this cue is sometimes misinterpreted to mean that the scapulae should be fixed in place and not allowed to move. To fix the scapulae is counter to the normal scapulohumeral rhythm and the desired upward rotation of the scapulae that accompanies overhead movements of the arms to the front or side. Focusing on the bottom of the shoulder blade (inferior angle) initially pulling slightly down and then out (scapular abduction)—well below the armpit—as the arms are raised can sometimes facilitate desired recruitment of the serratus anterior. Alternatively, thinking of the arms initially reaching slightly down and then out as they approach second position can sometimes help counter the habit of excessive scapular elevation.

horizontal abduction tends to be linked with adduction of the scapula (trapezius, rhomboids).

Special Considerations for the Shoulder Complex in Dance

In activities of daily living, many of the movements of the shoulder primarily function to position the hand. However, in dance, shoulder movements have aesthetic and gestural importance as well as functional importance. Different dance forms often utilize prescribed placement or carriage of the arms that can vary markedly between and within dance forms such as ballet, modern, jazz, and ethnic dance. This use of the arms is often subtle and may take years of concentrated training to master. Although the detailed use of the arms is beyond the scope of this book, a few general principles that apply to many dance forms are helpful to look at from a kinesiological perspective. These include avoiding excessive lifting of the shoulders, keeping the scapula wide, and connecting the arms to the torso. In addition, special demands are placed on the shoulder complex with partnering and use of positions in which the body weight is supported by the arms.

Lifting the Shoulders

One of the most common technique errors related to use of the arms in dance is excessive lifting or hiking of the shoulders, or in kinesiological terminology, excessive scapular elevation (figure 7.32A). In many forms of dance the goal is to emphasize upward rotation of the scapulae without visible scapular elevation when the arms are raised from the sides (figure 7.32B). Theoretically, this aesthetic can be achieved by appropriate use of the serratus anterior and lower trapezius—synergists that can assist with upward rotation but also produce scapular depression to counter the elevation of the upper trapezius (see figure 7.25, p. 402). However, many dancers have difficulty achieving this, and the tendency for excessive elevation can be countered by strengthening the lower trapezius and serratus anterior (see table 7.10C, p. 435) and by focusing on using more scapular depression. Cues such as (1) focusing on reaching the arms down and then out before raising them overhead, or (2) imagining that the scapulae have weights such that the medial border pulls down as the acromion process rotates up can sometimes help recruit the appropriate scapular depressors while still allowing the necessary upward rotation of the scapulae.

In certain movements, such as some floor work, dancers can avoid excessive elevation of the shoulders by contracting muscles that tend to depress the humerus in addition to using the muscles just discussed that depress the scapula. The latissimus dorsi and lower portion of the pectoralis major can function to help depress the humerus when the arms are down by the sides. You can feel this action of humeral and scapular depression when pressing down on the arms of a chair to come to standing if

---

DANCE CUES 7.3

"Connect Your Arms to Your Back"

Looking at the possible actions of the anterior deltoid, middle deltoid, and posterior deltoid (refer to figures 7.14-7.16 [pp. 387, 389, and 390] and table 7.2 [pp. 391-392]), one can see that all of the fundamental shoulder movements can be accomplished with these muscles alone. However, in dance there is the desire to use some of the larger muscles of the shoulder that connect the arms to the trunk rather than just the shoulder girdle. For example, the latissimus dorsi has extensive attachments, including onto the spine, pelvis, and lower ribs. When holding the arms in second position, dancers are sometimes directed to think of lightly pressing the arms down, even though the arms are remaining stationary in space. When following this directive, the latissimus dorsi and pectoralis major can often be seen or felt contracting—acting isometrically as shoulder adductors—while the shoulder abductors contract to maintain the arms at shoulder height. Such co-contraction can provide a different look and kinesthetic sensation of a greater "connection of the arms to the trunk" through use of muscles with more extensive attachments onto the trunk than that of the deltoid muscle.

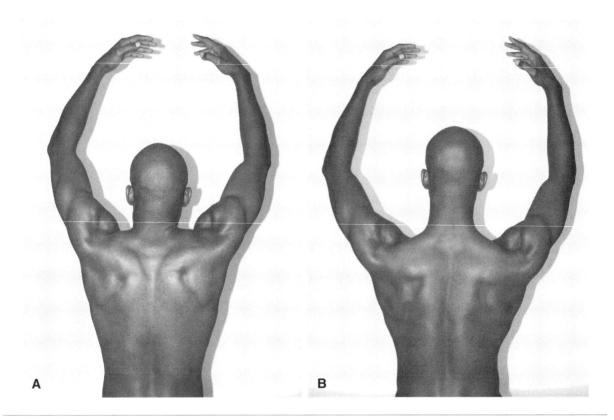

FIGURE 7.32   Elevation of the shoulders with overhead arm movements. (A) Excessive scapular elevation and (B) desired scapular upward rotation without elevation.

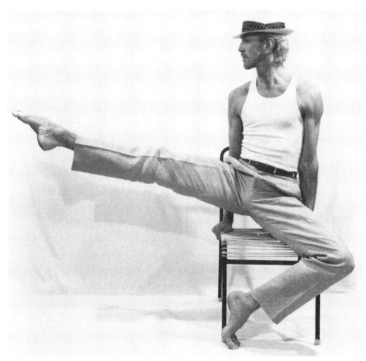

FIGURE 7.33   Use of depressors of the scapula and humerus when supporting the body weight with the arms.

Photo courtesy of Betsey Toombs. Dancer: Wade Madsen.

you focus on first pulling the scapula and humerus downward toward the chair (figure 7.33).

Wide Scapulae

Another common technique error in dance relates to positioning of the arms relative to the body. This problem is easiest to picture when the arms are being held out at shoulder height to the side (second position). If the arms are held too far back (excessive shoulder horizontal abduction), the scapulae are generally excessively "pinched together" (excessive scapular adduction) as seen in figure 7.34B. Conversely, if the arms are held too far forward (excessive shoulder horizontal adduction), the scapulae are generally excessively separated (excessive scapular abduction) as seen in figure 7.34C. Although different dance forms vary on the exact desired aesthetic, many utilize a position in which the scapulae are "wide" versus pinched but still lying flat along the back of the rib cage versus coming to the front of the body, as seen in figure 7.34A. This is basically a "neutral" position of the scapulae.

Thinking of keeping the elbows and scapulae pulling slightly to the side can sometimes help you find this position of the scapulae. This positioning is often accompanied by a sensation of slight co-

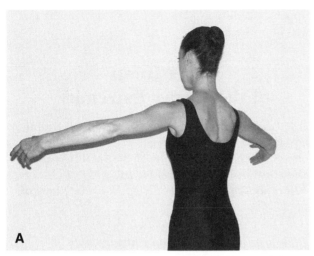

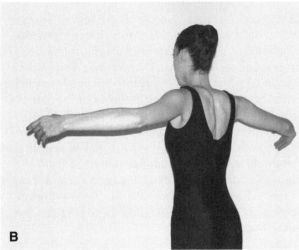

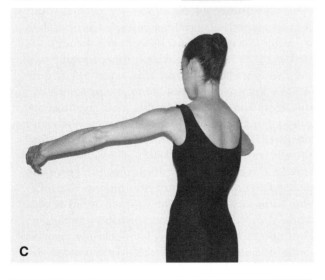

FIGURE 7.34   Arm placement will vary with the aesthetics of a given dance form but is generally close to (A) a neutral position of the scapulae and torso without (B) excessive scapular adduction and spinal hyperextension or (C) excessive scapular abduction and kyphosis.

contraction of the lower trapezius and serratus anterior. When the scapulae are in this position, the arms will be slightly in front of the coronal plane—that is, in the plane of the scapula (scaption). For dancers having difficulty finding this position, strengthening as well as utilizing cues to encourage use of the muscles that would correct the deviation can help (figure 7.34). For example, if the scapulae are excessively adducted, strengthening and developing better awareness of the scapular abductors (table 7.10K, p. 440) are recommended.

Connection of the Arms to the Torso

This positioning of the arms can also influence the positioning of the torso and vice versa. For example, when the arms are habitually held too far back, this is frequently accompanied by excessive arching of the low back (lumbar lordosis) and rib-leading, as well as excessive scapular adduction (figure 7.34B). Conversely, when the arms are habitually held too far forward, this is often accompanied by a rounding of the upper back (kyphosis) and "closing in" of the chest, as well as excessive scapular abduction (figure 7.34C). Instead, the goal is to be able to utilize a neutral positioning of the arms in which the torso is neutral and stabilized rather than distorted by arm placement. Then, the arms can be utilized to enhance the movement (allowing for more revolutions in turns, for example) rather than throwing the body off center. From this neutral position, the arms can also then be consciously utilized in "non-neutral" ways to meet a given choreographic goal; but it is important for dancers to know where their neutral position is, as well as how to make other choices without throwing off their balance.

Learning to use the arms in a manner that does not distort torso or shoulder alignment is a complex matter that incorporates many factors, including learning adequate torso stabilization, utilizing balanced synergies, and using muscles appropriately that connect the arms to the torso. In terms of this latter factor, focusing on using some of the larger muscles that connect the arms to the torso, such as the pectoralis major and latissimus dorsi, can sometimes help achieve more of a sense of connection of the arms to the torso and "center." As previously described, the pectoralis major and latissimus dorsi can be used to depress the humerus. Hence, focusing on reaching the arm down toward the floor before raising it forward or back can sometimes help you find these muscles. Since these muscles are located lower than some of the other prime movers such as the deltoids, you can sometimes feel these muscles working more if you think about using the muscles lower, by your armpit, rather than just on the upper shoulder.

Partnering and Arm Support

A lot of strength and proper mechanics are required to lift another dancer, to execute the partnering correctly and prevent injuries. In classical ballet schools, young men who are in the middle of growth spurts and not fully mature are often required to partner young female dancers who may be almost as tall or taller than they are. In many dance forms such as modern and jazz, contemporary choreographers may have women partner other women or men who may weigh more than they do. Many contemporary choreographers are also utilizing positions and movements requiring that the body weight be supported by the arms as in handstands, cartwheels, or back flips. The type of strength needed for such movements far exceeds that needed in a traditional dance class, and it is highly recommended that dancers perform supplemental upper extremity strengthening exercises, particularly for the shoulder flexors, extensors, and abductors (see table 7.10, p. 434). From an injury prevention perspective, it is also important to include exercises for the rotator cuff and muscles of scapular stabilization. The importance of these smaller muscles can be seen in figure 7.35; here the scapular muscles must be used to establish the scapulae as a stable platform in order for the other

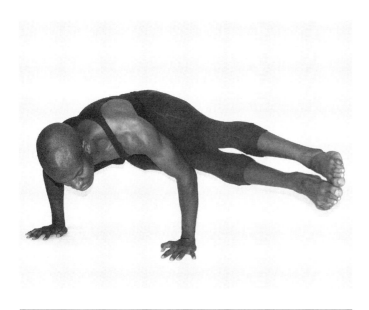

FIGURE 7.35   Sample dance movement with body weight supported by arms, requiring high levels of upper extremity strength and scapular stabilization.

upper extremity muscles to effectively support the weight of the body.

Other Joints of the Upper Extremity

Distal to the shoulder joint are the elbow joint, joints between the radius and ulna, wrist joint, and joints between the various bones of the hand. As these joints are discussed, consider the similarities and differences in relation to the comparable joints of the lower extremity.

Elbow Joint Structure and Movements

The elbow joint is composed of two different articulations (figure 7.36). More specifically, the distal end of the humerus widens and forms bony prominences—the medial epicondyle and lateral epicondyle. Between these epicondyles are a medial articular surface called the **trochlea** and a lateral articular surface called the **capitulum** (little head). The spool-shaped trochlea of the humerus articulates with a concave area on the proximal ulna called the **trochlear notch** (semilunar notch) to form the **humeroulnar joint,** while the spherical capitulum of the humerus articulates with the flattened proximal end of the radius, called the head, to form the **humeroradial joint.**

Due to ligamental binding of the radius to the ulna, the humeroulnar and humeroradial joints function together, and the elbow joint as a whole is considered a hinge joint. Its axis runs through the middle of the trochlea and capitulum, allowing only the movements of flexion and extension (figure 7.37A). The trochlear notch of the ulna terminates inferiorly and anteriorly with a small prominence called the **coronoid process,** and superiorly and posteriorly with a prominent process called the **olecranon process.** When the elbow is fully flexed, the head of the radius and the coronoid process fit into small indentations on the anterior humerus (radial fossa and coronoid fossa), while the olecranon process can be palpated as the "point" of the elbow. The olecranon process comes in contact with the table or floor when you lean on your elbows with the elbows bent and the forearms approximately vertical. Sometimes when you bump your elbow you get an odd tingling sensation running down to your little finger; this sensation is due to pressure on the ulnar nerve, which runs in the groove between the olecranon process and the medial epicondyle. When the elbow

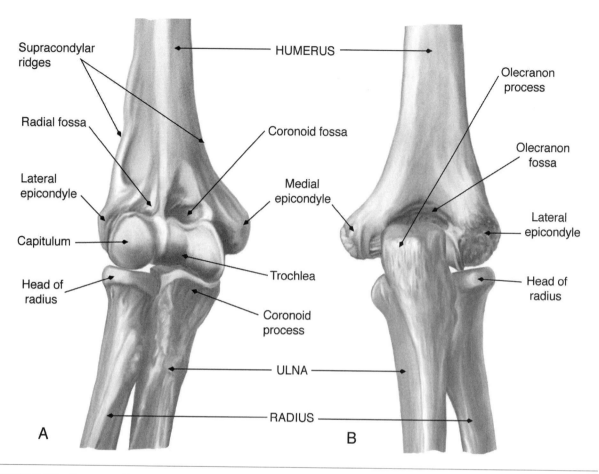

FIGURE 7.36   Bones and bony landmarks of the right elbow joint. (A) Anterior view, (B) posterior view.

goes into full extension, the olecranon process moves into a large indentation on the back of the lower humerus (olecranon fossa).

The bony configuration of the elbow joint makes it more stable than the shoulder. In addition, the paired articulations of the elbow joint are encased in a joint capsule that is thickened by various ligaments, including medial (or ulnar) and lateral (or radial) collateral ligaments, to add greater joint stability (figure 7.38). The ulnar collateral ligament is particularly key for stabilizing the elbow joint, and its medial location allows it to resist valgus stress associated with lifting heavy objects or the support of body weight. Many muscles of the elbow and the extrinsic muscles of the hand that cross the elbow joint have lines of pull that also provide considerable joint stability, in addition to joint movement (Kreighbaum and Barthels, 1996).

Alignment of the Elbow

As with the knee, the elbow can be hyperextended and can vary in its angulation. An understanding of

these deviations can help with achievement of the desired dance aesthetic.

Carrying Angle

The trochlea extends more distally than the capitulum. Hence in anatomical position with the elbow extended and forearm supinated, the forearm deviates slightly laterally relative to the humerus. This angulation is termed the **carrying angle,** or **cubital angle,** of the elbow (figure 7.39). Some have hypothesized that this angle functions to keep the hands from hitting the hips when a person is carrying something with the elbows by the sides, hence its name. The carrying angle varies markedly between individuals and tends to be greater in females versus males, and greater in adults versus children (Goldman and McCann, 1997). Normal values are considered to be 10° to 25° for females and 5° to 15° for males when the elbow is extended in anatomical position (Frankel and Nordin, 1980; Magee, 1997). An increase in this angle above normal due to greater lateral deviation of the forearm is termed **cubitus valgus,** while a decrease in this angle below norms is called **cubitus varus.**

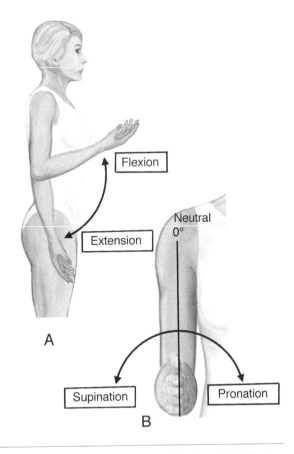

FIGURE 7.37   Movements of the (A) elbow joint (flexion-extension) and (B) radioulnar joints (pronation-supination).

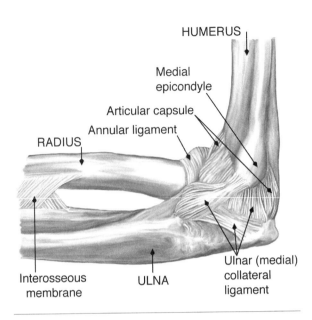

FIGURE 7.38   Medial view of the elbow showing capsule and medial ligaments (right elbow).

Due to the asymmetrical shape of the trochlea and the fact that the axis of the elbow joint angles slightly downward as it runs medially, the carrying angle decreases or even reverses when the elbow is flexed from anatomical position. One study showed a change from an average of 10° of valgus (lateral angulation of forearm relative to longitudinal axis of humerus) with the elbow fully extended to 8° of varus (medial angulation of forearm relative to longitudinal axis of humerus) with the elbow in full flexion. This is important to keep in mind when doing elbow flexion or extension strengthening exercises, and for most dancers, one should allow the forearm to deviate laterally versus trying to force the forearm to stay in line with the humerus when the elbow extends.

Elbow Hyperextension

While elbow flexion is often limited by contact of the soft tissues of the arm and forearm, extension can be limited by tightness of opposing ligaments or muscles, or by contact of the olecranon process of the ulna with the humerus. However, the point at which the elbow stops when it extends is quite variable

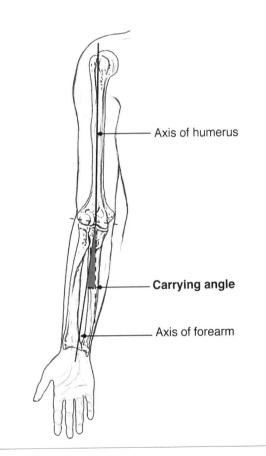

FIGURE 7.39   Carrying angle (right arm, anterior view).

between individuals; and many dancers, particularly female dancers, have the ability to extend the arm well beyond straight, that is, to hyperextend the elbow (figure 7.40). Whether due to ligamental laxity or a short olecranon process, dancers with marked **elbow hyperextension** often have to utilize muscular contraction of the elbow flexors in isolation or in coordination with the elbow extensors to avoid this undesired aesthetic, particularly in movements requiring arm support. As with knee hyperextension, it often takes a retraining of the kinesthetic sense with use of outside feedback, such as looking in the mirror, to relearn the position of straight versus hyperextended.

Description and Functions of Selected Individual Muscles of the Elbow

The muscles of the elbow are arranged so that those that cross anteriorly are in a position to cause elbow flexion and those that cross posteriorly are in a position to cause elbow extension. This arrangement is similar to that at the shoulder or hip, but opposite to that at the knee. (See Individual Muscles of the Elbow, pp. 416-422.)

Structure and Movements of the Radioulnar Joints

The radius and ulna are connected via two synovial joints—the proximal radioulnar joint and the distal radioulnar joint (figure 7.45). They are also connected via a ligamentous sheet (middle radioulnar joint).

The **proximal radioulnar joint** is a uniaxial, pivot joint lying within the capsule of the elbow joint. It is formed by the articulation between the side of the head of the radius and a notch on the ulna (radial notch) as seen in figure 7.45A. A strong ligament, the **annular ligament,** forms a three-quarters ring around the head of the radius, keeping it close to the ulna so that the desired rotation can occur without other undesired motions. You can feel the head of the radius moving under the skin by placing a finger about an inch below the lateral epicondyle of the right humerus and then slowly and repetitively bringing the palm of the right hand to face downward (forearm pronation) and then upward (supination).

The **middle radioulnar joint** is not a synovial joint, but rather a fibrous joint involving connection via a ligamentous sheet called the **interosseous membrane.** This joint functions to keep the radius and ulna from excessively separating or sliding apart

from each other in a longitudinal direction as seen in figure 7.45, A and B.

The **distal radioulnar joint** is a pivot joint formed between the head of the ulna and a concave surface of the radius (ulnar notch). Note that while the radius is the smaller bone proximally and terminates in a "head," the ulna is the smaller bone distally and terminates in a "head." This distal radioulnar joint allows that radius (with wrist and hand) to pivot around the head of the ulna (figure 7.45B). A triangular articular disc connects the radius and ulna and provides stability to the distal radioulnar joint.

Together, the radioulnar joints allow the radius to rotate relative to the ulna so that the palm is facing downward with the thumb positioned medially, termed pronation, or the palm is facing upward with the thumb positioned laterally, termed supination (figure 7.45C). The axis of this motion can be pictured as running between the head of the radius proximally and the head of the ulna distally (figure 7.45A). This motion is more complex than pure rotation about one bone, in that in a position of supination (e.g., anatomical position) the radius and ulna lie parallel to one another with the radius located lateral to the ulna. However, with pronation, although the proximal radius remains on the same side of the ulna as with supination, the distal radius crosses over to the medial side of the ulna. (See Individual Muscles of the Radioulnar Joints, pp. 423-424.)

(Text continues on p. 424.)

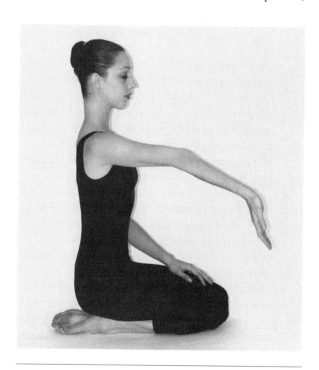

FIGURE 7.40   Elbow hyperextension.

Individual Muscles of the Elbow

Anterior Elbow Muscles

Three important anterior muscles that flex the elbow are the biceps brachii, brachialis, and brachioradialis. Some of the muscles of the forearm, wrist, and hand can also aid with elbow flexion but for purposes of simplicity will not be discussed here. Elbow flexion is important for lifting motions, movement involving bringing the hands toward the upper body, and gestural movements.

Attachments and Primary Actions of Biceps Brachii

Muscle	Proximal attachment(s)	Distal attachment(s)	Primary action(s)
Biceps brachii (BY-seps BRA-kee-eye)	Long head: just above glenoid cavity of scapula Short head: coracoid process of scapula	Tuberosity of radius via a common tendon	Elbow flexion Radioulnar supination (Shoulder flexion—long head) (Shoulder abduction when shoulder in external rotation—long head) (Shoulder adduction—long head)

Biceps Brachii

As its name implies, the **biceps brachii** (*biceps,* two heads + *brachium,* arm) has two heads. It is located superficially in the front portion of the upper arm (figure 7.41). The long head originates above the glenoid cavity on the scapula, and its tendon passes over the top of the humerus and then runs within the intertubercular groove of the humerus. Due to this location, the long head of the biceps brachii can depress the head of the humerus to help prevent impingement when forceful contraction of the biceps brachii is required such as in resisted elbow flexion (Schmitz and Ciullo, 1999; Smith, Weiss, and Lehmkuhl, 1996). The short head arises from the coracoid process of the scapula. In the proximal part of the upper arm these muscles exist as separate bellies, but about midway down the humerus they join to become one belly and attach to a tuberosity on the medial side of the radius (radial tuberosity) via a common tendon.

The biceps brachii is an important flexor of the elbow. With its attachment onto the tuberosity of the radius, when the forearm is pronated the biceps tendon will be twisted about halfway around the radius, and contraction of the biceps will produce supination of the forearm as well as elbow flexion. However, perhaps due to this wrapping around the radius, the biceps brachii makes only a minimal contribution to elbow flexion when the forearm is pronated (Hamill and Knutzen, 1995). Hence, performing a pull-up with the palms facing away from the body (forearm pronation) is more difficult than performing a pull-up with the palms facing the body, and the force generated by the elbow flexors in a maximal voluntary contraction has

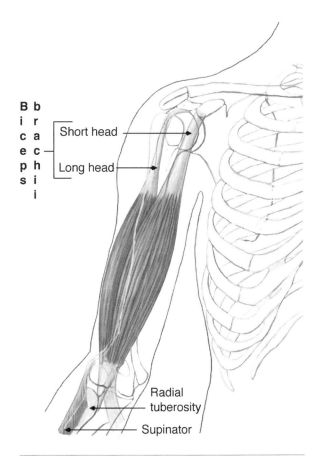

Biceps brachii

Short head
Long head

Radial tuberosity
Supinator

FIGURE 7.41   Biceps brachii and supinator (right arm, anterior view).

been shown to be least with the forearm pronated and most with the forearm supinated (Hamilton and Luttgens, 2002). At the shoulder, the biceps brachii can assist with shoulder flexion (and abduction when the shoulder is externally rotated with the elbow straight). Hence, performing elbow flexion with the shoulder in a position of flexion, such as in partnering or the kneeling biceps lift (table 7.10M, p. 442), will increase the difficulty for the biceps brachii, without influencing the difficulty for elbow flexors that do not cross the shoulder such as the brachialis. In addition, the biceps brachii can assist other muscles with adduction of the shoulder.

Palpation: The biceps brachii can be easily seen and palpated on the front of the upper arm. Sit with the fingers of the left hand on the front of your right upper arm, with the right elbow bent and the right palm under the top of a desk. You can feel the biceps brachii contracting when you press your right palm up against the desk as if to bend the elbow (isometric elbow flexion). Move your fingers distally on the biceps, and you will find its tendon standing out prominently at the fold of the elbow. Note that the biceps brachii attaches proximally on the scapula and attaches distally below the elbow, and has no actual attachment onto the humerus. Thus, when you relax this muscle, it can more readily be moved from side to side than the underlying brachialis, which has extensive attachments onto the humerus.

Attachments and Primary Actions of Brachialis

Muscle	Proximal attachment(s)	Distal attachment(s)	Primary action(s)
Brachialis (BRA-kee-al-is)	Anterior aspect of lower half of humerus	Upper ulna	Elbow flexion

Brachialis

The **brachialis** (*brachium,* arm) is located on the front of the arm beneath the biceps brachii (figure 7.42). It arises proximally from the anterior portion of the lower half of the humerus and attaches distally to the upper ulna. Due to its attachment on the ulna, the brachialis does not produce supination or pronation of the forearm and is not influenced by the position of the forearm. The brachialis is sometimes termed the "workhorse of the elbow" because it appears to work in almost all conditions of elbow flexion, regardless of speed, resistance, or forearm position.

Palpation: Sit with the fingers of the left hand on the front of your right arm (about 1 inch [2.5 centimeters] above the crease of the elbow and to the sides of the biceps brachii) while the right elbow is bent and the forearm pronated such that the right dorsum of the hand is under the top of a desk. You can feel the brachialis contracting just medial and lateral to the biceps when you press your right hand up against the desk as if to further bend the elbow (isometric elbow flexion).

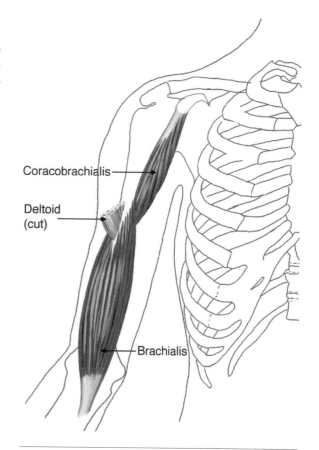

FIGURE 7.42   Brachialis and coracobrachialis (right arm, deep anterior view).

Attachments and Primary Actions of Brachioradialis

Muscle	Proximal attachment(s)	Distal attachment(s)	Primary action(s)
Brachioradialis (bra-kee-o-ra-dee-A-lis)	Above lateral epicondyle of humerus	Lateral aspect of styloid process of radius	Elbow flexion Radioulnar supination from pronation or vice versa to achieve midposition

Brachioradialis

As its name implies, the **brachioradialis** (*brachium,* arm + *radi,* radius) runs between the upper arm and the radius. This muscle arises above the lateral epicondyle of the humerus and runs down to attach distally to the lower radius just above the styloid process (figures 7.43 and 7.47, p. 425). It is the muscle that gives the rounded contour to the lateral forearm. When this muscle contracts it flexes the elbow. Due to its location, this muscle has been theorized to bring the forearm to a midposition (neutral position) from a position of either pronation or supination.

Palpation: Sit with the fingers of the left hand on the anterolateral aspect of the right forearm just distal to the crease of the elbow, with the right elbow bent and the right hand in a fist; have the thumb side of the fist under the top of a desk (forearm in a midposition between pronation and supination). You can see and feel the brachioradialis contracting when you press your right fist up against the desk. Move your fingers distally on the brachioradialis to the distal radius to follow its course.

Posterior Elbow Muscles

The posterior elbow muscles include the triceps brachii and the anconeus. Because these muscles attach distally to the ulna rather than the radius, their contribution is not influenced by the position of the forearm. Other extensors of the wrist and fingers that cross the elbow joint posteriorly can also contribute to elbow extension but have been omitted for purposes of simplicity.

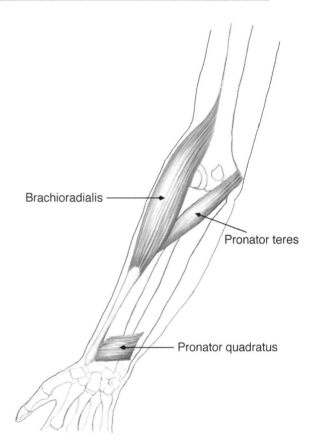

FIGURE 7.43 Brachioradialis, pronator teres, and pronator quadratus (right arm, anterior view).

Attachments and Primary Actions of Triceps Brachii

Muscle	Proximal attachment(s)	Distal attachment(s)	Primary action(s)
Triceps brachii (TRY-seps BRA-kee-eye)	Long head: just below glenoid cavity of scapula Lateral head: upper half of posterolateral humerus Medial head: lower two-thirds of posterior humerus	Olecranon process of ulna via a common tendon	Elbow extension (Shoulder extension—long head) (Shoulder adduction—long head)

Triceps Brachii

The **triceps brachii** (*triceps,* three heads + *brachi,* arm) is located superficially and makes up the muscle mass of the back of the arm (figure 7.44A). As its name suggests, this muscle contains three heads—the long, medial, and lateral heads. The long head arises proximally from just below the glenoid cavity of the scapula. The lateral head arises proximally from the posterolateral upper half of the humerus. The medial head originates from approximately the lower two-thirds of the posterior humerus. All three heads join and then attach distally via a strong flat tendon to the olecranon process of the ulna. The triceps is a powerful extensor of the elbow that is not influenced by pronation or supination of the forearm. However, the long head of the triceps brachii crosses the shoulder and so is influenced by the position of the shoulder. Its actions at the shoulder are extension and adduction. So, for example, performing elbow extension with the arm behind the body, as in triceps kick back (table 7.10E, p. 436), will put the long head at a disadvantage (length–tension principle) and provide greater overload.

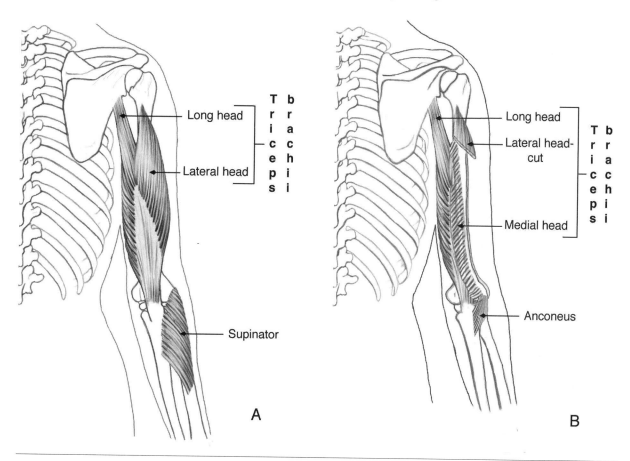

FIGURE 7.44   Triceps brachii, supinator, and anconeus (right arm, posterior view). (A) Superficial view, (B) deeper view.

Palpation: Sit in a chair with the fingers of the left hand placed midway on the posterior aspect of the right arm and the right palm resting on the right edge of the seat of the chair. The triceps brachii can be felt contracting under your fingers when the right hand presses down on the seat of the chair to lift the body (elbow extension).

Attachments and Primary Actions of Anconeus

Muscle	Proximal attachment(s)	Distal attachment(s)	Primary action(s)
Anconeus (an-KO-nee-us)	Posterior aspect of lateral epicondyle of humerus	Lateral aspect of olecranon process of ulna Upper posterior ulna	Assists with elbow extension

Anconeus

The **anconeus** (*ancon,* elbow) is a small muscle located just distal to the triceps brachii (figure 7.44B). It runs downward and medially from its proximal attachment on the lateral epicondyle of the humerus to its distal attachment on the posterior upper ulna. Its actions are to stabilize the elbow (Basmajian and DeLuca, 1985) and assist with elbow extension.

Palpation: Using the same movement as just described for palpation of the triceps brachii, you can feel the anconeus contracting when placing the fingertips of your left hand just lateral to the olecranon process of the ulna when the right hand presses down on the seat of the chair.

Summary of Elbow Muscle Attachments, Actions, and Roles in Movement

The muscles that cross the elbow joint serve to stabilize the joint as well as produce flexion and extension. A summary of attachments and actions of key muscles of the elbow are included in table 7.6, while the movements of the elbow and the muscles that can produce them are included in table 7.7. These tables also include key muscles and movements of the radioulnar joints, which will shortly be described in more detail in the text.

TABLE 7.6   Summary of Attachments and Primary Actions of the Muscles of the Elbow and Radioulnar Joints

Muscle	Proximal attachment(s)	Distal attachment(s)	Primary action(s)
Biceps brachii (BY-seps BRA-kee-eye)	Long head: just above glenoid cavity of scapula Short head: coracoid process of scapula	Tuberosity of radius via a common tendon	Elbow flexion Radioulnar supination (Shoulder flexion—long head) (Shoulder abduction when shoulder in external rotation—long head) (Shoulder adduction—long head)
Brachialis (BRA-kee-al-is)	Anterior aspect of lower half of humerus	Upper ulna	Elbow flexion
Brachioradialis (bra-kee-o-ra-dee-A-lis)	Above lateral epicondyle of humerus	Lateral aspect of styloid process of radius	Elbow flexion Radioulnar supination from pronation or vice versa to achieve midposition
Triceps brachii (TRY-seps BRA-kee-eye)	Long head: just below glenoid cavity of scapula Lateral head: upper half of posterolateral humerus Medial head: lower two-thirds of posterior humerus	Olecranon process of ulna via a common tendon	Elbow extension (Shoulder extension—long head) (Shoulder adduction—long head)
Anconeus (an-KO-nee-us)	Posterior aspect of lateral epicondyle of humerus	Lateral aspect of olecranon process of ulna Upper posterior ulna	Assists with elbow extension
Pronator teres (PRO-na-tor TE-reez)	Medial epicondyle of humerus Coronoid process of ulna	Lateral aspect of middle third of radius	Radioulnar pronation (Assists with elbow flexion)
Pronator quadratus (PRO-na-tor kwod-RA-tus)	Anterior aspect of lower quarter of ulna	Anterior aspect of lower quarter of radius	Radioulnar pronation
Supinator (soo-pi-NA-tor)	Lateral epicondyle of humerus Lateral aspect of upper ulna	Anterolateral aspect of upper radius	Radioulnar supination

TABLE 7.7   Movements of the Elbow and Radioulnar Joints and Key Muscles That Can Produce Them

Joint movement	Primary muscle(s)	Secondary muscle(s)
Elbow flexion	Biceps brachii Brachialis Brachioradialis	Pronator teres
Elbow extension	Triceps brachii	Anconeus
Radioulnar pronation	Pronator quadratus	Pronator teres Brachioradialis (to midposition)
Radioulnar supination	Supinator Biceps brachii	Brachioradialis (to midposition)

Looking at the role of these muscles in movement on the simplest level, if the movement is performed slowly and without a stylized quality, the following generalizations are germane. The elbow flexors—including the brachialis and biceps brachii—are most commonly used concentrically (in an open kinematic chain) to bring the forearm toward the upper arm against gravity such as when lifting something from the ground (e.g., a partner) or against other external resistance such as a dumbbell (concentration curl, table 7.10L, p. 441) or springs (kneeling biceps lift, table 7.10M, p. 442). The same elbow flexors would then be used eccentrically to control the lowering of the forearm (elbow extension). However, when the arm is fixed (closed kinematic chain), the elbow flexors can be used with the shoulder muscles to help bring the torso closer to the arms in pulling motions, such as in a pull-up or in rope climbing. In contrast, the elbow extensors—primarily the triceps brachii—can be used to straighten the elbow in open kinematic chain movements such as in the tennis serve or in an overarm throw. Strengthening exercises often incorporate elbow extension against external resistance, such as dumbbells (overhead triceps extension, table 7.10N, p. 443) or a spring (kneeling triceps kick back, table 7.10O, p. 444). When the hand is fixed, the elbow extensors are commonly used concentrically in closed kinematic chain pushing movements such as a push-up (table 7.10A, p. 434) or raising the torso from a chair (press-up, table 7.10C, p. 435) or the floor in dance. In dance, the elbow flexors and extensors are also commonly used gesturally to shape the arms in accordance with choreographic intent.

___ CONCEPT DEMONSTRATION 7.5 _____

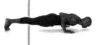

Change in Relative Positioning of the Distal Radius and Ulna With Pronation

Use the following exercise to demonstrate the influence of pronation and supination on the relative positioning of the radius and ulna.

Palpate the ulna with the fingertips of your left hand by following the border of this bone on your right arm from the olecranon down to the small projection at the wrist (**styloid process**). Keep the elbow bent to 90° and by your side. Then, pronate the forearm while keeping the fingertips on the styloid process, and note how the radius is now medial to the ulna, distally.

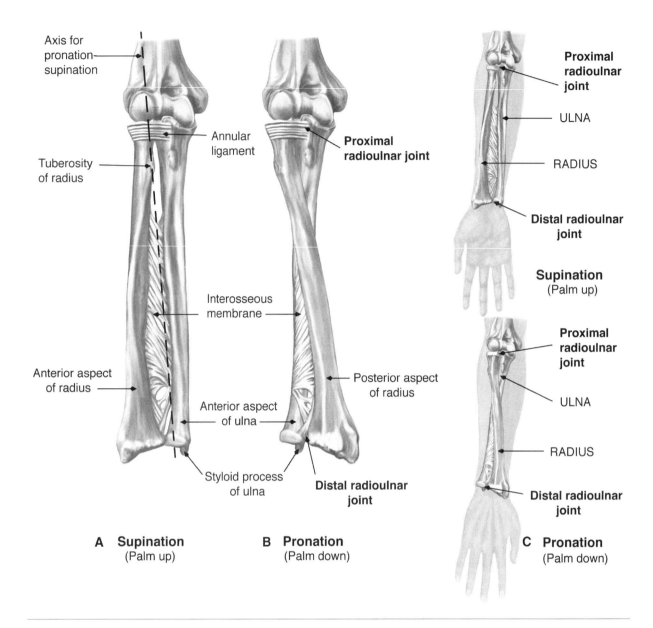

FIGURE 7.45 The radioulnar joints (right forearm). (A) Position of supination, (B) position of pronation, (C) change in hand position with supination and pronation.

CONCEPT DEMONSTRATION 7.6

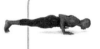

Combining Shoulder Rotation With Forearm Movements to Facilitate Positioning of the Hand

Use the following exercise to demonstrate how combining shoulder rotation with forearm pronation and supination can allow more range of motion for the hand.

Hold one arm out in second position with the palm facing up. Then, leading with the thumb, pronate the forearm and internally rotate the shoulder, and note where the thumb is facing in the end position. Next, just pronate the forearm without letting the shoulder internally rotate. Lastly, just internally rotate the shoulder without allowing any movement in the forearm. Compare the range of motion as evidenced by the facing of the thumb at the end position for each of these three conditions.

Individual Muscles of the Radioulnar Joints

Selected Muscles of the Radioulnar Joints

The two muscles that are the most important pronators of the forearm are the pronator teres and pronator quadratus. Two muscles that are particularly important supinators of the forearm are the biceps brachii and the supinator. The biceps brachii has already been described within the context of elbow flexion, and a description of the other muscles follows.

Attachments and Primary Actions of Pronator Teres and Pronator Quadratus

Muscle	Proximal attachment(s)	Distal attachment(s)	Primary action(s)
Pronator teres (PRO-na-tor TE-reez)	Medial epicondyle of humerus Coronoid process of ulna	Lateral aspect of middle third of radius	Radioulnar pronation (Assists with elbow flexion)
Pronator quadratus (PRO-na-tor kwod-RA-tus)	Anterior aspect of lower quarter of ulna	Anterior aspect of lower quarter of radius	Radioulnar pronation

Pronator Teres

The **pronator teres** (pronation, turning palm posteriorly, or down + *teres,* round) is a small muscle located anteriorly in the area of the elbow, partly covered by the brachioradialis (figure 7.43, p. 418). It runs laterally and obliquely from its proximal attachments on the medial epicondyle of the humerus and upper anterior ulna to its distal attachment on the lateral middle portion of the radius. As its name suggests, the primary action of this muscle is pronation of the forearm, which it accomplishes by pulling the radius over in front of the ulna. It can also assist with elbow flexion against resistance (Hamilton and Luttgens, 2002).

   Palpation: Sit with the fingers of the left hand placed on the anterior portion of the forearm, just lateral to the distal biceps brachii tendon and just below the crease of the right elbow while the elbow is flexed and the forearm is resting on your right thigh. You can feel the pronator teres contracting under your fingers when the forearm is pronated.

Pronator Quadratus

The **pronator quadratus** (pronation, turning palm posteriorly, or down + *quad,* square, four-sided) is located distally on the front of the forearm slightly proximal to the wrist (figure 7.43, p. 418). It is a thin, square-shaped muscle that runs transversely between the ulna and radius, deeply right next to these bones. As its name indicates, its action is to pronate the forearm, which it accomplishes by pulling the lower end of the radius over and across the ulna. Electromyographic studies suggest that the pronator quadratus is the major muscle responsible for pronation, with the pronator teres assisting, particularly when the pronation is resisted or rapid (Hall, 1999; Hamilton and Luttgens, 2002).

   Palpation: Due to its deep location, the pronator quadratus is difficult to palpate.

Attachments and Primary Actions of Supinator

Muscle	Proximal attachment(s)	Distal attachment(s)	Primary action(s)
Supinator (soo-pi-NA-tor)	Lateral epicondyle of humerus Lateral aspect of upper ulna	Anterolateral aspect of upper radius	Radioulnar supination

Supinator

The **supinator** (supination, turning palm anteriorly or upward) is a small, triangular-shaped muscle located deeply and posteriorly (figure 7.44, p. 419). It runs inferiorly and laterally from its proximal attachment posterolaterally on the lower humerus and upper ulna to wrap around the radius and attach to the anterolateral aspect of the upper radius (figure 7.41, p. 416). A way of picturing this action more clearly is to consider a position of pronation in which the radius would be moving forward and in front of the ulna. The supinator is in an appropriate position to pull the radius back (supination) toward anatomical position, in which the radius and ulna are approximately parallel. The supinator appears to actively produce supination of the forearm under all conditions (Hamilton and Luttgens, 2002).

Palpation: Sit with the fingertips of the left hand about 1 inch (2.5 centimeters) distal to the lateral epicondyle of the humerus while the right elbow is bent and resting against your waist. You can feel the supinator contracting under your fingertips when the forearm is slowly supinated.

Summary of Attachments, Actions, and Movement Roles of the Muscles of the Radioulnar Joints

A summary of the attachments and actions of the primary muscles that act to produce forearm pronation and supination was included in table 7.6. As with elbow flexion and extension, some of the other muscles whose primary action is at the wrist or hand can also assist with pronation and supination, but for purposes of simplicity they are not included in table 7.7.

In functional movement, the movements of pronation and supination are often used to appropriately position or assist with the action of the hand. For example, concentric contraction of the pronators—including the pronator quadratus and teres—is used in movements such as turning a screw counterclockwise (to loosen it) and dribbling a basketball. In dance, the pronators would be used in arm movements that involve facing the palm backward as in jazz. In contrast, concentric contraction of the supinators is used in tightening a screw, an underhand pitch, and a tennis backhand drive. In dance, the supinators—including the supinator and biceps brachii—would work when the dancer raises the arms from the sides with the palms facing upward.

In functional movement, the movements of the forearm are also often linked with motions at the shoulder joint. So, when the elbow is straight, forearm supination is often accompanied by external rotation of the shoulder, while forearm pronation is often linked with internal rotation of the shoulder. This combination allows a greater range of motion for the hand and more forceful movements such as used in turning a doorknob. In dance movements, these movements can also be combined to enhance range or provide a desired aesthetic, as in modern or jazz dance when the front arm is externally rotated with the palm facing up and the back arm is internally rotated with the palm facing back.

Note that this is a different arrangement than occurs in the lower leg, where the tibia and fibula are firmly connected and almost no motion is allowed between them. In the lower extremity, changing the facing of the foot occurs more distally within the bones of the feet rather than at the more proximal site of the forearm in the upper extremity.

Structure and Movements of the Wrist and Hand

The hand is a highly specialized structure that contains 27 bones and over 20 joints, and the wrist-hand complex involves the use of 25 key muscles. There are many parallels between the foot and hand, but one key distinction is that while the foot is designed primarily for strength to support the body weight, the hand is designed for manipulation.

The bones of the hand include eight **carpals** (which are arranged in two rows of four), five metacarpals (numbered from 1 through 5 starting from the thumb), and 14 phalanges as seen in figure 7.46. However, while there is a parallel with respect to the numbers and sequence of these bones, the tarsals and metatarsals of the foot are much larger than the corresponding carpals and metacarpals in the hand (to better serve their weight-bearing function), while in the hand the phalanges are larger than the phalanges in the foot (to better meet their manipulation function). The distal row of carpals articulates with the proximal end, or **base,** of the **metacarpals.** The shaft of the metacarpal is termed the **body;** and the distal rounded **head** of the metacarpal articulates anteriorly with its respective phalanges. The heads of the metacarpals can easily be palpated at the knuckles of the hand while the phalanges make up the digits of the fingers. The fingers are numbered like the corresponding metacarpals, with 1 corresponding to the thumb. They are also often designated as thumb, index finger, middle finger, ring finger, and little finger. The **phalanges** are termed the **proximal, middle,** and **distal** phalanges for fingers 2 through 5. The thumb is also termed the **pollex,** and like the hallux, it contains only two phalanges, the proximal and distal phalanges.

The hand is joined to the forearm at the wrist or **radiocarpal joint.** More specifically, the inferior concave surface of the radius and the adjacent triangular fibrocartilaginous disc articulate with the convex articular surface formed by the proximal row of carpals (scaphoid, lunate, and triquetrum bones) as shown in figure 7.47. Note that due to the presence of the fibrocartilage disc, the ulna does not directly participate in the wrist joint. However, this disc adds important stability to the wrist by binding the radius and ulna together distally (Magee, 1997). It also helps distribute the load between the radius and ulna. It has been estimated that the radius bears 60% of the load and the ulna 40% with the disc in place, in contrast to 95% for the radius and 5% for the ulna with the disc removed. The shape of the articular surfaces makes the wrist a biaxial condyloid joint. Hence, movements include flexion-extension and a specially designated form of abduction-adduction. Flexion refers to the motion of bringing the palm of the hand toward the front of the forearm, while the reverse movement of bringing the palm away is termed extension of the wrist as seen in figure 7.48. Abduction of the wrist refers to bringing the hand away from the midline such that the lateral surface of the hand (thumb) comes closer to the lateral

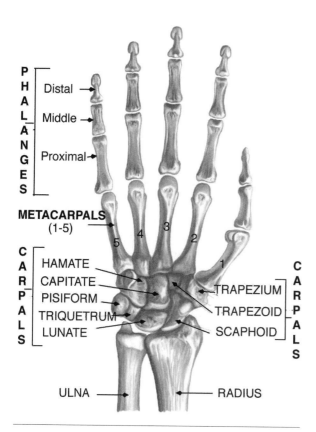

FIGURE 7.46   Bones of the hand (right hand, anterior or palmar view).

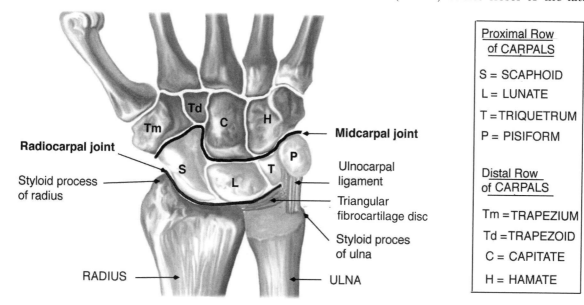

FIGURE 7.47   Radiocarpal and midcarpal joints (left hand, anterior or palmar view).

surface of the forearm. This motion is usually referred to with the specialized term **radial deviation.** The opposite motion of bringing the medial side of the hand (little finger) closer to the medial forearm is termed adduction or **ulnar deviation.**

However, these movements at the radiocarpal joint or wrist joint do not occur in isolation but rather also incorporate the **midcarpal joint.** The term midcarpal joint refers to the joint between the proximal and distal row of carpals. As with the foot, this "joint" actually incorporates several joints, and in the hand these joints are gliding in nature. However, the slight gliding movements of the midcarpal joint contribute additional range of motion and are automatically linked to movements of the radiocarpal joint.

Moving distally from the midcarpal joint, there are many additional joints that are important for allowing the complex movements of the hand. As with the feet, these joints are often named according to the bones that compose the joints, making learning the names easier and logical. The joints between the carpals and metacarpals 2 through 5 termed **carpometacarpal joints** are classified differently in different texts, but commonly as gliding joints (Hall, 1999; Magee, 1997). These joints are linked by strong ligaments such that almost no movement is allowed for joints 2 and 3, slight flexion is allowed with 4, and more flexion with 5. This arrangement facilitates the ability to cup the palm, which when combined with the motions of the first metacarpal facilitates the essential ability to grasp objects.

In contrast to the other carpometacarpal joints, the first carpometacarpal joint is a biaxial saddle joint, which allows for the specialized movement of opposition of the thumb to the fingers used to "grip" objects. **Opposition** refers to the ability to bring the palmar tip of the thumb toward the palmar surface of the other digits, and **reposition** is the reverse movement. This specialized movement of opposition is facilitated not only by the presence of this saddle joint and the cupping of the palm but also by the orientation of the joint relative to the other fingers. Unlike what occurs with the large toe in the foot, the thumb is separated from the second finger more widely than the other fingers are separated from one another and is turned on its axis so that it faces a plane perpendicular to that of the other fingers (Hamilton and Luttgens, 2002). In addition to the specialized movement of opposition-reposition, fundamental movements of the thumb include flexion-extension and abduction-adduction, shown in figure 7.48. Note that due to the rotated orientation of the thumb, these movements of the thumb occur in a plane perpendicular to the plane in which they classically occur. So, extension refers to a lateral movement of the thumb away from the index finger, while flexion is a return movement from extension; hyperflexion entails movement of the thumb across and parallel to the palm (i.e., in an almost frontal vs. sagittal plane). Abduction refers to movement of the thumb forward and away from the second finger in a plane perpendicular to the palm, while adduction would be the return movement to anatomical position (i.e., in an approximate sagittal vs. frontal plane). Given these movement descriptions, opposition can be seen as a combination of abduction and hyperflexion.

Moving further distally, the joint between the distal end of the first metacarpal bone and adjacent proximal phalange, termed the **metacarpophalangeal joint,** is a hinge joint allowing flexion and extension. However, the metacarpophalangeal joints for metacarpals 2 through 5 are biaxial condyloid joints—allowing flexion, extension, and slight abduction and adduction of the fingers. Flexion refers to bringing the anterior surface of the finger toward the palmar surface of the hand, while extension is the reverse movement of bringing the anterior surface of the finger away to return to anatomical position or slightly beyond (hyperextension) as seen in figure 7.48. Abduction and adduction occur relative to the middle finger, and abduction refers to movement of the second (index), fourth (ring), and fifth (little) fingers away from the third (middle) finger. The reverse motion of bringing the fingers back toward the middle finger is termed adduction. The side-to-side movements of the third finger are termed radial and ulnar flexion rather than abduction and adduction. Comparable to the situation with the wrist, radial flexion refers to lateral movement of the third finger toward the radial side of the forearm while ulnar flexion refers to medial movement of the third finger toward the ulnar side of the forearm. Lastly, the joints between all adjacent phalanges, the **interphalangeal joints,** are uniaxial hinge joints—allowing flexion and extension of the digits of the fingers and thumb. These movements of the fingers are comparable to those of the metacarpophalangeal joints, with flexion referring to approximating anterior surfaces of the digits of the fingers or bringing the anterior surface of the digits toward the palmar surface of the hand (or both). Extension would involve the reverse movement. In general, movements toward the palm of the hand (flexion) are of a larger range than movements toward the dorsum of the hand (extension).

Numerous strong ligaments interconnect the bones and reinforce the capsules of the many joints in the wrist-hand complex. Many muscles also act to

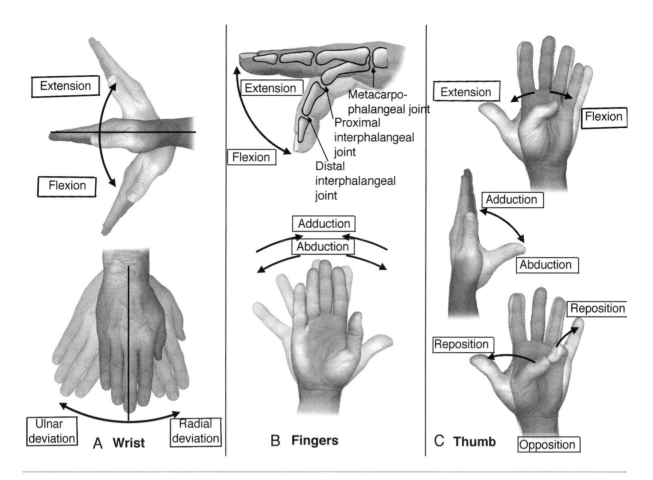

FIGURE 7.48   Movements of the (A) wrist, (B) fingers 2 through 5, and (C) thumb.

stabilize the joints and generate movements. As with the foot, there is a strong fascia that helps stabilize the joints (palmar aponeurosis) and maintain the cupped shape of the palm of the hand. The shape and arrangement of the carpals and difference in mobility of the carpometacarpal joints make the palm slightly concave anteriorly, vital for protection of the nerves, tendons, and blood vessels that cross the hand anteriorly. There are also retinacula that help keep the tendons in position. For example, the flexor retinaculum (composed of the palmar carpal and transverse carpal ligaments) helps hold the flexor tendons close to the wrist and prevents them from coming away from the bones when the wrist is flexed. Synovial sheaths surround many of the tendons in this area to help facilitate movement and diminish friction. Two small sesamoid bones are located on the palmar side of the metacarpophalangeal joint of the thumb, between which the long flexor of the thumb runs.

Muscles of the Wrist and Hand

There are approximately 25 primary muscles (some with multiple components) that perform functions

at the wrist and hand. Many of these muscles produce multiple actions, and an intricate coordination of muscles acting as prime movers, stabilizers, and synergists is often required to achieve the desired movements of the wrist and hand. A brief overview of these muscles follows. A summary of the attachments and actions of the extrinsic muscles of the wrist and hand is provided in table 7.8, while a summary of fundamental movements of the wrist and hand, and the extrinsic and intrinsic muscles that can produce them, is provided in table 7.9. Readers interested in a more thorough presentation are referred to the anatomy texts listed in the References and Resources at the back of the book.

Primary Muscles of the Wrist

There are six primary muscles that act on the wrist joint—flexor carpi radialis, palmaris longus, flexor carpi ulnaris, extensor carpi radialis longus, extensor carpi radialis brevis, and extensor carpi ulnaris (figures 7.49 and 7.50). There are also extrinsic muscles of the hands that cross the wrist joint and can assist with movements of the wrist as shown in table 7.8. As with the feet, many of the names of these muscles

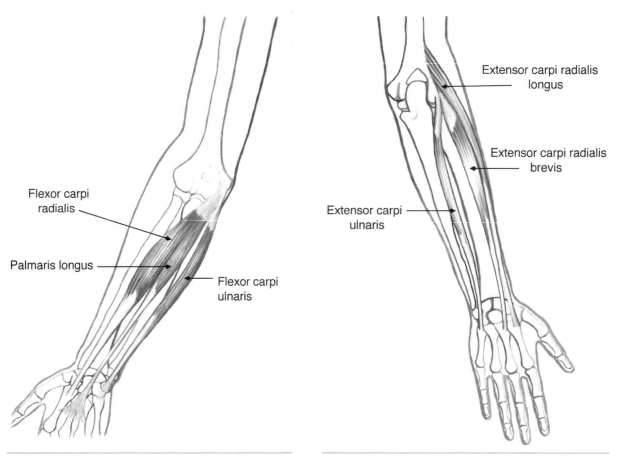

FIGURE 7.49   Primary flexors of the wrist (right forearm, anterior view).

FIGURE 7.50   Primary extensors of the wrist (right forearm, posterior view).

TABLE 7.8   Summary of Attachments and Primary Actions of Extrinsic Muscles of the Wrist and Hand

Muscle	Proximal attachment(s)	Distal attachment(s)	Primary action(s)
Muscles of the wrist			
Flexor carpi radialis (FLEK-sor KAR-pee ra-dee-A-lis)	Medial epicondyle of humerus	Base of 2nd and 3rd metacarpal	Wrist flexion Wrist radial deviation
Flexor carpi ulnaris (FLEK-sor KAR-pee ul-NA-ris)	Humeral head: medial epicondyle of humerus Ulnar head: olecranon and posterior border of ulna	Pisiform, hamate, and 5th metacarpal	Wrist flexion Wrist ulnar deviation
Palmaris longus (pahl-MA-ris LON-gus)	Medial epicondyle of humerus	Distal flexor retinaculum and palmar aponeurosis	Wrist flexion
Extensor carpi radialis longus (ek-STEN-sor KAR-pee ra-dee-A-lis LON-gus)	Lateral supracondylar ridge of humerus	Base of 2nd metacarpal	Wrist extension Wrist radial deviation
Extensor carpi radialis brevis (ek-STEN-sor KAR-pee ra-dee-A-lis BRE-vis)	Lateral epicondyle of humerus	Base of 3rd metacarpal	Wrist extension Wrist radial deviation
Extensor carpi ulnaris (ek-STEN-sor KAR-pee ul-NA-ris)	Lateral epicondyle of humerus and posterior ulna	Base of 5th metacarpal	Wrist extension Wrist ulnar deviation

Muscle	Proximal attachment(s)	Distal attachment(s)	Primary action(s)
Extrinsic muscles of fingers			
Flexor digitorum profundus (FLEK-sor di-ji-TOR-um pro-FUN-dus)	Proximal three-quarters of anterior and medial ulna	Base of distal phalanges of fingers 2 through 5	Flexion of fingers and hand (MP and distal IP joints of fingers 2-5) Assists with wrist flexion
Flexor digitorum superficialis (FLEK-sor di-ji-TOR-um soo-per-fish-ee-A-lis)	Medial epicondyle of humerus and proximal anterior radius	Middle phalanges of fingers 2 through 5	Flexion of fingers and hand (MP and proximal IP joints of fingers 2-5) Assists with wrist flexion
Extensor digitorum (ek-STEN-sor di-ji-TOR-um)	Lateral epicondyle of humerus	Base of distal and middle phalanges of fingers 2 through 5	Extension of fingers (MP, proximal IP, and distal IP joints of fingers 2-5) Assists with wrist extension
Extensor indicis (ek-STEN-sor IN-di-kis)	Distal posterior ulna	Extensor expansion of 2nd finger	Extension of 2nd finger (MP, proximal IP, and distal IP joints of 2nd finger) Assists with wrist extension
Extensor digiti minimi (ek-STEN-sor DI-ji-tie MI-ni-my)	Lateral epicondyle of humerus	Extensor expansion of 5th finger	Extension of 5th finger (MP, proximal IP, and distal IP joints of 5th finger) Assists with wrist extension
Extrinsic muscles of thumb (pollex)			
Flexor pollicis longus (FLEK-sor PAH-li-kis LON-gus)	Middle anterior radius	Base of distal phalanx of thumb	Flexion of thumb (CMC, MP, and IP joints of thumb) Assists with opposition of thumb and wrist flexion
Extensor pollicis longus (ek-STEN-sor PAH-li-kis LON-gus)	Middle posterior ulna	Base of distal phalanx of thumb	Extension of thumb (CMC, MP, and IP joints of thumb) Assists with wrist extension and radial deviation
Extensor pollicis brevis (ek-STEN-sor PAH-li-kis BRE-vis)	Middle posterior radius	Base of proximal phalanx of thumb	Extension of thumb (CMC and IP joints of thumb) Assists with abduction of thumb (CMC joint of thumb) Assists with wrist radial deviation
Abductor pollicis longus (ab-DUK-tor PAH-li-kis LON-gus)	Middle posterior ulna and radius	Radial side of base of 1st metacarpal	Abduction of thumb (CMC joint of thumb) Assists with extension of thumb (CMC joint of thumb), wrist flexion, and wrist radial deviation

indicate their action, location, or both. To aid with picturing the action of the muscles of the wrist and hand, remember to think about the line of pull of the respective muscles in reference to anatomical position with the forearm supinated and the palm facing forward. In this position, there is a logical arrangement of the muscles such that the flexors are located on the front while the extensors are located on the back of the forearm, wrist, and hand.

Another helpful organizational clue for the wrist is that the primary flexors of the wrist arise proximally from around the medial epicondyle of the humerus,

TABLE 7.9 Fundamental Movements of the Wrist and Hand and the Muscles That Can Produce Them

	Wrist				MP				PIP		DIP		CMC of thumb				
	Flexion	Extension	Radial deviation	Ulnar deviation	Flexion	Extension	Abduction	Adduction	Flexion	Extension	Flexion	Extension	Flexion	Extension	Abduction	Adduction	Opposition
Muscles of the wrist																	
Flexor carpi radialis	P		P														
Flexor carpi ulnaris	P			P													
Palmaris longus	P																
Extensor carpi radialis longus		P	P														
Extensor carpi radialis brevis		P	P														
Extensor carpi ulnaris		P		P													
Extrinsic muscles of the fingers and wrist																	
Flexor digitorum profundus	S				P				P		P						
Flexor digitorum superficialis	S				P				P								
Extensor digitorum		S				P				P		P					
Extensor indicis		S				P				P		P					
Extensor digiti minimi		S				P	S			P		P					
Intrinsic muscles of the fingers																	
Lumbricals					P					P		P					
Dorsal interossei					S		P			S		S					
Palmar interossei					S			P		S		S					
Abductor digiti minimi					S		P										
Flexor digiti minimi brevis					P												
Opponens digiti minimi					P		P										
Extrinsic muscles of the thumb (pollex)																	
Flexor pollicis longus	S				S				P		S		S				
Extensor pollicis longus		S	S			P				P				P			
Extensor pollicis brevis			S			P								P	S		
Abductor pollicis longus	S		S											S	P		
Intrinsic muscles of the thumb (pollex)																	
Flexor pollicis brevis													P				S
Opponens pollicis																	P
Adductor pollicis																P	
Abductor pollicis brevis															P		S

P = primary action(s) of muscle; S = secondary action(s) of muscle; MP = metacarpophalangeal joint; PIP = proximal interphalangeal joint (for thumb PIP equivalent to interphalangeal joint; DIP = distal interphalangeal joint; CMC = carpometacarpal joint of thumb.

430

while the extensors arise proximally from around the lateral epicondyle of the humerus. Depending on their distal attachment and resultant line of pull, they also can contribute to ulnar or radial deviation of the wrist. For example, the flexor carpi radialis and the extensor carpi radialis longus and brevis attach distally to the second and third metacarpals and so can produce radial deviation as well as their respective flexion or extension of the wrist. In contrast, the flexor carpi ulnaris and extensor carpi ulnaris have distal attachments that include the fifth metacarpal and so can produce ulnar deviation as well as their respective flexion or extension of the wrist.

Primary Muscles of the Fingers

There are five muscles that have proximal attachments in the forearm (extrinsic muscles) that can be used to flex and extend the fingers. Three of these act on all four fingers at once, two to produce flexion of the fingers (flexor digitorum superficialis, flexor digitorum profundus) and one to produce extension (extensor digitorum) of the fingers. The remaining two muscles act selectively on the fingers, one to extend the index finger (extensor indicis) and the other to extend the little finger (extensor digiti minimi). In addition, there are 14 smaller muscles located within the hand (intrinsic muscles). Eleven of these muscles work to flex, extend, abduct, and adduct the four fingers. They are arranged in three groups called the lumbricals (four muscles), dorsal interossei (four muscles), and palmar interossei (three muscles). Three additional intrinsic muscles act selectively on the little finger (abductor digiti minimi, flexor digiti minimi brevis, and opponens digiti minimi) to flex, abduct, or aid in bringing the little finger across the palm for important movement of opposition with the thumb. Both the flexors and extensors of the digits have complex splitting and attachments of tendon slips onto various positions on the phalanges to allow for isolated or combined movements of the various digits of the fingers.

Primary Muscles of the Thumb

In addition, there are four muscles that originate in the forearm (extrinsic muscles) that can be used to flex, extend, abduct, or assist with opposition of the thumb (flexor pollicis longus, extensor pollicis longus, extensor pollicis brevis, abductor pollicis longus). Four other intrinsic muscles can also produce movements of the thumb (flexor pollicis brevis, opponens pollicis, abductor pollicis brevis, adductor pollicis). These muscles form the rounded contour that can be felt below and medial to the thumb (thenar eminence).

Key Considerations for the Upper Extremity in Whole Body Movement

In the upper extremities as a whole, a complex interplay of muscles is often utilized to allow for isolated movement and stabilization of the relevant joints. It is often necessary to utilize synergies to achieve the desired movements and to avoid positions of active insufficiency or passive insufficiency when multijoint muscles are involved. Furthermore, in functional movement, movements of the various upper extremity joints are often linked, and a meaningful movement analysis should take into account the contributions of relevant joints.

Actions of Multijoint Upper Extremity Muscles

Many of the muscles of the upper extremity, and particularly the hand, cross two or more joints and have actions or potential actions over each of these joints. Because the tendency of a multijoint muscle is to produce movement at all of the joints it crosses, other muscles are often required to act as stabilizers and synergists so that the movement occurs at just the desired joints and in the desired direction for a given task. For example, when the desired action of the biceps brachii is only supination, the elbow extensors (triceps brachii and anconeus) can contract simultaneously (acting as synergists) to prevent the undesired action of the biceps (elbow flexion). Thus, when turning a doorknob (supination), the elbow can be appropriately positioned in extension to complete the task, rather than having the elbow flex and the hand pull away from the doorknob as supination is attempted.

In dance, synergies are often used to neutralize or control the magnitude of secondary muscle actions so that the desired aesthetics can be achieved. For example, when the dancer raises the arms from second to high fifth, the triceps brachii can again work to limit elbow flexion while the biceps brachii is working to produce the desired supination of the forearm. At the wrist, simultaneous contraction of the flexor carpi radialis and flexor carpi ulnaris allows desired slight flexion of the wrist while the respective radial deviation and ulnar deviation are neutralized.

Also, remember that with multijoint muscles, motion at one joint alters muscle length, which in turn affects the muscle's ability to produce force or be stretched across the other joint(s) it crosses. For example, components of the biceps brachii and triceps brachii cross both the shoulder joint and the elbow joint. Functionally, movements often utilize joint motion combinations that simultaneously lengthen the muscle at one joint and shorten the muscle at the other joint such that active insufficiency is avoided and effective force production can proceed. For example, during pulling motions, the extension at the shoulder lengthens the biceps brachii (across the shoulder joint) so that sufficient tension can be generated as the elbow flexes (which shortens the biceps). However, in other cases such as when lifting a dancer to the front with an underhand grip, the biceps brachii will be shortened across both the elbow and shoulder joints and active insufficiency can become operative. Both active and passive insufficiency also come into play with the extrinsic muscles of the hands, and appropriate positioning of the wrist is often used to avoid these potential limitations.

Coordinated Movements of Multiple Upper Extremity Joints

In functional movement, there is often an intricate coordination between the hand, wrist, radioulnar, elbow, and shoulder joints to facilitate successful execution of the desired movement. In open kinematic chain movements, many joints often contribute to effective positioning of the hand for manipulation of objects. For example, the later phase of overhead throwing often involves wrist flexion and ulnar deviation, complemented by forearm pronation, internal shoulder rotation, and scapular abduction (Kreighbaum and Barthels, 1996). In dance, aesthetic criteria are often more operative, and characteristic placement and use of the arms are often associated with different forms and schools of dance. For example, classical ballet often uses a slight internal rotation at the shoulder joint, flexion of the elbow, supination of the forearm, and flexion of the wrist to achieve the desired line of the arm when held out to the side such as seen in the opening photo for chapter 1 (p. 1). An example of stylized use of the upper extremity for flamenco dance can be seen in figure 7.31 (p. 408), the Graham modern dance technique in figure 7.51A, and African dance in figure 7.51B. Development of the intricate coordination required to achieve the given dance aesthetic may take years of training to perfect.

Conditioning Exercises for the Upper Extremity

Unlike some of the other joints previously discussed, for many dancers, adequate flexibility is less of an issue in the upper extremity than strength. Because the shoulder is designed for mobility, adequate strength in the surrounding muscles is key for stability and injury prevention. Furthermore, many dance classes do not provide movements that progressively develop strength for the upper extremity as is done for the lower extremity. Hence, strengthening performed outside of class is often necessary to successfully achieve dance movements requiring high levels of strength such as partnering or inverted positions.

Strength Exercises for the Upper Extremity

Selected strength exercises for the shoulder, scapula, and elbow are provided in table 7.10, and a brief description of their importance follows. Interested readers are referred to texts by Kraemer and Fleck (2005); Peterson, Bryant, and Peterson (1995); and other resources available through the National Strength and Conditioning Association for a more comprehensive coverage of upper extremity strengthening exercises. When performing strength exercises for the shoulder, it is important to note that the resistance arm is very long when lifting a weight with the elbow straight. Due to this relationship, the muscle force required to support the limb at 90° of shoulder abduction has been calculated to be about 8.2 times the weight of the limb (Soderberg, 1986). This means that holding a 10-pound (4.5-kilogram) weight in the hand would require about 82 pounds (37 kilograms) of muscle force to support that weight. Hence, to achieve the desired benefits and avoid injury, particular care should be taken to perform such exercises slowly, in a controlled manner, with correct technique, in a range in which no joint discomfort is experienced, and with gradual increases of resistance in small increments as strength gains allow. It is also important to realize that there are great individual differences in upper extremity strength in accordance with many factors, including gender and body type. So, for example, a male dancer with proportionally shorter arms might be able to safely lift a much heavier weight than a female dancer with proportionally longer arms. In light of these factors, many of the sample exercises given in table 7.10 utilize body weight, bands, or relatively light dumbbells for resistance. However, dancers interested in developing greater strength are encouraged to work with a qualified exercise specialist so that appropriate progressions can be made.

(Text continues on p. 444.)

Passive Insufficiency With Finger Flexion

Fully flex the fingers with the wrist held in a neutral position of extension. Now, slowly flex the wrist and notice how the fingers start extending slightly, and notice that it is not possible to maintain full flexion of the fingers. This is due to passive insufficiency of the extensor digitorum. The extensor digitorum is not long enough to stretch over all of the joints it crosses, including the wrist, midcarpal, metacarpophalangeal, and interphalangeal joints. Under normal conditions when one makes a fist, the wrist extensors (extensor carpi ulnaris and extensor carpi radialis longus and brevis) hold the wrist in extension, acting as synergists to neutralize flexion of the wrist produced by the extrinsic flexors of the fingers so that full lexion of the fingers can occur. The optimal position for grip function appears to be about 20° to 30° of wrist extension (Soderberg, 1986), and forcefully flexing the wrist of someone holding a weapon can be used in combat to force the person to loosen the grip on the weapon.

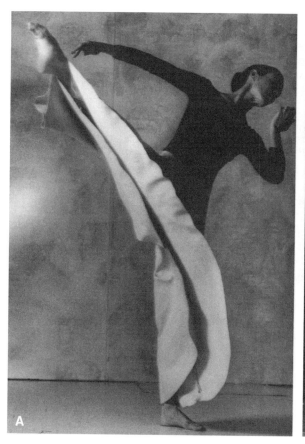

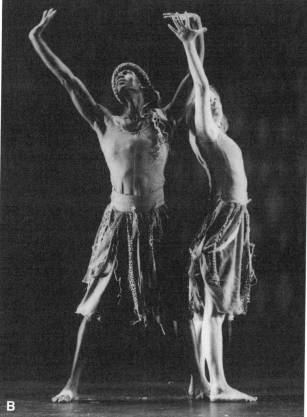

FIGURE 7.51   An example of stylized use of the upper extremity in (A) the Graham-based movement and (B) African dance.

Figure 7.51A: Photo courtesy of Scott Peterson. Dancer: Susan McLain.
Figure 7.51B: Photo courtesy of Keith Ian Polakoff. CSULB dancers Delyer Anderson and Dwayne Worthington.

TABLE 7.10 Selected Strength Exercises for the Upper Extremity

Exercise name (Resistance)	Description (Technique cues)	Progression
Muscle groups: Shoulder flexors and elbow extensors **Muscles emphasized: Pectoralis major**		
Joint movement: Shoulder flexion with elbow extension		
A. Push-up with elbows in (Body weight) *Variation 1*	Support body weight on knees or feet and hands in accordance with current strength level, with hands about shoulder-width apart. Slowly bend the elbows and return to the starting position. (Maintain a neutral position of the pelvis and avoid arching the low back; aim to create a straight line along the side of the shoulder, hip, and knee; keep the elbows close to the sides as they bend and straighten.) *Variation 1:* Push-up plus—After returning to the starting position with the elbows straight, continue pressing against the floor so that the shoulder blades come toward the sides of the rib cage and the upper back rounds. As skill improves, isolate the movement to just scapular abduction while the upper spine stays in its neutral extended position.	1. Lower chest closer to floor. 2. Progress to feet if performing on knees. 3. Perform with knees or feet on a ball or step.
Muscle group: Shoulder flexors **Muscles emphasized: Anterior deltoid and pectoralis major (sternal)**		
Joint movement: Shoulder flexion with elbow extension maintained		
B. Front arm raise (Dumbbell) 	Stand with feet hip-width apart and a dumbbell in one hand with the palm facing down. Slowly raise the arm to the front in a pain-free range to a maximum of about shoulder height, pause, and slowly return to the starting position. (Keep abdominals firmly contracted to maintain a neutral pelvis and avoid leaning the torso back as the arm raises. Bend the knees slightly if necessary to avoid knee hyperextension.) *Variation 1:* Perform with both arms raising and lowering simultaneously.	1. Gradually increase dumbbell from about 3 pounds to 10 pounds.

Exercise name (Resistance)	Description (Technique cues)	Progression

Muscle groups: Shoulder flexors, scapular depressors, and elbow extensors
Muscles emphasized: Lower trapezius and serratus anterior

Joint movement: Shoulder flexion with elbow extension and scapular depression

C. Press-up (Body weight) 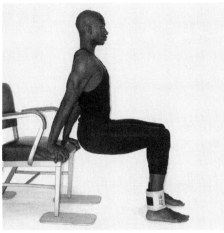 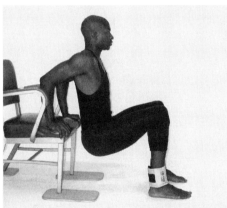	Sit at the very edge of a chair (with the chair securely positioned by placing its back against a wall) with the hands at the edge of the seat and the fingers facing forward. Then press down into the seat of the chair so that the elbows straighten, and shift the pelvis forward so that it is just in front of the chair seat. Then slowly bend the elbows and lower the trunk, pause, and straighten the elbows to return to the starting position. (Focus on firmly pulling the shoulder blades down in the starting position, and only work in a range in which slight scapular depression and adduction can be maintained and no shoulder discomfort is experienced; keep the elbows close to your sides as they bend and straighten.) *Variation 1:* Perform with the hands at the edge of the seat but with the fingers facing to the side and the elbows bending to the side to focus on strengthening the shoulder adductors.	1. Perform with more body weight supported on one arm. 2. Perform with one arm.

Muscle groups: Shoulder extensors and scapular adductors
Muscles emphasized: Latissimus dorsi and lower trapezius

Joint movements: Shoulder extension and scapular adduction with elbow flexion maintained

D. Sitting row (elbows in) (Elastic band) 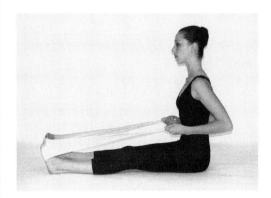	Sit with the legs outstretched to the front with the middle of the band passing under the balls of the feet, one end of each band in each hand, and the elbows extended. Then pull the elbows backward, pause, and slowly return to the starting position. (Focus on pulling the shoulder blades slightly downward and together as the elbows pull back.) *Variation 1:* Perform sitting on a box on the Reformer facing the straps with one strap in each hand. *Variation 2:* Sitting row (elbows out)—Perform with the elbows at shoulder height (shoulder horizontal abduction) and the palms facing down.	1. Pull the elbows farther backward while still maintaining good form. 2. Hold farther forward on the band. 3. Use a heavier band.

(continued)

Exercise name (Resistance)	Description (Technique cues)	Progression
Muscle groups: Shoulder extensors and elbow extensors **Muscles emphasized: Latissimus dorsi and triceps brachii**		
Joint movement: Shoulder extension with elbow extension		
E. Lunge triceps kick back (Dumbbell)	Stand in a lunge with the left foot forward, the torso partially supported by the right hand on the left thigh and the left arm hanging toward the floor with the elbow extended and a dumbbell in the left hand. Then slowly bend and raise the left elbow up toward the ceiling, extend the elbow, pause, slowly bend the elbow, and return to the starting position. Repeat on the other side. (Focus on keeping the elbow high as it extends to a straight but not hyperextended position; maintain firm trunk stabilization.)	1. Gradually increase dumbbell from 5 pounds to 10 pounds.

Exercise name (Resistance)	Description (Technique cues)	Progression
Muscle group: Shoulder abductors **Muscles emphasized: Middle deltoid and supraspinatus**		
Joint movement: Shoulder abduction with elbow extension		
F. Side arm raise (Dumbbell) 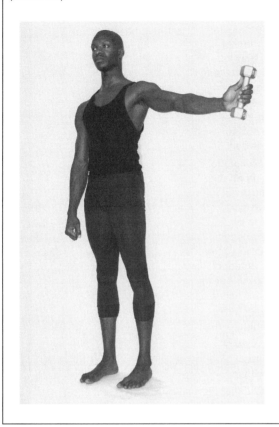	Stand with feet hip-width apart and a dumbbell in one hand. Slowly raise the arm to the side to a maximum of shoulder height, pause, and slowly return to the starting position. Externally rotate the shoulder as the arm raises so that the thumb ends facing up toward the ceiling, and maintain the arm slightly forward of the frontal plane in scaption. Repeat on the other side. (Focus on allowing the scapula to upwardly rotate as the arm raises without excessive elevation; use a low enough weight and range of motion that no shoulder discomfort is experienced.) *Variation 1:* Perform the exercise without external rotation so that the palm stays facing downward and in the frontal plane, but limit the range to about 60° abduction (pain free). *Variation 2:* Perform either version of the exercise with a dumbbell in each hand and both arms raising simultaneously.	1. Gradually increase dumbbell from 3 pounds to 8 or 10 pounds.

(continued)

Exercise name (Resistance)	Description (Technique cues)	Progression
Muscle group: Shoulder abductors and elbow extensors **Muscles emphasized: Middle deltoid**		
Joint movement: Shoulder abduction with elbow extension		
G. Sitting overhead press (Elastic band) *Variation 2*	Sit with the knees bent and feet on the floor while each hand holds the end of a band that passes under the knees. Start with the palms facing forward in front of each shoulder and the elbows bent close to the sides. Then slowly extend the elbows as the hands reach toward the ceiling, pause, and slowly bend the elbows to return to the starting position. (Focus on the elbows reaching to the side and the scapulae rotating without excessive elevation as the arms go overhead; extend the elbows with control to a straight but not hyperextended position; use co-contraction of the abdominals to avoid an anterior pelvic tilt or rib-leading as the arms go overhead.) *Variation 1:* Perform sitting with light dumbbells in the hands. *Variation 2:* Kneeling overhead press—Perform kneeling on the Reformer, starting with the sternum above the footbar and the elbows facing outward. Then press against the footbar as the elbows extend so that the carriage moves backward. *Variation 3:* Perform any of these versions with the elbows facing forward instead of sideward to emphasize the shoulder flexors instead of the shoulder abductors.	1. Shorten the band by gripping it with the hands closer together. 2. Use a heavier band.

Exercise name (Resistance)	Description (Technique cues)	Progression

Muscle groups: Shoulder external rotators and scapular adductors
Muscles emphasized: Infraspinatus, teres minor, and lower trapezius

Joint movement: Shoulder external rotation with scapular adduction

| H. Kneeling scarecrow (Dumbbells) 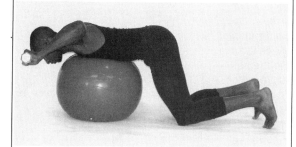 | Kneel on the floor or a mat with the torso supported on an exercise ball and the elbows bent to about 90°, with a dumbbell held in each hand such that the fists face the floor. Tighten the abdominals firmly to stabilize the lumbar spine, raise the elbows up toward the ceiling, externally rotate the upper arms at the shoulder joint so that the hands raise forward and up, hold 4 counts, and then slowly derotate the arms to bring them back to the starting position.

(Focus on pulling the shoulder blades slightly together as you raise the elbows higher than your back. Then focus on keeping the shoulder blades slightly down and together as the arms externally rotate.)

Variation 1: Perform sitting, facing toward the back of a chair with the upper chest resting against the back of the chair (shown previously in figure 3.26A on p. 99).

Variation 2: Perform sitting with an elastic band, one arm at a time, as the other arm anchors the band in front of the body (figure 7.20C, p. 396). | 1. After full external rotation of the shoulders, extend the elbows and reach the hands overhead in line with the shoulders and above the height of the ears.
2. After full external rotation of the shoulders, arch the upper back.
3. After full external rotation of the shoulders, arch the upper back and then extend the elbows as the hands reach overhead. |

Muscle group: Shoulder external rotators
Muscles emphasized: Infraspinatus and teres minor

Joint movement: Shoulder external rotation with scapular adduction

| I. Double-shoulder external rotation (Elastic band) 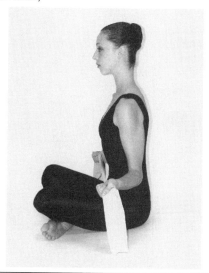 | Sit with the knees bent and the legs crossed or the feet on the floor while each hand holds the end of a band, with the palms facing upward and the elbows bent to about 90° and close to the sides. Then externally rotate the arms at the shoulder joint, bringing the thumbs backward.

(Keep the elbows close to the sides; focus on pulling the shoulder blades slightly together and down as the arms externally rotate.)

Variation 1: Perform sitting on the box or kneeling, facing the straps of a Reformer, with one strap in each hand and the palms facing upward while the elbows are bent to about 90° by the sides. | 1. Rotate further so that the hands come back further.
2. Place the hands closer together on the band.
3. After external rotation of the arms, arch the upper back while firmly pulling up from the lower attachment of the abdominals to limit anterior tilting of the pelvis.
4. After external rotation of the arms, arch the upper back and extend the elbows, reaching the hands out to the sides and slightly behind the back. |

(continued)

Exercise name (Resistance)	Description (Technique cues)	Progression
Muscle group: Shoulder internal rotators **Muscles emphasized: Subscapularis**		
Joint movement: Shoulder internal rotation with elbow flexion maintained		
J. Single-shoulder internal rotation (Reformer) 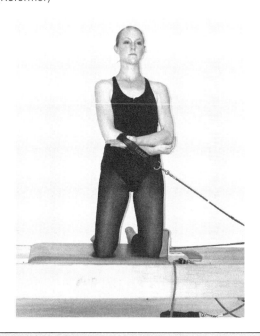	Kneel on a Reformer with the knees about shoulder-width apart and the left knee against the shoulder rest, with the left side facing the straps. Hold one strap in the left hand with the palm facing up, the elbow bent to about 90°, and the shoulder externally rotated while the right hand supports the left elbow. Then slowly internally rotate the left arm at the shoulder joint, bringing the little finger toward the right elbow, pause, and slowly externally rotate the arm to return to the starting position. Repeat on the other side. (Keep the elbow close to the side as the arm rotates, and focus on keeping the shoulder blade slightly down and back so that the shoulder does not roll forward.) *Variation 1:* Perform using an elastic band or tubing that is secured to a barre.	1. Use heavier springs. 2. Use slightly shorter straps.
Muscle group: Scapular abductors **Muscles emphasized: Serratus anterior**		
Joint movement: Scapular abduction with shoulder flexion and horizontal adduction combined		
K. Arm across (Elastic band) 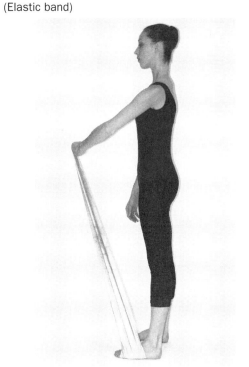	Stand with the feet about shoulder-width apart and one end of a band secured under the left foot and the other end held in the left hand, which is positioned just in front of the left thigh with the left elbow extended. Then slowly raise the arm on a diagonal such that the movement ends with the hand in front of the right shoulder, pause, and slowly lower the arm to the starting position. Repeat on the other side. (Focus on reaching the arm forward and across the body such that scapular abduction is emphasized. Maintain the elbow close to fully extended but not hyperextended throughout the movement.)	1. Grip further up on the band. 2. Use a heavier band.

Exercise name (Resistance)	Description (Technique cues)	Progression

Muscle group: Elbow flexors
Muscles emphasized: Biceps brachii and brachialis

Joint movement: Elbow flexion

L. Concentration curl (Dumbbell) 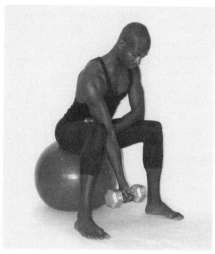 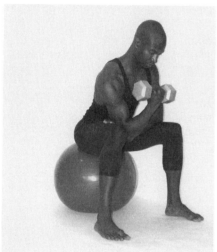	Sit on an exercise ball or chair with the right elbow resting against the right inner thigh and the right hand holding a dumbbell, while the left forearm rests on the left thigh to help support the torso and the left hand helps to stabilize the right arm. Then slowly bend the right elbow, bringing the right hand toward the right shoulder, pause, and slowly lower the hand to the starting position. Repeat on the other side. (Focus on keeping the tip of the elbow stationary as the elbow flexes and extends; slowly return to a straight but not hyperextended position of the elbow.)	1. Gradually increase dumbbells from 5 pounds to 10 pounds.

(continued)

Exercise name (Resistance)	Description (Technique cues)	Progression
Muscle groups: Elbow flexors and shoulder flexors **Muscles emphasized: Biceps brachii and pectoralis major (clavicular)**		
Joint movements: Elbow flexion and shoulder flexion		
M. Kneeling biceps lift (Reformer) 	Kneel on a Reformer, facing the springs, with the soles of the feet against the shoulder rests. Hold one strap in each hand with the palms facing front and the elbows slightly bent and positioned behind the torso. Then slowly flex the elbows and bring the arms forward and up to about the height of the forehead, pause, and gradually return the arms to the starting position. Time the elbow movement so that the elbows reach about 90° flexion when they are by the sides, and then extend in the upper ranges of shoulder flexion so that tension is maintained in the straps. (Focus on keeping the trunk stationary and allowing the scapulae to rotate and slightly abduct without excessive elevation as the arms raise.) *Variation 1:* Perform standing with your back to a barre with the middle of an elastic band looped around the barre and one end of the band held in each hand.	1. Increase springs. 2. Slightly shorten straps.

Exercise name (Resistance)	Description (Technique cues)	Progression
Muscle group: Elbow extensors **Muscles emphasized: Triceps brachii**		
Joint movement: Elbow extension with shoulder abduction maintained		
N. Overhead triceps extension (Dumbbell) 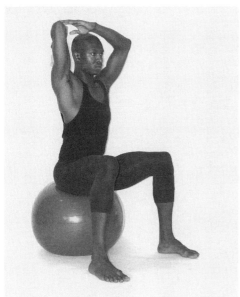 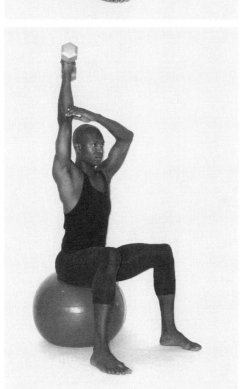	Sit on an exercise ball or chair with the right elbow pointing up toward the ceiling and the right hand holding a dumbbell while the left hand helps stabilize the right arm. Then slowly extend the right elbow, bringing the right hand directly up toward the ceiling, pause, and slowly bend the elbow to return to the starting position. Repeat on the other side. (Focus on keeping the torso and upper arm stationary as the elbow slowly extends to a straight but not hyperextended position; carefully control the flexion of the elbow during the return movement.)	1. Gradually increase the dumbbell from 5 pounds to 10 pounds.

(continued)

TABLE 7.10   Selected Strength Exercises for the Upper Extremity *(continued)*

Exercise name (Resistance)	Description (Technique cues)	Progression
Muscle groups: Elbow extensors and shoulder extensors **Muscles emphasized: Triceps brachii and latissimus dorsi**		
Joint movement: Elbow extension with shoulder extension		
O. Kneeling triceps kick back (Reformer)	Kneel on the Reformer, facing the straps, with the thighs against the shoulder rests. Begin holding one strap in each hand with the arms positioned to the front at about 45° of shoulder flexion and the elbows extended. Then pull the elbows back behind the torso, slowly extend the elbows, pause, and slowly bend the elbows to return to the starting position. (Focus on keeping the elbows high as they extend to a straight but not hyperextended position; keep palms facing forward as elbows extend; maintain firm trunk stabilization.)	1. Increase springs. 2. Slightly shorten straps.

Shoulder Flexors

Developing strength in the shoulder flexors is particularly important for choreography requiring body support by the arms. The push-up (table 7.10A) is a helpful exercise for developing this strength and the skill to stabilize the torso while using the arms. Push-up tests are commonly used to assess shoulder flexor strength and primarily endurance. Many female dancers test below average on this test, perhaps due to limited upper extremity conditioning provided in many dance classes, the prevalence of the long-limbed body type (at least in the ballet world), and the common occurrence of rapid weight loss (from dieting) with associated upper extremity muscle loss. The press-up (table 7.10C) is another useful exercise for developing the strength to support the body weight with the arms in floor work. Adequate shoulder flexor strength is also essential for lifting or holding a partner, and the front arm raise (table 7.10B) and sitting overhead press (table 7.10G, variation 3) can help develop this strength.

However, such overhead positions, like that used in the overhead press, can create shoulder injury such as impingement and should only be used if no shoulder pain is experienced and after building strength with exercises using lower ranges of should flexion, such as push-ups and the front arm raise (limited to 60° or 90° flexion).

Shoulder Extensors

Strengthening the shoulder extensors is important for pulling movements and for muscle balance. Many athletes overemphasize strengthening the shoulder flexors relative to the shoulder extensors, and the resultant muscle imbalance can lead to a rolled shoulder posture. The shoulder extensors are classically strengthened with the calisthenic of pull-ups. However, many dancers have insufficient strength to perform pull-ups or lack access to appropriate apparatus on which to perform them. The sitting row (table 7.10D) and triceps kick back (table 7.10, E and O) provide alternatives for strengthening the extensors.

Shoulder Abductors

Adequate strength in the shoulder abductors is important for being able to hold the arms up in second position, as well as some types of partnering or lifting. The side arm raise (table 7.10F) is particularly helpful for holding the arms, while the sitting overhead press is more useful for overhead partnering (table 7.10G). A push-up can also be carefully advanced in stronger dancers by progressively lifting the hips more over the hands until the dancer can perform the exercise in a handstand position with the legs resting against the wall and the elbows bending to the side on the down-phase. However, overhead positions involving shoulder abduction hold a high risk for impingement, and these types of exercises should be performed only if they are pain free and after a base of strength and good mechanics have been developed through performance of exercises like the side arm raise.

TESTS AND MEASUREMENTS 7.1

Push-Up Test

Perform the following test with another dancer to assess the strength and endurance of key upper extremity muscles (shoulder flexors and elbow extensors).

   Start in a push-up position with either your knees or feet (with the toes tucked under/metatarsophalangeal hyperextension) as the pivotal point in accordance with strength level. The hands are placed approximately shoulder-width apart and directly under the shoulders with the fingers facing straight forward or slightly inward. A partner places a fist on the ground under your chest and counts the number of times you can consecutively lower your body while maintaining the back straight until you touch the fist and then return to the starting position.

   Goals: Goals vary by gender, age group, and study performed. For ages 20 to 29, the norms given by the Canadian Physical Activity, Fitness and Lifestyle Appraisal (as cited in Nieman, 1999) are as follows:

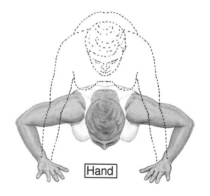

	Male (from toes)	Female (from knees)
Excellent	≥36	≥30
Average	22-28	15-20

Shoulder Adductors

Since the shoulder adductors are not a separate muscle group, but rather reflect a pairing of flexors and extensors working together, specific exercises are not included for shoulder adduction in this text. Due to the large muscles capable of producing this movement, the greatest force can be generated with shoulder adduction—often about twice the force that can be generated with shoulder abduction (Hamill and Knutzen, 1995). However, in the gym, exercises for the shoulder adductors include lat pull-downs and pull-downs performed with high wall pulleys. The press-up (table 7.10C, p. 435) can also be modified by facing the fingers and bending the elbows to the sides to encourage use of shoulder adductors. Similarly, strengthening of the shoulder adductors can easily be included with the curl-up performed on the Reformer (previously described in table 3.4D on p. 135) by pulling the arms down from shoulder height to the sides in the frontal plane—that is, shoulder adduction versus shoulder flexion.

Shoulder External Rotators

Strengthening the shoulder external rotators should also be a priority due to their importance in promoting correct shoulder mechanics and in preventing rolled shoulders, impingement syndrome, and other shoulder injuries. Everyday activity does not necessarily provide the desired strength for the external rotators, and they are generally able to produce less torque than the internal rotators or any other muscle group of the shoulder. Furthermore, one study showed that the ratio of internal rotation to external rotation was about 30% higher in the dominant versus the nondominant shoulders of 15 normal subjects, due to higher internal rotation in the dominant versus the nondominant arm and approximately the same external rotation in the dominant and nondominant arm (Warner et al., 1990). The kneeling scarecrow (table 7.10H, p. 439) offers an effective exercise for the shoulder external rotators that can be performed with weights, while double-shoulder external rotation (table 7.10I, p. 439) can be performed with an elastic band.

Performing the latter exercise with the elbow slightly in front of the torso (with the shoulder in the plane of the scapula) will allow greater conformity between the head of the humerus and glenoid fossa, greater force production due to a more optimal length of the shoulder external rotators, and more range of motion due to slackening of the joint capsule (Greenfield et al., 1990). Gently pressing your elbow inward against your opposite hand (shoulder adduction in the plane of the scapula) may also allow

less use of the posterior deltoid and greater use of the rotator cuff for external rotation.

Shoulder Internal Rotators

Strengthening the shoulder internal rotators is advisable for balance if a lot of exercises are being performed for the shoulder external rotators or if there is a history of shoulder injury. The shoulder internal rotators (particularly the subscapularis) are considered key for shoulder stability. Single-shoulder internal rotation (table 7.10J, p. 440) provides an exercise that can easily be performed on the Reformer or using an elastic band or tubing. However, with the prevalence of rolled shoulder, often it is advisable to at least initially emphasize strengthening the shoulder external rotators exclusively.

Scapular Adductors and Scapular Depressors

Adequate strength in the scapular adductors is important for preventing rolled shoulders and for promoting correct arm placement during dance. Due to the natural linking of scapular adduction with external rotation, focusing on pulling the shoulder blades together when performing the exercises for the shoulder external rotators (kneeling scarecrow [table 7.10H, p. 439] or double-shoulder external rotation [table 7.10I, p. 439]) is a good way to strengthen both of these muscle groups with one exercise. The use of scapular adduction with shoulder horizontal abduction while the torso is inclined (such as is commonly used with rows in a gym setting) has also been shown to be a very effective way of overloading the trapezius muscle (Brunnstrom, 1972). When performing any of these exercises, adding an upper back arch provides a way to counter all of the elements that tend to be associated with rolled shoulder posture (shoulder internal rotation, scapular abduction, and kyphosis) with one exercise. Furthermore, when executing these exercises, focusing on pulling the shoulder blades down is a good way to emphasize strengthening the lower trapezius (scapular depressor), which is important in dance for preventing excessive elevation of the shoulders during arm movements and shoulder impingement injury. In addition, the press-up (table 7.10C, p. 435), previously described for strengthening the shoulder flexors, offers an effective exercise for both learning to activate and strengthening the scapular depressors.

Scapular Abductors

Adequate strength in the scapular abductors that is balanced with strength of the scapular adductors is important for preventing winging of the scapulae and for promoting proper arm placement during dance.

Adequate strength in the serratus anterior is also important for preventing shoulder impingement. One can strengthen the scapular abductors by focusing on keeping the scapulae wide (abducted) during push-ups, rather than letting the scapulae come together on the down-phase of the push-up, and including slight additional scapular abduction at the end of the up-phase of the push-up, termed a push-up plus (table 7.10A, variation 1, p. 434). Similarly, in the gym, one can strengthen the scapular abductors by reaching the arms forward at the end of a bench press so that the scapulae abduct ("lock out"). Arm across (table 7.10K, p. 440) is another exercise that can be performed for the scapular abductors that uses an elastic band for resistance. Focusing on keeping the shoulder blade down as the scapula moves forward will also help strengthen the depression function of the serratus anterior.

Other Scapular Muscles

Because of the multiple functions of the scapular muscles and their linked action with movements of the shoulder, various scapular muscles are recruited in any strengthening exercises for the shoulder complex. However, a study using electromyography concluded that the combination of scaption with external rotation, rowing, push-up plus, and press-up would challenge all of the scapular muscles and provide a core program for rehabilitation and prevention of shoulder injuries (Johnson, Gauvin, and Fredericson, 2003; Moseley et al., 1992).

Elbow Flexors

Strengthening the elbow flexors is important for types of partnering that involve holding or supporting another dancer with one elbow or both elbows flexed. Strengthening these muscles will also provide more tone and definition along the front of the arm. The concentration curl (table 7.10L, p. 441) is an effective exercise that is performed with dumbbells, while the kneeling biceps lift (table 7.10M, p. 442) can be performed on the Reformer or with an elastic band for resistance. Remember that forearm position will influence the relative contribution of the elbow flexors. So, performing elbow flexion with the forearm supinated should encourage use of the biceps brachii, the forearm in midposition should emphasize use of the brachioradialis, and the forearm pronated should deemphasize biceps brachii contribution.

Elbow Extensors

The attachment of the triceps brachii is closer to the axis of the elbow joint for flexion-extension than that of the biceps brachii, giving it a smaller moment arm and a relative disadvantage in terms of production of torque (Hall, 1999). Furthermore, the elbow flexors are more readily used in everyday activities such as lifting and carrying objects. Thus, in general the elbow flexors are almost twice as strong as the elbow extensors (Hamill and Knutzen, 1995), making it important to place emphasis on strengthening the elbow extensors. In dance, adequate strength in the elbow extensors is important for overhead partnering and for floor work that involves pressing the body up or supporting the body weight with the arms. Strength in the elbow extensors can also improve the tone and contour of the back of the arm and help prevent the undesired "sag" that some dancers experience in this area.

The elbow extensors can be strengthened with many exercises, including the push-up (table 7.10A, p. 434), press-up (table 7.10C, p. 435), lunge triceps kick back (table 7.10E, p. 436), sitting overhead press (table 7.10G, p. 438), overhead triceps extension (table 7.10N, p. 443), and kneeling triceps kick back (table 7.10O, p. 444). While the position of the forearm does not influence the ability of the elbow extensors to produce force, position of the shoulder will influence the contribution of the long head of the triceps brachii. For example, putting the shoulder in extension, such as with the triceps kick back, shortens the long head across the shoulder and makes the exercise more demanding than if the shoulder was not extended.

Compound Strengthening Exercises

Other exercises including multiple joints and incorporating movement patterns similar to those used in activity are useful for developing functional strength in the upper extremity, such as bench presses and cleans. Male dancers or female dancers who have to perform highly demanding partnering or body support may want to consider progressing from some of the basic exercises described in this text to more advanced exercises using Pilates apparatus, weight apparatus, or free weights as their strength develops. Working with a qualified Pilates instructor, personal trainer, kinesiologist, or strength coach to supervise and design a safe and effective program for your needs is recommended.

Flexibility Exercises for the Upper Extremity

Table 7.11 provides average range of motion for the fundamental movements of the shoulder in the general population, as well as the primary constraints to these movements. Many dancers exhibit adequate shoulder flexibility or even excessive mobility, and supplemental stretching is not necessary or probably

TABLE 7.11   Normal Range of Motion and Constraints for Fundamental Movements of the Shoulder (Non-Dance Populations)

Shoulder joint movement	Normal range of motion*	Normal passive limiting factors
Flexion	0-180°	Joint capsule: posterior portion Ligaments: coracohumeral (posterior band) Muscles: shoulder extensors and external rotators
Extension	0-60°	Joint capsule: anterior portion Ligaments: coracohumeral (anterior band) Muscles: pectoralis major (clavicular portion)
Abduction	0-180°	Joint capsule: inferior portion Ligaments: glenohumeral (middle and inferior bands) Muscles: shoulder adductor muscles
Adduction	0-45°**	Apposition with trunk

External rotation
   Arm 90° abduction
   Arm by side
	
	0-90°
	0-60°
		Joint capsule: anterior portion
		Ligaments: glenohumeral and coracohumeral
		Muscles: shoulder internal rotator muscles (subscapularis, pectoralis major, teres major, and latissimus dorsi)

Internal rotation
   Arm 90° abduction
   Arm by side
	
	0-70°
	0-80°
		Joint capsule: posterior portion
		Muscles: shoulder external rotator muscles (infraspinatus and teres minor)

*From American Academy of Orthopaedic Surgeons (1965).
**From Gerhardt and Rippstein (1990). This measure allows the arm to pass in front of the body.

advisable until there is a better understanding of the potential relationship between shoulder range of motion and shoulder instability (Rodeo et al., 1998; Sauers et al., 2001). Some other dancers may have tightness in specific areas that require supplemental stretching to achieve the desired ranges for dance. A few areas that are more frequently tight and that are particularly important for dance are described in the remainder of this section and in table 7.12.

When one performs these and other stretches for the shoulder area, it is very important to stabilize the torso. When the arm approaches the end of its range in a given direction, it is easy to adjust the torso to get more range of the distal end of the arm, reducing the effectiveness for the targeted shoulder muscle.

Shoulder Flexors

Adequate flexibility in the shoulder flexors is important for allowing the arm to be brought backward behind the body (shoulder hyperextension). If inadequate flexibility is present, the shoulder is often rounded forward with the scapula elevated, an undesired aesthetic in dance, in an effort to get more range. The arms back shoulder stretch (table 7.12A) is a stretch for the shoulder flexors that can be performed with a bar, dowel, ballet barre, or towel.

Shoulder Extensors

Adequate flexibility in the shoulder extensors is important for allowing the arms to be brought fully overhead or even slightly past overhead, necessary for movements such as partnering or ballet port de bras. If inadequate shoulder flexibility is present, the back is often arched (hyperextended) to allow the arms to be moved farther back. This can put undue stress on the low back as well as disrupt the desired aesthetic or "line." One can quickly evaluate the flexibility of the shoulder extensors by bringing the arm forward in flexion and checking that it can reach an overhead position without distorting torso alignment, as seen in Tests and Measurements 7.2. Two stretches for the shoulder extensors are provided in table 7.12. The kneeling arms overhead shoulder stretch (table 7.12B) is a stretch that can be performed with a chair or ballet barre, while the sitting arms overhead shoulder stretch (table 7.12C) can be performed sitting upright to work on maintaining correct torso positioning or sitting with the back supported by an exercise ball to provide a position in which gravity will assist with providing a stretch to the shoulders (table 7.12C, variation 1).

TABLE 7.12   Selected Stretches for the Shoulder

Exercise name (Method of stretch)	Description (Technique cues)	Progression
Muscle group: Shoulder flexors **Muscles emphasized: Pectoralis major (clavicular) and anterior deltoid**		
Joint position: Shoulder extension with elbow extension		
A. Arms back shoulder stretch (Static) 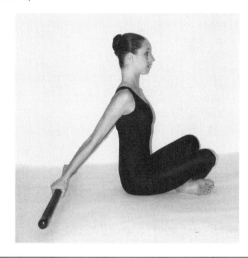	Grasp a bar, dowel, or towel behind the back with the hands slightly wider than shoulder-width apart and the palms facing forward. Slowly raise the arms backward and upward until a stretch is felt across the front of the shoulders. (Emphasize keeping the scapulae slightly down and together, and only raise the arms as high as it is possible while maintaining this positioning of the scapulae.)	1. Lift bar higher while maintaining good form. 2. Move hands closer toward each other on the bar, dowel, or towel.
Muscle group: Shoulder extensors **Muscles emphasized: Pectoralis major (sternal) and latissimus dorsi**		
Joint position: Shoulder flexion		
B. Kneeling arms overhead shoulder stretch (Static) 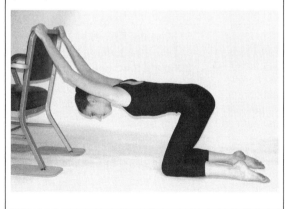	Kneel about 4 feet (1.2 meters) away from the back of a chair or a ballet barre with the hands slightly wider than shoulder-width apart. Slowly flex at the hips and allow the torso to fall through the arms until a stretch is felt across the front of the shoulders. (Firmly contract the abdominals, focusing on pulling the lower ribs down and back and the pubic bone up such that hyperextension of the back and rib-leading are avoided, and the stretch occurs at the desired site of the shoulders.)	1. Allow more of the weight of the torso to hang on the arms. 2. Start kneeling slightly farther away from the chair or barre.

(continued)

449

TABLE 7.12 **Selected Stretches for the Shoulder** *(continued)*

Exercise name (Method of stretch)	Description (Technique cues)	Progression
Muscle group: Shoulder extensors **Muscles emphasized: Pectoralis major (sternal) and latissimus dorsi**		
Joint position: Shoulder flexion		
C. Sitting arms overhead shoulder stretch (Static) 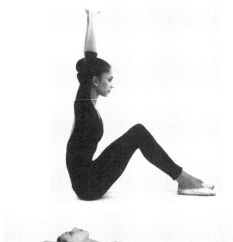 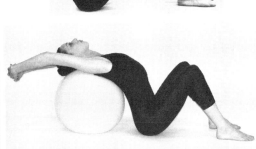 *Variation 1*	Sit with the legs to the front with the knees bent and the feet flat on the floor while the arms are clasped overhead. Slowly bring the arms backward until a stretch is felt in the lower or posterior area of the shoulder. (Initially contract the abdominals firmly to maintain slight flexion of the lumbar and lower thoracic spine as the arms are brought backward. As stabilization skill improves, utilize a neutral position of the spine but avoid any spinal hyperextension or rib-leading as the arms move backward.) *Variation 1:* Perform sitting with the arms overhead, the elbows bent or straight, and the upper back supported by an exercise ball so that gravity assists with providing a greater shoulder stretch.	1. Bring the arms further back.
Muscle group: Shoulder horizontal adductors **Muscles emphasized: Pectoralis major and anterior deltoid**		
Joint position: Shoulder horizontal abduction		
D. Wall shoulder stretch (Static) 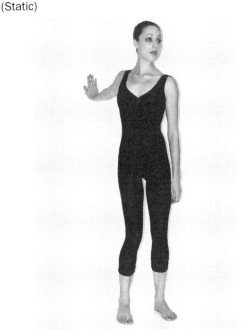	Stand with your right side facing the wall and your right palm on the wall, with the fingers facing up toward the ceiling. Slowly rotate your torso to the left away from the wall until a stretch is felt across the front of the shoulder. Repeat on the other side. (Keep the right shoulder externally rotated and the scapula pulled downward as the torso is rotated.)	1. Move the arm slightly farther back on the wall. 2. Rotate the torso further, slightly away from the arm.

Exercise name (Method of stretch)	Description (Technique cues)	Progression
Muscle group: Shoulder horizontal abductors **Muscles emphasized: Posterior deltoid**		
Joint position: Shoulder horizontal adduction with elbow flexion		
E. Supine elbow across shoulder stretch (Static) 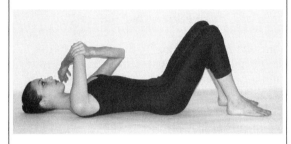	Lie supine on the floor with the right elbow bent facing outward at shoulder height and the left hand on the elbow. Use the left hand to pull the right elbow across the chest until a stretch is felt across the back of the shoulder. Repeat on the other side. (Keep the scapulae slightly together, and avoid letting the scapula come forward as the arm is brought across the body.)	1. Move the arm slightly farther across the chest.

TESTS AND MEASUREMENTS 7.2

Screening Test for Shoulder Extensor Flexibility

A test is shown for measuring passive shoulder flexion, a motion that will generally reflect the flexibility of the shoulder extensors in healthy dancers. While the dancer is sitting with both knees bent and the feet on the floor, the examiner stabilizes the torso with one hand while the dancer brings one arm as far overhead as possible without distorting torso alignment.

The axis of the goniometer is placed at the approximate axis of the shoulder joint, while the stationary arm is vertical and in line with the side of the torso and the moving arm is along the midline of the upper humerus. A position with the arm straight overhead is considered "0," and the number of degrees the arm can be brought back beyond this point are considered a positive number. The ability to easily achieve "0" degrees is important to allow for overhead positions, as used with partnering, without undesired compensations of the trunk. However, many dancers exhibit much greater range of motion in this direction, and the author considers a minimum of 10° desirable to help achieve the aesthetics of various port de bras and gestural movements used in dance. If a goniometer is not available, one can use a rough guide of being able to bring the elbow approximately 3 inches (7.6 centimeters) behind the middle of the ear while vertical alignment of the head and torso are maintained.

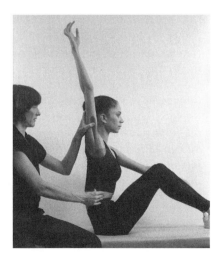

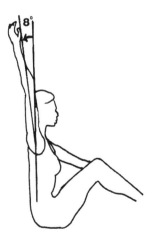

Shoulder Horizontal Adductors

Adequate flexibility in the shoulder horizontal adductors is necessary to allow the arms to be adequately "open" when held in second position and to help prevent rolled shoulders. The wall shoulder stretch (table 7.12D) is a stretch for this muscle group.

Shoulder Horizontal Abductors and Posterior Capsule

Recent studies suggest that tightness in the posterior capsule and posterior rotator cuff may be an associated factor with some shoulder injuries (such as the impingement syndrome). The supine elbow across shoulder stretch (table 7.12E) is designed to provide a stretch to this area. However, to be effective, the scapula must be stabilized through conscious use of the scapular adductors to maintain the scapula close to the spine so that a stretch is applied to the posterior shoulder versus the scapular adductors.

Upper Extremity Injuries in Dancers

Because dance is primarily weight bearing with the lower extremity, the reported incidence of injury in the upper extremity has been historically much lower than in the lower extremity. In fact, many reports of female ballet dance injuries do not even include upper extremity injuries, and there are a very limited number of studies addressing upper extremity injuries in dancers. However, some forms of dance such as break dancing (Washington, 1987) show a higher incidence of upper extremity injuries, and the incidence of upper extremity injuries in some modern, ballet, and jazz dancers appears to be on the rise.

In terms of increasing incidence, demands for the upper extremity have markedly increased in some choreography with more use of nonclassical partnering by men, women partnering other women or men, floor work, and demanding movements requiring support of the body by the arms. In the modern arena, contact improvisation can produce additional stresses to the upper extremity when unanticipated movements require rapid use of the arms to support the body weight of the dancer or another dancer. In jazz, the trend to incorporate acrobatic types of movements and hip-hop/break dancing choreography has markedly increased the stresses to the upper extremity. One older study of 50 male break dancers showed that about 23% of the total injuries occurred in the hand, 7.5% in the wrist, and about 9% in the shoulder (Washington, 1987). After reviewing 20 years of ballet injuries at the Lewisham Hospital, Millar (1987) noted a slow but steady increase in injuries to the neck and upper extremities that he attributed to the greater and more varied choreographic demands placed on ballet dancers who have to perform modern ballets.

Prevention of Upper Extremity Injuries

A common mechanism of injury to the upper extremity involves falling on an outstretched arm; but in dance, injuries more commonly relate to performing repetitive overhead movements or demanding movements in which the upper extremity is supporting the weight of the dancer or another dancer. When forces exceed the passive mobility, stability, and dynamic control of the shoulder joint, injury can occur (Warner et al., 1990).

Dancers can lower the risk of injury by developing adequate and balanced strength, developing and maintaining adequate flexibility, properly warming up, avoiding fatigue, and focusing on good technique. In regard to strength, performing supplemental strength training two to three times per week can develop a base of upper extremity strength. Then, when unaccustomed choreography places high demands on the upper body, injury is less likely to occur. Including exercises for the rotator cuff and scapular muscles, as well as the large shoulder muscles, will provide greater joint stability and foster proper shoulder and scapular mechanics necessary for avoiding impingement syndromes. Lastly, focusing on correct arm placement with an appropriate scapulohumeral rhythm can reduce shoulder stress.

Rehabilitation of Shoulder Injuries

Although different injuries often require specific treatments, some general principles follow for treatment of the shoulder. For more specific treatment protocols, interested readers are referred to the related references provided at the back of this book.

As with injuries to other joints, initial recommended treatment usually involves the use of ice, anti-inflammatories, and relative rest/protected movement to control pain, swelling, and inflammation (Goldman and McCann, 1997). When symptoms are adequately controlled, various other physical therapy modalities such as ultrasound, electrical stimulation, or phonophoresis are often prescribed to help restore normal range of motion and to promote healing. However, unlike the situation with other joints, there is a greater priority on maintaining range of motion in the early stages of a shoulder injury because the shoulder is particularly prone to contractures, capsulitis, and severe loss of movement if it is immobilized. Hence, early treatment often involves exercises that are aimed at maintaining range of motion without aggravating the condition, performed several to many times per day.

When symptoms allow, progressive resistance exercises are gradually added. These strengthening exercises should include exercises for (1) the rotator cuff, vital for shoulder stability and the SIT force couple; (2) the scapular muscles, key for restoring an appropriate scapulohumeral rhythm; and (3) the other major glenohumeral muscles, important for shoulder joint stability and movements.

Evaluation and, if necessary, correction of shoulder mechanics are also essential for successful rehabilitation and the prevention of injury recurrence of the shoulder. With many shoulder injuries, the scapulohumeral rhythm tends to become disrupted (scapular dyskinesis), and excessive elevation accompanied by inadequate or delayed upward rotation of the scapula occurs. Use of technique cues and reeducation, in conjunction with selective strengthening of necessary muscles such as the serratus anterior and lower trapezius, is often necessary to restore proper mechanics. As with other joints previously discussed, progression to exercises involving support of the body weight (closed kinematic chain exercises) and proprioceptive challenges (such as performing exercises with single- or double-arm support on a foam roller, ball, or balance board) is also desired.

Common Injuries of the Upper Extremity

A brief discussion of some of the more common injuries that involve the upper extremity follows. Although there is limited research related to upper extremity injuries in dancers, interested readers are referred to the vast number of studies of sports in which upper extremity injuries are common such as swimming, throwing sports, racket sports, and gymnastics.

Acromioclavicular Sprain (Acromioclavicular Separation)

An **acromioclavicular sprain,** acromioclavicular separation, or "shoulder separation" refers to a sprain and often dislocation of the acromioclavicular joint. It involves a tearing of the ligaments and frequently the capsule of the joint. This injury often occurs from a fall on the point of the shoulder or on an outstretched hand (Hall-Craggs, 1985).

An acromioclavicular sprain is characterized by severe pain that is aggravated by movements of the arm and by localized tenderness and swelling directly over the acromioclavicular joint (Roy and Irvin, 1983). Less severe sprains are associated with a subluxation, while more severe sprains are associated with a complete dislocation of the acromioclavicular joint as seen in figure 7.52. With more severe sprains, the ligaments that connect the clavicle to the coracoid process of the scapula (coracoclavicular ligaments: coronoid and trapezoid ligaments) are torn; the distal end of the clavicle is raised relative to the acromion and may even ride above the acromion process (figure 7.52B). The shoulder tends to fall away from the clavicle, due to the weight of the arm, and appears to droop relative to the other shoulder. The acromion of the scapula also appears more prominent on the injured side (Moore and Agur, 1995).

Recommended treatment often involves use of a snug arm sling designed to support the weight of the arm (Yamaguchi, Wolfe, and Bigliani, 1997). Since the stability of this joint is dependent on the ligaments and the surrounding muscles do little for stability, the focus of initial treatment is generally more oriented toward trying to prevent excessive motion of the acromioclavicular joint so that ligamental healing can occur. With severe dislocations it is often difficult to maintain the desired alignment of the acromion and scapula without the clavicle's overriding the acromion; and for elite athletes, some physicians recommend surgery to stabilize the joint.

Shoulder Dislocation

Due to the design of the shoulder for mobility and its inherent instability, the shoulder (glenohumeral joint) is vulnerable to dislocation. Although there are four types of dislocation that can occur, inferior and particularly anterior dislocations occur most frequently in forming athletes (Moore and Agur, 1995). In **anterior** or **subcoracoid dislocations** (figure 7.53B), as the head of the humerus moves forward, the joint capsule, inferior glenohumeral ligament, and sometimes the glenoid labrum can be torn from their anterior attachment onto the glenoid cavity. Common mechanisms for this injury include an abducted and externally rotated arm position, or less frequently an arm position involving extreme shoulder extension with external rotation. In contrast, the mechanism of injury for **inferior** or **subglenoid dislocation** (figure 7.53C) is a blow or large downward force applied to the arm when it is fully abducted in

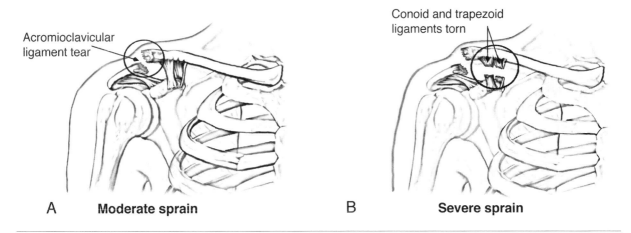

FIGURE 7.52   (A) Moderate and (B) severe sprain of the acromioclavicular joint (right shoulder, anterior view).

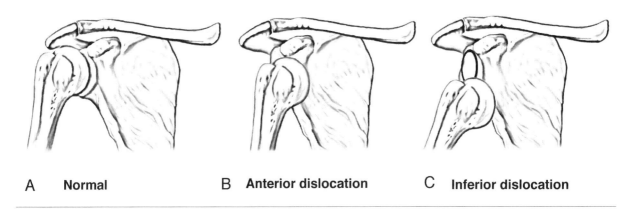

FIGURE 7.53   Two common types of shoulder dislocations (right shoulder, anterior view). (A) Normal positioning of the head of the humerus, (B) anterior (subcoracoid) dislocation, (C) inferior (subglenoid) dislocation.

an overhead position. In dance, shoulder dislocations occur infrequently. When they do occur, potential mechanisms include falls, mistakes with partnering or contact improvisation, or demanding positions of body support by an arm.

Anterior dislocation of the shoulder is visually apparent, as the rounded appearance of the shoulder due to the greater tubercle of the humerus disappears and a cavity can be felt below the acromion while the acromion appears more prominent (Roy and Irvin, 1983). The initial dislocation of the shoulder is associated with intense pain. Pain with movement is severe, and the dancer may attempt to support the injured arm with the opposite arm. Tingling and numbness may be present down the arm to the hand.

This is a medical emergency, and a qualified medical professional should be summoned or the medical emergency system activated (call 911). In some cases, the humerus will go back into its socket by itself (spontaneous reduction), but in other cases a

specific reduction maneuver has to be performed by a qualified physician as nerves and blood vessels can be injured if the procedure is performed incorrectly. Furthermore, additional injury such as fractures and rotator cuff tears can be associated with a dislocation and must be ruled out by a qualified medical professional before reduction is performed.

The arm is often initially placed in a sling (Park, Blaine, and Levine, 2002) as initial symptoms are controlled. When rehabilitation occurs, a particularly strong emphasis is placed on building the strength of the rotator cuff muscles. Emphasis on strengthening the deltoid and scapular muscles, as well as progressing to proprioceptive exercises and functional open and closed kinematic chain movement patterns, is important for restoring correct mechanics and stability (Shea, 2001). Unfortunately, traumatic shoulder dislocations often involve disruption of the glenoid labrum and inferior glenohumeral ligament, as well as deformation of the joint capsule. This damage can readily lead to shoulder instability, and reports of shoulder dislocation recurrence rates in athletes vary from 50% to 90% (Yamaguchi, Wolfe, and Bigliani, 1997). Hence, corrective surgery may be necessary, often involving the repair of any avulsion of the glenoid labrum, ligaments, or capsule from the rim of the glenoid fossa and "tightening" of the joint capsule (Levine et al., 2000; Nelson and Arciero, 2000; Steinbeck and Jerosch, 1998).

External Shoulder Impingement Syndrome

External shoulder impingement syndrome (subacromial impingement) is classically used to describe a pinching or impingement of inflamed or tender soft tissues between the head of the humerus and the overlying coracoacromial ligament, acromion process, or both. The space inferior to the coracoacromial arch and superior to the head of the humerus, termed the subacromial space, is only about 0.4 inches (1 centimeter) when the arm is down by the side (Kreighbaum and Barthels, 1996). External impingement syndrome can be further subdivided into primary and secondary impingement. **Primary impingement** occurs when this subacromial space is mechanically narrowed by factors such as a hooked acromion, bone spurs, a thickened rotator cuff, or fibrotic subacromial bursa (Myers, 1999). In contrast, **secondary impingement** occurs when the subacromial space is functionally narrowed by factors such as scapular or rotator cuff muscle weakness and fatigue, posterior capsule tightness, or glenohumeral instability. These latter

factors have the effect of allowing the head of the humerus to migrate upward or not stay centered in the glenoid cavity during shoulder flexion and abduction, producing impingement. Secondary impingement occurs more frequently in individuals under 35 years of age (Cavallo and Speer, 1998), while primary impingement occurs more commonly in older individuals.

Given that the supraspinatus tendon runs right over the top of the humerus to attach onto the upper portion of the greater tubercle (figure 7.54), it is not surprising that the most common inflamed structure "pinched" with external shoulder impingement syndrome is the external surface of the supraspinatus tendon. However, other structures located in this area that can be involved include the tendon of the biceps brachii and the subacromial bursa.

The impingement syndrome is particularly prevalent in sports that utilize repetitive shoulder flexion and abduction, particularly overhead motions such as in baseball, swimming, gymnastics, and weightlifting (Briner and Benjamin, 1999; Cavallo and Speer, 1998; Kammer, Young, and Niedfeldt, 1999; Warner et al., 1990). As many as 50% of competitive swimmers report impingement-type shoulder pain (Nuber et al., 1986). In dance, similar stresses can occur with overhead partnering, choreography that requires very rapid and percussive use of the arms, and movements that require support of the body weight by the arms such as handstands, cartwheels, and handsprings.

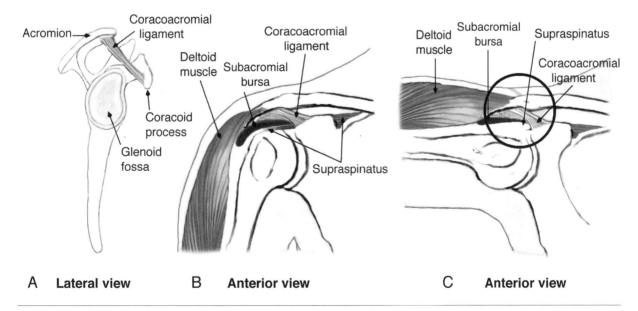

A   Lateral view   **B   Anterior view**   **C   Anterior view**

FIGURE 7.54   Impingement syndrome (right shoulder). (A) Lateral view of coracoacromial arch. (B) With arm down by side, adequate space is present between the humerus and coracoacromial arch, but (C) with shoulder abduction the space is reduced and impingement can occur.

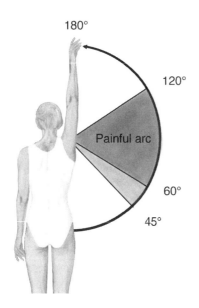

180°

120°

Painful arc

60°

45°

FIGURE 7.55   Classic arc of pain during shoulder abduction with external impingement syndrome.

External impingement syndrome is characterized by pain in the anterior, superior, or lateral shoulder (Wolin and Tarbet, 1997) that is aggravated by overhead movements, particularly between 60° and 120° of shoulder abduction as seen in figure 7.55. Due to the mechanics of the shoulder, the initial range of abduction does not approximate the involved structures sufficiently to produce impingement. However, usually at about 60° (although sometimes as early as 45°) the inflamed tendons or bursa is impinged against the overlying coracoacromial arch, producing pain. Blood supply to the supraspinatus tendon may also be compromised in this range of motion (Kreighbaum and Barthels, 1996). In some cases, a snapping sensation or crepitus may also accompany the pain occurring in this arc. Sometimes the pain is severe enough to prohibit further raising of the arm, but if not, the pain usually diminishes after about 120° when external rotation of the humerus places the greater tubercle behind the acromion so that impingement no longer occurs. Due to pain, the use of the shoulder joint is often limited, and muscle inhibition, weakness, and atrophy often follow.

During initial phases of treatment, shoulder abduction and overhead movements are often limited or avoided. Dancers can temporarily modify use of the arms to below shoulder height (or whatever range is pain free) or perform some combinations with and some without arms so that fatigue and associated pain are avoided. Stretching to maintain normal range of motion is often recommended, as low range of motion in shoulder horizontal abduc-

tion (Greipp, 1985), shoulder external rotation, shoulder internal rotation, and shoulder horizontal adduction (Warner et al., 1990) may increase the risk for impingement. The latter decrease in range is often due to tightness in the posterior capsule and is theorized to produce undesired anterior glide and elevation of the head of the humerus during shoulder flexion.

When symptoms allow, strengthening exercises are initiated. Particular emphasis is placed on strengthening the rotator cuff due to its important role in helping prevent excessive upward movement of the head of the humerus (SIT force couple). Furthermore, the impingement syndrome has been shown to be associated with low strength in the external rotators relative to the internal rotators (Warner et al., 1990), suggesting that greater emphasis should be placed on strengthening shoulder external rotation. However, positions for strengthening the rotator cuff often have to be modified to avoid 60° to 120° of abduction, and a position in which the arm is slightly raised (30° of abduction in the scapular plane) so that blood flow is not decreased and impingement risk is low is often recommended. Strengthening of the scapular depressors and upward rotators (lower trapezius and serratus anterior) is also essential for restoring a normal scapulohumeral rhythm when the arm is raised overhead. With normal mechanics, upward rotation of the scapula moves the acromion process out of the way as the humerus approaches it during abduction (Kreighbaum and Barthels, 1996). However, individuals with impingement appear to exhibit inhibition and disrupted recruitment patterns of the serratus anterior and lower trapezius (Cools et al., 2003), with increased activity of the rhomboids (Johnson, Gauvin, and Fredericson, 2003) or upper trapezius (Kibler, McMullen, and Uhl, 2001). This disruption of scapular synergies can lead to excessive scapular elevation, or hiking of the shoulder when raising the arm, perhaps to compensate for decreased glenohumeral motion but tending to drive the humeral head upward and increase impingement risk. Thus, restoration of adequate strength and shoulder mechanics is necessary for avoidance of impingement and resolution of symptoms. Correction of rolled shoulder and kyphosis, when indicated, may also be prudent due to the decrease in subacromial space associated with these postural problems (DePalma and Johnson, 2003).

Rotator Cuff Tear

In some cases, injury to the rotator cuff may not involve only inflammation (tendinitis) but rather an incomplete or complete tear of the rotator cuff. Such an injury most commonly involves the supraspinatus (figure 7.56) at its musculotendinous junction where blood supply is poor but may also include the infraspinatus tendon. In the younger athlete, this tear is often associated with a traumatic event such as a fall on an outstretched hand or forceful deceleration of internal rotation as in throwing (Duda, 1985; Yamaguchi, Wolfe, and Bigliani, 1997). During the acceleration phase of throwing, shoulder internal rotation can reach velocities of 9,000° per second in male intercollegiate baseball players (Brindle et al., 1999). Following the release of the ball, the rotator cuff works eccentrically to quickly decelerate this high-velocity internal rotation, leaving it vulnerable for injury. A rotator cuff tear can also follow weakening of the tendon from tendinitis and impingement. Millar (1987) states that rotator cuff strains are the most common shoulder injury in dancers and especially in male dancers.

The signs and symptoms of a **rotator cuff tear** are often very similar to those of the impingement syndrome, with tenderness near the insertion of the supraspinatus and aching pain that is magnified by shoulder abduction, especially between 60° and 120°. Pain is often persistent at rest and even at night (Wolin and Tarbet, 1997) and is often referred to the distal attachment of the deltoid. Furthermore, wasting of the supraspinatus may be present; and with more serious tears there may be the inability to abduct the arm against resistance or hold the arm in abduction (Caillet, 1996), probably due to pain. One test used, the drop arm test (Tests and Measurements 7.3) involves trying to hold the arm in abduction after it has been passively raised to about 90° (Magee, 1997; Mercier, 1995).

Recommended initial treatment may involve use of a sling and limitation of abduction, with additional treatment similar to that used with the shoulder impingement syndrome, including careful strength-

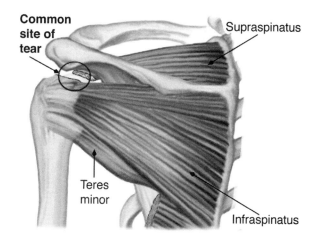

FIGURE 7.56   Rotator cuff tear (left shoulder, posterior view).

ening of the rotator cuff, proprioceptive exercises, and restoration of proper shoulder mechanics. However, in cases of a complete tear or when conservative treatment is unsuccessful, surgical repair may be recommended (Mercier, 1995; Yamaguchi, Wolfe, and Bigliani, 1997).

Bursitis

Bursitis is an inflammation of a bursa, and the subacromial bursa is most commonly involved at the shoulder (figure 7.54). As described with the shoulder impingement syndrome, the subacromial bursa's location inferior to the coracoacromial arch and superior to the supraspinatus tendon allows it to become readily inflamed due to impingement. Bursitis can also result from irritation by calcium deposits in the rotator cuff tendons (Wolf III, 1999) that occur in response to degenerative changes in these tendons or secondary to other injuries of the shoulder or acromioclavicular joint. As with impingement,

---

__ TESTS AND MEASUREMENTS 7.3 __

Drop Arm Test for a Rotator Cuff Tear

This test is performed by a physician or physical therapist when a tear of the rotator cuff is suspected. The examiner lifts the patient's arm to 90° abduction and then lets go. The patient attempts to hold the arm in this position and then slowly lower it back down to the side. The inability to hold this position alone or against slight resistance, or the inability to lower the arm in a smooth, controlled manner without extreme pain, is considered a drop sign and suggests that a tear of the rotator cuff is present.

bursitis is particularly common in individuals utilizing repetitive overhead movements.

Bursitis is often associated with a generalized ache around the shoulder that is aggravated by full abduction, as well as external or internal rotation in abduction (Magee, 1997; McCarthy, 1989; Millar, 1987). It is also generally aggravated by sleeping with the arm overhead. Tenderness may also be present over the front and lateral aspect of the shoulder joint.

Recommended treatment often involves modification of activity to avoid lifting or overhead arm movements that aggravate the condition, modalities including ice or heat, anti-inflammatory medications, and, when symptoms allow, rehabilitation emphasizing strengthening the rotator cuff and correcting any technique/training errors (McCarthy, 1989). Careful injection of corticosteroids into the bursa (avoiding the closely aligned tendons) is also recommended by some physicians in cases that do not respond to these former treatments (Mercier, 1995; Millar, 1987).

Frozen Shoulder (Adhesive Capsulitis)

A **frozen shoulder,** or **adhesive capsulitis,** involves chronic inflammation and fibrosis of the glenohumeral capsule. In later stages it often involves adhesions between the capsule and articulating surfaces, as well as inflammation of the subacromial bursa and coracohumeral ligament. These changes result in a situation in which shoulder motion is dramatically reduced (e.g., inability to raise the arm overhead), hence the term "frozen shoulder." The etiology is not well understood, but frozen shoulder generally occurs after inactivity of the shoulder consequent to an injury or inflammation of the shoulder complex. Although it is rare in young active individuals, it can occur in older dancers, and particularly in women versus men (Mercier, 1995).

Adhesive capsulitis is generally associated with progressive loss of shoulder motion and an insidious onset of pain, localized to the area of the rotator cuff. This pain often interferes with sleep, prevents lying on the affected shoulder, and is progressive in nature. Tenderness is often present around the rotator cuff and biceps tendon. In terms of range of motion, there tends to be a generalized loss of both passive and active range of motion, and universally a loss of external rotation (Yamaguchi, Wolfe, and Bigliani, 1997). Although the person is often comfortable when moving within the restricted range, severe pain is often experienced with accidental movement beyond this range.

Treatment often involves anti-inflammatory medications and physical therapy that focuses on stretching and restoring range of motion. However, if

conservative approaches fail, corticosteroids or more aggressive measures such as breaking of the adhesions under local anesthesia or surgical release of the capsule by an orthopedic surgeon may be required, followed by aggressive rehabilitation to avoid adhesion (Caillet, 1996; Pearsall and Speer, 1998).

Biceps Tendinitis and Rupture

The biceps brachii tendon can become inflamed, resulting in tendinitis (figure 7.57). This most commonly involves the tendon of the long head of the biceps brachii and its sheath (tenosynovitis). This tenosynovitis most often occurs in adults over 40 or in younger athletes whose sports demand repetitive arm movements (Mercier, 1995). Factors including a narrow intertubercular groove, repetitive subluxing of the tendon, or impingement under the coracoacromial arch may precipitate this injury.

Biceps tendinitis is characterized by pain that extends down the anterior aspect of the upper arm, lower than usually experienced with involvement of the supraspinatus tendon. Tenderness is also generally present over the bicipital groove when palpated. The intertubercular groove and associated biceps tendon can be easily palpated on the anterior shoulder when the arm is abducted 90° and the elbow is flexed 90°. The pain can often be replicated through utilization of maneuvers that place the biceps tendon on a stretch such as shoulder hyperextension with the elbow extended.

Recommended treatment often involves the usual limitation of motion to pain-free ranges, anti-

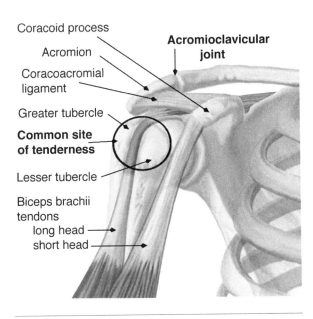

FIGURE 7.57 Biceps tendinitis (right shoulder, anterior view).

inflammatory medications, and physical therapy. However, successful treatment also needs to address potential underlying causes such as technique or shoulder impingement syndrome. If inadequately treated, chronic tendinitis, similar to that described at the ankle-foot, can result in an area of degeneration within the tendon that may precipitate complete rupture of the tendon (Mercier, 1995). Rupture usually follows a forceful contraction of the biceps and may be accompanied by the sensation of a "snap" and ensuing pain and weakness of the arm. Increased size and a distorted shape of the retracted biceps are often visible.

Lateral Epicondylitis or Tennis Elbow

Lateral epicondylitis involves injury in the area of the lateral epicondyle that is thought to entail inflammation and small tears of the proximal tendinous attachments of the extensors of the wrist (Moore and Agur, 1995; Soderberg, 1986). Lateral epicondylitis is an overuse injury that is common in athletes utilizing the wrist extensors repetitively, such as pitchers and tennis players. In fact, this injury is so common in tennis that it is often termed "tennis elbow." Approximately 45% of tennis players who play daily develop tennis elbow (Weldon, 1988). In dancers, lateral epicondylitis is likely related to partnering and support of the body weight by the arms and has been reported to be the most common injury to the elbow (Millar, 1987).

Lateral epicondylitis is characterized by pain over the lateral aspect of the elbow, usually 0.4 to 0.8 inches (1-2 centimeters) distal to the lateral epicondyle (Goldman and McCann, 1997) as seen in figure 7.58. The pain is initially associated with activity and relieved by rest. Pain can generally be reproduced with passive wrist flexion or by resisting wrist exten-

sion (Magee, 1997) and tends to be aggravated by movements involving active wrist extension, rotation of the forearm (such as turning a doorknob or lid of a jar), or grasping of objects. If activity is continued, the pain often radiates down into the forearm and progresses such that it occurs during rather than only after activity.

Initial recommended treatment generally involves cessation or modification of aggravating movements, oral anti-inflammatory medications, and physical therapy modalities such as heat, cold, electric stimulation, and ultrasound (Kulund et al., 1979; Nirschl and Kraushaar, 1996a). Some physicians advocate the injection of corticosteroids in individuals who do not respond to other measures (Ciccotti and Charlton, 2001; Roberts, 2000). When symptoms allow, balanced strength and flexibility of the elbow and forearm muscles are developed with emphasis on strength and flexibility of the wrist extensors. Technique should also be evaluated and correction made, if indicated. Some dancers may benefit from wearing a band (counter brace) 1 inch (2.5 centimeters) or more below the elbow (Barclay, 2004; Goldman and McCann, 1997) during rehearsals or classes that involve movements placing repetitive or large stresses on this area. Elbow counterforce braces have been shown to decrease elbow angular acceleration and reduce activity of the wrist extensors (Groppel and Nirschl, 1986), valuable for the treatment of lateral epicondylitis.

Carpal Tunnel Syndrome

The carpal tunnel is a narrow tunnel found in the hand. Its floor is formed by selected carpals that create a concave surface, and its roof is formed by a fibrous band formed by the flexor retinaculum or transverse carpal ligament (figure 7.59). Hence, this tunnel is termed a fibro-osseous tunnel ("osseous" meaning bone). The carpal tunnel extends about 1.2 inches (3 centimeters) and is traversed by the nine tendons of the flexors of the fingers and the median nerve (Caillet, 1996; Kreighbaum and Barthels, 1996). Due to the limited space available in this canal, the carpal tunnel becomes a common site for nerve compression, termed **carpal tunnel syndrome** (CTS).

Although the cause of this condition is poorly understood, a higher risk is associated with occupations involving repetitive finger or wrist flexion (such as with computer keyboards), repetitive gripping, or prolonged exposure to vibration. Similarly, athletes engaged in activities with repetitive flexion or gripping such as racquetball players, golfers, and rock climbers tend to sustain CTS (Rosenwasser and

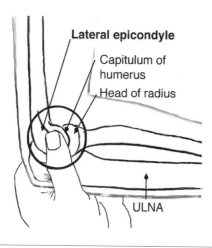

FIGURE 7.58 Lateral epicondylitis (right elbow, lateral view).

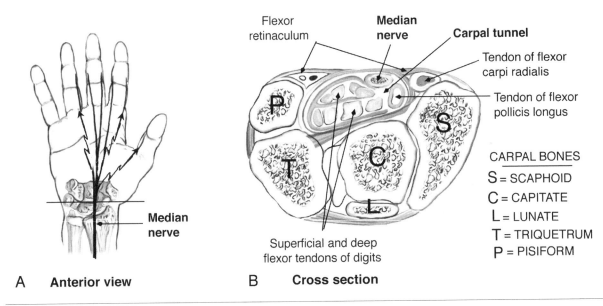

Flexor retinaculum   **Median nerve**   **Carpal tunnel**

Tendon of flexor carpi radialis

Tendon of flexor pollicis longus

CARPAL BONES
S = SCAPHOID
C = CAPITATE
L = LUNATE
T = TRIQUETRUM
P = PISIFORM

Median nerve

Superficial and deep flexor tendons of digits

A   **Anterior view**   B   **Cross section**

FIGURE 7.59   Carpal tunnel with flexor retinaculum and carpals and containing the median nerve and flexors of the fingers. (A) Anterior view of the tunnel, (B) cross section of tunnel.

Wilson, 1997). In dance, choreography demanding repetitive support of the body by the arms, especially in dancers not accustomed to such activity, may increase the risk for CTS. During pregnancy, the associated fluid retention tends to cause compression of the median nerve; and as many as 20% of pregnant women may experience carpal tunnel symptoms, which tend to go away after delivery (Magee, 1997; Mercier, 1995).

Carpal tunnel syndrome is characterized by numbness and tingling in the middle and index fingers, or these plus the thumb and the lateral half of the ring finger (Moore and Agur, 1995). The tingling of the fingers can often be reproduced or worsened if the wrist is held in a position of maximum flexion for a period of at least 1 minute (Phalen's test). Carpal tunnel syndrome is also often accompanied by night pain, which has been conjectured to be due to wrist flexion or the slight swelling associated with decreased activity during sleeping (Mercier, 1995). In severe cases, the pain associated with CTS may radiate into the forearm, arm, and even shoulder. If compression persists, motor function may also be affected, leading to weakness of wrist flexion; finger flexion; and flexion, abduction, and opposition of the thumb. With more advanced cases this weakness may be evidenced by the lack of fine coordination, loss of grip strength, tendency to drop things, and difficulty turning the lids on jars.

Treatment often involves the use of a splint that prevents extreme wrist flexion or extension, and modification or elimination of the movements

that aggravate the condition. Anti-inflammatory medications and physical therapy modalities such as ultrasound may reduce the symptoms (O'Connor, Marshall, and Massy-Westropp, 2004). When symptoms allow, flexibility and strength exercises for the wrist-hand complex are often recommended. However, initially, flexion-extension exercises of the wrist or fingers can increase pressures in the canal and aggravate the condition, and the effectiveness of exercise for this condition is controversial. In cases that do not respond to conservative treatment and in which symptoms are severe or motor weakness is developing, surgical release of the transverse carpal ligament is sometimes recommended and has been shown to generally have good outcomes (Barclay, 2002; Kao, 2003).

Summary

The upper extremity has many structural parallels to the lower extremity and also some important differences. Many of these differences are necessary to meet the primary demand of the upper extremity for mobility and manipulation of objects, in contrast to the demand for stability, support, and locomotion of the lower extremity. A summary of the bones and joints of the upper extremity can be seen in figure 7.60, while figure 7.61 shows the superficial muscles of the arm. Refer back to figures 7.17 and 7.18 (pp. 393-394) for a summary of additional muscles of the shoulder complex. The ringlike shoulder girdle hangs on the axial skeleton, connected to the axial

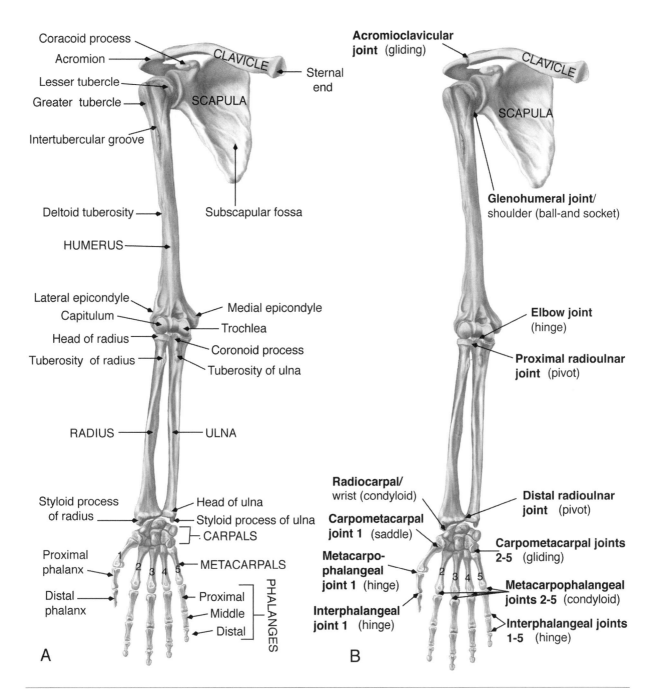

FIGURE 7.60   (A) Bones and (B) joints of the upper extremity (right side, anterior view).

skeleton only at the sternoclavicular joint. This very mobile structure can perform elevation, depression, abduction, adduction, upward rotation, and downward rotation in order to optimize the relationship of the glenoid cavity to the head of the humerus during the desired movement of the humerus. The shoulder joint is the most mobile ball-and-socket joint in the human body, naturally allowing for a large range of motion in flexion, extension, abduction, adduction, external rotation, and internal rotation. Many

muscles assist with these movements and can be functionally divided into three groups: the scapular muscles, rotator cuff, and other major glenohumeral muscles. In addition to producing the movements of the shoulder, these muscles function to give this structurally weak joint stability, maintain correct alignment, and foster correct mechanics for the SIT force couple and the scapulohumeral rhythm.

Moving distally from the shoulder joint, the elbow joint functions as a hinge joint allowing flexion and

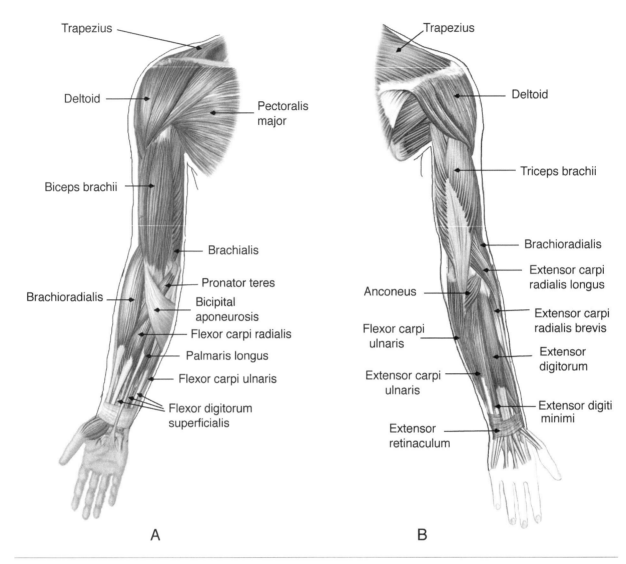

FIGURE 7.61   Superficial muscles of the right arm. (A) Anterior view, (B) posterior view.

extension. The proximal and distal radioulnar joints are pivot joints that allow the crossing over of the distal end of the radius relative to the distal ulna in the specialized movements of pronation and supination of the forearm. The wrist joint is a condyloid joint allowing flexion, extension, radial deviation, and ulnar deviation. One of the primary functions of these joints as a group is to position the hand. The hand is designed for rapid mobility and precision with its complex array of joints and muscles. One of the unique properties of the hand is the ability to perform opposition, a function essential for grasping and manipulation of objects. Many muscles cross these joints to produce movement; and due to the many multijoint muscles in this region, relative positioning of the joints crossed by these muscles will influence which muscles are used and

the amount of torque the muscle can generate in a given movement.

With the relatively weak structural design of the upper extremity, muscular strength is essential not only for providing stability but also for helping prevent injuries in this region. Although the prevalence of upper extremity injuries in many dancers is markedly less than that for the lower extremity, injury incidence is on the rise, at least in some dance forms. With increased choreographic demands on the upper extremity, it is important that dancers perform supplemental strengthening to both enhance their technique and lower the risk of injury. In some cases, performing stretches for the shoulder is also desirable. When injuries do occur, a good medical diagnosis and treatment are important to prevent frozen shoulder, chronic conditions, and injury recurrence.

Study Questions and Applications

1. Locate the following bones and bony landmarks on a skeleton and then on your own body: (a) Scapula and sternoclavicular joint; (b) spine, acromion process, supraspinous fossa, infraspinous fossa, coracoid process, and glenoid cavity of the scapula; (c) clavicle and acromioclavicular joint; (d) lesser tubercle, greater tubercle, medial epicondyle, lateral epicondyle, trochlea, and capitulum of the humerus; (e) ulna and olecranon process of ulna; (f) radius and head of radius; (g) metacarpals; (h) phalanges (proximal, middle, and distal).

2. Draw the following muscles on a skeletal chart and use an arrow to indicate the line of pull of each muscle. Then, next to each muscle, list its actions: (a) Pectoralis major, (b) latissimus dorsi, (c) teres major, (d) supraspinatus, (e) trapezius, (f) rhomboids, (g) serratus anterior, (h) biceps brachii, (i) brachialis, (j) triceps brachii.

3. Locate the following muscles on your partner or your own body, perform or have your partner perform actions that these muscles produce, and palpate their contraction during these movements: (a) Pectoralis major, (b) deltoid, (c) latissimus dorsi, (d) biceps brachii, (e) triceps brachii.

4. Observe a partner and note his or her carrying angle. How would this angle change when performing a concentration curl (table 7.10L, p. 441)?

5. Working with a partner, demonstrate the fundamental movements of the scapula, and observe and describe how these scapular motions are linked with the following movements at the shoulder joint: (a) Shoulder flexion, (b) shoulder abduction, (c) shoulder horizontal adduction, (d) shoulder external rotation.

6. Analyze the following movements, accounting for the joint movement, muscle group, and muscles used on the up-phase and down-phase at the scapula, glenohumeral joint, and elbow joint. Be sure to consider the effect of gravity: (a) Pull-up, (b) push-up, (c) pulling a dancer toward you, (d) bringing arms sideways from low fifth to second position.

7. Diagram the SIT force couple and describe its function and relationship to the impingement syndrome. Describe two strengthening exercises that could be performed to promote use of this force couple.

8. Demonstrate an exercise for strengthening the following muscles: (a) Pectoralis major, (b) middle deltoid, (c) latissimus dorsi, (d) biceps brachii, (e) triceps brachii.

9. Describe how one could attempt to correct a dancer who has rolled shoulders and holds his or her arms too far forward when in second position, including (a) strength exercises, (b) flexibility exercise(s), and (c) technique cues.

10. A dancer excessively elevates the scapulae when bringing the arms sideways from low to high fifth position. What corrections could be given in terms of (a) strengthening exercises and (b) technique cues?

CHAPTER EIGHT

Analysis of Human Movement

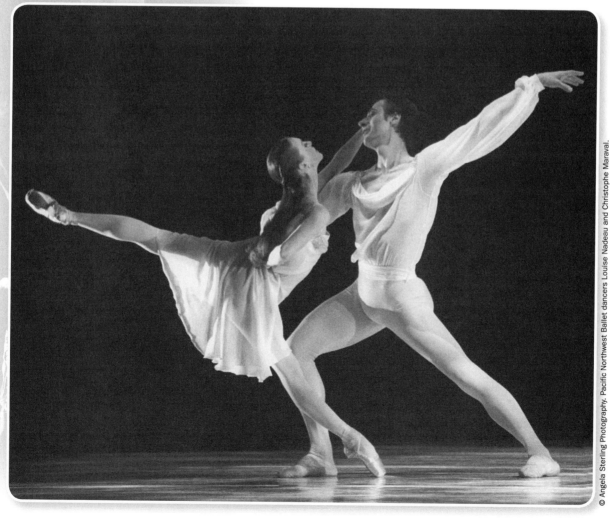

© Angela Sterling Photography. Pacific Northwest Ballet dancers Louise Nadeau and Christophe Maraval.

Prior chapters of this text have addressed the anatomy and mechanics of specific joints of the human body. This chapter will focus on looking at movement of the body as a whole. When we examine movements used in dance, they generally involve many joints moving in multiple planes as exemplified by the photo on page 465 involving partnering. This pose involves an intricate coordination of prime movers, stabilizers, and synergists at numerous joints to achieve balance with such limited support, as well as aesthetic challenges such as the desired lines and emotive qualities. Being able to analyze such movements will allow for a better understanding of the primary muscles responsible for the generation and control of the movement, potential flexibility constraints, strength demands, and cues that can be used to encourage optimal technique and reduce joint stress. Topics covered in this chapter include the following:

• Anatomical movement analysis of whole body movements

• Other methods for movement analysis

• Research-supported movement analysis

• Optimal performance models

• Movement cues

Anatomical Movement Analysis of Whole Body Movements

A schema for simplified anatomical movement analysis was provided in chapter 2 (table 2.5, p. 64) and applied in the Study Questions and Applications at the ends of chapters 3 through 7 for analysis of simple movements involving a limited number of joints. Now this schema will be expanded to incorporate additional elements for use in analyzing movements that are less isolated and that involve simultaneous use of more joints of the whole body.

Key Concepts for Anatomical Movement Analysis

While the principles used in a simplified analysis of focusing on joint movements and prime movers are still operative, the movement analysis process is often complicated—when we look at more complex movements—by the involvement of more joints, more phases, changes in the relationship to gravity, and intricate technique issues. A brief discussion of key concepts follows.

Divide Movement Into Phases

Divide a movement into phases based on change in movement direction or different functional goals. For example, in simple movements previously examined such as isolation strength exercises or pliés, using the terminology up-phase and down-phase reflects a change in movement direction that will facilitate movement analysis. However, in movements like walking, the phases have a more functional origin, with stance phase referring to the phase when the foot is in contact with the ground and must support the weight of the body, versus swing phase, referring to when the foot loses contact with the ground and moves forward in space to position the foot appropriately for the next step. In movements that have been rigorously researched such as walking, running, and jumping, there are various standardized terms that have been adopted for these phases, while for many other, less-studied movements, analysts are free to develop their own phases in a logical manner, generally in accordance with movement direction or function.

For some movements that have an apparent beginning and end, termed discrete movements, dividing the movement functionally into a preparation phase, execution phase, and recovery or follow-through phase can be helpful (Kreighbaum and Barthels, 1996). Examples of dance movements that can be effectively divided into these phases include jumps, leaps, pirouettes, and falls. In contrast, some movements, termed continuous movements, involve repeated cycles, and these cycles become a functional unit that is divided into logical phases. Examples of continuous dance movements that can be effectively divided into phases within cycles are walks, runs, triplets, and prances.

In analysis of more complex movements, further subdivisions may be necessary. For example, with walking, the direction of joint movement and the type of muscle contraction of the prime movers change more than once during the stance phase, leading to one classic approach of further subdividing the stance phase into contact, midstance, and propulsion periods as presented in chapter 6. These further divisions can be termed phases, subphases, or periods or just given numbers. Furthermore, in many movements, the two limbs may not be performing the same movements simultaneously but rather doing different things within a given phase. In such cases, the movements of both limbs must be accounted for. For example, in a fondu développé front (devant), the support leg and gesture leg must be listed separately for accurate description of the movement.

Select Key Joints

Select the joints where visible movement occurs. With more complex movements, add more focus on the joints that are particularly key for correct generation of the movement, versus joint movements that may be more gestural or supplementary in nature.

Identify Key Joint Movements

Identify the joint movements that occur in each of the key joints in each phase of the movement. Remember that movement terms refer to the direction of movement and not a joint position or angle. For example, when you begin to rise from a parallel first-position plié, the hip would be described as undergoing extension because that is the direction of the movement, even though if you stopped the movement before its completion, the hip would be in a position of flexion (relative to anatomical position).

Identify Type of Muscle Contraction

Identification of the type of muscle contraction requires an appraisal of external forces relative to internal forces and the resultant direction of movement (chapter 2). In dance, concentric contractions are generally used to move the body or its segments in a direction against gravity and to accelerate limbs. Conversely, eccentric contractions are generally used to move the body or its segments in the same direction as gravity and to decelerate limbs. Additionally, isometric contractions are used to maintain the position of the body or its segments with no apparent joint movement occurring.

Identify Prime Movers

Once the type of muscle contraction has been identified, the prime movers can be easily determined. Remember that with a concentric contraction the prime movers will be the muscle group whose action is in the same direction as the observed joint movement, while with an eccentric contraction, the active muscles are those whose action is opposite to the observed joint movement. If you are having trouble delineating the prime movers, imagine what joint movements would occur if all the muscles around the joints under observation relaxed. The prime movers would then be the muscle groups that would have to function to create or control movement in the desired direction at each joint. If the goal is to have no movement occur at a given joint but relaxation results in movement, the muscle group with an action opposing this movement would be working isometrically to maintain the desired joint position.

As done in previous movement analyses, when delineating the prime movers, first list them in terms of the functional group (e.g., hip flexors) and then provide specific examples (e.g., iliopsoas, rectus femoris) obtained from figures 8.1 and 8.2 and table 8.1. Including the functional muscle group is recommended because it provides a simple way of trying to accurately reflect the muscles that would have to work without having to refer to studies that investigate the relative contribution of specific muscles with factors such as the speed of motion, changes in line of pull relative to the relevant axis of rotation in different ranges of motion, secondary actions of agonists, and the amount of resistance to the given motion. Then, when providing specific sample muscles, choosing primary muscles versus secondary muscles for the given joint movement (table 8.1) will generally help provide muscles that are responsible for generating a large percentage of the necessary force and that are operative under many conditions. However, if more accuracy is necessary, referring to EMG and other research studies can be helpful.

Identify Key Stabilizers (Optional)

Remember that when a muscle contracts as discussed in chapter 2, the muscle unpreferentially tends to bring both of its attachments toward one another (law of approximation). In many movements, isometric co-contraction of many muscles is occurring to stabilize segments of the body and prevent unwanted movement due to this law of approximation or due to movement of body segments away from the center of mass of the body. For example, when movements such as brushes (dégagés) are performed, co-contraction of many muscles of the hip and spine works to prevent undesired compensations of the pelvis or torso.

To simplify movement analysis, emphasis is usually placed on the body segments that are moving. However, it is important to realize that appropriate functioning of these muscles of stabilization is key for technique and injury prevention. In recognition of their role, one approach is to include one or two stabilizers that are essential to prevent common technique/alignment errors and allow proper execution of the movement. Another approach is to address stabilizers with technique considerations only if a technique error is occurring that relates to inappropriate use of a stabilizer. For example, if one were analyzing a movement, the function of the abdominal muscles as stabilizers to prevent hyperlordosis (figure 8.3, p. 471) could be listed in a section titled "stabilizers" or in a section addressing "alignment and technique considerations" if excessive arching of the low back was noted.

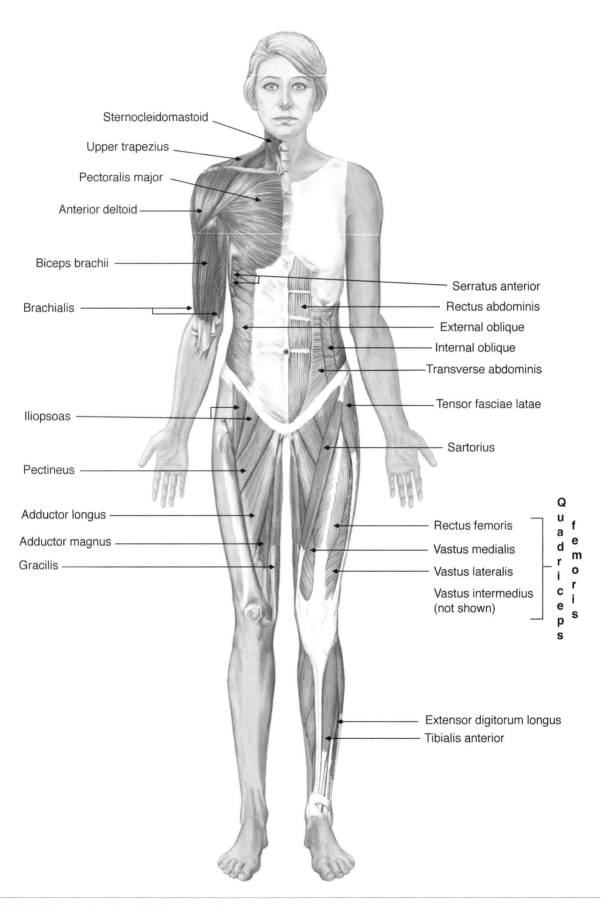

Sternocleidomastoid

Upper trapezius

Pectoralis major

Anterior deltoid

Biceps brachii

Brachialis

Iliopsoas

Pectineus

Adductor longus

Adductor magnus

Gracilis

Serratus anterior

Rectus abdominis

External oblique

Internal oblique

Transverse abdominis

Tensor fasciae latae

Sartorius

Rectus femoris

Vastus medialis

Vastus lateralis

Vastus intermedius
(not shown)

Quadriceps femoris

Extensor digitorum longus

Tibialis anterior

FIGURE 8.1   Anterior view of primary muscles.

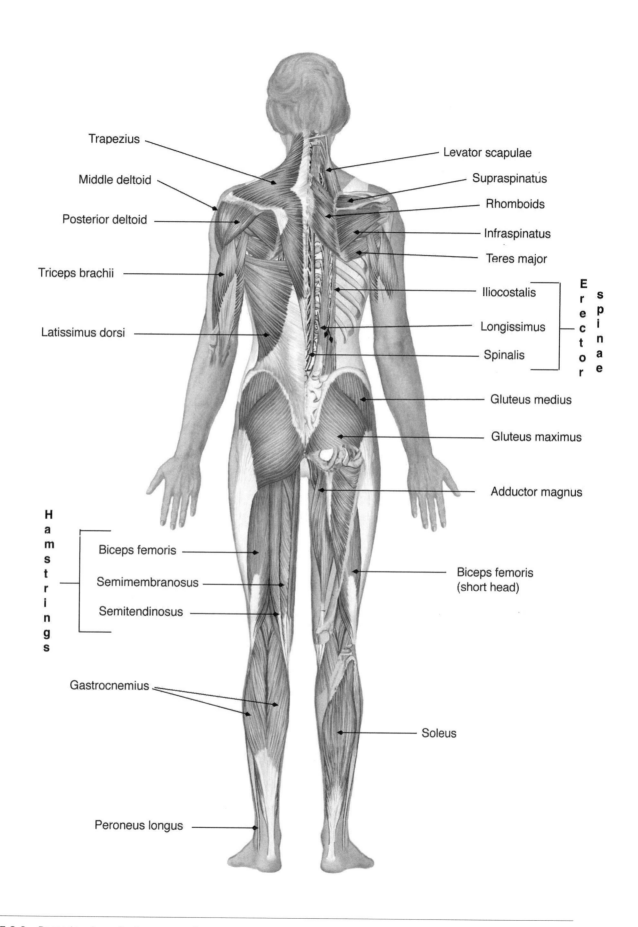

Trapezius

Middle deltoid

Posterior deltoid

Triceps brachii

Latissimus dorsi

Levator scapulae

Supraspinatus

Rhomboids

Infraspinatus

Teres major

Iliocostalis

Longissimus

Spinalis

Erector spinae

Gluteus medius

Gluteus maximus

Adductor magnus

Hamstrings

Biceps femoris

Semimembranosus

Semitendinosus

Biceps femoris (short head)

Gastrocnemius

Soleus

Peroneus longus

FIGURE 8.2   Posterior view of primary muscles.

TABLE 8.1   Summary of Fundamental Movements of Major Joints and the Primary Muscles That Can Produce Them

Major joint	Movement	Prime mover	Major joint	Movement	Prime mover
Spine	Flexion	Rectus abdominis External oblique Internal oblique	Ankle-foot	Plantar flexion	Gastrocnemius Soleus
	Extension	Erector spinae		Dorsiflexion	Tibialis anterior Extensor digitorum longus
	Rotation	External oblique Internal oblique Erector spinae		Inversion	Tibialis anterior Tibialis posterior
	Lateral flexion	Quadratus lumborum External oblique Internal oblique Erector spinae		Eversion	Peroneus longus Peroneus brevis
Hip	Flexion	Iliopsoas Rectus femoris Sartorius	Shoulder	Flexion	Pectoralis major (clavicular) Anterior deltoid
	Extension	Hamstrings Gluteus maximus		Extension	Pectoralis major (sternal) Latissimus dorsi Teres major Posterior deltoid
	Abduction	Gluteus medius Gluteus minimus		Abduction	Middle deltoid Supraspinatus
	Adduction	Adductor longus Adductor brevis Adductor magnus Gracilis		Adduction	Pectoralis major and latissimus dorsi* Anterior deltoid and posterior deltoid*
	External rotation	Gluteus maximus Deep outward rotators		External rotation	Infraspinatus Teres minor
	Internal rotation	Gluteus medius Gluteus minimus		Internal rotation	Subscapularis Teres major
Knee	Flexion	Hamstrings	Elbow	Flexion	Biceps brachii Brachialis
	Extension	Quadriceps femoris		Extension	Triceps brachii

*Adduction is produced by simultaneous action of these paired muscles.

Identify Key Synergists (Optional)

As just discussed, when a muscle contracts, it tends to produce all of its possible joint movements. If some of these actions are not being used in the analyzed movement, it is likely that one or more synergists are being used to neutralize the undesired action(s). To simplify movement analysis, the action of these synergists is often ignored. However, as with stabilizers, more sophisticated analysis may include one or more synergists that are key for correct execution of the movement, or this area can be selectively addressed with technique considerations if a related error is observed. For example, in movements where the arms are overhead, the scapular depressors can act as synergists to prevent undesired excessive elevation of the shoulders (figure 8.4) and could be listed in a section titled "stabilizers" or in a section addressing "alignment and technique considerations" if undesired scapular elevation was noted.

Identify Any Requirements for Extreme Range of Motion (Movement Specific)

Some movements performed in dance require extreme ranges of motion in one or more directions and joints. In such cases, it is important that a movement analysis note this, as it may be relevant

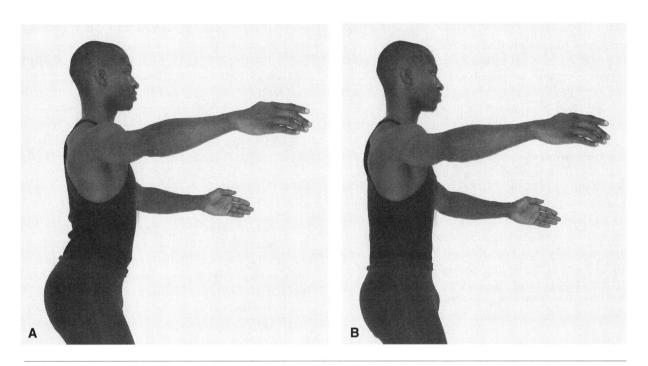

FIGURE 8.3   Use of the abdominal muscles as stabilizers to prevent arching of the low back. (A) Excessive spinal hyperextension, (B) desired spinal stabilization.

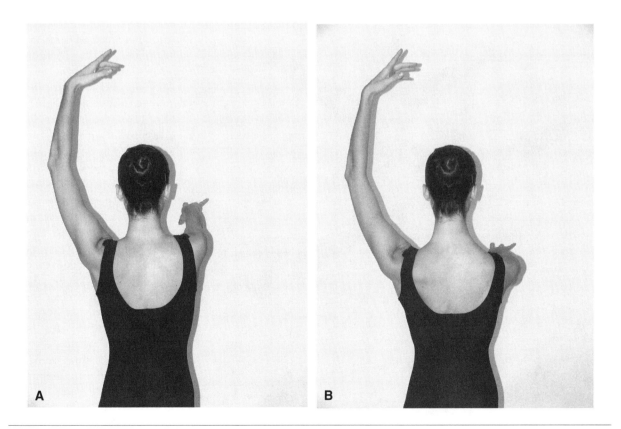

FIGURE 8.4   Use of the scapular depressors to prevent undesired elevation of the scapulae. (A) Excessive scapular elevation, (B) desired positioning of the scapulae.

for optimal performance of the movement. These extremes of motion may represent points in the movement where either inadequate strength or inadequate flexibility can prohibit achieving the desired position. For example, performing the jump shown in figure 8.5 (sissone ouverte) requires high levels of hip flexor strength and hip extensor (hamstring) flexibility for the front leg, and high levels of hip extensor strength and hip flexor flexibility for the back leg. This concept is particularly relevant with multijoint muscles in which active insufficiency or passive insufficiency can readily limit potential range of motion or when movements require ranges far exceeding those used in activities of daily living, such as in the pictured jump (figure 8.5) or the extreme ankle-foot plantar flexion desired for pointe work.

Identify Any Requirements for Marked Strength or Power (Movement Specific)

Some movements performed in dance require marked strength or power (ability to generate a large amount of force in a small amount of time) that may limit performance capacity not related to using extreme range of motion. Examples of dance movements that particularly rely on lower extremity strength are movements that involve projecting the body through space such as jumps and leaps and movements involving lowering the body weight toward the floor such as hinges and falls (figure 8.6). Examples that rely more on upper extremity strength are partnering and movements requiring arm support such as handstands or cartwheels (figure 8.7).

Body Alignment and Technique Considerations

After determining the joint movements and key muscles involved in the movement under analysis, one should look more closely at the performance of the movement in terms of alignment, joint mechanics, and special dance considerations discussed in previous chapters on specific joints. For example, in performance of some more stationary movements at the barre or center floor, the goal is frequently to maintain an approximately neutral positioning of many joints, avoiding excessive pronation of the foot, hyperextension of the knee, tilting of the pelvis, or elevation of the shoulders.

However, in more dynamic movement, some of these movements naturally occur, and the concern becomes one of magnitude. For example, pronation is a normal part of walking and running movements that is important for shock absorption, but excessive pronation can increase risk for certain types of injuries. Similarly, some anterior tilting of the pelvis and increased spinal hyperextension must occur with an arabesque in order to achieve the desired height of the leg, but excessive amounts without coordinated co-contraction of abdominal muscles can increase injury risk to the low back and are considered undesired from an aesthetic perspective. In some cases, it may be necessary to obtain an understanding of what "normal" values are from reading research studies, observing "correct" performances of movement, or practical knowledge gained

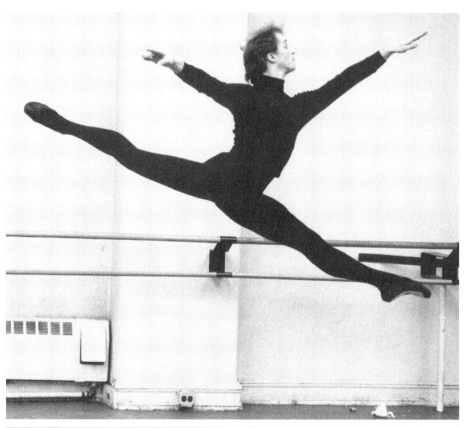

FIGURE 8.5 Sample dance movement requiring extreme range of motion of the hamstrings and hip flexors.

Photo courtesy of Myra Armstrong. Dancer: Lorin Johnson with American Ballet Theatre.

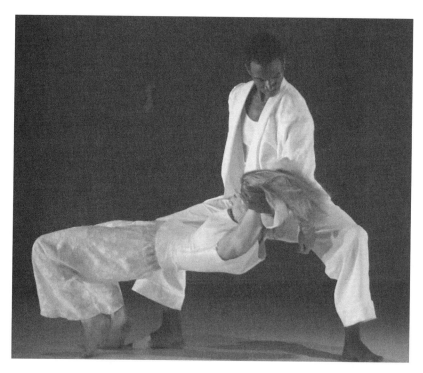

FIGURE 8.6 Sample dance movement demanding high levels of strength of the knee extensors.

Photo courtesy of Patrick Van Osta. CSULB dancers Shana Menaker and Dwayne Worthington.

only is a knowledge of "normal" required but also a skillful analysis is necessary so that appropriate corrections can be generated that will enhance performance and not just create new problems. One important aspect of this skill is the ability to distinguish a causal relationship between errors and decide if something is a problem in itself or is an effect resulting from another more fundamental problem. Another important consideration is the ability to prioritize problems and decide which areas to address first. One key factor that influences this prioritization is how much improvement would be expected from the correction of a problem.

Although there are many approaches that can be taken, one approach commonly used by the author is to begin with more central or proximal corrections, as these corrections often positively impact performance, as well as influence more distal problems. For example, when addressing a dancer performing a

from personal experience of incorrect and correct execution of a given movement before one can make an appraisal of "excessive." In other cases, "normal" is more intuitively obvious or is set by the aesthetic of a given school of dance.

Some examples of common problems to look for are provided in table 8.2. These errors can come from many sources including inadequate stabilization of prime movers, inadequate use of synergists to neutralize undesired secondary actions of muscles, unbalanced co-contraction of antagonist muscles, inadequate muscle contraction to counter external forces, and inappropriate weight placement (or combinations of these). In some cases the problems may be linked to inadequate or imbalanced strength or flexibility in select muscles, while in other cases the problems may relate more to neural control factors and suboptimum coordination of muscles to produce desired movements. When movement analysis is being performed, key alignment and technique errors should be noted; and if the analyst has sufficient knowledge, brief suggestions for improving these problems can be given. Sample strength exercises, stretches, mechanics, and cues that may help improve these problems are provided in table 8.2.

However, if recommendations are to be given in an effort to correct these technique problems, not

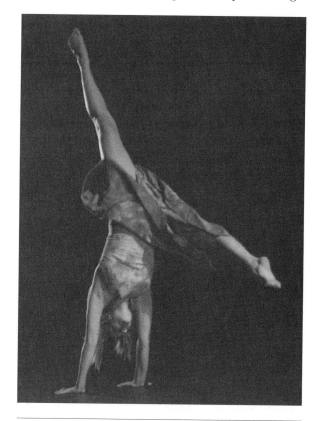

FIGURE 8.7 Sample dance movement demanding high levels of upper extremity strength.

Photo courtesy of Patrick Van Osta. CSULB dancer Delyer Anderson.

TABLE 8.2 Key Alignment/Technique Problems and Potential Corrective Measures

Joint alignment/ technique problem (Common terminology)	Corrective measures			
	Strengthen	Stretch	Mechanics	Sample cues
Spine				
Excessive cervical lordosis (Forward head, leading with chin)	Neck flexors (example: figure 3.29B, p. 103)	Neck extensors (example: figure 3.29C, p. 103)	Use the flexors of the head and neck to decrease cervical extension.	Bring the bottom of the chin back, and imagine being suspended from behind the ears or just behind the midpoint of the top of the head.
Excessive thoracolumbar extension (Rib-leading)	Abdominals (upper emphasis) (examples: table 3.4, B-D, pp. 134-135)	Spinal extensors (lower and middle) (examples: table 3.7, A and B, p. 144)	Contract the abdominals with emphasis on the upper attachment bringing the ribcage down and back.	Pull the bottom of the front of the rib cage down and back toward the spine as the upper back lifts up and slightly forward.
Excessive lumbar lordosis (Arched low back)	Abdominals (lower emphasis) (examples: table 3.4, E and F, pp. 135-136 and figure 3.25A, p. 97)	Spinal extensors (lower) Hip flexors (examples: figure 3.25, B and C, p. 97)	Contract the abdominals to posteriorly tilt the pelvis and reduce lumbar extension until a neutral position of the pelvis and normal lumbar curve are obtained.	Pull the pubic bone and bottom of the front of the rib cage toward each other.
Kyphosis (Collapsed, rounded, slumped, upper back)	Upper back extensors (example: figure 3.26A, p. 99)	Anterior shoulder muscles (examples: table 7.12, B-D, pp. 449-450) Abdominals (examples: figure 3.26B, p. 99, and table 3.7D, p. 145)	Contract the thoracic spinal extensors to decrease thoracic flexion.	Lift the upper back up and slightly forward toward the ceiling.
Pelvis				
Anterior pelvic tilt (Released pelvis)	Abdominals (lower emphasis) (examples: table 3.4, A-C and E, pp. 134 and 135)	Hip flexors (examples: table 4.7, A and B, p. 224) Spinal extensors (lower)	Use the abdominals (with inferior attachment onto pelvis moving) or abdominal–hamstring force couple to posteriorly tilt the pelvis until the pubic symphysis and ASIS are in vertical alignment.	Pull up the pubic symphysis to create a neutral position of the pelvis.
Posterior pelvic tilt (Tucked pelvis)	Spinal extensors Hip flexors (examples: table 4.5, A-C, pp. 213-214)	Abdominals (examples: table 3.7, C and D, pp. 144-145)	Use the hip flexors or spinal extensors to anteriorly tilt the pelvis until the ASIS and pubic symphysis are vertically aligned, and use the spinal extensors to reduce flexion of the lumbar spine.	Bring the top of the pelvis forward, and lift the lower spine up.

Joint alignment/ technique problem (Common terminology)	Corrective measures			
	Strengthen	Stretch	Mechanics	Sample cues
Hip				
Not achieving or maintaining hip external rotation (Losing turnout)	Deep outward rotators (examples: table 4.5, M-O, pp. 219-220)	Hip internal rotators, hip joint capsule, and anterior ligaments (example: figure 3.42, p. 126) Hip flexors (example: table 4.7A, p. 224) Hip adductors (example: table 4.7J, p. 228)	Emphasize use of the lower DOR to keep the femur externally rotated in the acetabulum, particularly when extending the knees.	Bring the greater trochanter toward the sitz bones, and wrap the back of the thigh inward.
Knee				
Valgus position of knee (Knees facing inward, knees falling inside feet)	Deep outward rotators (examples: table 4.5, M-O, pp. 219-220)	Hip internal rotators (if indicated) (example: figure 4.32, p. 198)	Prevent internal rotation of the femur or tibia relative to the foot via contraction of the hip external rotators, knee external rotators, or positioning of the foot.	Maintain rotation at the hip, and guide the knee over the foot during knee flexion.
Knee hyperextension (Pressing knees back, locking knees)	Quadriceps (examples: table 5.3, C and D, pp. 275-276) Hamstrings (example: table 5.3F, p. 277) Deep outward rotators (examples: table 4.5, N and O, p. 220)		Use the DOR to limit internal rotation of the femur associated with the final stages of knee extension, or stop knee extension before hyperextension via co-contraction of the hamstrings and quadriceps or relative positioning of body segments.	Keep the knees facing forward and just in front of the ankle bones (lateral malleoli) as the knees extend.
Ankle-foot				
Excessive pronation (Rolling in)	Foot inverters (examples: table 6.6, E-G, pp. 346-347)	Triceps surae (examples: table 6.8, A-D, pp. 356-357)	Maintain adequate rotation at the hip, and contract the biceps femoris as needed to prevent undesired internal rotation of the tibia and associated pronation. Use the foot inverters to limit pronation, and keep adequate weight on the lateral metatarsal heads (toes).	Lift up the inner border of the foot to achieve a neutral position of the foot and maintain appropriate rotation at the hip for proper knee-foot alignment.
Excessive supination (Rolling out)	Foot everters (examples: table 6.6, H and I, p. 348)		Avoid excessive rotation of the tibia or varus position of the knee and associated supination. Maintain adequate weight on the hallux.	Lift up the outer border of the foot to achieve a neutral position of the foot and maintain appropriate knee-foot alignment.

(continued)

TABLE 8.2   Key Alignment/Technique Problems and Potential Corrective Measures *(continued)*

Joint alignment/ technique problem (Common terminology)	Strengthen	Stretch	Mechanics	Sample cues
Ankle-foot *(continued)*				
Inadequate plantar flexion (Stiff foot, inadequate point)	Ankle-foot plantar flexors (examples: table 6.6, A and B, pp. 343-344) Stirrup muscles (examples: table 6.6, F, H, and N, pp. 347, 348, and 351) Intrinsic muscles that support medial longitudinal arch (examples: table 6.6, J and K, p. 349)	Ankle-foot dorsiflexors and other passive constraints to plantar flexion (examples: table 6.8, E and F, p. 358)	Maximize plantar flexion of the intertarsal and tarsometatarsal joints, not just talocrural joints. Shift the body weight forward adequately to facilitate optimal plantar flexion.	Pull up and forward with the stirrup muscles.
Shoulder				
Rolled shoulders (Rounded shoulders, closed chest) Often accompanied by kyphosis	Scapular adductors Shoulder external rotators Thoracic spinal extensors (examples: table 7.10, H and I, p. 439)	Shoulder internal rotators and horizontal adductors (example: table 7.12D, p. 450)	Prevent undesired "rolled position" of the shoulders by contracting the shoulder external rotators and scapular adductors.	Bring the shoulder blades slightly together and down as the shoulders reach sideward.
Excessive scapular elevation (Lifted shoulders)	Scapular depressors (example: table 7.10C, p. 435)	Upper trapezius (example: figure 3.29C, p. 103)	Use the scapular depressors to prevent undesired elevation during the desired upward rotation of the scapula that accompanies shoulder abduction or flexion.	Reach the arm down, out, and around as the scapula rotates, without excessive lifting, when raising the arm overhead.
Excessive scapular adduction (Pinched shoulders) Often accompanied by thoracolumbar extension	Scapular abductors (example: table 7.10K, p. 440)	Scapular adductors Thoracic spinal extensors (example: table 3.7B, p. 144)	Use the scapular abductors to prevent undesired scapular adduction, and use the abdominals to prevent undesired thoracolumbar spinal extension.	Reach the elbows away and slightly forward so that the hands are visible in the peripheral vision when the arms are at the sides or overhead.

second-position plié, correction of excessive lumbar lordosis and an anterior pelvic tilt will often correct the associated functional valgus position of the knees and excessive foot pronation. So, using various cues (and supplemental exercises if indicated) to aid the dancer in establishing a neutral position of the spine and pelvis should be prioritized, as this will also have positive effects on distal joints. Similarly, providing cues and exercises to aid the dancer in achieving and maintaining appropriate external rotation at the hip will often positively influence distal joints as discussed in previous chapters. Adding sufficient external rotation at the hip can correct relative functional tibial internal rotation and the associated pronation of the foot.

CONCEPT DEMONSTRATION 8.1

Influence of Spinal-Pelvic Alignment on Distal Joint Mechanics

Stand in a turned-out second position in front of a mirror.

• **Valgus and varus position of the knee.** Perform a demi-plié in a second position, focusing on guiding the middle of your kneecap over your second toe as your knees bend. Then, purposely slowly anteriorly tilt the pelvis, letting the top of the pelvis rotate forward. Notice the associated tendency for your knees to move inward, creating a valgus position of the knee. Now, purposely slowly posteriorly tilt the pelvis, bringing the bottom of the pelvis forward while the top of the pelvis rotates back. Notice the associated tendency for your knees to move outward, perhaps even to a position where they are behind the axis of the foot (varus position of the knee). Lastly, establish a neutral position of the pelvis where the top of the anterior pelvis (anterior superior iliac spines) is vertically aligned above the bottom of the anterior pelvis (pubic symphysis) and see if you can more readily position the midpoint of your patellas over your second toes.

• **Foot pronation and supination.** Again, perform a demi-plié in second position, focusing on guiding the middle of your kneecap over your second toe, with the foot in neutral alignment. Then, purposely slowly anteriorly tilt the pelvis, and notice that as the knees fall inward, the feet also tend to roll in, creating a pronated position of the feet. Next, posteriorly tilt (tuck) the pelvis, and notice that as your knees tend to move outward, the feet also tend to roll out, creating a supinated position of the foot. Lastly, establish a neutral position of the pelvis, and see if you can position the mid-patella approximately over the second toe such that the foot is in a neutral position with slightly more weight placed over the base of the big toe versus the little toe, and a formed longitudinal arch.

• **Changes in muscle use.** Again, while maintaining a second-position plié, anteriorly tilt your pelvis, and this time also let your torso slightly lean forward. Notice if you feel any difference in muscle use with this misaligned position than when in a neutral position. Go back and forth between these positions several times to check your observation. Some dancers experience a greater sense of work in the quadriceps femoris and tensor fasciae latae in the misaligned position and more ability to feel the hamstrings working in the correctly aligned position.

In contrast, correcting the distal foot pronation by contracting the foot inverters, without addressing the underlying more fundamental alignment of the spine and pelvis, will often not provide the desired corrections proximally and may result in muscle fatigue and potentially shin splints if positioning of proximal segments are producing large internal rotation forces of the tibia that are countered by only relatively small muscles of the foot. It is also generally not possible to maintain this distal correction in dynamic movement, which requires complex adjustment of the joints of the feet including relative pronation and supination to meet the demands of shock absorption and propulsion in locomotor movements. However, it is important to note that in athletes that wear shoes (such as runners), distal correction with well-designed arch supports or orthotics, rather than superimposed contraction of the inverters, can often be helpful for improving technique.

Special Considerations

In faster movements, movement analysis can become more complex. Rather than the more sustained use of a prime mover with a certain type of contraction throughout most or all of a phase, bursts of muscle activity, the use of momentum, and quick changes in contraction type play a more prominent role. For example, as the thigh swings forward during low leg swings, the hip flexors are briefly used concentrically to initiate the motion; next, momentum becomes primary; and then toward the end of the forward motion, the hip extensors are used eccentrically to decelerate the thigh and then concentrically to initiate the swing of the leg in a backward direction in the next phase of the movement. This eccentric use of muscles to aid with changing the direction of movement of a limb does not invalidate classic movement analysis, which would suggest that the hip flexors

Influence of Movement Quality on Muscle Use

While standing or sitting in a chair, perform shoulder flexion and extension with your right arm according to the following directions.

· **Slow raise and lower.** Slowly raise your arm to the front to shoulder height, pause, and then slowly lower it. Note the predominance of muscle activity in the anterior shoulder muscles (including the anterior deltoid), working concentrically when raising and eccentrically when lowering the arm.

· **Resisted raise and lower.** Slowly raise and then lower your arm as if moving through tar or molasses. Note the muscle work on both sides of the shoulder (including the anterior and posterior deltoid) as the antagonist creates internal resistance (eccentric contraction) while the agonist acts concentrically as the prime mover.

· **Slow raise and released lower.** Slowly raise your arm to shoulder height, pause, and then relax the muscles and just let the arm drop as gravity effects the movement. Now, just add a very small amount of muscle contraction to decelerate and control the movement toward the end of the drop.

"Use Your Bones, Not Your Muscles"

In contemporary dance techniques emphasizing a "released quality of movement," teachers will sometimes cue students to "use your bones, not your muscles." This cue is not consistent with anatomical principles since bones cannot produce movement, and if the muscles were not used during movement the dancer would collapse to the floor. One possible interpretation of the intent of this cue is to relax muscles during portions of a movement, allowing gravity and momentum to play a more prominent role in generation of movement of the limb or body part utilized. However, some muscle contraction would be necessary toward the end of a given movement to decelerate the body segment to prevent collapsing or to change the direction of movement. Rewording the movement cue to incorporate muscle contribution with phrases such as "release and recover" or "fall and recover" would be more consistent with anatomical and biomechanical principles.

work as prime movers to swing the thigh forward and that the hip extensors work as prime movers to swing the thigh backward. Rather, it just demonstrates additional contribution of muscles revealed from EMG studies of rapidly reversing reciprocal motions that would not necessarily be predicted from a pure anatomical analysis of the movement.

In addition to speed, dance often utilizes very subtle and specific execution directives that can influence muscle use. For example, many movements can be purposely varied to provide an "accent," or emphasis, at different times during the movement, as in emphasizing the "out" or "in" phase of the

movement when performing a high kick to the front (grand battement). If the emphasis is "in," the hip extensors (hamstrings) can be felt working concentrically sooner to close the leg back in to the starting position on the down-phase of the movement; when the accent is "out," the hip flexors can be felt working eccentrically longer in the down-phase of the movement. Similarly, other differences in qualities or efforts of movement can influence muscle use. Laban (Hodgson, 2001) uses words such as "light" and "strong" or "free" and "bound" to describe the "efforts" associated with movement. With bound movements, internal resistance is often created

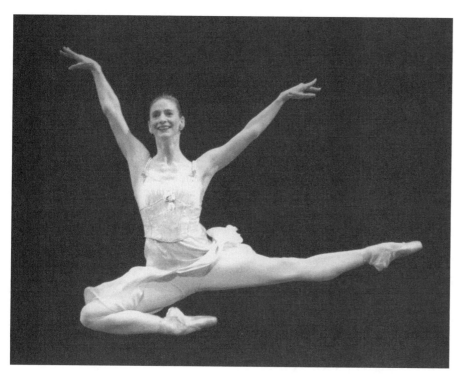

FIGURE 8.8   Performance of a jump with an appearance of effortlessness.
© Angela Sterling Photography. Pacific Northwest Ballet dancer Lisa Apple.

with co-contraction of antagonists and agonists. In contrast, with some types of free movements (e.g., "release"), momentum is allowed to make a greater contribution, with muscular contraction often occurring more briefly to accelerate and decelerate body segments, rather than working in a more continuous manner to control movement.

A related and subtle special consideration has to do with the external appearance of effort and movement economy. In many dance forms, part of the dance aesthetic is to perform demanding movements without an undue appearance of effort and without disrupting the expressive quality desired by the choreographer (figure 8.8). One aspect of achieving this appearance likely relates to movement economy. The desire is often to achieve the objective of the movement without any unnecessary work, effort, or apparent movements of body segments not designed to be part of the movement. This requires very skilled activation of muscles with appropriate magnitude and timing and may involve less activation of muscles in general, and specifically less reliance on co-contraction for movement accuracy.

Analysis Check

If possible, perform the movement under analysis with your own body and palpate the muscles you think should be working, or internally key in to which muscles you feel working, or do both. Use this to check your analysis. If your body check is not consistent with your theoretical analysis, rethink your analysis and make sure the effect of gravity is being appropriately accounted for. Also, make sure that the sensation you are keying in to in your body is one of muscle contraction, and not one from stretching the antagonist. In addition, remember that you may feel muscles working that are not prime movers, but rather stabilizers and synergists.

Schema for Anatomical Movement Analysis

A schema for analyzing movements that incorporates the concepts just discussed is provided in table 8.3. This schema will be used to analyze sample movements in this section. Readers are also encouraged to develop analysis skills by applying this schema to many other movements. Research indicates that both practice of movement analysis in general and practice in distinguishing the critical features of a given skill can markedly improve analysis ability (Hall, 1999). For readers new to this process, having the subject wear body-conforming attire such as a leotard and the use of a background that facilitates observation (such as one with a grid, vertical lines, or colors contrasting with those on the subject) can aid in the observation process. In some cases, adding sticky markers (such as dots) to key landmarks, or having the subject wear an elastic belt that contrasts in color to the leotard and background, will make alignment considerations easier to evaluate. For more complex or faster movements, using a video recording that can be repetitively observed or watched at a slower speed can help with observation and train observation skills.

Sample Anatomical Movement Analyses

An anatomical analysis of two sample dance movements follows. These movements were selected to provide an example of lower limb movement occurring primarily in the sagittal plane and lower limb movement occurring primarily in the frontal plane.

TABLE 8.3 Movement Analysis Schema

Basic analysis	Supplemental analysis
1. **Divide the movement into phases** based on movement direction or functional goals.	6. **Identify key muscles acting as stabilizers** that are important for correct technique (optional).
2. **Select the key joint(s)** where visible movement occurs and that are particularly important for correct execution of the movement.	7. **Identify key muscles acting as synergists** that are important for correct technique (optional).
3. **Identify the key joint movements** that occur in each phase.	8. **Identify any requirements for extreme range of motion** (movement specific).
4. **Identify the type of muscle contraction** in each of the phases or phase subdivisions. In more simple movement analysis, the entire phase generally involves the same type of muscle contraction. With more complex movements, multiple types of muscle contractions may exist within a given phase. A. *Identify concentric muscle contractions/phases.* Concentric muscle contractions act in the opposite direction to gravity or other external forces where the action of the given muscle group is in the same direction as the direction of the observed movement. B. *Identify eccentric muscle contractions/phases* (if present). Eccentric muscle contractions act in the same direction as gravity or other external forces to decelerate or control movement, such as on the down-phase of a given movement. The action of the active muscle group is in the opposite direction to the direction of the observed movement. C. *Identify key isometric muscle contractions/phase(s)* (if present). Isometric muscle contractions exactly balance opposing forces so that there is no change in joint angle and no visible movement is observed.	9. **Identify any requirements for marked strength or power** (movement specific).
5. **Identify the primary muscle group(s) (and sample prime movers)** that produce/control the joint movement(s) in each phase. Where appropriate: A. *Begin with the primary muscle group that produces the joint movement on the concentric phase(s)* (muscles whose primary action is the joint movement observed during the concentric phase). B. *Then identify the primary muscle group that produces the joint movement on the eccentric phase(s)* (muscles whose primary action is opposite to the joint movement observed—often the same muscle group as used in the concentric phase is used in the eccentric phase to control the opposite joint action).	10. **Identify any body alignment and technique problems** (dancer specific).
	11. **Identify special considerations** that influence muscle use (movement specific).
	12. **Check your analysis** by performing the movement and rethinking the logic used.

Front Kick (Grand Battement Devant) From a Lunge

With the front kick (table 8.4), the hip flexors work concentrically on the gesture leg (right leg) in the beginning of the up-phase (subphase A to B) to bring the leg forward, while the knee extensors keep the knee extended and the ankle-foot plantar flexors point the foot. At the same time, the hip extensors and knee extensors of the support leg (left leg) work concentrically to bring their respective joints from a position of flexion to the "extended position" used in normal standing and in anatomical position. The ankle-foot plantar flexors also work concentrically to decrease dorsiflexion by pulling the tibia backward (ankle-foot plantar flexion with proximal segment—the tibia—moving). These actions result in appropriate positioning of the hip, knee, and ankle to provide a stable support leg for the next two subphases of the movement. In the next subphase (subphase B to C), the hip extensors, knee extensors, and ankle plantar flexors of the support leg work isometrically to maintain their position, while the hip flexors of the gesture leg concentrically contract in a forceful manner to raise the leg high to the front. Simultaneously, the knee extensors work to keep the knee extended, and generally the plantar flexors contract concentrically to produce a slightly greater pointed position of the gesture ankle and foot.

Now, to reverse the movement, the hip flexors of the gesture leg work eccentrically to control the lowering of the leg during the initial part of the down-phase (subphase C to D), while the knee extensors and ankle-foot plantar flexors work isometrically to maintain their positions. In the final portion of the down-phase (subphase D to E), the hip extensors of the gesture leg work concentrically to bring the leg behind the body, while the knee extensors work isometrically to keep the knee straight. At the end of this subphase, ankle-foot dorsiflexion of this leg can be produced by a combination of concentric contraction of the ankle-foot dorsiflexors and the passive effect of shifting the body weight back so that the gesture leg now helps support the body weight. During this subphase, the support leg is also undergoing joint movements to return to the starting position. In this case, the hip extensors, knee extensors, and ankle-foot plantar flexors all work eccentrically to control hip flexion, knee flexion, and ankle dorsiflexion, respectively.

Because this movement is performed in a turned-out versus parallel position, the hip external rotators are working in an approximately isometric manner throughout the movement on both the support and gesture legs. In different phases of the movement, changes in joint angle and other factors will influence the relative contribution of specific hip external rotators and the degree to which they are activated.

Looking at the upper extremity and simplifying the analysis to the shoulders, the right and left shoulder flexors work concentrically to raise the arms to the front to different heights on the up-phase of the movement. On the down-phase, gravity would tend to make the arms rapidly fall back down to the sides, and so the shoulder flexors work eccentrically to control the lowering of the arms (shoulder extension). A more detailed analysis of this movement would take into account the subtle rotation that occurs at the shoulder to help position the elbow and forearm in accordance with this classical aesthetic.

Looking at the movement more specifically, because of the challenge of balancing on one leg and the large weight of the leg being displaced, many muscles throughout the body would have to work in an approximately isometric manner as stabilizers to maintain the desired "aligned" upright position of the body with the body weight appropriately

maintained over the support leg. One particularly key muscle group acting as stabilizers are the hip external rotators on the support leg. If these are not appropriately used, the pelvis will tend to rotate toward the support leg (left pelvic rotation resulting in relative hip internal rotation of the support leg) as the gesture leg is lifted. Cueing dancers to focus on maintaining turnout on the hip of the support leg is key for helping to limit pelvic rotation to a degree that is accepted by the aesthetic of the particular school of dance. In terms of synergists, the hip adductors would theoretically act as helping synergists on the gesture leg to neutralize the undesired abduction action of lateral hip flexors, such as the tensor fasciae latae and sartorius, so as to keep the leg appropriately positioned in front of the body. Focusing on the end of the up-phase of the movement, it can be ascertained that inadequate hamstring flexibility (passive insufficiency) or inadequate hip flexor strength (active insufficiency), or both, could limit the dancer's ability to achieve the desired height of the leg.

In terms of technique, one common error is bending the knee of the support leg as the gesture leg is lifted to the front. As described in chapter 4, posteriorly tilting the pelvis will change the facing of the acetabulum and allow for less relative shortening of the iliopsoas, both of which would facilitate greater height of the gesture leg. One study showed that an average of 30° of posterior tilting of the pelvis (beginning at about 45° thigh displacement) and an average of 82° of hip flexion were combined to effect the end position of a grand battement devant (Ryman and Ranney, 1979). However, an excessive degree of posterior tilting of the pelvis or tight hip flexors will bring the femur forward and cause undesired flexion of the knee on the support leg.

Preventing this undesired knee flexion can be accomplished in many ways, including emphasizing using the quadriceps femoris to maintain the knee in an extended position (often encouraged through cueing to "pull up the thigh of the support leg"), using an appropriately balanced co-contraction of the hip flexors and extensors on the support leg to limit hip hyperextension and associated posterior tilting of the pelvis (often encouraged through cueing to "reach the sitz bones down toward the floor on the support leg"), or limiting the backward lean of the torso and associated hip hyperextension and posterior pelvic tilt (often encouraged through cueing to "keep the torso directly above the pelvis"). Although there is a natural slight backward shift of the torso as the leg kicks (Ryman and Ranney, 1979) to offset the forward leg displacement and put the hip flexors in a better position in terms of their length for force generation, excessive backward lean is undesired from an aesthetic perspective. In terms of special considerations, if the movement is performed rapidly, there is likely use of the hip extensors eccentrically to help decelerate the leg toward the end of the up-phase. There is also likely use of the hip extensors concentrically at the end of the down-phase to help close the leg back into the starting position.

TABLE 8.4   Anatomical Analysis of a Front Kick (Grand Battement Devant) From a Lunge (hip, knee, ankle-foot, shoulder)

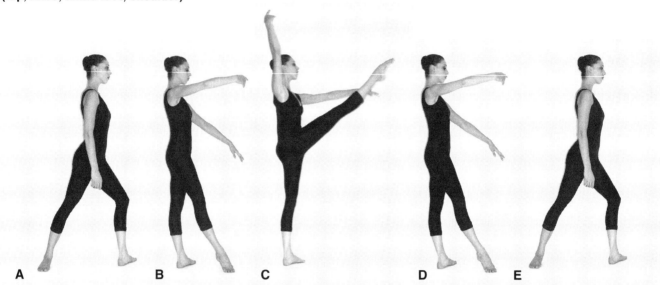

A   B   C   D   E

Movement phases	Joint movements	Contraction type	Prime movers: muscle group (sample muscles)
Up-phase			
Subphase: A to B			
Right hip	Hip flexion	Concentric	Hip flexors (iliopsoas, rectus femoris)
	(Hip external rotation maintained)	Isometric	Hip external rotators (deep outward rotators)
Right knee	(Knee extension maintained)	Isometric	Knee extensors (quadriceps femoris)
Right ankle-foot	A-F plantar flexion	Concentric	A-F plantar flexors (gastrocnemius, soleus)
Left hip	Hip extension	Concentric	Hip extensors (hamstrings, gluteus maximus)
	(Hip external rotation maintained)	Isometric	Hip external rotators (deep outward rotators)
Left knee	Knee extension	Concentric	Knee extensors (quadriceps femoris)
Left ankle-foot	A-F plantar flexion	Concentric	A-F plantar flexors (gastrocnemius, soleus)
Right shoulder	Shoulder flexion	Concentric	Shoulder flexors (anterior deltoid, pectoralis major)
Left shoulder	Shoulder flexion	Concentric	Shoulder flexors (anterior deltoid, pectoralis major)
Subphase: B to C			
Right hip	Hip flexion	Concentric	Hip flexors (iliopsoas, rectus femoris)
	(Hip external rotation maintained)	Isometric	Hip external rotators (deep outward rotators)
Right knee	(Knee extension maintained)	Isometric	Knee extensors (quadriceps femoris)
Right ankle-foot	A-F plantar flexion	Concentric	A-F plantar flexors (gastrocnemius, soleus)
Right shoulder	Shoulder flexion	Concentric	Shoulder flexors (anterior deltoid, pectoralis major)
Left shoulder	Shoulder flexion	Concentric	Shoulder flexors (anterior deltoid, pectoralis major)

Movement phases	Joint movements	Contraction type	Prime movers: muscle group (sample muscles)
Down-phase			
Subphase: C to D			
Right hip	Hip extension (Hip external rotation maintained)	Eccentric Isometric	Hip flexors (iliopsoas, rectus femoris) Hip external rotators (deep outward rotators)
Right knee	(Knee extension maintained)	Isometric	Knee extensors (quadriceps femoris)
Right ankle-foot	(A-F plantar flexion maintained)	Isometric	A-F plantar flexors (gastrocnemius, soleus)
Right shoulder	Shoulder extension	Eccentric	Shoulder flexors (anterior deltoid, pectoralis major)
Left shoulder	Shoulder extension	Eccentric	Shoulder flexors (anterior deltoid, pectoralis major)
Subphase: D to E			
Right hip	Hip extension (Hip external rotation maintained)	Concentric Isometric	Hip extensors (hamstrings, gluteus maximus) Hip external rotators (deep outward rotators)
Right knee	(Knee extension maintained)	Isometric	Knee extensors (quadriceps femoris)
Right ankle-foot	A-F dorsiflexion	Concentric	A-F dorsiflexors (extensor digitorum longus, tibialis anterior)
Left hip	Hip flexion (Hip external rotation maintained)	Eccentric Isometric	Hip extensors (hamstrings, gluteus maximus) Hip external rotators (deep outward rotators)
Left knee	Knee flexion	Eccentric	Knee extensors (quadriceps femoris)
Left ankle-foot	A-F dorsiflexion	Eccentric	A-F plantar flexors (gastrocnemius, soleus)
Right shoulder	Shoulder extension	Eccentric	Shoulder flexors (anterior deltoid, pectoralis major)
Left shoulder	Shoulder extension	Eccentric	Shoulder flexors (anterior deltoid, pectoralis major)

Lateral Tilt

With the lateral tilt (table 8.5), the hip abductors work concentrically on the gesture leg (right leg) to raise the leg (hip abduction with distal segment—femur—moving) in the beginning of the tilt phase (subphase A to B), while the knee extensors work isometrically to keep the knee extended and the ankle-foot plantar flexors work concentrically to point the foot. Then, as the torso tilts "up and over" the support leg (subphase B to C), the hip adductors work eccentrically on the support leg (left leg) to help control the lateral tilt of the trunk via the pelvis (hip abduction with proximal segment—pelvis—moving). Once the torso is no longer vertically aligned relative to the support leg, gravity would tend to make the trunk rapidly fall to the left, and it is the eccentric contraction of the hip adductors of the support leg (and the isometric contraction of the right lateral flexors of the spine) that are vital for controlling this off-center movement and achieving the desired dance aesthetic.

Now, to reverse the movement, the hip adductors of the support leg now work concentrically (hip adduction with proximal segment—pelvis—moving) to help return the trunk to vertical in the initial part of the return phase (subphase C to D). The right hip abductors, knee extensors, and ankle-foot plantar flexors continue to act isometrically to maintain the desired positioning of the gesture leg. Then, in the later portion of the return phase (subphase D to E), generally the hip abductors of the gesture leg briefly work eccentrically to control the lowering of the leg until the toe contacts the floor, at which point the hip adductors work concentrically to draw the leg back to the starting position while the knee extensors continue to work isometrically to maintain the knee in extension. After the toe contacts the ground, concentric contraction of the ankle-foot dorsiflexors and the passive effect of shifting the body weight back over the right leg also act to produce the desired dorsiflexion of the right ankle.

Looking at the upper extremity and simplifying the analysis to the shoulders, the shoulder abductors work concentrically to simultaneously abduct the right and left shoulder on the tilt phase of the movement. On the return phase, gravity would tend

TABLE 8.5 Anatomical Analysis of a Lateral Tilt (hip, knee, ankle-foot, shoulder)

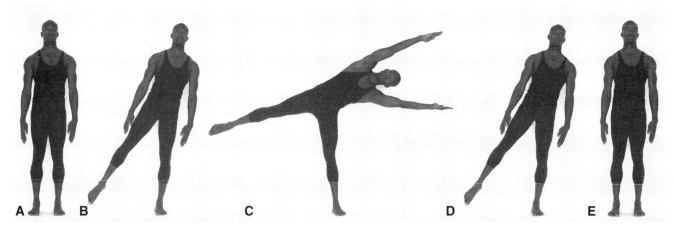

Movement phases	Joint movements	Contraction type	Prime movers: muscle group (sample muscles)
Tilt phase			
Subphase: A to B			
Right hip	Hip abduction	Concentric	Hip abductors (gluteus medius, gluteus minimus)
Right knee	(Knee extension maintained)	Isometric	Knee extensors (quadriceps femoris)
Right ankle-foot	A-F plantar flexion	Concentric	A-F plantar flexors (gastrocnemius, soleus)
Subphase: B to C			
Left hip	Hip abduction	Eccentric	Hip adductors (adductor longus, adductor magnus)
Right hip	(Hip abduction maintained)	Isometric	Hip abductors (gluteus medius, gluteus minimus)
Right knee	(Knee extension maintained)	Isometric	Knee extensors (quadriceps femoris)
Right ankle-foot	(A-F plantar flexion maintained)	Isometric	A-F plantar flexors (gastrocnemius, soleus)
Right and left shoulders	Shoulder abduction	Concentric	Shoulder abductors (middle deltoid, supraspinatus)
Return phase			
Subphase: C to D			
Left hip	Hip adduction	Concentric	Hip adductors (adductor longus, adductor magnus)
Right hip	(Hip abduction maintained)	Isometric	Hip abductors (gluteus medius, gluteus minimus)
Right knee	(Knee extension maintained)	Isometric	Knee extensors (quadriceps femoris)
Right ankle-foot	(A-F plantar flexion maintained)	Isometric	A-F plantar flexors (gastrocnemius, soleus)
Right and left shoulders	Shoulder adduction	Eccentric	Shoulder abductors (middle deltoid, supraspinatus)
Subphase: D to E			
Right hip	Hip adduction	Concentric	Hip adductors (adductor longus, adductor magnus)
Right knee	(Knee extension maintained)	Isometric	Knee extensors (quadriceps femoris)
Right ankle-foot	A-F dorsiflexion	Concentric	A-F dorsiflexors (tibialis anterior, extensor digitorum longus)

to make the arms rapidly fall back down to the sides, and so the shoulder abductors work eccentrically to control the lowering of the arms. A more detailed analysis of this movement would take into account the more specific effects of gravity. For example, as the right arm passes a vertical position, such as seen in table 8.5C, gravity would actually tend to produce shoulder abduction rather than adduction, and the right shoulder adductors would actually be used eccentrically in the brief portion of the range of motion to bring the arms to the full overhead position, isometrically if position C was maintained, and concentrically for the brief portion of the return phase until the arm passes a vertical position.

Looking at the movement more specifically, because of the challenge of balancing on one leg as the trunk moves laterally and the large weight of the gesture leg, many muscles work as stabilizers in a highly coordinated manner to achieve desired positioning of the segments of the body. One important example of stabilization occurs with the spine. In the starting position, co-contraction of the spinal flexors and extensors can be used to achieve the desired approximately neutral alignment of the trunk with the desired lift or presentation of the torso. However, as the trunk moves laterally, gravity now plays a key role, tending to produce lateral flexion of the trunk. Now, as previously stated, the right lateral flexors have to work approximately isometrically to keep the desired neutral extended position of the spine. Cueing students to "reach the spine out long and in line with the middle of the sacrum" (vs. letting it fall sideways—laterally tilt) as the trunk tilts primarily from the hip joint can sometimes help achieve the desired positioning.

In terms of synergists, the oblique abdominal muscles have been shown to be key lateral flexors of the spine. However, contraction of the right internal oblique would also tend to produce undesired right rotation and flexion of the spine. The right external oblique could be used as a synergist to neutralize undesired rotation, and the spinal extensors could be used as synergists to neutralize undesired flexion of the spine.

Considering strength and flexibility and focusing on the end of the up-and-over phase of the movement, it can be ascertained that inadequate hip adductor flexibility, as well as inadequate hip abductor strength, could limit the dancer's ability to achieve the desired height of the leg. If performed turned out, inadequate hamstring flexibility and inadequate hip flexor and hip external rotator strength could also limit the height of the gesture leg. Lastly, adequate strength and flexibility as well

as skilled activation of many muscles of the support leg are vital for successful execution of this movement.

In terms of technique, one common error is failure to keep the trunk movement primarily in the frontal plane. The trunk is commonly flexed at the hip joint, with the bottom of the pelvis going back while the ribs project forward (excessive thoracolumbar extension). In such a case, cueing to "keep the sitz bones down and forward over the support leg" (neutral position of hip extension via use of the abdominal–hamstring force couple) while "the front of the lower ribs are pulled down and slightly back" (neutral position of the spine) can help achieve the desired positioning.

In terms of special considerations, this movement can be performed with many variations, including off-center positions of the trunk and allowing marked lateral tilt of the pelvis to maximize leg height. In the latter case, marked right lateral flexion of the spine is required in the tilt position to bring the shoulders and eyes to an approximately horizontal position. This demands marked spinal flexibility and strength of the lateral flexors of the spine.

Potential Benefits of Anatomical Movement Analysis

Anatomical movement analysis can be used to help improve performance of a given movement in various ways. First, such an analysis results in the determination of which muscles are acting as prime movers. An understanding of the muscles acting as prime movers can help with appropriate generation of movement cues and strengthening exercises. For example, in the front kick from a lunge, many dancers aim to improve the height to which they can lift the leg. Anatomical analysis and reference to EMG studies reveal that the hip flexors, and especially the iliopsoas, are key for performance of this movement in high ranges of motion. Hence, cues aimed at emphasizing use of the iliopsoas, as well as supplemental exercises that focus on strengthening and activation of this muscle in a range of motion similar to that required by the movement, should result in improvement in leg height.

Anatomical analysis also yields potential flexibility constraints for a given movement; and when inadequate flexibility is operative, improving the flexibility of these muscles can improve performance of the given movement. So, in the front kick, anatomical analysis reveals that adequate flexibility of the hamstrings is key for maximizing the height to which the leg can be lifted to the front, and

Comparison of Passive and Active Range of Motion for a Grand Battement

Perform the screening test for hamstring flexibility described in chapter 4 (Tests and Measurements 4.4, p. 205) on yourself by using one hand to lightly bring one leg toward your shoulder while the back of the other leg stays in contact with the floor, as shown in the figure (A). Compare the angle of hip flexion derived passively with this hamstring test to the range of hip flexion exhibited when actively raising the leg to the front at a relatively slow speed (B). An easy way to practically compare these measurements is to note the height of your foot relative to your head and trunk. If the passive hamstring test results (hip angle) are low relative to desired values for dancers and the foot height is close to the level achieved actively, the hamstrings are likely serving as constraints, and hamstring stretching would be recommended to help improve battement height. However, many dancers achieve a much greater range passively than they can achieve actively, especially in movements such as slow front extensions in which momentum cannot be of much help. In such cases, the hamstrings are likely not the primary limiting constraint, and focus should move to strengthening the hip flexors (iliopsoas emphasis) and optimizing technique.

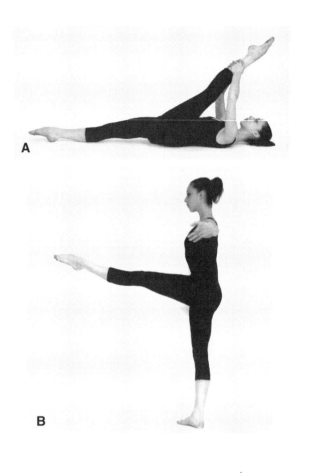

improving hamstring flexibility with supplemental stretching exercises could improve performance if hamstring tightness is a limiting factor. One way to quickly ascertain if strength or flexibility is a limiting factor is to compare passive range of motion to the range used by the dancer during execution of the movement (Tests and Measurements 8.1). If passive range of motion is close to that achieved actively, this suggests that improving flexibility would likely help improve the range utilized in the movement. However, if the range achieved passively is markedly higher than achieved in the movement, this suggests that flexibility is not limiting and that strength or activation patterns, or both, are more likely implicated.

Analysis of potential muscle constraints can also be useful for predicting and lowering injury risk.

Multijoint muscles such as the hamstrings that are required to undergo extreme elongation appear to be at greater risk for being strained. Although this is a complex and controversial area, performing supplemental exercises for these muscles to develop adequate flexibility, adequate strength, balanced strength between right and left sides for the same muscle, and balanced strength between the muscle of concern and its antagonist will likely reduce injury risk.

Lastly, evaluation of alignment and technique factors can reveal factors that, when corrected, can enhance performance, help develop general dance skills, and in some cases reduce injury risk. For example, analysis might reveal that a dancer is excessively arching his or her back during the front kick. This movement pattern, considered undesired aesthetically in many dance forms, can interfere with allowing the normal slight posterior tilting of the pelvis that accompanies higher ranges of hip flexion and hence limit the height of the leg, interfere with establishing relationships of the center of mass of body segments desired for complex balancing, produce increased shear forces in the low lumbar spine, create an undesired increase in spinal extensor activity, and negatively affect the biomechanics of distal weight-bearing joints. Hence, correction of this error can have significant impact on both dance performance and injury risk. However, as previously stated, this aspect of anatomical analysis requires a keen understanding of the desired movement characteristics, as well as a skillful analysis of the causes of technique problems when they are present. For example, is the lumbar lordosis just described related to hip flexor tightness, low back tightness, abdominal weakness, or suboptimal muscle activation patterns?

Other Methods for Movement Analysis

Despite the potential value, it is also important to realize that a basic anatomical movement analysis represents a gross simplification of what is actually going on, used for practical purposes. Anatomical analysis relies on determination of joint movement (direction) through observation combined with theoretical actions of key muscles to predict the muscles that are primarily responsible for a given movement. Hence, one can enhance its accuracy, precision, and depth by referring to studies that utilize quantitative analysis to substantiate or reject theoretical predictions and by applying some basic principles of mechanics.

Quantitative Versus Qualitative Analysis

The anatomical movement analysis presented in this chapter utilizes a qualitative method of analysis. **Qualitative analysis** involves a direct, subjective, non-numerical evaluation by the senses, most commonly a visual analysis. In contrast, **quantitative analysis** involves objective numerical measurements of the whole human body or its parts. These measurements are generally not direct but rather are taken from recordings of the movement performance. Quantitative analysis can involve measurements that relate to describing motion without reference to the forces that produce the motion, termed **kinematic data,** or relate to the forces associated with

movement, termed **kinetic data.** Many tools can be utilized to measure kinematic quantities, including timing devices, computer-linked film analysis (computerized cinematography), computer-linked video analysis (computerized videography), devices that are attached to joints to provide joint angle recordings during movement (electrogoniometry), and use of very small electric lights (light-emitting diodes, or LEDs) or electromagnetic markers interfaced with cameras and computers (optoelectronic systems).

Examples of information obtained from kinematic quantitative analysis include the displacement of the center of gravity or landmarks of concern, joint angles at different phases of movement, and the rate or duration of motion of body segments. Figure 8.9 shows the use of body landmark markers and the application of a special type of goniometer (electrogoniometer, or elgon) that is hooked up to a recorder so that it can monitor changes in joint angle during the movement being studied.

Tools for obtaining kinetic data include devices used to measure applied forces for strength analysis (dynamometers and tensiometers), pressure platforms in shoes, or devices that can be attached to a foot to provide graphical or digital information

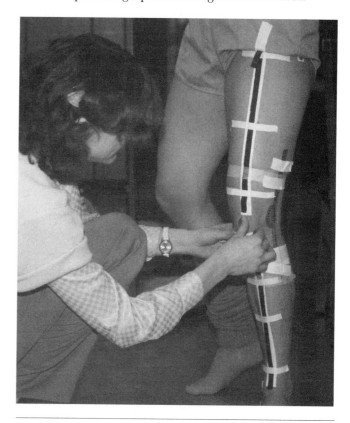

FIGURE 8.9   Use of body landmark markers and an elgon to study the plié.

regarding the pressures on the plantar surface of the foot. Force platforms are used to provide information about the ground reaction forces in vertical, mediolateral, and anteroposterior directions (dynamography). When the foot presses against the ground during movement, the ground applies equal and opposite forces on the foot and body (Newton's third law) termed **ground reaction forces.** The recordings of ground reaction forces from force platforms can be used to determine many important aspects of movement, such as weight placement, pronation, the forces associated with takeoff, and the forces associated with landing (impact). Figure 8.10 provides an example of the vertical ground reaction force associated with landing from a forward leap (grand jeté devant) by an elite ballet dancer (Clippinger and Novak, 1981). One way to get a more practical idea of the meaning of this information is to compare the forces to body weight. In this example, the dancer's maximum vertical ground reaction force in landing from this jeté was almost 5 times (485%) her body weight.

Although electromyography (EMG) is not a direct measure of muscle force, some texts also consider EMG a source of kinetic data. Electromyography can provide information about the onset, duration, and peak of muscle activity, as well as the relative activity of the same muscle in different phases of a movement or with different trials of a given movement. Examples of EMG records when standing in first position were given in chapter 2 (Tests and Measurements 2.1, p. 64), and examples of

EMG records when performing a second-position plié were given in chapter 5 (figure 5.28 and 5.29, p. 273). Because factors such as electrode placement dramatically influence the records, these records are often presented as a percentage of that seen with a maximum voluntary contraction of a given muscle so that more meaningful comparisons can be made between muscles and between subjects. EMG data are often used in conjunction with other data such as joint angles and positions of key body landmarks. In figure 8.11, a camera, mirrors, and a control frame were used to allow a three-dimensional analysis (3-D cinematography) of the knee with special consideration to muscle activation and patellar positioning in different angles of a plié. EMG studies can also be used to support or refute muscle activity predicted from qualitative movement analyses.

Mechanical Analysis

While beyond the scope of this book, integration of concepts related to the laws of motion and kinetic data provides very valuable information that can be utilized in biomechanical analysis of movement. Interested readers are referred to the books by Kreighbaum and Barthels (1996), Hall (1999), Laws (2002), and Hamilton and Luttgens (2002). The latter authors use a recommended approach in which an anatomical analysis is followed by a brief mechanical analysis and brief discussion of mechanical principles as they relate to optimizing performance of the movement being analyzed.

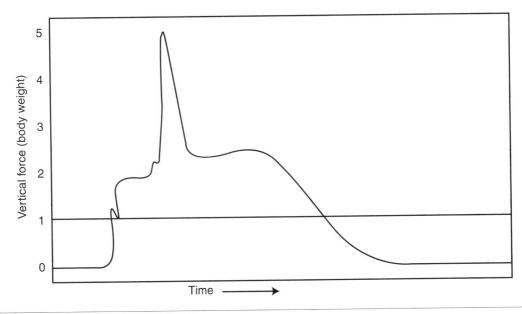

FIGURE 8.10   Example of use of recordings from a force platform to investigate forces associated with landing from a grand jeté.

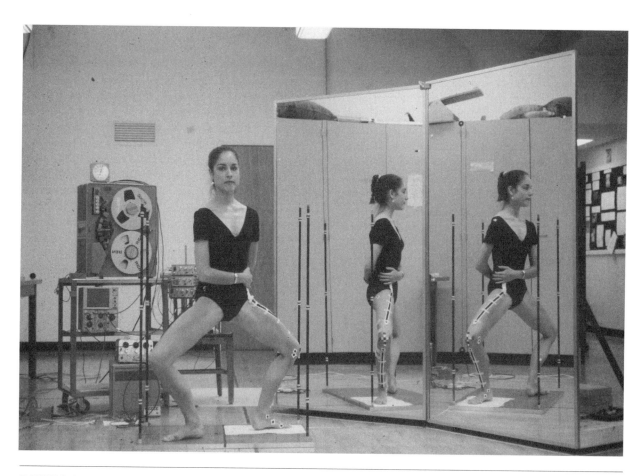

FIGURE 8.11   Use of EMG, body markers, and 3-D cinematography to investigate the plié.

Research-Supported Movement Analysis

Whether one is performing an anatomical movement analysis or an analysis that integrates more mechanical principles, reading related research will allow the analyst to develop a much more in-depth and accurate model of what is normal or desired for a particular movement, as well as an appreciation of the magnitude and type of variability seen between individuals. This will allow the observer to better focus on critical criteria and have a clearer idea of how performance can be improved. For example, extensive research on walking gait has revealed factors that are particularly key to allow walking to proceed with a limited displacement of the center of mass of the body, such that movement economy is fostered, while still serving the primary goal of effectively moving the body through space (determinants of gait). In keeping with these determinants of gait, very specific magnitudes and timings of joint motions such as ankle dorsiflexion, knee flexion, pelvic rotation, and trunk rotation have been discerned that

are valuable for gait modification in rehabilitation settings, as well as for the design of lower extremity prosthetics.

Similarly, extensive research has been done on running. Factors that contribute to optimal performance, running economy, and injury risk with runners ranging from endurance runners to sprinters have been rigorously investigated. A simple analysis of running that integrates selected research findings follows. This was selected because of the common use of running, albeit often shaped by choreographic criteria, in dance.

Unfortunately, scientific investigation of dance-specific vocabulary is much more limited. The leap was selected as a sample dance movement for analysis because there have been some scientific investigations of this movement and because much of the research on jumps from other arenas is relevant for developing a better understanding of optimal performance and injury risk. In keeping with the focus of this text, this analysis will emphasize an anatomical basis but bring in selected particularly key mechanical principles and data.

Running

Running gait, like walking, can be classified as a continuous movement involving a sequential pattern of movement that is repeated. To aid with description, the analysis involves only one leg as it goes through a complete cycle of motion from the time that foot strikes the ground until the same foot again strikes the ground, termed a **stride.** Running is different from walking in that there is a brief period when the body is totally suspended and both feet lose contact with the ground (flight phase), and there is no point during the cycle when both feet are in contact with the ground. Although researchers often use a more complex subdivision of phases into periods, running is divided here into a support phase, a driving or propulsion phase, and a recovery phase as seen in table 8.6 (Hay, 1993; Jensen, Schultz, and Bangerter, 1983).

The **support phase** begins when the foot strikes the ground. The primary function of the muscles in the support phase is to control and arrest the downward motion of the body caused by gravity, absorbing the downward force of the runner and creating stabilization (Elliott and Blanksby, 1979), similar to what occurs in landing from a jump. This phase contains eccentric contraction of the hip extensors, knee extensors, and ankle plantar flexors to control the respective hip flexion, knee flexion, and ankle dorsiflexion produced by gravity and, at the ankle, also passively due to forward movement (momentum) of the body over the foot. This phase also allows the runner to move into position for the next phase.

As the center of gravity of the body moves in front of the foot, the **propulsion phase** (table 8.6) begins. The primary function of the muscles during this phase is to generate the forces that will propel the body. This phase is accompanied by hip exten-

TABLE 8.6   Anatomical Analysis of Running (hip, knee, ankle-foot)

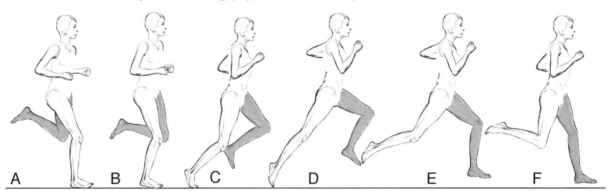

Movement phases	Joint movements	Contraction type	Prime movers: muscle group (sample muscles)
Support phase: Right leg A to B			
Right hip	Hip flexion	Eccentric	Hip extensors (hamstrings, gluteus maximus)
Right knee	Knee flexion	Eccentric	Knee extensors (quadriceps femoris)
Right ankle-foot	A-F dorsiflexion	Eccentric and passive	A-F plantar flexors (gastrocnemius, soleus)
Propulsion phase: Right leg C to D			
Right hip	Hip extension	Concentric	Hip extensors (hamstrings, gluteus maximus)
Right knee	Knee extension	Concentric	Knee extensors (quadriceps femoris)
Right ankle-foot	A-F plantar flexion	Concentric	A-F plantar flexors (gastrocnemius, soleus)
Recovery phase: Right leg E to F and left leg A to E			
Right and left hip	Hip flexion	Concentric	Hip flexors (iliopsoas, rectus femoris)
Right knee	Knee flexion (early in phase)	Largely passive and seconpdarily concentric	490
Right ankle-foot	A-F dorsiflexion	Concentric	Ankle dorsiflexors (tibialis anterior, extensor digitorum longus)

sion, knee extension, and ankle plantar flexion to help produce the backward push of the foot against the ground, which combined with rapid forward swing of the opposite leg will help propel the body upward and forward (Hay, 1993; Mann, Moran, and Dougherty, 1986).

The next phase, the **recovery phase,** begins as the foot leaves the ground (table 8.6E, right leg). The primary function of the muscles in this phase is to bring the leg forward in preparation for the beginning of the next cycle in which the foot again comes in contact with the ground. This phase can be pictured by looking at the right leg in table 8.6, E and F, and then realizing that it would continue to swing forward until just before it contacts the ground, as pictured with the left leg in table 8.6, A through E. So, the recovery phase is accompanied by hip flexion produced by concentric contraction of the hip flexors. At the beginning of this phase, the knee flexes (largely passively due to the transfer of inertial force) and the ankle dorsiflexes via concentric contraction of the ankle-foot dorsiflexors. This knee flexion and ankle-foot dorsiflexion shorten the distance from the hip to the toes (functionally reducing limb length), allowing the leg to clear the ground and swing forward more rapidly (decreased moment of inertia). Later in the recovery phase, when the hip has almost reached full flexion, the knee rapidly undergoes extension (left leg—table 8.6, D to just before foot contact in F), allowing a longer distance to be covered (increased stride length). The initial extension is passive (transfer of momentum) as the thigh decelerates, followed by concentric contraction of the knee extensors.

To understand the relationship between the right and left legs during running, one must know that for the sake of simplicity table 8.6 only shows one half of a stride. So, to picture a full stride, one must realize that following what is pictured in table 8.6F, the left leg (shown in gray) would now go through what is shown for the right leg (shown in white) in A through F. Similarly, after what is pictured in table 8.6F, the right leg would now go through what is shown for the left leg in A through F. Some key points that clarify the relationship between the right and left leg during running follow. When one leg is in the early part of the recovery phase, the body is airborne (table 8.6E for the right leg) with both feet out of contact with the ground (flight phase). When knee flexion brings the recovery knee almost to the center of mass of the body (table 8.6A for the left leg), the opposite leg contacts the ground and enters its support phase; and when the recovery hip reaches about maximum hip flexion in the late recovery phase (table 8.6, just

following D for the left leg), the opposite leg enters its recovery phase and the body is again airborne (Slocum and James, 1968).

Although useful information can be gathered from this simplified analysis, research has demonstrated additional elements that complement these basic elements. For example, at the end of the recovery phase and very beginning of the support phase, the hip actually undergoes a very brief period of concentric hip extension and the knee a very brief period of concentric flexion. This helps decrease the undesired braking force that would tend to push the body backward if the hip was still undergoing flexion and the knee still undergoing extension as the foot contacted the ground. At the beginning of the support phase this concentric contraction of the hip extensors, especially the hamstrings, then serves to pull the body over the point of contact of the foot with the ground; and in sprinting, the strength of these muscles to effect this motion is considered essential for success (Kyrolainen, Belli, and Komi, 2001; Mann et al., 1984). Brief ankle plantar flexion controlled by eccentric contraction of the dorsiflexors has also been noted just as the foot strikes the ground to help position the foot at the same time the ankle plantar flexors are co-contracting for stability (Elliot and Blanskby, 1979).

Similarly, at the very beginning of the recovery phase, concentric contraction of the hip extensors continues briefly and the hip flexors actually work eccentrically first, to decelerate hip extension, prior to working concentrically to bring the leg forward. At the ankle, the concentric contraction of the ankle plantar flexors at the end of the support phase is followed by a brief eccentric contraction of the ankle dorsiflexors to decelerate this plantar flexion of the foot prior to the previously described concentric contraction of the dorsiflexors in the support phase (McGinnis, 2005). And at the end of the recovery phase the hip extensors (hamstrings) work eccentrically to decelerate hip flexion and knee extension, prior to working concentrically briefly at foot strike as previously described. So, an eccentric contraction is commonly used to decelerate a limb, just prior to reversal of the direction of movement. This common use of an eccentric contraction immediately preceding a concentric contraction (i.e., the stretch–shortening cycle discussed in chapter 2) makes running much more efficient, requiring markedly less energy than if it were composed of only sequential concentric muscle contractions (Biewener and Roberts, 2000; Ito et al., 1983; Kram, 2000).

For simplicity this analysis has been limited to sagittal plane movements at the hip, knee, and ankle.

These joints and selected movements are particularly key in running. The action of the arms appears to function primarily to counterbalance the off-center thrust of the legs (Adrian and Cooper, 1989). However, a more complete analysis would include the smaller movements of abduction-adduction and external rotation-internal rotation of the hip and knee, as well as movements of the pelvis (tilts and rotations), spine, upper extremity, and key joints of the foot. Although these movements may be smaller or less fundamental for moving the body through space, they are essential for running mechanics, and deviations in these movements are often implicated with common technique errors and overuse injuries.

In terms of stabilizers, one key muscle group is the hip abductors. During the stance phase, these muscles play a key role in preventing excessive undesired lateral tilt of the pelvis (Trendelenburg sign) or lateral excursion of the pelvis relative to the support foot. In terms of flexibility, although a visual evaluation of running does not display requirements for extreme ranges of motion commonly seen in dance movements, many runners exhibit suboptimal levels of flexibility at various joints, and inadequate range of ankle dorsiflexion can result in compensatory excessive pronation during the support phase. Similarly, tight hip flexors can produce an undesired excessive anterior tilt of the pelvis and limit the desired positioning of the pelvis as the leg swings forward such that stride length is negatively affected. Although still controversial, adequate hamstring flexibility may also have a positive effect on running performance and reduced injury risk (Hreljac, Marshall, and Hume, 2000; Koceja, Burke, and Kamen, 1991). In terms of strength, research has shown that adequate "knee lift" (requiring hip flexor strength) and high levels of hip extensor strength are key for high-level sprinting performance. The latter element of strength is key for increasing the power of the leg drive for greater acceleration of the runner.

In terms of technique, one common error is to swing the gesture leg around (circumduction) during the recovery phase. Cueing the runner to "swing the knee forward on a slight diagonal line" (slightly toward the midline) versus "swinging the knee around in a small semicircle" can help achieve desired positioning. Unnecessary lateral motions decrease the efficiency of running and decrease forward propulsion (Hamilton and Luttgens, 2002). Similarly, cueing to drive the back leg downward and backward at push-off with correct timing and positioning of the trunk can help achieve optimal forward propulsion. The desire is to produce a ground reaction force with a large horizontal component that will propel the runner forward without excessive vertical movement of the body. Positioning of the foot when it contacts the ground at the beginning of stance phase is also key for determining the ground reaction forces generated. Since the ground reaction force is equal in magnitude but opposite in direction to the force produced by the foot when it contacts the ground, having the lower leg still moving forward or having the foot land well in front of the line of gravity (extending vertically from the center of mass of the whole body) will produce a forward force on the floor resulting in a ground reaction force that pushes the body backward, termed a braking force. Avoiding swinging the leg too far forward ("overstriding") and cueing runners to think of "pulling the ground toward them" when the foot strikes can help reduce braking forces and enhance running economy.

In terms of special considerations, the goal of running in athletics (such as long-distance running vs. sprinting) will also influence optimal mechanics, supplemental conditioning, and appropriate cues. For example, research has demonstrated that a successful endurance runner is characterized by less vertical oscillation, slightly longer strides, less change in velocity during the ground contact, and a lower first peak in the vertical component of the ground reaction force, associated with a tendency to have smaller braking forces (Kyrolainen, Belli, and Komi, 2001). These characteristics are associated with greater running economy or efficiency, and the lower peak vertical forces (impact forces) that are less rapid in development may also reduce injury risk in runners (Ferber et al., 2002; Hreljac, 2004; Hreljac, Marshall, and Hume, 2000).

In dance, the goal often has more to do with meeting the aesthetics of the choreography versus optimizing economy or speed. For example, a choreographer may desire that running be performed low to the ground, maintaining the knees in flexion and emphasizing horizontal movement of the body. In another case, the choreographer may desire more of a "prance," emphasizing vertical movement of the body at the expense of horizontal movement. So, although many of the principles just discussed with running are still relevant, the movement will often be shaped by aesthetic versus biomechanical criteria.

Leap (Grand Jeté en Avant)

In kinesiology, a leap is defined as a locomotor movement that involves taking off from one leg and landing on the opposite leg, while a jump involves takeoff and landing on both feet. The leap analyzed in table 8.7 follows these criteria. However, in many forms of dance, the term "jump" is used more loosely and includes single and double takeoffs or landings or both.

This grand jeté movement can be divided into the following phases: preparation, takeoff, flight, and landing. For purposes of simplicity, this discussion will focus on the hip, knee, and ankle. The **preparation phase** involves hip flexion, knee flexion, and ankle dorsiflexion of the takeoff leg (right leg in table 8.7A). Since this movement is primarily produced by gravity, eccentric contraction of the opposite muscles, the hip extensors, knee extensors, and ankle plantar flexors, is necessary to control these movements. This movement is important to bring the center of gravity of the body over the foot of the support leg (Adrian and Cooper, 1989), and a moderate amount of hip and knee flexion is necessary to allow time to generate sufficient force (impulse) during takeoff for an effective jump (Ryman, 1978).

During the **takeoff phase,** as with running, the takeoff leg (right leg) undergoes rapid hip extension, knee extension, and ankle plantar flexion, against gravity, via concentric contraction of the hip extensors, knee extensors, and ankle plantar flexors, respectively. Proper timing and adequate force generation associated with these joint movements are essential for producing the forces that will propel the body. As the right leg extends, the left leg swings forward, utilizing concentric contraction of the hip flexors to bring the thigh forward, isometric contraction of the knee extensors to maintain the knee in extension, and concentric contraction of the ankle-foot plantar flexors to help point the foot. The right arm also swings forward (concentric contraction of the shoulder flexors) as the left arm raises to the side (concentric contraction of the shoulder abductors). These movements of the right leg (takeoff leg via the resultant ground reaction force), combined with the forward movements of the left leg (lead leg) and right arm, propel the center of gravity of the body up and forward for the flight phase. The takeoff phase ends just before the foot of the takeoff leg loses contact with the ground (just before B in table 8.7, where the toes would still be in contact with the ground).

When the takeoff leg no longer is in contact with the ground, the **flight phase** (table 8.7, just prior to B through D) begins. This takeoff leg is rapidly brought backward and upward, ideally to the height of the lead leg, via rapid concentric contraction of the hip extensors. The knee of this back leg (right leg) is maintained in extension by utilizing a contraction of the knee extensors, while concentric contraction of the right ankle-foot plantar flexors serves to slightly increase the "point" of the foot. For many dancers, the initial flight phase is also accompanied by a very brief continuation of the forward motion of the lead leg (left leg) produced by concentric contraction of the hip flexors while the knee extensors contract isometrically to maintain knee extension and the ankle-foot plantar flexors contract isometrically to help keep the foot pointed. Then, further forward motion of the leg is arrested, and this hip angle is maintained isometrically by the hip flexors while transfer of momentum from the leg to the torso facilitates desired forward motion of the center of gravity of the body.

During the flight phase, the center of mass of the body follows a parabolic path (as shown in table 8.7). The shape of this trajectory is determined by the angle (angle of projection), speed, and height of the body at takeoff. Hence, one of the key determinants of achieving the desired height or distance in a given jump is maximizing the velocity of the body at takeoff.

In accordance with the laws of physics, once in the air the center of mass of the body must follow this given parabolic path. However, to achieve the illusion of "suspension," skilled dancers often manipulate the relative position of the center of mass within the body by lifting or lowering the limbs. For example, during a grand jeté, a well-timed extra lift of the legs or lift of the arms near the peak of the jump will cause the center of mass to move up within the body and allow a very brief moment in which the head and torso move approximately horizontally, giving the illusion of floating (Laws, 2002; Ryman, 1978).

During the **landing phase** (similar to the support phase in running), the primary function of the muscles is to control and arrest the downward motion of the body caused by gravity, with eccentric contraction of the hip extensors, knee extensors, and ankle plantar flexors to control the respective hip flexion, knee flexion, and ankle dorsiflexion produced by gravity on the landing leg (left leg in table 8.7E). This phase is also important for appropriately positioning the body for the next movement in the given choreography. If the body changes direction or stays in place, this landing phase also functions to halt the forward motion of the body; and on landing, the center of gravity needs to be behind the body so that the push of the landing foot on the floor slows the forward motion of the body. This is different from what occurs in sprinting or dance choreography such as repetitive forward leaps in which the goal is to have the center of gravity almost over the foot so that forward motion is maximized. As with sprinting, it appears that some dancers may use the hamstrings

TABLE 8.7 Anatomical Analysis of a Forward Leap (Grand Jeté en Avant)

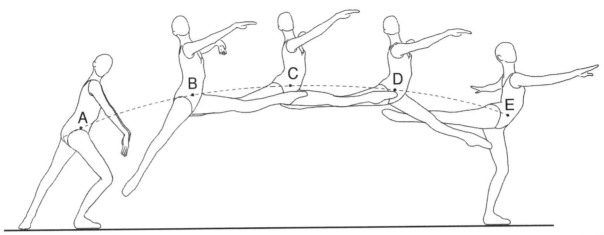

Movement phases and selected joints	Joint movements	Contraction type	Prime movers: muscle group (sample muscles)
Preparation phase: A			
Right hip	Hip flexion	Eccentric	Hip extensors (hamstrings, gluteus maximus)
Right knee	Knee flexion	Eccentric	Knee extensors (quadriceps femoris)
Right ankle-foot	A-F dorsiflexion	Eccentric and passive as body moves forward over foot	A-F plantar flexors (gastrocnemius, soleus)
Takeoff phase: A to just before B			
Right hip	Hip extension	Concentric	Hip extensors (hamstrings, gluteus maximus)
Right knee	Knee extension	Concentric	Knee extensors (quadriceps femoris)
Right ankle-foot	A-F plantar flexion	Concentric	A-F plantar flexors (gastrocnemius, soleus)
Left hip	Hip flexion	Concentric	Hip flexors (iliopsoas, rectus femoris)
Left knee	Knee extension	Isometric	Knee extensors (quadriceps femoris)
Left ankle-foot	A-F plantar flexion	Concentric	A-F plantar flexors (gastrocnemius, soleus)
Right shoulder	Shoulder flexion	Concentric	Shoulder flexors (anterior deltoid, pectoralis major)
Left shoulder	Shoulder abduction	Concentric	Shoulder abductors (middle deltoid, supraspinatus)
Flight phase: just before B to D			
Right hip	Hip extension	Concentric	Hip extensors (hamstrings, gluteus maximus)
Right knee	(Knee extension maintained)	Isometric	Knee extensors (quadriceps femoris)
Right ankle-foot	A-F plantar flexion	Concentric	A-F plantar flexors (gastrocnemius, soleus)
Left hip	Hip flexion	Concentric	Hip flexors (iliopsoas, rectus femoris)
Left knee	(Knee extension maintained)	Isometric	Knee extensors (quadriceps femoris)
Left ankle-foot	(A-F plantar flexion maintained)	Isometric	A-F plantar flexors (gastrocnemius, soleus)

Movement phases and selected joints	Joint movements	Contraction type	Prime movers: muscle group (sample muscles)
Landing phase: E			
Left hip	Hip flexion	Eccentric	Hip extensors (hamstrings, gluteus maximus)
Left knee	Knee flexion	Eccentric	Knee extensors (quadriceps femoris)
Left ankle-foot	A-F dorsiflexion	Eccentric and passive as body moves forward over foot	A-F plantar flexors (gastrocnemius, soleus)
Right hip	Hip extension	Concentric	Hip extensors (hamstrings, gluteus maximus)
Right knee	(Knee extension maintained)	Isometric	Knee extensors (quadriceps femoris)
Right ankle-foot	(A-F plantar flexion maintained)	Isometric	A-F plantar flexors (gastrocnemius, soleus)

in the early portion of this phase to initiate knee flexion so that braking forces are minimized and the tendency for the femur to translate anteriorly on the tibia (knee shear forces) is lessened (Simpson and Kanter, 1997; Simpson and Pettit, 1997).

While the landing leg plays the vital role of controlling the downward motion of the body and preparing for the ensuing direction of motion of the body's center of gravity, the right leg may stay behind in an arabesque as shown in table 8.7E. With this variation of a grand jeté en avant, the hip extensors of the back leg must contract rigorously with an isometric or slight concentric contraction to prevent the leg from dropping and to achieve the desired aesthetic of the arabesque position. The knee extensors work isometrically to maintain the knee in extension while the ankle-foot plantar flexors work isometrically to help maintain the point of the foot.

In terms of stabilization, the complex co-contraction of the spinal extensors and flexors is again key to achieve the desired aesthetic of the movement. The desire is to keep the upper torso relatively vertical during the flight phase of the movement. Some dancers get an undesired visible flexion and extension of the trunk during the movement. One reason the torso often flexes forward is that the pelvis must be tilted anteriorly to allow the back leg to reach the desired height. However, as discussed in connection with an arabesque in chapter 4, the back extensors can contract to bring the upper torso back to vertical and to prevent the undesired forward motion of the whole torso.

Anatomical analysis also reveals that extreme range of motion is required at the hips to achieve the split position in the air. A quick test that can be used to help determine if hip flexibility is a limiting factor is a passive split (Tests and Measurements 8.2).

If a split position cannot easily be accomplished, this suggests that muscular constraints would offer internal resistance to the desired split position in the grand jeté, making it more difficult or not possible to achieve (depending on the extent of limitation). To more specifically determine the soft tissue constraints, tests presented in chapter 4 can be used. Hamstring flexibility (Tests and Measurements 4.4 on p. 205) can be tested to see if these muscles are limiting the desired height of the front leg, while hip flexor flexibility (Tests and Measurements 4.5 on p. 212) can be tested to see if these muscles are limiting the desired height of the back leg.

Analysis of the grand jeté also reveals that there are high strength demands for the hip extensors, knee extensors, and ankle plantar flexors of the takeoff leg (right leg) to overcome the weight of the body and project the body in space during the takeoff phase. As with running, the greater the force generated by the body against the floor at takeoff, the greater the ground reaction force that will propel the body, and the greater the acceleration of the body. During the flight phase, moderate levels of hip flexor strength are needed to lift the lead leg, and moderate levels of hip extensor strength are needed to lift the back leg to the desired split position. During the landing phase, there are high strength demands on the support leg (left leg) of the hip extensors, knee extensors, and ankle plantar flexors in order to decelerate the body and absorb the large forces associated with landing. A preliminary investigation of three elite ballet dancers found vertical maximum forces of approximately 3 to 6 times body weight associated with landing from a grand jeté devant (Clippinger and Novak, 1981).

In terms of technique considerations, one common error in beginning dancers is to not achieve

Quick Check for Limitations Due to Passive Hip Constraints in a Grand Jeté en Avant

Perform a passive split with the torso vertical and compare this position of the legs to the position seen when executing a grand jeté. If a dancer cannot achieve or has difficulty achieving the passive split position, this suggests that the hamstrings or hip flexors are likely limiting the desired positioning of the legs in the grand jeté.

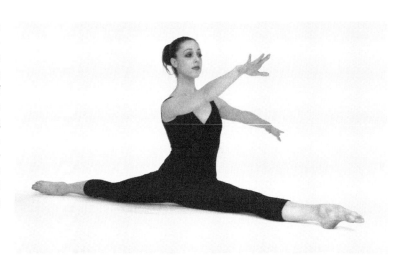

the desired position of the back leg (almost parallel to the floor) in the flight phase. This can relate to hip flexor tightness of the back leg, hamstring tightness of the front leg, limited range in spinal hyperextension, inadequate hip extensor strength of the back leg, inadequate spinal extensor strength, or inappropriate timing and activation of key muscles. Another important technique consideration is skilled use of flexion of the support leg (hip flexion, knee flexion, and ankle dorsiflexion) during the preparation phase to provide a prestretch of the extensors (hip extensors, knee extensors, and ankle plantar flexors) that will markedly enhance the ability of the muscle to generate force (stretch-shortening cycle) in the takeoff phase. While some dancers appear to display a natural use of this potential enhancement, other dancers do not fully utilize this mechanism due to errors such as making the preparatory movement too large or too small and excessively delaying the reversal from flexion to extension. One study showed that 36% of young ballet dancers were not able to use this elastic potential of muscle correctly and were able to jump higher from a semi-squatting position without a countermovement than when a countermovement (preparatory plié) was used (Poggini et al., 1997). However, another study of skilled dancers showed a consistent submaximal depth of demi-plié prior to various movements, suggesting a preset motor program (Clarkson, Kennedy, and

Flanagan, 1984; McNitt-Gray, Koff, and Hall, 1992) that may relate to stretch-shortening optimization and movement economy. Experienced dancers have also been shown to utilize a faster reaction time in the preparatory plié prior to a sauté than in other movements requiring less power (relevé or pointe) or than non-dance controls (Clarkson, Kennedy, and Flanagan, 1984). Hence, encouraging dancers to use a moderate depth of preparatory plié (Ryman, 1978) and to make a rapid reversal from flexion to extension can help some dancers reap potential stretch-shortening cycle benefits and enhance jump height or distance.

Similarly, the timing and magnitude of flexion of the support leg during the landing phase are also important. In this case, the issue is primarily one of absorption of forces versus generation of forces, essential for injury prevention as well as achieving dance aesthetic criteria. Increasing the time used to decelerate the body when landing from a jump will decrease the magnitude of the peak forces borne by the body. An eccentric contraction of the extensors of the hip, extensors of the knee, and plantar flexors of the ankle to allow greater flexion at their respective joints can be used to provide more time for absorption of forces. So, soft landings are associated with lower peak vertical ground reaction forces that remain elevated for a longer period of time, while hard landings are associated with higher peak vertical

"Don't Stop Your Plié"

When dancers are performing a preparatory plié prior to a demanding movement such as a jump or turn, the cue to "not stop your plié" is sometimes given. Often a further explanation of this cue is to "avoid hesitating or stopping" at the bottom of the plié. From a mechanical perspective, hesitating or delaying at the bottom of the plié will lessen the benefits of the stretch-shortening cycle. The potential enhancement from the prestretch of key muscles such as the calf muscles, quadriceps femoris, hamstrings, and gluteus maximus rapidly declines if there is much delay between the eccentric and the following concentric contraction. So dancers should be encouraged to make a very rapid reversal from the down- to the up-phase of the movement. The commonly used counting technique of "and *one*," with the "and" rapid and the "one" emphasized, versus an even count of "one" for the down-phase of the plié and "two" for the up movement, can also be helpful in encouraging the desired quick reversal of direction without a hesitation.

"Land Softly"

The instruction to "land softly" is often used by teachers in an effort to reduce the forces associated with landing. From a biomechanical perspective, soft versus stiff landings are associated with lower vertical ground reaction forces; greater absorption of forces by the hip and knee muscles; slightly less absorption of forces by the ankle plantar flexors; and greater hip flexion, greater knee flexion, and slightly less plantar flexion at the beginning of floor contact (Devita and Skelly, 1992; Kovacs et al., 1999; Self and Paine, 2001). In soft versus stiff landings from a vertical fall of 23 inches (59 centimeters), Devita and Skelly found that overall the muscular system absorbed 19% more of the body's kinetic energy, thereby reducing impact stress to other tissues. While just using the cue of landing "softly" may be sufficient to elicit the desired response from a dancer, some dancers are unclear as to how to achieve this type of landing. For example, one study found that providing video feedback with specific verbal analysis of how to land more softly was more effective in reducing peak vertical forces both directly following instructions and one week later than simply instructing subjects to key into the sensation of landing and try to land more softly (Onate, Guskiewicz, and Sullivan, 2001). Similarly, using more abstract images has been found to be less effective than providing more concrete directives related to changes in joint angles or the sound of landing (McNair, Prapavessis, and Callender, 2000). One approach is to emphasize some of the biomechanical criteria associated with soft versus stiff landings. Practically, these can be encouraged by directing dancers to think of slightly flexing the knees and hips just before landing and then using a slightly deeper but slower plié to decelerate the body. This directive can also be valuable for preventing knee hyperextension when landing, the classic mechanism for anterior cruciate ligament tears in dancers.

ground reaction forces that stay elevated for a shorter period of time (Dufek and Bates, 1990).

Also in line with these principles, a study of traveling dance jumps showed that the quadriceps femoris was particularly important in attenuating impact forces as jump distance and vertical ground reaction

forces increased (Simpson and Kanter, 1997). Two additional studies showed that trained dancers had significantly greater degrees of knee flexion and hip flexion (deeper pliés) when landing from vertical jumps than non-dancers (Clarkson, Kennedy, and Flanagan, 1984; McNitt-Gray, Koff, and Hall, 1992),

"Go Through Your Foot"

The instruction to "go through your foot" is often used by teachers when landing from a jump to achieve a certain aesthetic and prevent injuries. Toe-heel versus flat-foot landing has been shown to be advantageous in terms of force absorption. For example, one study found peak vertical ground reaction forces of about four times body weight with toe-heel landing in contrast to six times body weight with flat-foot landing (Dufek and Bates, 1990). Another study found that toe-heel landings were associated with a greater time to reach peak forces (Kovacs et al., 1999). Both of these factors are considered important for reducing the risk of lower extremity injuries. Hence, cueing to go through the foot in a toe-heel manner can be useful for reducing impact. This mechanism appears to be developed in dancers, as trained dancers exhibit a significantly longer time to reach minimum ankle position and use a markedly larger ankle range of motion than nondancers when landing from jumps (McNitt-Gray, Koff, and Hall, 1992). However, given the preponderance of ankle-foot injuries in dancers, this cue is best combined with encouraging a soft landing with adequate flexion of the knees and hips because the contribution of the plantar flexors has been shown to drop from 50% in stiff landings to 37% in soft landings, with knee and hip extensors now providing greater absorption (Devita and Skelly, 1992; Self and Paine, 2001).

while another study demonstrated that experienced dancers utilized a longer time to reach the maximum positions of flexion of the ankle (dorsiflexion) and knee and hip (Ryman, 1978). Practically, these concepts are often encouraged by such directives as "land softly," feel your body "yield" as you land, or "use your plié" when you land. These directives are often used to discourage "stiff" landings with inadequate flexion of lower extremity joints.

Another mechanism that can be used to soften landings is well-timed use of the ankle-foot plantar flexors. The calf complex plays a critical role in absorbing the impact associated with landing from jumps, and the ankle plantar flexors have been estimated to be responsible for 44% (on average), 34% (the knee), and 22% (the hip) of the total muscular work done when landing from a vertical fall of 23 inches (59 centimeters) (Devita and Skelly, 1992). Directives encouraging a toe-heel versus a flat-foot landing such as "go through your foot" are often used to encourage use of this mechanism. However, although optimal use of the plantar flexors is important, it appears that with soft landings involving greater jump height the contribution of the hip extensors and knee extensors becomes more substantial (Zhang, Bates, and Dufek, 2000).

Another important technique consideration is placement of the knee relative to the foot when landing from jumps. In leaps, stability must be present on one leg to allow for development and

absorption of large forces without injury. Thus, directives to promote good alignment and avoid excessive rotation or medial-lateral movements, such as cueing to think of the knees as hinges and guide the knee over the ball of the foot (Roniger, 2002) or second toe can be helpful. Furthermore, when stability is a problem, providing supplemental coordination training such as balancing on one leg with a balance board or foam roller, utilizing quick movements of the gesture leg while standing on one leg, and jumps can be helpful. A conditioning program developed by Dr. Mandelbaum including strengthening exercises, agility drills, and plyometrics reinforcing soft landings with bent knees and hips was found to reduce anterior cruciate tears by 88% in female soccer players when compared to controls in a 12-week playing season, while another program with similar emphasis was shown to reduce maximum vertical ground reaction forces by 22% and abduction and adduction moments by 50% (Hewett et al., 1996).

In terms of special considerations, there are many variations in the way a leap is executed with respect to positioning of the legs, torso, and arms that will affect muscle use and movement analysis. For example, the lead leg can swing forward straight or with a developing movement; there can be an extra "split" motion of the legs at the peak of the movement; or the back leg can bend. In addition, aesthetic criteria play a key role and may dictate a leap that emphasizes height (vertical component), distance (horizontal component), or other criteria.

When providing cues or considering the addition of supplemental conditioning exercises, it is very important to keep the specificity of these goals in mind. For example, several studies practicing jumps in various environments showed no gains in jump height or gains lower than reported for other athletes in jump height (McLain, Carter, and Abel, 1997; Poggini et al., 1997). Instead, it appears that dancers may naturally tend to favor emphasizing improvement in technique, efficiency of movement (Harley et al., 2002), or constraining peak impact forces. One would theorize that if increased jump height was the goal, a program should be utilized that integrates key lower extremity strengthening exercises to allow greater absorption of forces as jump height increased, as well as cues and functional movement patterns emphasizing jump height. The specificity of motor control strategies is demonstrated by studies showing a greater contribution of the hip with greater jump height (Vanrenterghem et al., 2004), adjustment of lower extremity tension (stiffness) upon landing in accordance with jump height and floor force absorption characteristics (Devita and Skelly, 1992; Hamilton and Luttgens, 2002), and significant improvement in dancers' vertical jump height off two feet and off the right foot (but not the left) after a plyometric training program (Griner, Boatwright, and Howell, 2003). This latter finding is particularly interesting given the tendency for many right-handed ballet dancers to prefer jumping off their left legs (Golomer and Fery, 2001).

The process of improving jumps is also complicated by aesthetic requirements. For example, greater hip flexion obtained by more forward lean of the torso will allow markedly greater force production in the takeoff phase of jumping, probably largely related to the ability of the gluteus maximus to produce more force in this position. Similarly, greater hip flexion obtained by more forward lean of the torso will also allow for lower impact forces upon landing (Devita and Skelly, 1992), probably in part due to bringing the center of mass of the torso closer to the knees (decreased moment arm of resistance). However, dance generally encourages a more vertical positioning of the torso, and aesthetics will limit the amount of forward lean of the torso that is permitted.

Optimal Performance Models

So, anatomical and biomechanical analysis of movement can provide vital information that can deepen our understanding of a given movement. However, whether this information can be used to develop an optimal performance model is controversial and complex. Such models will need to take into account individual differences and the observation that with complex movement, different movement strategies can be developed to achieve the same movement outcome. The strategy that works for one elite athlete may not necessarily be optimal for another due to many variables such as body type, lever length, muscle fiber type, strength and power in key muscles, flexibility in key joint ranges of motion, and other neuromuscular factors. Still, when studies of multiple elite strategies are combined with theoretical anatomical and biomechanical analyses, a pattern usually emerges that is consistent with scientific principles of movement. From such models, recommendations can be generated for instructing and improving skill in a given movement task, taking into consideration the differences between individuals.

In dance, this issue of generating models of optimal performance is made more complex by the tremendous variety of movements used. In contrast to walking, running, hurdling, or high jumping, where there is one movement pattern or sequence to be studied, dance contains many basic movement categories including walks, runs, leaps, slides, skips, jumps, lunges, swings, pliés, rises, reaches, brushes, kicks, drops, isolations, contractions, turns, and falls, as well as countless variations and combinations of these and other movement vocabulary.

Generating models of optimal performance in dance is also made more difficult by the need to meet aesthetic criteria. In many forms of athletics, the primary goal is to accomplish a movement outcome that can be measured quantitatively. For example, in the high jump, the goal is to jump as high as possible over a bar, and the success of the outcome is basically determined by how high a bar can be cleared. In contrast, dance is heavily guided by meeting aesthetic criteria not only in the outcome but also throughout the process of achieving the outcome. With regard to turns, for example, in many schools of dance there may be a quantitative component in that it is desirable, and considered a sign of greater skill, to be able to perform multiple repetitions of a given turn. However, the preparation for the turn and the manner in which the turn is performed are considered vitally important, not just the number of revolutions accomplished. This emphasis has led to the statement by some that when compared to many forms of athletics, dance is process as well as product oriented. Furthermore, while some of these aesthetic criteria involved in the "process" of moving may be shared by many dance forms, others differ between and within given dance forms. Some examples of aesthetic issues that may be important are movement quality, movement economy, lack of visible undesired compensations associated with limb movements, placement or alignment of various body segments, desired "shaping" of various joints or body parts in standard vocabulary (e.g., plantar flexed and everted foot, neutral foot, dorsiflexed and inverted foot), emotional expressiveness, and the desired relationship of the movement in time (rhythmicity).

However, despite these difficulties, it is essential that more research be performed on dance movements and that information gained from research on similar movements be applied to dance. While the qualitative anatomical analysis and knowledge of joint mechanics presented in this text can provide a very beneficial basic understanding of dance movements, specific research will test our assumptions and deepen and clarify our knowledge. This knowledge can then be used to help the dancer accomplish technical proficiency within the context of the desired aesthetic. While the variety of aesthetics present in the dance world will likely preclude a single model for optimal performance of a given movement, research should help reveal fundamental principles that can be adjusted in accordance with the specific aesthetic, as well as clarify key aspects that distinguish aesthetics.

Movement Cues

There is a need to take the knowledge of movement obtained from anatomical and biomechanical analysis and apply it in the classroom in a manner that can be readily used by dancers to achieve desired movement outcomes. One common approach is for teachers to use movement cues when describing or correcting movements. Some of these cues have a biomechanical basis that is logical. For example, cues described in chapter 3 oriented toward utilizing sufficient abdominal stabilization could reduce undue stress on the low back and improve spinal-pelvic alignment. Other cues are more oriented toward the laws of motion. Such cues may foster skill improvement through taking fuller advantage of physics and Newton's laws of motion. For example, the cue to emphasize pressing down into the floor just prior to rising to relevé can increase the upward vertical force (vertical component of the ground reaction force), making it easier to rise.

Some cues, however, have been passed down through generations of teaching but do not stand up to scientific scrutiny. They may suggest that dancers do things that are not possible or that do not actually occur with a given movement. Sometimes such cues persist because parts of them fit with sensation or a dancer's sense of truth while some other part of the description is inaccurate. For example, as described in chapter 4, for a kick to the side (battement à la seconde), the cue to lift the leg from underneath is inaccurate in that the hamstrings cannot lift the leg. However, when the movement is performed correctly, there is a sensation of the proximal femur (greater trochanter) coming down and under just before the distal femur and leg rises up. A cue that describes this drop of the trochanter without implying that the hamstrings lift the leg would be more accurate and less confusing to students. So, teachers and students are encouraged to closely evaluate the anatomical and mechanical basis and accuracy of cues used in dance, and teachers should be sure that they do not perpetuate misconceptions or ask students to do something that is not physically possible. Examples of cues have been given throughout this text. Often a subtle change in wording will allow the cue to evoke the desired sensation or action and at the same time be supported by, versus countered by, anatomical and biomechanical principles.

Summary

Despite the wide array and complexity of dance movements, current technology makes analysis of movement tremendously easier than it was just a decade or two ago. There is a dire need to supplement qualitative anatomical analysis with information gained from well-designed research studies addressing a wide variety of dance movements so that we can better understand the relevant muscles, forces, and neural factors involved in a given movement. In turn, this information can be used for evaluation of current teaching cues and strategies and the design of new approaches, where relevant. Such information will also be useful for better understanding of injury mechanisms and prevention.

Study Questions and Applications

1. Perform a basic anatomical analysis (table 8.3, steps 1-5, p. 480) of the following:

   a. A roll-down

   b. A tendu side

   c. A penché

2. Perform an anatomical analysis of a développé to the front (développé a la quatrième devant) (table 8.3, steps 1-12). Contrast and compare this with a grand battement to the front as analyzed in table 8.4 (p. 482).

3. Perform an anatomical analysis of a développé to the side (développé à la seconde) (table 8.3, steps 1-12). Contrast and compare this with a développé to the front.

4. Perform a basic anatomical analysis (table 8.3, steps 1-5) of a rise onto the ball of the foot preceded by a plié (relevé). How does this differ from a rise performed with a straight knee (elevé) and from a jump in parallel first position?

5. Observe a dancer performing the movements analyzed in question 3. Note any technique problems. Theorize what could be done to correct any noted problems, and see if applying these theorized corrections on the dancer results in the desired improvement.

6. Perform a basic anatomical analysis (table 8.3, steps 1-5) of a short movement sequence that is regularly used at the barre or in the warm-up section of your dance technique class.

7. Select a movement from dance class that you are having difficulty performing with optimal technique. Perform an anatomical analysis of this movement and provide four strength exercises, two flexibility exercises, and three technique cues that could be used to help improve your performance of this movement.

8. Design a movement sequence that involves all the fundamental movements of the shoulder, spine, hip, knee, and ankle. Orally identify the movements as they occur.

9. Select three cues commonly used in dance classes to aid with performing given movements. Evaluate their anatomical or biomechanical base in terms of accuracy. Is there a way each cue could be stated that would be more consistent with scientific principles?

10. A dancer wants to improve her Russian splits.

    a. Using the schema presented in table 8.3, analyze the movement in terms of the ankle, knee, and hip joints.

    b. What muscles serve as prime movers? What are the extreme range of motion requirements in the split position, and what muscles should be stretched to improve this range? What are the key strength demands of this movement, and what muscles should be strengthened to meet these demands?

    c. What cues could be used to enhance benefits from use of the stretch-shortening cycle just prior to takeoff?

References and Resources

Chapter 1

Abernethy, B., Hanrahan, S., Kippers, V., Mackinnon, L., and Pandy, M. (2005). *The biophysical foundations of human movement.* 2nd ed. Champaign, IL: Human Kinetics.

American College of Sports Medicine (ACSM). (1997). Position stand: The female athlete triad. *Medicine and Science in Sports and Exercise,* 29(5): i-ix.

Andreoli, A., Monteleone, M., Van Loan, M., Promenzio, L., Tarantino, U., and Lorenzo, A. (2001). Effects of different sports on bone density and muscle mass in highly trained athletes. *Medicine and Science in Sports and Exercise,* 33(4): 507-511.

Beck, B., and Shoemaker, R. (2000). Osteoporosis: Understanding key risk factors and therapeutic options. *The Physician and Sportsmedicine,* 28(2): 69-84.

Bennell, K.L., Malcolm, S.A., Thomas, S.A., Reid, S.J., Bruckner, P.D., Ebeling, P.R., and Wark, J.D. (1996). Risk factors for stress fractures in track and field athletes. A twelve-month prospective study. *American Journal of Sport Medicine,* 24: 810-818.

Browning, K. (2001). Hip and pelvis injuries in runners. *The Physician and Sportsmedicine,* 29(1): 23-24.

Brukner, P. (2000). Exercise-related lower leg pain: An overview. *Medicine and Science in Sports and Exercise,* 32(3 Suppl.): S1-S3.

Brukner, P., Bradshaw, C., and Bennell, K. (1998). Managing common stress fractures: Let risk level guide treatment. *The Physician and Sportsmedicine,* 26(8): 39-47.

Burr, D. (1997). Bone, exercise and stress fractures. *Exercise and Sport Sciences Reviews,* 25: 171-194.

Clark, N. (1997). *Nancy Clark's sports nutrition guidebook.* 2nd ed. Champaign, IL: Leisure Press.

Clarkson, P. (1998). An overview of nutrition for female dancers. *Journal of Dance Medicine and Science,* 2(1): 32-39.

Clippinger, K. (1999). Smoking in young dancers. *Journal of Dance Medicine and Science,* 1(3): 115-125.

Dudek, S. (1997). *Nutrition handbook for nursing practice.* Philadelphia: Lippincott.

Enoka, R. (2002). *Neuromechanics of human movement.* 3rd ed. Champaign, IL: Human Kinetics.

Frost, H.M. (2000). Muscle, bone, and the Utah paradigm: A 1999 overview. *Medicine and Science in Sports and Exercise,* 32(5): 911-917.

Goss, C.M., ed. (1980). *Gray's anatomy of the human body.* Philadelphia: Lea & Febiger.

Guyton, A. (1976). *Textbook of medical physiology.* Philadelphia: W.B. Saunders.

Hall, S.J. (1999). *Basic biomechanics.* Boston: McGraw-Hill.

Hall-Craggs, E.C.B. (1985). *Anatomy as a basis for clinical medicine.* Baltimore: Urban & Schwarzenberg.

Hamill, J., and Knutzen, K.M. (1995). *Biomechanical basis of human movement.* Philadelphia: Lippincott Williams & Wilkins.

Hamilton, N., and Luttgens, K. (2002). *Kinesiology: Scientific basis of human motion.* New York: McGraw-Hill.

Hershman, E., and Mailly, T. (1990). Stress fractures. *Clinics in Sports Medicine,* 9(1): 183-214.

Huwyler, J.S. (1999). *The dancer's body: A medical perspective on dance and dance training.* McLean, VA: International Medical.

Kadel, N., Teitz, C., and Kronmal, R. (1992). Stress fractures in ballet dancers. *The American Journal of Sports Medicine,* 20(4): 446-449.

Kaufman, J. (2000). Osteoporosis tests. http://orthoinfo. aaos.org/fact/thr_report.cfm?Thread_ID=176&topcateg ory=Osteoporosis.

Kenney, R. (1982). *Physiology of aging: A synopsis.* Chicago: Year Book Medical.

Khan, K., Green, R., Saul, A., Bennell, K., Crichton, K., Hopper, J., and Wark, J. (1996). Retired elite female ballet dancers and nonathletic controls have similar bone mineral density at weightbearing sites. *Journal of Bone and Mineral Research,* 11(10): 1566-1574.

Khan, K., McKay, A., Stiehl, A., Warren, M., and Wark, J. (1999). Bone mineral density in active and retired ballet dancers. *Journal of Dance Medicine and Science,* 3(1): 15-23.

Kreighbaum, E., and Barthels, K.M. (1996). *Biomechanics: A qualitative approach for studying human movement.* 4th ed. Needham Heights, MA: Allyn & Bacon.

Levangie, P.K., and Norkin, C.C. (2001). *Joint structure and function: A comprehensive analysis.* Philadelphia: Davis.

Lundon, K., Melcher, L., and Bray, K. (1999). Stress fractures in ballet: A twenty-five year review. *Journal of Dance Medicine and Science,* 3(3): 101-107.

Marieb, E. (1995). *Human anatomy and physiology.* New York: Benjamin/Cummings.

Matheson, G., Clement, D., McKenzie, D., Taunton, J., Lloyd-Smith, D., and MacIntyre, J. (1987). Stress fractures in athletes: A study of 320 cases. *American Journal of Sports Medicine,* 15(1): 46-58.

McCarthy, P. (1989). Managing bursitis in the athlete: An overview. *The Physician and Sportsmedicine,* 17(11): 115-125.

Mercier, L. (1995). *Practical orthopedics.* St. Louis: Mosby.

Micheli, L., and Solomon, R. (1990). Stress fractures in dancers. In R. Solomon, S. Minton, and J. Solomon (eds.), *Preventing dance injuries: An interdisciplinary perspective* (pp. 133-153). Reston, VA: American Alliance for Health, Physical Education, Recreation and Dance.

Moore, K., and Agur, A. (1995). *Essential clinical anatomy.* Baltimore: Williams & Wilkins.

Myszkewycz, L., and Koutedakis, Y. (1998). Injuries, amenorrhea and osteoporosis in active females: An overview. *Dance Medicine and Science,* 2(3): 88-94.

Rasch, P. (1989). *Kinesiology and applied anatomy.* Philadelphia: Lea & Febiger.

Rasch, P., and Burke, R. (1978). *Kinesiology and applied anatomy.* Philadelphia: Lea & Febiger.

Roy, R., Baldwin, K., and Edgerton, V.R. (1996). Response of the neuromuscular unit to spaceflight: What has been learned from the rat model. *Exercise and Sport Sciences Reviews,* 24: 399-425.

Smith, L., Weiss, E., and Lehmkuhl, L. (1996). *Brunnstrom's clinical kinesiology.* Philadelphia: Davis.

Stewart, A., and Hannan, J. (2000). Total and regional bone density in male runners, cyclists, and controls. *Medicine and Science in Sports and Exercise,* 32(8): 1373-1377.

Taube, R., and Wadsworth, L. (1993). Managing tibial stress fractures. *The Physician and Sportsmedicine,* 21(4): 123-130.

Taunton, J.E., Clement, D.B., and Webber, D. (1981). Lower extremity stress fractures in athletes. *The Physician and Sportsmedicine,* 9: 77-86.

U.S. Department of Agriculture. (1981). Nutritive value of foods. Home and Garden Bulletin No. 72.

Warren, M., Brooks-Gunn, J., Hamilton, L., Warren, F., and Hamilton, W. (1986). Scoliosis and fractures in young ballet dancers. *New England Journal of Medicine,* 314(21): 1348-1353.

Whiting, W.C., and Zernicke, R.F. (1998). *Biomechanics of musculoskeletal injury.* Champaign, IL: Human Kinetics.

Williams, N. (1998). Reproductive function and low energy availability in exercising females: A review of clinical and hormonal effects. *Journal of Dance Medicine and Science,* 2(1): 19-31.

Zernicke, R.F., Vailas, A.C., and Salem, G.J. (1990). Biomechanical response of bone to weightlessness. *Exercise and Sport Sciences Reviews,* 18: 167-192.

Chapter 2

Alter, M. (2004). *Science of flexibility.* 3rd ed. Champaign, IL: Human Kinetics.

American College of Sports Medicine (ACSM). (1998). Position stand: The recommended quantity and quality of exercise for developing and maintaining cardiorespiratory and muscular fitness, and flexibility in healthy adults. *Medicine and Science in Sports and Exercise,* 30(6): 975-991.

American College of Sports Medicine (ACSM). (2001). *ACSM's resource manual for guidelines for exercise testing and prescription.* Philadelphia: Lippincott Williams & Wilkins.

Asmussen, E., and Bonde-Petersen, F. (1974). Storage of elastic energy in skeletal muscles in man. *Acta Physiologica Scandinavica,* 91: 385-392.

Basmajian, J., and DeLuca, C. (1985). *Muscles alive—Their functions revealed by electromyography.* Baltimore: Williams & Wilkins.

Behnke, R. (2006). *Kinetic anatomy.* 2nd ed. Champaign, IL: Human Kinetics.

Bosco, A., and Komi, P.V. (1979). Potentiation of the mechanical behavior of the human skeletal muscle through pre-stretching. *Acta Physiologica Scandinavica,* 106: 467-472.

Cronin, J.B., McNair, P.J., and Marshall, R.N. (2000). The role of maximal strength and load on initial power production. *Medicine and Science in Sports and Exercise,* 32(10): 1763-1769.

Dye, S., and Vaupel, G. (2000). Functional anatomy of the knee: Bony geometry, static and dynamic restraints, sensory and motor innervation. In S. Lephart and F. Fu (eds.), *Proprioception and neuromuscular control in joint stability* (pp. 59-76). Champaign, IL: Human Kinetics.

Enoka, R. (2002). *Neuromechanics of human movement.* 3rd ed. Champaign, IL: Human Kinetics.

Garrett, W. (1990). Muscle strain injuries: Clinical and basic aspects. *Medicine and Science in Sports and Exercise,* 22: 436-443.

Garrett, W. (1996). Muscle strain injuries. *The American Journal of Sports Medicine,* 24: S2-S8.

Gordon, T., and Pattullo, M.C. (1993). Plasticity of muscle fiber and motor unit types. *Exercise and Sport Sciences Reviews,* 21: 331-362.

Gowitzke, B., and Milner, M. (1988). *Understanding the scientific bases of human movement.* Baltimore: Williams & Wilkins.

Hall, S.J. (1999). *Basic biomechanics.* Boston: McGraw-Hill.

Hamill, J., and Knutzen, K.M. (1995). *Biomechanical basis of human movement.* Philadelphia: Lippincott Williams & Wilkins.

Hamilton, N., and Luttgens, K. (2002). *Kinesiology: Scientific basis of human motion.* New York: McGraw-Hill..

Hay, J., and Reid, J. (1982). *The anatomical and mechanical bases of human motion.* Englewood Cliffs, NJ: Prentice Hall.

Huxley, H.E. (1969). The mechanism of muscular contraction. *Science,* 164: 1356.

Irrgang, J., and Neri, R. (2000). The rationale for open and closed kinematic chain activities for restoration of proprioception and neuromuscular control following injury. In S. Lephart and F. Fu (Eds.), *Proprioception and neuromuscular control in joint stability* (pp. 363-374). Champaign, IL: Human Kinetics.

Jeon, H., Trimble, M., Brunt, D., and Robinson, M. (2001). Facilitation of quadriceps activation following a concentrically controlled knee flexion movement: The influence of transition rate. *Journal of Orthopaedic Sports Physical Therapy,* 31(4): 122-132.

Komi, P.V. (1979). Neuromuscular performance: Factors influencing force and speed production. *Scandinavian Journal of Sports Science,* 1: 2-15.

Kreighbaum, E., and Barthels, K.M. (1996). *Biomechanics: A qualitative approach for studying human movement.* 4th ed. Needham Heights, MA: Allyn & Bacon.

Lephart, S., and Fu, F. (2000). *Proprioception and neuromuscular control in joint stability.* Champaign, IL: Human Kinetics.

Levangie, P.K., and Norkin, C.C. (2001). *Joint structure and function: A comprehensive analysis.* Philadelphia: Davis.

McGinnis, P.M. (2005). *Biomechanics of sport and exercise.* 2nd ed. Champaign, IL: Human Kinetics.

Netter, F. (1995). *Interactive atlas of human anatomy* (CD-ROM). Summit, NJ: Ciba-Geigy, Medical Education and Publications.

Nieman, D. (1999). *Exercise testing and prescription.* Mountain View, CA: Mayfield.

Pitt-Brooke, J. (1998). *Rehabilitation of movement.* Philadelphia: Saunders.

Platzer, W. (1978). *Color atlas and textbook of human anatomy, volume 1: Locomotor system.* Chicago: Year Book Medical.

Powers, S.K., and Howley, E.T. (1990). *Exercise physiology.* Dubuque, IA: Brown.

Rasch, P. (1989). *Kinesiology and applied anatomy.* Philadelphia: Lea & Febiger.

Rasch, P., and Burke, R. (1978). *Kinesiology and applied anatomy.* Philadelphia: Lea & Febiger.

Shrier, I., and Gossal, K. (2000). Myths and truths of stretching: Individualized recommendations for healthy muscles. *The Physician and Sportsmedicine,* 28(8): 57-63.

Smith, L., Weiss, E., and Lehmkuhl, L. (1996). *Brunnstrom's clinical kinesiology.* Philadelphia: Davis.

Soderberg, G. (1986). *Kinesiology: Application to pathological motion.* Baltimore: Williams & Wilkins.

Takashi, A., Kumagai, K., and Brechue, W. (2000). Fascicle length of leg muscles is greater in sprinters than distance runners. *Medicine and Science in Sports and Exercise,* 32(6): 1125-1129.

Tanigawa, M. (1972). Comparison of hold-relax procedures and passive mobilization on increasing muscle length. *Physical Therapy,* 52: 725-734.

Taylor, D., Dalton, J., Seaber, A., and Garrett, W. (1990). Viscoelastic properties of muscle-tendon units: The biomechanical effects of stretching. *American Journal of Sports Medicine,* 18(3): 300-309.

Thys, H., Cavagna, G., and Margaria, R. (1975). The role played by elasticity in an exercise involving movements of small amplitude. *Pflugers Archives,* 354: 281-286.

Wallin, D., Ekblom, B., Grahn, R., and Nordinborg, T. (1985). Improvement of muscle flexibility: A comparison between two techniques. *American Journal of Sports Medicine,* 13(4): 263-268.

Wells, K., and Luttgens, K. (1976). *Kinesiology: Scientific basis of human motion.* Philadelphia: Saunders.

Wilmore, J., and Costill, D. (2004). *Physiology of sport and exercise.* 3rd ed. Champaign, IL: Human Kinetics.

Chapter 3

Adams, M., Dolan, P., and Hutton, W. (1988). The lumbar spine in backward bending. *Spine,* 13(9): 1019-1026.

Adams, M., and Hutton, W. (1982). Prolapsed intervertebral disc: A hyperflexion injury. *Spine,* 7(3): 184-191.

Aggrawal, N., Kaur, R., and Kumar, S. (1979). A study of changes in the spine in weight lifters and other athletes. *British Journal of Sports Medicine,* 13: 58-61.

Akella, P., Warren, M., Jonnavithula, S., and Brooks-Gunn, J. (1991). Scoliosis in ballet dancers. *Medical Problems of Performing Artists,* 6(3): 84-86.

American Academy of Orthopaedic Surgeons. (1965). *Joint motion: Method of measuring and recording.* Chicago: American Academy of Orthopaedic Surgeons.

Andersson, G., Ortengren, R., and Nachemson, A. (1977). Intradiskal pressure, intra-abdominal pressure and myoelectric back muscle activity related to posture and loading. *Clinical Orthopaedics and Related Research,* 129(Nov-Dec): 156-164.

Axler, C., and McGill, S. (1997). Low back loads over a variety of abdominal exercises: Searching for the safest abdominal challenge. *Medicine and Science in Sports and Exercise,* 29(6): 804-810.

Azegami, H., Murachi, S., Kitoh, J., Ishida, Y., Kawakami, N., and Makino, M. (1998). Etiology of idiopathic scoliosis. *Clinical Orthopaedics and Related Research,* 357: 229-236.

Bartelink, D. (1957). The role of the intra-abdominal pressure in relieving the pressure on the lumbar intervertebral disc. *Journal of Bone and Joint Surgery,* 39B: 718-725.

Basmajian, J., and DeLuca, C. (1985). *Muscles alive—Their functions revealed by electromyography.* Baltimore: Williams & Wilkins.

Becker, J. (1986). Scoliosis in swimmers. *Clinics in Sports Medicine,* 5: 149-158.

Beimborn, D., and Morrissey, M. (1988). A review of the literature related to trunk muscle performance. *Spine,* 13(6): 655-660.

Bejjani, F., Halpern, N., and Pavlidis, L. (1990). Spinal motion and strength measurements in flamenco dancers. *Medical Problems of Performing Artists,* 5(3): 121-126.

Beuerlein, M., Raso, V.J., Hill, D.L., Moreau, M.J., and Mahood, J.K. (2003). Changes in alignment of the scoliotic spine in response to lateral bending (abstract). *Spine,* 28(7): 693-698.

Bradford, F., and Spurling, R. (1945). *The intervertebral disc.* Springfield, IL: Charles C Thomas.

Bronner, S., Ojofeitimi, S., and Rose, D. (2003). Injuries in a modern dance company: Effect of comprehensive management on injury incidence and time loss. *American Journal of Sports Medicine,* 31(3): 365-373.

Burton, A., Tillotson, K., and Troup, J. (1989a). Prediction of low-back trouble frequency in a working population. *Spine,* 14(9): 939-946.

Burton, A., Tillotson, K., and Troup, J. (1989b). Variation in lumbar sagittal mobility with low-back trouble. *Spine,* 14(6): 584-590.

Caillet, R. (1996). *Soft tissue pain and disability.* Philadelphia: Davis.

Carpenter, D., Graves, J., Pollock, M., Leggett, S., Foster, D., Holmes, B., and Fulton, M. (1990). Effect of 12 and 20 weeks of training on lumbar extension strength (abstract). *Medicine and Science in Sports and Exercise,* 22(2 Suppl.): S19.

Chaffin, D. (1974). Human strength capability and low-back pain. *Journal of Occupational Medicine,* 16(4): 248-254.

Clippinger-Robertson, K. (1985). Prevention of low back injuries in athletes: Putting theory into practice. In J. Terauds and J. Barham (eds.), *Proceedings of the International Symposium of Biomechanics in Sports* (pp. 407-413). Del Mar, CA: Research Center for Sports.

Clippinger-Robertson, K. (1991). Flexibility in different level female ballet dancers. Presented at the International Association of Dance Medicine and Science annual meeting, Baltimore, June 23.

Clippinger-Robertson, K.S., Hutton, R.S., Miller, D.I., and Nicholas, T.R. (1986). Mechanical and anatomical factors relating to the incidence and etiology of patellofemoral pain in dancers. In C. Shell (ed.), *The dancer as athlete: The 1984 Olympic Scientific Congress Proceedings* (vol. 8, pp. 53-72). Champaign, IL: Human Kinetics.

Deckey, J., and Weidenbaum, M. (1997). The thoracic and lumbar spine. In G. Scuderi, P. McCann, and P. Bruno (eds.),

Sports medicine: Principles of primary care (pp. 202-219). St. Louis: Mosby.

De Troyer, A., Estenne, M., Ninane, V., Gansbeke, D., and Gorini, M. (1990). Transversus abdominis muscle function in humans. *Journal of Applied Physiology*, 68(3): 1010-1016.

Dolan, P., Adams, M., and Hutton, W. (1988). Commonly adopted postures and their effect on the lumbar spine. *Spine*, 13(2): 197-201.

Donisch, E., and Basmajian, J. (1972). Electromyography of deep back muscles in man. *American Journal of Anatomy*, 133: 25-36.

Drezner, J., and Herring, S. (2001). Managing low-back pain: Steps to optimize function and hasten return to activity. *The Physician and Sportsmedicine*, 29(8): 37-44.

Eck, J., and Riley, L. (2004). Return to play after lumbar spine conditions and surgeries. *Clinics in Sports Medicine*, 23(3): 367-379.

Eie, N. (1966). Load capacity of the low back. *Journal of the Oslo City Hospitals*, 16(4): 74-98.

Eie, N., and Wehn, P. (1962). Measurements of the intra-abdominal pressure in relation to weight bearing of the lumbosacral spine. *Journal of the Oslo City Hospitals*, 12: 205-217.

Evans, R.W., Evans, R.I., and Carvajal, S. (1996). A survey of injuries among Broadway performers: Types of injuries, treatments and perceptions of performers. *Medical Problems of Performing Artists*, 11(1): 15-19.

Fehlandt, A., and Micheli, L. (1993). Lumbar facet stress fracture in a ballet dancer. *Spine*, 18(16): 2537-2539.

Fiorini, G., and McCammond, D. (1976). Forces on lumbo-vertebral facets. *Annals of Biomedical Engineering*, 4: 354-363.

Flint, M., and Gudgell, J. (1965). Electromyographic study of abdominal muscular activity during exercise. *Research Quarterly*, 36(1): 29-37.

Floyd, W., and Silver, P. (1950). Electromyographic study of patterns of activity of the anterior abdominal wall muscles in man. *Journal of Anatomy*, 84: 132-145.

Frankel, V., and Nordin, M. (1980). *Basic biomechanics of the skeletal system*. Philadelphia: Lea & Febiger.

Garrick, J., and Requa, R. (1993). Ballet injuries: An analysis of epidemiology and financial outcome. *American Journal of Sports Medicine*, 21(4): 586-590.

Gerbino, P., and Micheli, L. (1995). Back injuries in the young athlete. *Clinics in Sports Medicine*, 14(3): 571-590.

Godfrey, K., Kindig, L., and Windell, J. (1977). Electromyographic study of duration of muscle activity in sit-up variations. *Archives of Physical Medicine and Rehabilitation*, 58: 132-135.

Goldberg, B., and Boiardo, R. (1984). Profiling children for sports participation. *Clinics in Sports Medicine*, 3: 153.

Grabiner, M. (1989). The vertebral column. In P. Rasch (ed.), *Kinesiology and applied anatomy* (pp. 169-192). Philadelphia: Lea & Febiger.

Grabiner, M., Koh, T., and Ghazawi, E. (1992). Decoupling of bilateral paraspinal excitation in subjects with low back pain. *Spine*, 17(10): 1219-1223.

Gracovetsky, S., Kary, M., Pitchen, I., Levy, S., Eng, B., and Said, R. (1989). The importance of pelvic tilt in reducing compressive stress in the spine during flexion-extension exercises. *Spine*, 14(4): 412-416.

Granhed, H., and Morelli, B. (1988). Low back pain among retired wrestlers and heavyweight lifters. *American Journal of Sports Medicine*, 16(5): 530-533.

Graves, J., Pollock, M., Carpenter, D., Leggett, S., Jones, A., MacMillan, M., and Fulton, M. (1990). Quantitative assessment of full range-of-motion isometric lumbar extension strength. *Spine*, 15: 289-294.

Graves, S., Pollock, M., Leggett, S., Carpenter, D., Fix, C., and Fulton, M. (1990). Nonspecificity of limited range-of-motion lumbar extension strength training (abstract). *Medicine and Science in Sports and Exercise*, 22(2 Suppl.): S19.

Grieve, D. (1978). The dynamics of lifting. *Exercise and Sport Sciences Reviews*, 5: 157-179.

Grillner, S., Nilsson, J., and Thorstensson, A. (1978). Intra-abdominal pressure changes during natural movements in man. *Acta Physiologica Scandinavica*, 103: 275-283.

Guimaraes, A., Vaz, M., Campos, M., and Marantes, R. (1991). The contribution of the rectus abdominis and rectus femoris in twelve selected abdominal exercises. *Journal of Sports Medicine and Physical Fitness*, 31(2): 222-230.

Gutin, B., and Lipetz, S. (1971). An electromyographic investigation of the rectus abdominis in abdominal exercises. *Research Quarterly*, 42(3): 256-263.

Hall, S.J. (1999). *Basic biomechanics*. Boston: McGraw-Hill.

Hall, S., Lee, J., and Wood, T. (1990). Evaluation of selected sit-up variations for the individual with low back pain. *Journal of Applied Sport Science Research*, 4(2): 42-46.

Hall, S., and Lindoo, J. (1985). Torque and myoelectric activity in the lumbar region during selected aerobic dance exercise. Presented at the 32nd annual ACSM meeting, Nashville.

Hall-Craggs, E.C.B. (1985). *Anatomy as a basis for clinical medicine*. Baltimore: Urban & Schwarzenberg.

Halpern, A., and Bleck, E. (1979). Sit-up exercises: An electromyographic study. *Clinical Orthopaedics and Related Research*, 145: 172-178.

Hamill, J., and Knutzen, K.M. (1995). *Biomechanical basis of human movement*. Philadelphia: Lippincott Williams & Wilkins.

Hamilton, L., Hamilton, W., Warren, M., Keller, K., and Molnar, M. (1997). Factors contributing to the attrition rate in elite ballet students. *Journal of Dance Medicine and Science*, 1(4): 131-138.

Hamilton, N., and Luttgens, K. (2002). *Kinesiology: Scientific basis of human motion*. Boston: McGraw-Hill.

Harvey, J., and Tanner, S. (1991). Low back pain in young athletes: A practical approach. *Sports Medicine*, 12(6): 394-406.

Hay, J., and Reid, J. (1982). *The anatomical and mechanical bases of human motion*. Englewood Cliffs, NJ: Prentice Hall.

Herman, J., Pizzutillo, P., and Cavalier, R. (2003). Spondylolysis and spondylolisthesis in the child and adolescent athlete. *Orthopedic Clinics of North America*, 34(3): 461-467.

Hides, J., Stokes, M., Saide, M., Jull, G., and Cooper, D. (1994). Evidence of lumbar multifidus muscle wasting ipsilateral to symptoms in patients with acute/subacute low back pain. *Spine*, 19(2): 165-172.

Hodges, P. (2003). Core stability exercise in chronic low back pain. *Orthopedic Clinics of North America*, 34(2): 245-254.

Hodges, P., and Richardson, C. (1996). Inefficient muscular stabilization of the lumbar spine associated with low back pain. *Spine*, 21(22): 2640-2650.

Hodges, P., and Richardson, C. (1997). Contraction of the abdominal muscles associated with movement of the lower limb. *Physical Therapy,* 77(2): 132-144.

Hutton, W., Cryon, B., and Stott, J. (1979). The compressive strength of lumbar vertebrae. *Journal of Anatomy,* 129(4): 753-758.

Imamura, K., Ashida, H., Ishikawa, T., and Fujii, M. (1983). Human major psoas muscle and sacrospinalis muscle in relation to age: A study by computed tomography. *Journal of Gerontology,* 38(6): 678-681.

Ireland, M., and Micheli, L. (1987). Bilateral stress fracture of the lumbar pedicles in a ballet dancer. *Journal of Bone and Joint Surgery,* 69A(1): 140-142.

Jeong, G.K., and Errico, T.J. (2002). Spinal deformity update: The Lenke classification of adolescent idiopathic scoliosis. *Medscape Orthopaedics and Sports Medicine,* 6(2). www.medscape.com/viewarticle/445056.

Kelley, D. (1982). Exercise prescription and the kinesiological imperative. *Journal of Health, Physical Education, Recreation and Dance,* 53(1): 18-20.

Kelsey, J., White, A., Pastides, H., and Bisbee, G. (1979). The impact of musculoskeletal disorders on the population of the United States. *Journal of Bone and Joint Surgery,* 61A: 959-964.

Kendall, F., McCreary, E., and Provance, P. (1993). *Muscles: Testing and function.* Baltimore: Williams & Wilkins.

Klausen, K., Nielsen, B., and Madsen, L. (1981). Form and function of the spine in young males with and without "back troubles." In A. Morecki, K. Fidelus, K. Kedzior, and A. Wit (eds.), *Biomechanics VII-A, Proceedings of the Seventh International Congress of Biomechanics, Warsaw, Poland* (pp. 174-180). Baltimore: University Park Press.

Kollmitzer, J., Ebenbichler, G., Sabo, A., Kerschan, K., and Bochdansky, T. (2000). Effects of back extensor strength training versus balance training on postural control. *Medicine and Science in Sports and Exercise,* 32(10): 1770-1776.

Kotani, P., Ichikawa, N., Wakabayashi, W., Yoshii, T., and Koshimune, M. (1970). Studies of spondylolysis found among weight-lifters. *British Journal of Sports Medicine,* 6: 4-8.

Kreighbaum, E., and Barthels, K.M. (1996). *Biomechanics: A qualitative approach for studying human movement.* 4th ed. Boston: Allyn & Bacon.

Kujala, U., Taimela, S., Erkintalo, M., Salminen, J., and Kaprio, J. (1996). Low-back pain in adolescent athletes. *Medicine and Science in Sports and Exercise,* 28(2): 165-170.

Kumar, S., and Davis, P. (1978). Interrelationship of physiological and biomechanical parameters during stoop lifting. In F. Landry and W. Orban (eds.), *Biomechanics of sports and kinanthropometry.* Miami: Symposium Specialists Inc.

LaBan, M., Raptou, A., and Johnson, E. (1965). Electromyographic study of function of iliopsoas muscle. *Archives of Physical Medicine and Rehabilitation,* Oct.: 676-679.

LaFreniere, J. (1985). *The low-back patient: Procedures for treatment by physical therapy.* New York: Masson.

Lange, C., Unnithan, V., Larkam, E., and Latta, P. (2000). Maximizing the benefits of Pilates-inspired exercise for learning functional motor skills. *Journal of Bodywork and Movement Therapies,* 4(2): 99-108.

Laskowski, E., Newcomer-Aney, K., and Smith, J. (1997). Refining rehabilitation with proprioception training: Expediting return to play. *The Physician and Sportsmedicine,* 25(10): 89-102.

Levangie, P., and Norkin, C. (2001). *Joint structure and function.* Philadelphia: Davis.

Liederbach, M. (2000). General considerations for guiding dance injury rehabilitation. *Journal of Dance Medicine and Science,* 4(2): 54-65.

Liederbach, M., Spivak, J., and Rose, D. (1997). Scoliosis in dancers: A method of assessment in quick-screen settings. *Journal of Dance Medicine and Science,* 1(3): 107-112.

Lipetz, S., and Gutin, B. (1970). An electromyographic study of four abdominal exercises. *Medicine and Science in Sports,* 2(1): 35-38.

Livanelioglu, A., Otman, S., Yakut, Y., and Uygur, F. (1998). The effects of classical ballet training on the lumbar region. *Journal of Dance Medicine and Science,* 2(2): 52-55.

Liyang, D., Yinkan, X., Wenming, Z., and Zhihua, Z. (1989). The effect of flexion-extension motion of the lumbar spine on the capacity of the spinal canal. *Spine,* 14(5): 523-525.

Magee, D. (1997). *Orthopedic physical assessment.* Philadelphia: W.B. Saunders.

McGill, S. (2001). Low back stability: From formal description to issues for performance and rehabilitation. *Exercise and Sport Sciences Review,* 29: 26.

McKenzie, R. (1981). *The lumbar spine: Mechanical diagnosis and therapy.* Upper Hunt, New Zealand: Wright and Carman Limited.

McMeeken, J., Tully, E., Nattrass, C., and Stillman, B. (2002). The effect of spinal and pelvic posture and mobility on back pain in young dancers and non-dancers. *Journal of Dance Medicine and Science,* 6(5): 79-85.

Mercier, L. (1995). *Practical orthopedics.* St. Louis: Mosby.

Michele, A. (1960). The iliopsoas muscle: Its importance in disorders of the hip and spine. *Clinical Symposia,* 12(3): 67-101.

Micheli, L. (1983). Back injuries in dancers. *Clinics in Sports Medicine,* 2(3): 473-484.

Micheli, L. (1988). Dance injuries: The back, hip, and pelvis. In P. Clarkson and M. Skrinar (eds.), *Science of dance training* (pp. 193-207). Champaign, IL: Human Kinetics.

Micheli, L., Solomon, R., Solomon, J., and Gerbino, P. (1999). Low back pain in dancers. *Medscape General Medicine,* 1(3). www.medscape.com/viewarticle/408509.

Micheli, L., and Wood, R. (1995). Back pain in young athletes. *Archives of Pediatric and Adolescent Medicine,* 149(1): 5-8.

Miller, M., and Medeiros, J. (1987). Recruitment of internal oblique and transversus abdominis muscles during the eccentric phase of the curl-up exercise. *Physical Therapy,* 67(8): 1213-1217.

Moeller, J., and Rifat, S. (2001). Spondylolysis in active adolescents: Expediting return to play. *The Physician and Sportsmedicine,* 29(12): 27-32.

Mohan, A.L., and Das, K. (2003). History of surgery for the correction of spinal deformity. *Journal of Neurosurgery,* 14(1): 1-5.

Molnar, M., and Esterson, J. (1997). Screening students in a pre-professional ballet school. *Journal of Dance Medicine and Science,* 1(3): 118-121.

Mooney, V., Gulick, J., and Pozos, R. (2000). A preliminary report on the effect of measured strength training in adolescent idiopathic scoliosis (abstract). *Journal of Spinal Disorders,* 13(2): 102-107.

Moore, K., and Agur, A. (1995). *Essential clinical anatomy.* Baltimore: Williams & Wilkins.

Moore, K., and Dalley, A. (1999). *Clinically oriented anatomy.* Philadelphia: Lippincott Williams & Wilkins.

Morris, J., Lucas, D., and Bresler, B. (1961). Role of the trunk in stability of the spine. *Journal of Bone and Joint Surgery,* 43A: 327-351.

Mutoh, Y. (1978). Low back pain in butterfliers. *Swimming Medicine,* IV: 115-123.

Myklebust, J., Pintar, F., Yoganandan, N., Cusick, J., Maiman, D., Myers, T., and Sances, A. (1988). Tensile strength of spinal ligaments. *Spine,* 13(5): 526-531.

Nachemson, A. (1966). Electromyographic studies on the vertebral portion of the psoas muscle. *Acta Orthopaedica Scandinavica,* 37: 177-190.

Nachemson, A. (1981). Disc pressure measurements. *Spine,* 6(1): 93-97.

Nachemson, A., and Morris, J. (1964). In vivo measurements of intradiscal pressure. *Journal of Bone and Joint Surgery,* 46A: 1077-1092.

Napier, J. (1967). The antiquity of human walking. *Scientific American,* April: 216-256.

Nault, M., Allard, P., Hinse, S., LeBlanc, R., Caron, O., and Sadeghi, H. (2002). Relations between standing stability and body posture parameters in a scoliosis. *Spine,* 27(17): 1911-1917.

Ng, J., Kippers, V., Parnianpour, M., and Richardson, K. (2002). EMG activity normalization for trunk muscles in subjects with and without back pain. *Medicine and Science in Sports and Exercise,* 34(7): 1082-1086.

Nixon, J. (1983). Injuries to the neck and upper extremities of dancers. *Clinics in Sports Medicine,* 2(3): 459-472.

Ohlen, G., Wredmark, T., and Spangfort, E. (1989). Spinal sagittal configuration and mobility related to low-back pain in the female gymnast. *Spine,* 14: 847-850.

Omey, M.L., Micheli, L.J., and Gerbino, P.G. (2000). Idiopathic scoliosis and spondylolysis in the female athlete. *Clinical Orthopaedics and Related Research,* 372: 74-84.

Ortengren, R., and Andersson, G. (1977). Electromyographic studies of trunk muscles, with special reference to the functional anatomy of the lumbar spine. *Spine,* 2(1): 44-52.

Palmer, L., and Epler, M. (1990). *Clinical assessment procedures in physical therapy.* Philadelphia: Lippincott.

Panjabi, M., Abumi, K., Duranceau, J., and Oxland, T. (1989). Spinal stability and intersegmental muscle forces. A biomechanical model. *Spine,* 14(2): 194-199.

Panjabi, M., Tech, D., and White III, A. (1980). Basic biomechanics of the spine. *Neurosurgery,* 7(1): 76-93.

Parnianpour, M., Nordin, M., Kahanovitz, N., and Frankel, V. (1988). The triaxial coupling of torque generation of trunk muscles during isometric exertions and the effect of fatiguing isoinertial movements on the motor output and movement patterns. *Spine,* 13(9): 982-992.

Pauly, J. (1966). An electromyographic analysis of certain movements and exercises. Some deep muscles of the back. *Anatomy Record,* 155: 223-234.

Pitt-Brooke, J. (1998). *Rehabilitation of movement.* Philadelphia: Saunders.

Plowman, S. (1992). Physical activity, physical fitness, and low back pain. *Exercise and Sport Sciences Reviews,* 20: 221-242.

Pollock, M., Leggett, S., Graves, J., Jones, A., Fulton, M., and Cirulli, J. (1989). Effect of resistance training on lumbar extension strength. *American Journal of Sports Medicine,* 17(5): 624-629.

Porter, R., Adams, M., and Hutton, W. (1989). Physical activity and the strength of the lumbar spine. *Spine,* 14(2): 201-203.

Quinney, H., Smith, D., and Wenger, H. (1984). A field test for the assessment of abdominal muscular endurance in professional ice hockey players. *Journal of Orthopaedic and Sports Physical Therapy,* 6: 30-33.

Quirk, R. (1983). Ballet injuries: The Australian experience. *Clinics in Sports Medicine,* 2(3): 507-514.

Ramel, E., Moritz, U., and Jarnlo, G. (1999). Recurrent musculoskeletal pain in professional ballet dancers in Sweden: A six-year follow-up. *Journal of Dance Medicine and Science,* 3(3): 93-101.

Rasch, P., and Burke, R. (1978). *Kinesiology and applied anatomy.* Philadelphia: Lea & Febiger.

Ricci, B., Marchetti, M., and Figura, F. (1981). Biomechanics of sit-up exercises. *Medicine and Science in Sports and Exercise,* 13(1): 54-59.

Richardson, C., Hodges, P., and Hides, J. (2004). *Therapeutic exercise for lumbopelvic stabilization.* New York: Churchill Livingstone.

Robertson, L., Cunningham, M., Changsut, R., Himmelsbach, J., and Koenig, P. (1988). Statistical and practical issues affecting the acceptability of timed and untimed conditions for a new abdominal fitness test. *Journal of Human Movement Studies,* 14: 255-268.

Rovere, G., Webb, L., Gristina, A., and Vogel, J. (1983). Musculoskeletal injuries in theatrical dance students. *American Journal of Sports Medicine,* 11(4): 195-198.

Roy, S., DeLuca, C., and Casavant, D. (1989). Lumbar muscle fatigue and chronic lower back pain. *Spine,* 14(9): 992-1001.

Roy, S., and Irvin, R. (1983). *Sports medicine: Prevention, evaluation, management, and rehabilitation.* Englewood Cliffs, NJ: Prentice Hall.

Saal, J. (1988a). Rehabilitation of football players with lumbar spine injury (part 1 of 2). *The Physician and Sportsmedicine,* 16(9): 61-67.

Saal, J. (1988b). Rehabilitation of football players with lumbar spine injury (part 2 of 2). *The Physician and Sportsmedicine,* 16(10): 117-123.

Salter-Pedersen, M., and Wilmerding, V. (1998). Injury profiles of student and professional flamenco dancers. *Journal of Dance Medicine and Science,* 2(3): 108-114.

Sammarco, J. (1984). Diagnosis and treatment in dancers. *Clinical Orthopaedics and Related Research,* 187(July/Aug.): 176-187.

Sarti, M., Monfort, M., Fuster, M., and Villaplana, L. (1996). Muscle activity in upper and lower rectus abdominus during abdominal exercises. *Archives of Physical Medicine and Rehabilitation,* 77: 1293-1297.

Schnebel, B., Simmons, J., Chowning, J., and Davidson, R. (1988). A digitizing technique for the study of movement of intradiscal dye in response to flexion and extension of the lumbar spine. *Spine,* 13(3): 309-312.

Schnebel, B., Watkins, R., and Dillin, W. (1989). The role of spinal flexion and extension in changing nerve root compression in disc herniations. *Spine,* 14(8): 835-837.

Seitsalo, S., Antila, H., Karrinaho, T., Riihimaki, H., Schlenzka, D., Osterman, K., and Ahonen, J. (1997). Spondylolysis in ballet dancers. *Journal of Dance Medicine and Science,* 1(2): 51-54.

Sheffield, F. (1962). Electromyographic study of the abdominal muscles in walking and other movements. *American Journal of Physical Medicine*, 41(4): 142-147.

Smidt, G., Blanpied, P., and White, R. (1989). Exploration of mechanical and electromyographic responses of trunk muscles to high-intensity resistive exercise. *Spine*, 14(8): 815-830.

Smidt, G., Herring, T., Amundsen, L., Rogers, M., Russell, A., and Lehmann, T. (1983). Assessment of abdominal and back extensor function: A quantitative approach and results for chronic low-back pain patients. *Spine*, 8: 211-219.

Smith, C. (1977). Physical management of muscular low back pain in the athlete. *CMA Journal*, 117: 632-635.

Smith, L., Weiss, E., and Lehmkuhl, L. (1996). *Brunnstrom's clinical kinesiology*. Philadelphia: Davis.

Soderberg, G. (1986). *Kinesiology: Application to pathological motion*. Baltimore: Williams & Wilkins.

Solomon, R., and Micheli, L. (1986). Technique as a consideration in modern dance injuries. *The Physician and Sportsmedicine*, 14(8): 83-90.

Sparling, P. (1997). Field testing for abdominal muscular fitness. *ACSM's Health and Fitness Journal*, 1(4): 30-33.

Stanforth, D., Stanforth, P., Hahn, S., and Phillips, A. (1998). A 10-week training study comparing resistaball and traditional trunk training. *Journal of Dance Medicine and Science*, 2(4): 134-140.

Stanish, W. (1979). Low back pain in middle-aged athletes. *American Journal of Sports Medicine*, 7(6): 367-369.

Stanitski, C. (1982). Low back pain in young athletes. *The Physician and Sportsmedicine*, 10(10): 77-91.

Suzuki, N., and Endo, S. (1983). A quantitative study of trunk muscle strength and fatigability in the low-back pain syndrome. *Spine*, 8(1): 69-74.

Sward, L. (1992). The thoracolumbar spine in young elite athletes. Current concepts on the effects of physical training. *Sports Medicine*, 13: 357-364.

Sward, L., Hellstrom, M., Jacobsson, B., Hyman, R., and Peterson, L. (1991). Disc degeneration and associated abnormalities of the spine in elite gymnasts: A magnetic resonance imaging study. *Spine*, 16: 437-443.

Taft, E., and Francis, R. (2003). Evaluation and management of scoliosis. *Journal of Pediatric Health Care*, 17(1): 42-44.

Trepman, E., Gellman, R., Solomon, R., Murthy, K.R., Micheli, L.J., and De Luca, C.J. (1994). Electromyographic analysis of standing posture and demi-plié in ballet and modern dancers. *Medicine and Science in Sports and Exercise*, 26(6): 771-782.

Trepman, E., Walaszek, A., and Micheli, L. (1990). Spinal problems in the dancer. In R. Solomon, S. Minton, and J. Solomon (eds.), *Preventing dance injuries: An interdisciplinary perspective* (pp. 103-131). Reston, VA: American Alliance for Health, Physical Education, Recreation and Dance.

Troup, J. (1970). The risk of weight training and weight lifting in young people. *British Journal of Sports Medicine*, 5(1): 27-33.

Wallmann, H. (1998). Low back pain: Is it really all behind you? *ACSM's Health and Fitness Journal*, 2(5): 30-35.

Warren, M., Brooks-Gunn, J., Hamilton, L., Warren, F., and Hamilton, W. (1986). Scoliosis and fractures in young ballet dancers. *New England Journal of Medicine*, 314(21): 1348-1353.

Watson, A. (1995). Sports injuries in footballers related to defects of posture and body mechanics. *Journal of Sports Medicine and Physical Fitness*, 35(4): 289-293.

Weiker, G. (1982). The dancer's spine. *Emergency Medicine*, 14(10): 28-32.

Welsh, T., Jones, G., Lucker, K., and Weaver, B. (1998). Back strengthening for dancers: A within-subject experimental analysis. *Journal of Dance Medicine and Science*, 2(4): 141-148.

White III, A., and Panjabi, M. (1978). *Clinical biomechanics of the spine*. Philadelphia: Lippincott.

Whiting, W., and Zernicke, R. (1998). *Biomechanics of musculoskeletal injury*. Champaign, IL: Human Kinetics.

Wolf, S., Basmajian, J., Russe, T., and Kutner, M. (1979). Normative data on low back mobility and activity levels. *American Journal of Physical Medicine*, 58(5): 217-229.

Woodhull, A., Maltrud, K., and Mello, B. (1985). Alignment of the human body in standing. *European Journal of Applied Physiology*, 54: 109-115.

Woodhull-McNeal, A., Clarkson, P., James, R., Watkins, A., and Barrett, S. (1990). How linear is dancers' posture? *Medical Problems of Performing Artists*, 5(4): 151-154.

Chapter 4

American Academy of Orthopaedic Surgeons. (1965). *Joint motion: Method of measuring and recording*. Chicago: American Academy of Orthopaedic Surgeons.

Barclay, L., and Vega, C. (2004). Exercise improves pelvic girdle pain after pregnancy. *Medscape Medical News*, www.medscape.com/viewarticle/470431.

Basmajian, J., and DeLuca, C. (1985). *Muscles alive—Their functions revealed by electromyography*. Baltimore: Williams & Wilkins.

Bauman, P., Singson, R., and Hamilton, W. (1994). Femoral neck anteversion in ballerinas. *Clinical Orthopaedics and Related Research*, 302: 57-63.

Bechtel, R. (2001). Physical characteristics of the axial interosseous ligament of the human sacroiliac joint. *The Spine Journal*, 1: 255-259.

Best, T., and Garrett, W. (1996). Hamstring strains: Expediting return to play. *The Physician and Sportsmedicine*, 24(8): 37-44.

Bronner, S., Brownstein, B., Worthen, L., and Ames, S. (2000). Skill acquisition and mastery in performance of a complex dance movement (abstract). *Journal of Dance Medicine and Science*, 4(4): 139.

Brown, T., and Micheli, L. (1998). Where artistry meets injury. *Biomechanics*, 5(9): 12-25.

Browning, K. (2001). Hip and pelvis injuries in runners. *The Physician and Sportsmedicine*, 29(1): 23-34.

Burkett, L.N. (1970). Causative factors in hamstring strains. *Medicine and Science in Sports and Exercise*, 2: 39-42.

Caillet, R. (1996). *Soft tissue pain and disability*. Philadelphia: Davis.

Chen, Y., Fredericson, M., and Smuck, M. (2002). Sacroiliac joint pain syndrome in active patients. *The Physician and Sportsmedicine*, 30(11): 30-37.

Cheng, J., and Song, J. (2003). Anatomy of the sacrum. *Nuerosurgery Focus*, 15(2): 1-4.

Clarkson, H.M., and Gilewich, G.B. (1989). *Musculoskeletal assessment: Joint range of motion and manual muscle strength.* Baltimore: Williams & Wilkins.

Clement, D., Ammann, W., Tauton, J., Lloyd-Smith, R., Jesperson, D., McKay, H., Goldring, J., and Matheson, G. (1993). Exercise-induced stress injuries to the femur. *International Journal of Sports Medicine,* 14(6): 347-352.

Clippinger-Robertson, K. (1984). Incidence and etiology of patellofemoral complaints in dancers. Submitted in partial fulfillment of the requirement for the degree of master of science in physical education. Department of Kinesiology, University of Washington, Seattle.

Clippinger-Robertson, K. (1991). Flexibility in different level female ballet dancers. Presented at the International Association of Dance Medicine and Science annual meeting. Baltimore, June 23.

Clippinger-Robertson, K.S., Hutton, R.S., Miller, D.I., and Nichols, T.R. (1986). Mechanical and anatomical factors relating to the incidence and etiology of patellofemoral pain in dancers. In C. Shell (ed.), *The dancer as athlete: The 1984 Olympic Scientific Congress Proceedings* (vol. 8, pp. 53-72). Champaign, IL: Human Kinetics.

Colliton, J. (1999). Managing back pain during pregnancy. *Medscape General Medicine,* 1(2). www.medscape.com/viewarticle/408838.

Desiderio, V. (1988). Hamstring injuries. In P. Taylor and D. Taylor (eds.), *Conquering athletic injuries* (pp. 144-145). Champaign, IL: Leisure Press.

DiTullio, M., Wilczek, L., Paulus, D., Kiriakatis, A., Pollack, M., and Eisenhardt, J. (1989). Comparison of hip rotation in female classical ballet dancers versus female nondancers. *Medical Problems of Performing Artists,* 4(4): 154-158.

DonTigny, R. (1990). Anterior dysfunction of the sacroiliac joint as a major factor in the etiology of idiopathic low back pain syndrome. *Physical Therapy,* 70(4): 250-265.

Dorman, P. (1971). A report of 140 hamstring injuries. *Australian Journal of Sports Medicine,* 4: 30-36.

Dujardin, F., Roussignol, X., Hossenbaccus, M., and Thomine, J. (2002). Experimental study of the sacroiliac joint micromotion in pelvic disruption. *Journal of Orthopaedic Trauma,* 16(2): 99-103.

Ekstrand, J., and Gillquist, J. (1982). The frequency of muscle tightness and injuries in soccer players. *American Journal of Sports Medicine,* 10(2): 75-78.

Emery, C., and Meeuwisse, W. (2001). Risk factors for groin injuries in hockey. *Medicine and Science in Sports and Exercise,* 33(9): 1423-1432.

Estwanik, J., Sloane, B., and Rosenberg, M. (1990). Groin strain and other possible causes of groin pain. *The Physician and Sportsmedicine,* 18(2): 54-65.

Frankel, V., and Nordin, M. (1980). *Basic biomechanics of the skeletal system.* Philadelphia: Lea & Febiger.

Fredericson, M., Guillet, M., and DeBenedictis, L. (2000). Quick solutions for iliotibial band syndrome. *The Physician and Sportsmedicine,* 28(2): 169-175.

Garrett, W., Califf, J., and Bassett III, F. (1984). Histochemical correlates of hamstring injuries. *The American Journal of Sports Medicine,* 12: 98-103.

Garrick, J., and Requa, R. (1993). Ballet injuries: An analysis of epidemiology and financial outcome. *American Journal of Sports Medicine,* 21(4): 586-590.

Garrick, J., and Requa, R. (1994). Turnout and training in ballet. *Medical Problems of Performing Artists,* June: 43-49.

Gerhardt, J., and Rippstein, J. (1990). *Measuring and recording of joint motion: Instrumentation and techniques.* Toronto: Hofgrefe & Huber.

Godge, J., Varnum, D., and Sanders, K. (2002). Impairment-based examination and disability management of an elderly woman with sacroiliac region pain. *Physical Therapy,* 82: 812-821.

Grossman, G., and Wilmerding, V. (2000). The effect of conditioning on the height of dancer's extension in a la seconde. *Journal of Dance Medicine and Science,* 4(4): 117-121.

Hall, S.J. (1999). *Basic biomechanics.* Boston: McGraw-Hill.

Hamill, J., and Knutzen, K. (1995). *Biomechanical basis of human movement.* Philadelphia: Lippincott Williams & Wilkins.

Hamilton, L., Hamilton, W., Warren, M., Keller, K., and Molnar, M. (1997). Factors contributing to the attrition rate in elite ballet students. *Journal of Dance Medicine and Science,* 1(4): 131-138.

Hamilton, W., Hamilton, L., Marshall, P., and Molnar, M. (1992). A profile of the musculoskeletal characteristics of elite professional ballet dancers. *American Journal of Sports Medicine,* 20(3): 267-273.

Harper, M., Schaberg, J., and Allen, W. (1987). Primary iliopsoas bursography in the diagnosis of disorders of the hip. *Clinical Orthopaedics and Related Research,* 221: 238-241.

Honorio, B., Katz, J., Benzon, H., and Iqbal, M. (2003). Piriformis syndrome: Anatomic considerations, a new injection technique, and a review of the literature. *Anesthesiology,* 98(6): 1442-1448.

Hooper, A.C.B. (1977). The role of the iliopsoas muscle in femoral rotation. *Irish Journal of Medical Science,* 146(4): 108-112.

Jacobson, T., and Allen, W. (1990). Surgical correction of the snapping iliopsoas tendon. *American Journal of Sports Medicine,* 18(5): 470-474.

Jonhagen, S., Nemeth, G., and Eriksson, E. (1994). Hamstring injuries in sprinters: The role of concentric and eccentric hamstring muscle strength and flexibility. *American Journal of Sports Medicine,* 22(2): 262-266.

Kagan II, A. (1999). Rotator cuff tears of the hip. *Clinical Orthopaedics and Related Research,* 368: 135-140.

Kendall, F.P., McCreary, E.K., and Provance, P.G. (1993). *Muscles: Testing and function.* Baltimore: Williams & Wilkins.

Khan, K., Brown, J., Way, S., Vass, N., Crichton, K., Alexander, R., Baxter, A., Butler, M., and Wark, J. (1995). Overuse injuries in classical ballet. *Sports Medicine,* 19(5): 341-357.

Khan, K., Roberts, P., Nattrass, C., Bennell, K., Mayes, W., Way, S., Brown, J., McMeeken, J., and Wark, J. (1997). Hip and ankle range of motion in elite classical ballet dancers and controls. *Clinical Journal of Sports Medicine,* 7: 174-179.

Kreighbaum, E., and Barthels, K.M. (1996). *Biomechanics: A qualitative approach for studying human movement.* 4th ed. Boston: Allyn & Bacon.

Kushner, S., Saboe, L., Reid, D., Penrose, T., and Grace, M. (1990). Relationship of turnout to hip abduction in professional ballet dancers. *American Journal of Sports Medicine,* 18(3): 286-291.

Lacroix, V. (2000). A complete approach to groin pain. *The Physician and Sportsmedicine,* 28(1): 14-28.

Levangie, P., and Norkin, C. (2001). *Joint structure and function.* Philadelphia: F.A. Davis.

Lieberman, G., and Harwin, S. (1997). Pelvis, hip and thigh. In G. Scuderi, P. McCann, and P. Bruno (eds.), *Sports medicine: Principles of primary care* (pp. 306-335). St. Louis: Mosby.

Liemohn, W. (1978). Factors related to hamstring strains. *American Journal of Sports Medicine,* 18: 71-76.

Luke, A., and Micheli, L. (2000). Management of injuries in the young dancer. *Journal of Dance Medicine and Science,* 4(1): 6-15.

Marshall, W., and Waddell, D. (2000). Nonoperative management of osteoarthritis of the knee. From a special report: Osteoarthritis of the knee. www.physsportsmed.com/asr/knee/marshall.htm.

Mellin, G. (1988). Correlations of hip mobility with degree of back pain and lumbar spinal mobility in chronic low-back pain patients. *Spine,* 13(6): 668-670.

Mercier, L.R. (1995). *Practical orthopedics.* 4th ed. St. Louis: Mosby.

Michele, A. (1960). The iliopsoas muscle. *Clinical Symposia,* 12(3): 67-101.

Mierau, D., Cassidy, J., and Yong-Hing, K. (1989). Low-back pain and straight leg raising in children and adolescents. *Spine,* 14(5): 526-528.

Miller, E., Schneider, H., Bronson, J., and McLain, D. (1975). A new consideration in athletic injuries: The classical ballet dancer. *Clinical Orthopaedics and Related Research,* 111: 181-191.

Moore, K., and Dalley, A. (1999). *Clinically oriented anatomy.* Philadelphia: Lippincott Williams & Wilkins.

Palmer, M.L., and Epler, M.E. (1990). *Clinical assessment procedures in physical therapy.* Philadelphia: Lippincott.

Papadopoulos, E., and Khan, S. (2004). Piriformis syndrome and low back pain: A new classification and review of the literature. *Orthopedic Clinics of North America,* 35(1): 65-71.

Quirk, R. (1983). Ballet injuries: The Australian experience. *Clinics in Sports Medicine,* 2(3): 507-514.

Rasch, P.J. (1989). *Kinesiology and applied anatomy.* Philadelphia: Lea & Febiger.

Rasch, P.J., and Burke, R.K. (1978). *Kinesiology and applied anatomy.* 6th ed. Philadelphia: Lea & Febiger.

Reid, D.C., Burnham, R.S., Saboe, L.A., and Kushner, S.F. (1987). Lower extremity flexibility patterns in classical ballet dancers and their correlation to lateral hip and knee injuries. *American Journal of Sports Medicine,* 15(4): 347-351.

Rich, B., and McKeag, D. (1992). When sciatica is not disk disease. *The Physician and Sportsmedicine,* 20(10): 105-115.

Roy, S., and Irvin, R. (1983). *Sports medicine: Prevention, evaluation, management, and rehabilitation.* Englewood Cliffs, NJ: Prentice Hall.

Ruane, J., and Rossi, T. (1998). When groin pain is more than "just a strain": Navigating a broad differential. *The Physician and Sportsmedicine,* 26(4): 78-103.

Safran, M., Garrett, W., Seaber, A., Glisson, R., and Ribbeck, B. (1988). The role of warmup in muscular injury prevention. *American Journal of Sports Medicine,* 16(2): 123-129.

Sammarco, J. (1983). The dancer's hip. *Clinics in Sports Medicine,* 2(3): 485-498.

Sammarco, J. (1987). The dancer's hip. In A. Ryan and R. Stephens (eds.), *Dance medicine: A comprehensive guide* (pp. 220-242). Chicago: Pluribus Press.

Sayson, S., Ducey, J., Maybrey, J., Wesley, R., and Vermilion, D. (1994). Sciatic entrapment neuropathy associated with an anomalous piriformis muscle. *Pain,* 59: 149-152.

Schaberg, J., Harper, M., and Allen, W. (1984). The snapping hip syndrome. *American Journal of Sports Medicine,* 12(5): 361-365.

Schafle, M., Requa, R., and Garrick, J. (1990). A comparison of patterns of injury in ballet, modern and aerobic dance. In R. Solomon, S.C. Minton, and J. Solomon (eds.), *Preventing dance injuries: An interdisciplinary perspective* (pp. 1-14). Reston, VA: American Alliance for Health, Physical Education, Recreation and Dance.

Smith, L., Weiss, E., and Lehmkuhl, L. (1996). *Brunnstrom's clinical kinesiology.* Philadelphia: Davis.

Soderberg, G. (1986). *Kinesiology: Application to pathological motion.* Baltimore: Williams & Wilkins.

Solomon, R., and Micheli, L. (1986). Technique as a consideration in modern dance injuries. *The Physician and Sportsmedicine,* 14(8): 83-90.

Stone, D. (2001). Hip problems in dancers. *Journal of Dance Medicine and Science,* 5(1): 7-10.

Sturesson, B., Selvik, G., and Uden, A. (1989). Movements of the sacroiliac joints: A roentgen stereophotogrammetric analysis. *Spine,* 14(2): 162-165.

Taylor, D., Dalton, J., Seaber, A., and Garrett, W. (1990). Viscoelastic properties of muscle-tendon units: The biomechanical effects of stretching. *American Journal of Sports Medicine,* 18(3): 300-309.

Teitz, C. (2000). Hip and knee injuries in dancers. *Journal of Dance Medicine and Science,* 4(1): 23-29.

Thomasen, E. (1982). *Diseases and injuries of ballet dancers.* Arhus, Denmark: Universitetsforlaget.

Trepman, E., Gellman, R., Solomon, R., Murthy, K., Micheli, L., and DeLuca, C. (1994). Electromyographic analysis of standing posture and demi-plié in ballet and modern dancers. *Medicine and Science in Sports and Exercise,* 26(6): 771-782.

Tyler, T., Nicholas, S., Campbell, R., and McHugh, M. (2001). The association of hip strength and flexibility with the incidence of adductor muscle strains in professional ice hockey players. *American Journal of Sports Medicine,* 29: 124-128.

Warren, C., Lehmann, J., and Koblanski, J. (1971). Elongation of rat tail tendon: Effect of load and temperature. *Archives of Physical Medicine and Rehabilitation,* 52: 465-474.

Warren, C., Lehmann, J., and Koblanski, J. (1976). Heat and stretch procedures: An evaluation using rat tail tendon. *Archives of Physical Medicine and Rehabilitation,* 57: 122-126.

Welsh, T., Jones, G., Lucker, K., and Weaver, B. (1998). Back strengthening for dancers: A within-subject experimental analysis. *Journal of Dance Medicine and Science,* 2(4): 141-148.

Wiesler, E., Hunter, D., Martin, D., Curl, W., and Hoen, H. (1996). Ankle flexibility and injury patterns in dancers. *American Journal of Sports Medicine,* 24(6): 754-757.

Worrell, T. (1994). Factors associated with hamstring injuries: An approach to treatment and preventative measures. *Sports Medicine,* 17(5): 338-345.

Young, S., Aprill, C., and Laslett, M. (2003). Correlation of clinical examination characteristics with three sources of chronic low back pain. *The Spine Journal,* 3: 460-465.

Chapter 5

American Academy of Orthopaedic Surgeons. (1965). *Joint motion: Method of measuring and recording.* Chicago: American Academy of Orthopaedic Surgeons.

Barnes, M., Dip, T., Krasnow, D., Tupling, S., and Thomas, M. (2000). Knee rotation in classical dancers during the grand plie. *Medical Problems of Performing Artists,* 15: 140-147.

Barrack, R., Skinner, H., and Buckley, S. (1989). Proprioception in the anterior cruciate deficient knee. *American Journal of Sports Medicine,* 17(1): 1-6.

Basmajian, J., and DeLuca, C. (1985). *Muscles alive—Their functions revealed by electromyography.* Baltimore: Williams & Wilkins.

Bergfeld, J. (1982). The dancer's knee. *Emergency Medicine,* 14(10): 32-41.

Besier, T., Lloyd, D., Ackland, T., and Cochrane, J. (2001). Anticipatory effects on knee joint loading during running and cutting maneuvers. *Medicine and Science in Sports and Exercise,* 33(7): 1176-1181.

Besier, T., Lloyd, D., Cochrane, J., and Ackland, T. (2001). External loading of the knee joint during running and cutting maneuvers. *Medicine and Science in Sports and Exercise,* 33(7): 1168-1175.

Blazina, M., Kerlan, R., Jobe, F., Carter, V., and Carlson, G. (1973). Jumper's knee. *Orthopedic Clinics of North America,* 4(3): 665-678.

Boden, B., Griffin, L., and Garrett, W. (2000). Etiology and prevention of noncontact ACL injury. *The Physician and Sportsmedicine,* 28(4): 53-60.

Brown, S., and Clippinger, K. (1996). Rehabilitation of anterior cruciate ligament insufficiency in a dancer using the clinical reformer and a balanced body exercise method. *Work,* 7: 109-114.

Butler, D., Noyes, F., and Grood, E. (1980). Ligamentous restraints to anterior-posterior drawer in the human knee. *Journal of Bone and Joint Surgery,* 62: 259-270.

Caillet, R. (1996). *Soft tissue pain and disability.* Philadelphia: Davis.

Chmelar, R., Shultz, B., Ruhling, R., Fitt, S., and Johnson, M. (1988). Isokinematic characteristics of the knee in female, professional and university, ballet and modern dancers. *Journal of Orthopaedic and Sports Physical Therapy,* 9(12): 410-418.

Clippinger, K. (2002). Complementary use of open and closed kinetic chain exercises. *Journal of Dance Medicine and Science,* 6(3): 77-78.

Clippinger, K. (2005). Biomechanical considerations in turnout. In R. Solomon, J. Solomon, and S.C. Minton (eds.), *Preventing dance injuries: An interdisciplinary perspective* (2nd ed., pp. 75-102). Champaign, IL: Human Kinetics.

Clippinger-Robertson, K. (1991). Flexibility among different levels of ballet dancers. Presented at the International Association of Dance Medicine and Science annual meeting, Baltimore, June 23.

Clippinger-Robertson, K.S., Hutton, R.S., Miller, D.I., and Nichols, T.R. (1986). Mechanical and anatomical factors relating to the incidence and etiology of patellofemoral pain in dancers. In C. Shell (ed.), *The dancer as athlete: The 1984 Olympic Scientific Congress Proceedings* (vol. 8, pp. 53-72). Champaign, IL: Human Kinetics.

Cook, J., Khan, K., Maffulli, N., Purdam, C., and Phty, D. (2000). Overuse tendinosis, not tendinitis; part 2: Applying the new approach to patellar tendinopathy. *The Physician and Sportsmedicine,* 28(6): 31-46.

Diduch, D., Scuderi, G., and Scott, W. (1997). Knee injuries. In G. Scuderi, P. McCann, and P. Bruno (eds.), *Sports medicine: Principles of primary care* (pp. 336-374). St. Louis: Mosby.

Dowson, D., and Wright, V. (1981). *An introduction to the biomechanics of joints and joint replacement.* London: Mechanical Engineering Publications.

Dye, S., and Vaupel, G. (2000). Functional anatomy of the knee: Bony geometry, static and dynamic restraints, sensory and motor innervation. In S. Lephart and F. Fu (eds.), *Proprioception and neuromuscular control in joint stability* (pp. 59-76). Champaign, IL: Human Kinetics.

Escamilla, R. (2001). Knee biomechanics of the dynamic squat exercise. *Medicine and Science in Sports and Exercise,* 33(1): 127-141.

Escamilla, R., Francisco, A., Kayes, A., Speer, K., and Moorman, C. (2002). Electromyographic analysis of sumo and conventional style deadlifts. *Medicine and Science in Sports and Exercise,* 34(4): 682-688.

Evans, N., Chew, H., and Stanish, W. (2001). The natural history and tailored treatment of ACL injury. *The Physician and Sportsmedicine,* 29(9): 19-34.

Evans, R.W., Evans, R.I., and Carvajal, S. (1996). A survey of injuries among Broadway performers: Types of injuries, treatments and perceptions of performers. *Medical Problems of Performing Artists,* 11(1): 15-19.

Ferland, G., Gardiner, L., and Lèbe-Néron, L. (1983). Analysis of the electromyographic profile of the rectus femoris and biceps femoris during the demi-plie in dance. Abstract of poster presentation. *Medicine and Science in Sports and Exercise,* 15: 159.

Frankel, V., and Nordin, M. (1980). *Basic biomechanics of the skeletal system.* Philadelphia: Lea & Febiger.

Garrick, J. (1989). Anterior knee pain (chondromalacia patellae). *The Physician and Sportsmedicine,* 17(1): 75-84.

Garrick, J. (1999). Early identification of musculoskeletal complaints and injuries among female ballet students. *Journal of Dance Medicine and Science,* 3(2): 80-83.

Garrick, J., and Requa, R. (1993). Ballet injuries: An analysis of epidemiology and financial outcome. *American Journal of Sports Medicine,* 21(4): 586-590.

Garrick, J., and Requa, R. (1994). Turnout and training in dance. *Medical Problems of Performing Artists,* 9(2): 43-49.

Gillquist, J., and Messner, K. (1999). Anterior cruciate ligament reconstruction and the long term incidence of gonarthrosis. *Sports Medicine,* 27: 143-156.

Grabiner, M., Koh, T., and Draganich, L. (1994). Neuromechanics of the patellofemoral joint. *Medicine and Science in Sports and Exercise,* 26(1): 10-21.

Haffajee, D., Moritz, V., and Svantesson, G. (1972). Isometric knee extension strength as a function of joint angle, muscle length and motor unit activity. *Acta Orthopaedica Scandinavica,* 43: 138-147.

Hall, S.J. (1999). *Basic biomechanics.* Boston: McGraw-Hill.

Hall-Craggs, E.C.B. (1985). *Anatomy as a basis for clinical medicine.* Baltimore: Urban & Schwarzenberg.

Hamill, J., and Knutzen, K. (1995). *Biomechanical basis of human movement.* Philadelphia: Lippincott Williams & Wilkins.

Hamilton, L., Hamilton, W., Warren, M., Keller, K., and Molnar, M. (1997). Factors contributing to the attrition rate in elite ballet students. *Journal of Dance Medicine and Science,* 1(4): 131-138.

Hamilton, W., Hamilton, L., Marshall, P., and Molnar, M. (1992). A profile of the musculoskeletal characteristics of elite professional ballet dancers. *American Journal of Sports Medicine,* 20(3): 267-273.

Hewett, T., Riccobene, J., Lindenfeld, T., and Noyes, E. (1999). The effect of neuromuscular training on the incidence of knee injury in female athletes: A prospective study. *American Journal of Sports Medicine,* 27(6): 699-706.

Hopkins, J., Ingersoll, C., Krause, B., Edwards, J., and Cordova, M. (2001). Effect of knee joint effusion on quadriceps and soleus motoneuron pool excitability. *Medicine and Science in Sports and Exercise,* 33(1): 123-126.

Hungerford, D., and Barry, M. (1979). Biomechanics of the patellofemoral joint. *Clinical Orthopaedics,* 144: 9-15.

Hurley, M., Jones, D., and Newham, D. (1994). Arthrogenic quadriceps inhibition and rehabilitation of patients with extensive traumatic knee injuries. *Clinical Science,* 86: 305-310.

Insall, J., Bullough, P., and Burstein, A. (1979). Proximal "tube" realignment of the patella for chondromalacia patella. *Clinics in Orthopaedics and Related Research,* 144: 63-69.

Ireland, M. (2000). Proprioception and neuromuscular control related to the female athlete. In S. Lephart and F. Fu (eds.), *Proprioception and neuromuscular control in joint stability* (pp. 291-297). Champaign, IL: Human Kinetics.

Irrgang, J. (1993). Modern trends in anterior cruciate ligament rehabilitation: Nonoperative and postoperative management. *Clinics in Sports Medicine,* 12(4): 797-813.

Irrgang, J., and Neri, R. (2000). The rationale for open and closed kinematic chain activities for restoration of proprioception and neuromuscular control following injury. In S. Lephart and F. Fu (eds.), *Proprioception and neuromuscular control in joint stability* (pp. 363-374). Champaign, IL: Human Kinetics.

Jenkinson, D., and Bolin, D. (2001). Knee overuse injuries in dance. *Journal of Dance Medicine and Science,* 5(1): 16-20.

Kennedy, J., Alexander, I., and Hayes, K. (1982). Nerve supply of the human knee and the functional importance. *American Journal of Sports Medicine,* 10(6): 329-335.

Khan, K., Brown, J., Way, S., Vass, N., Crichton, K., Alexander, R., Baxter, A., Butler, M., and Wark, J. (1995). Overuse injuries in classical ballet. *Sports Medicine,* 19(5): 341-357.

Khan, K., Roberts, P., Nattrass, C., Bennell, K., Mayes, W., Way, S., Brown, J., McMeeken, J., and Wark, J. (1997). Hip and ankle range of motion in elite classical ballet dancers and controls. *Clinical Journal of Sport Medicine,* 7: 181-187.

Kirkendall, D., Bergfeld, J., Calabrese, L., Lombardo, J., Street, G., and Weiker, G. (1984). Isokinetic characteristics of ballet dancers and the response to a season of ballet training. *Journal of Orthopaedic and Sports Physical Therapy,* 5(4): 207-211.

Koutedakis, Y., Agrawal, A., and Sharp, C. (1998). Isokinematic characteristics of knee flexors and extensors in male dancers, Olympic oarsmen, Olympic bobsleighers, and non-athletes. *Journal of Dance Medicine and Science,* 2(2): 63-67.

Koutedakis, Y., Khaloula, M., Pacy, P., Murphy, M., and Dunbar, G. (1997). Thigh peak torques and lower-body injuries in dancers. *Journal of Dance Medicine and Science,* 1(1): 12-15.

Kreighbaum, E., and Barthels, K. (1996). *Biomechanics: A qualitative approach for studying human movement.* 4th ed. Boston: Allyn & Bacon.

Levangie, P., and Norkin, C. (2001). *Joint structure and function.* Philadelphia: Davis.

Lieb, F., and Perry, J. (1968). Quadriceps functions. *Journal of Bone and Joint Surgery,* 50A: 1535-1538.

Liederbach, M., and Dilgen, F. (1998). A descriptive study of the mechanics and outcome of anterior cruciate ligament injuries in dancers (abstract). *Journal of Dance Medicine and Science,* 2(4): 153.

Lombard, W.P., and Abbott, F.M. (1907). The mechanical effects produced by the contraction of individual muscles of the thigh of the frog. *American Journal of Physiology,* 20: 1-60.

Loosli, A., and Herold, D. (1992). Knee rehabilitation for dancers using a Pilates-based technique. *Kinesiology and Medicine for Dance,* 14(2): 1-12.

Luke, A., and Micheli, L. (2000). Management of injuries in the young dancer. *Journal of Dance Medicine and Science,* 4(1): 6-15.

Magee, D. (1997). *Orthopedic physical assessment.* Philadelphia: Saunders.

Mercier, L.R. (1995). *Practical orthopedics.* 4th ed. St. Louis: Mosby.

Micheli, L. (1987). The traction apophysitises. *Clinics in Sports Medicine,* 6(2): 389-404.

Molnar, M., and Esterson, J. (1997). Screening students in a pre-professional ballet school. *Journal of Dance Medicine and Science,* 1(3): 118-121.

Mostardi, R. (1986). Musculoskeletal and cardiopulmonary evaluation of professional ballet dancers. In C. Shell (ed.), *The dancer as athlete: The 1984 Olympic Scientific Congress proceedings* (vol. 8, pp. 101-107). Champaign, IL: Human Kinetics.

Mostardi, R., Porterfield, J., Greenberg, B., Goldberg, B., and Lea, M. (1983). Musculoskeletal and cardiopulmonary characteristics of the professional ballet dancer. *The Physician and Sportsmedicine,* 11(12): 53-61.

Palmer, L.P., and Epler, M.E. (1990). *Clinical assessment procedures in physical therapy.* Philadelphia: Lippincott.

Perrin, D., and Shultz, S. (2000). Models for clinical research involving proprioception and neuromuscular control. In S. Lephart and F. Fu (eds.), *Proprioception and neuromuscular control in joint stability* (pp. 349-362). Champaign, IL: Human Kinetics.

Perry, J., Antonelli, D., and Ford, W. (1975). Analysis of knee-joint forces during flexed knee stance. *Journal of Bone and Joint Surgery,* 57A(7): 961-967.

Poggini, L., Losasso, S., and Iannone, S. (1999). Injuries during the dancer's growth spurt: Etiology, prevention, and treatment. *Journal of Dance Medicine and Science,* 3(2): 73-79.

Powers, C., Shellock, F., Beering, T., Garrido, D., Goldbach, R., and Molnar, T. (1999). Effect of bracing on patellar kinematics in patients with patellofemoral joint pain. *Medicine and Science in Sports and Exercise*, 31(12): 1714-1720.

Quirk, R. (1983). Ballet injuries: The Australian experience. *Clinics in Sports Medicine*, 2(3): 507-514.

Quirk, R. (1987). The dancer's knee. In A. Ryan and R. Stephens (eds.), *Dance medicine: A comprehensive guide* (pp. 177-219). Chicago: Pluribus Press.

Quirk, R. (1988). Knee injuries in classical dancers. *Medical Problems of Performing Artists*, 3(2): 52-59.

Rasch, P.J. (1989). *Kinesiology and applied anatomy*. Philadelphia: Lea & Febiger.

Rasch, P., and Burke, R. (1978). *Kinesiology and applied anatomy*. Philadelphia: Lea & Febiger.

Reid, D.C. (1988). Prevention of hip and knee injuries in ballet dancers. *Sports Medicine*, 6(5): 295-307.

Reid, D.C. (1993). The myth, mystic, and frustration of anterior knee pain. *Clinical Journal of Sports Medicine*, 3: 139-143.

Reid, D.C., Burnham, R.S., Saboe, L.A., and Kushner, S.F. (1987). Lower extremity flexibility patterns in classical ballet dancers and their correlation to lateral hip and knee injuries. *American Journal of Sports Medicine*, 15(4): 347-351.

Reider, B., Marshall, J., and Warren, R. (1981). Clinical characteristics of patellar disorders in young athletes. *American Journal of Sports Medicine*, 9(4): 270-274.

Reilly, D.J., and Martens, M. (1972). Experimental analysis of the quadriceps muscle function and patellofemoral joint reaction force for various activities. *Acta Orthopaedica Scandinavica*, 43: 126-137.

Rovere, G., Webb, L., Gristina, A., and Vogel, J. (1983). Musculoskeletal injuries in theatrical dance students. *American Journal of Sports Medicine*, 11(4): 195-198.

Roy, S., and Irvin, R. (1983). *Sports medicine: Prevention, evaluation, management, and rehabilitation*. Englewood Cliffs, NJ: Prentice Hall.

Schafle, M., Requa, R., and Garrick, J. (1990). A comparison of patterns of injury in ballet, modern and aerobic dance. In R. Solomon, S.C. Minton, and J. Solomon (eds.), *Preventing dance injuries: An interdisciplinary perspective* (pp. 1-14). Reston, VA: American Alliance for Health, Physical Education, Recreation and Dance.

Scioscia, T., Giffin, J.R., and Fu, F. (2001). Knee ligament and meniscal injuries in dancers. *Journal of Dance Medicine and Science*, 5(1): 11-15.

Sheehan, F., and Drace, J. (1999). Quantitative MR measures of three-dimensional patellar kinematics as a research and diagnostic tool. *Medicine and Science in Sports and Exercise*, 31(10): 1399-1405.

Silver, D., and Campbell, P. (1985). Arthroscopic assessment and treatment of dancers' knee injuries. *The Physician and Sportsmedicine*, 13(11): 74-82.

Smith, L., Weiss, E., and Lehmkuhl, L. (1996). *Brunnstrom's clinical kinesiology*. Philadelphia: Davis.

Soderberg, G.L. (1986). *Kinesiology: Application to pathological motion*. Baltimore: Williams & Wilkins.

Solomon, R., and Micheli, L. (1986). Technique as a consideration in modern dance injuries. *The Physician and Sportsmedicine*, 14(8): 83-90.

Stanitski, C. (1993). Combating overuse injuries: A focus on children and adolescents. *The Physician and Sportsmedicine*, 21(1): 87-106.

Suter, E., and Herzog, W. (2000). Does muscle inhibition after knee injury increase the risk of osteoarthritis? *Exercise and Sport Sciences Reviews*, 28(1): 15-18.

Teitz, C. (1990). Knee problems in dancers. In R. Solomon, S. Minton, and J. Solomon (eds.), *Preventing dance injuries: An interdisciplinary perspective* (pp. 39-73). Reston, VA: American Alliance for Health, Physical Education, Recreation and Dance.

Thomasen, E. (1982). *Diseases and injuries of ballet dancers*. Arhus, Denmark: Universitetsforlaget.

Trepman, E., Gellman, R., Solomon, R., Murthy, K., Micheli, L., and DeLuca, C. (1994). Electromyographic analysis of standing posture and demi-plie in ballet and modern dancers. *Medicine and Science in Sports and Exercise*, 26(6): 771-782.

Urbach, D., Nebelung, W., Weiler, H., and Awiszus, F. (1999). Bilateral deficit of voluntary quadriceps muscle activation after unilateral ACL tear. *Medicine and Science in Sports and Exercise*, 31(12): 1691-1696.

Weiker, G. (1988). Dance injuries: The knee, ankle, and foot. In P. Clarkson and M. Skrinar (eds.), *Science of dance training* (pp. 147-192). Champaign, IL: Human Kinetics.

Wiesler, E., Hunter, D., Martin, D., Curl, W., and Hoen, H. (1996). Ankle flexibility and injury patterns in dancers. *American Journal of Sports Medicine*, 24(6): 754-757.

Williams, J. (1974). Vastus medialis re-education in the management of chondromalacia patella. *Medical Aspects of Sports*, 16: 19-24.

Winslow, J., and Yoder, E. (1995). Patellofemoral pain in female ballet dancers: Correlation with iliotibial band tightness and tibial external rotation. *Journal of Orthopaedic and Sports Physical Therapy*, 22(1): 18-21.

Wittenbecker, N., and DiNitto, L. (1989). Successful treatment of patellofemoral dysfunction in a dancer. *Journal of Orthopaedic and Sports Physical Therapy*, 10(7): 270-273.

Worthen, L., Patten, C., and Hamill, J. (1998). A kinematic analysis of internal/external rotation at the knee joint during two ballet movements (abstract). *Journal of Dance Medicine and Science*, 2(4): 153.

Chapter 6

American Academy of Orthopaedic Surgeons. (1965). *Joint motion: Method of measuring and recording*. Chicago: American Academy of Orthopaedic Surgeons.

Basmajian, J., and DeLuca, C. (1985). *Muscles alive—Their functions revealed by electromyography*. Baltimore: Williams & Wilkins.

Baxter, D. (1994). Treatment of bunion deformity in the athlete. *Orthopedic Clinics of North America*, 25(1): 33-39.

Blackman, P. (2000). A review of chronic exertional compartment syndrome in the lower leg. *Medicine and Science in Sports and Exercise*, 32(3 Suppl.): S4-S10.

Bolin, D. (2001). Evaluation and management of stress fractures in dancers. *Journal of Dance Medicine and Science*, 5(2): 37-42.

Brodsky, A., and Khalil, M. (1986). Talar compression syndrome. *American Journal of Sports Medicine*, 14(6): 472-476.

Brown, S.E., and Clippinger, K. (1996). Rehabilitation of anterior cruciate ligament insufficiency in a dancer using the clinical reformer and a balanced body exercise method. *Work,* 7: 109-114.

Brukner, P. (2000). Exercise-related lower leg pain: An overview. *Medicine and Science in Sports and Exercise,* 32(3 Suppl.): S1-S3.

Brukner, P., Bradshaw, C., and Bennell, K. (1998). Managing common stress fractures: Let risk level guide treatment. *The Physician and Sportsmedicine,* 26(8): 39-47.

Brukner, P., Bradshaw, C., Kahn, K., White, S., and Crossley, K. (1996). Stress fractures: A review of 180 cases. *Clinical Journal of Sports Medicine,* 6(2): 86-89.

Bryk, E., and Grantham, A. (1983). Shin splints: A chronic deep posterior ischemic compartmental syndrome of the leg? *Orthopaedic Review,* 12(4): 29-40.

Burr, D. (1997). Bone, exercise, and stress fractures. *Exercise and Sport Sciences Reviews,* 25: 171-194.

Burton, P., and Amaker, B. (1994). Stress fracture of the great toe sesamoid in a ballerina: MRI appearance. *Pediatric Radiology,* 24: 37-38.

Clippinger-Robertson, K. (1991). Flexibility in different level female ballet dancers. Presented at the International Association of Dance Medicine and Science annual meeting, Baltimore, June 23.

Conti, S., and Wong, Y. (2001). Foot and ankle injuries in the dancer. *Journal of Dance Medicine and Science,* 5(2): 43-50.

Couture, C., and Karlson, K. (2002). Tibial stress injuries: Decisive diagnosis and treatment of "shin splints." *The Physician and Sportsmedicine,* 30(6): 29-36.

Cross, J., Crichton, K., Gordon, H., and Mackie, I. (1988). Peroneus brevis rupture in the absence of the peroneus longus muscle and tendon in a classical ballet dancer: A case report. *American Journal of Sports Medicine,* 16(6): 677-678.

Devita, P., and Skelly, W. (1992). Effect of landing stiffness on joint kinetics and energetics in the lower extremity. *Medicine and Science in Sports and Exercise,* 24(1): 108-115.

DiFiori, J. (1999). Stress fracture of the proximal fibula in a young soccer player: A case report and a review of the literature. *Medicine and Science in Sports and Exercise,* 31(7): 926-928.

Drez, D., Young, J., Johnston, R., and Parker, W. (1980). Metatarsal stress fractures. *American Journal of Sports Medicine,* 8(2): 123-125.

Dufek, J., and Bates, B. (1990). The evaluation and prediction of impact forces during landings. *Medicine and Science in Sports and Exercise,* 22(3): 370-377.

Dyal, C., and Thompson, F. (1997). The foot and ankle. In G. Scuderi, P. McCann, and P. Bruno (eds.), *Sports medicine: Principles of primary care* (pp. 386-412). St. Louis: Mosby.

Eils, E., and Rosenbaum, D. (2001). A multi-station proprioceptive exercise program in patients with ankle instability. *Medicine and Science in Sports and Exercise,* 33(12): 1991-1998.

Ende, L., and Wickstrom, J. (1982). Ballet injuries. *The Physician and Sportsmedicine,* 10(7): 101-118.

Femino, J., Trepman, E., Chisholm, K., and Razzano, L. (2000). The role of the flexor hallucis longus and peroneus longus in the stabilization of the ballet foot. *Journal of Dance Medicine and Science,* 4(3): 86-89.

Fernández-Palazzi, F., Rivas, S., and Mujica, P. (1990). Achilles tendinitis in ballet dancers. *Clinical Orthopaedics and Related Research,* 257 (Aug.): 257-261.

Fiolkowski, P., and Bauer, J. (1997). The effects of different dance surfaces on plantar pressures. *Journal of Dance Medicine and Science,* 1(2): 62-66.

Fitt, S. (1990). Strengthening and stretching the muscles of the ankle and tarsus to prevent common dance injuries. In R. Solomon, S.C. Minton, and J. Solomon (eds.), *Preventing dance injuries: An interdisciplinary perspective* (pp. 223-259). Reston, VA: American Alliance for Health, Physical Education, Recreation and Dance.

Fond, D. (1983). Flexor hallucis longus tendinitis—a case of mistaken identity and posterior impingement syndrome in dancers: Evaluation and management. *Journal of Orthopaedic and Sports Physical Therapy,* 5(4): 204-206.

Frankel, V., and Nordin, M. (1980). *Basic biomechanics of the skeletal system.* Philadelphia: Lea & Febiger.

Frey, C., and Shereff, M. (1988). Tendon injuries about the ankle in athletes. *Clinics in Sports Medicine,* 7(1): 103-118.

Gans, A. (1985). The relationship of heel contact in ascent and descent from jumps to the incidence of shin splints in ballet dancers. *Physical Therapy,* 65(8): 1192-1196.

Garrick, J. (1999). Early identification of musculoskeletal complaints and injuries among female ballet students. *Journal of Dance Medicine and Science,* 3(2): 80-83.

Garrick, J., and Requa, R. (1988). The epidemiology of foot and ankle injuries in sports. *Clinics in Sports Medicine,* 7(1): 29-36.

Garrick, J., and Requa, R. (1997). The relationship between age and sex and ballet injuries. *Medical Problems of Performing Artists,* 12(3): 79-82.

Garth, W. (1981). Flexor hallucis tendinitis in a ballet dancer. *Journal of Bone and Joint Surgery,* 63A(9): 1489.

Geary, S., and Kelly, M. (1997). The leg. In G. Scuderi, P. McCann, and P. Bruno (eds.), *Sports medicine: Principles of primary care* (pp. 376-385). St. Louis: Mosby.

Gehlsen, G., and Seger, A. (1980). Selected measures of angular displacement, strength, and flexibility in subjects with and without shin splints. *Research Quarterly,* 51(3): 478-485.

Goodman, P., Heaslet, M., Pagliano, J., and Rubin, B. (1985). Stress fracture diagnosis by computer-assisted thermography. *The Physician and Sportsmedicine,* 13(4): 114-132.

Hall, S.J. (1999). *Basic biomechanics.* Boston: McGraw-Hill.

Hall-Craggs, E.C.B. (1985). *Anatomy as a basis for clinical medicine.* Baltimore: Urban & Schwarzenberg.

Hamill, J., and Knutzen, K. (1995). *Biomechanical basis of human movement.* Philadelphia: Lippincott Williams & Wilkins.

Hamilton, L., Hamilton, W., Warren, M., Keller, K., and Molnar, M. (1997). Factors contributing to the attrition rate in elite ballet students. *Journal of Dance Medicine and Science,* 1(4): 131-138.

Hamilton, N., and Luttgens, K. (2002). *Kinesiology: Scientific basis of human motion.* Boston: McGraw-Hill.

Hamilton, W. (1982). The dancer's ankle. *Emergency Medicine,* May 30: 42-49.

Hamilton, W. (1988). Foot and ankle injuries in dancers. *Clinics in Sports Medicine,* 7(1): 143-173.

Hamilton, W. (1991). Orthopaedic aspects of dance medicine. In L. Micheli, R. Solomon, and J. Solomon (eds.), *Soviet-American dance medicine: Proceedings of the 1990 Glasnost Dance Medicine Conference and Workshops* (pp. 16-20). Reston, VA: American Alliance for Health, Physical Education, Recreation and Dance.

Hamilton, W., Geppert, M., and Thompson, F. (1996). Pain in the posterior aspect of the ankle in dancers. *Journal of Bone and Joint Surgery,* 78A(10): 1491-1500.

Hamilton, W., Hamilton, L., Marshall, P., and Molnar, M. (1992). A profile of the musculoskeletal characteristics of elite professional ballet dancers. *American Journal of Sports Medicine,* 20(3): 267-273.

Hardaker, W. (1989). Foot and ankle injuries in classical ballet dancers. *Orthopedic Clinics of North America,* 20(4): 621-627.

Hardaker, W., Colosimo, A., Malone, T., and Meyers, M. (1988). Ankle sprains in theatrical dancers. *Medical Problems of Performing Artists,* Dec.: 146-150.

Hardaker, W., and Moorman, C. (1986). Foot and ankle injuries in dance and athletics: Similarities and differences. In C. Shell (ed.), *The dancer as athlete: The 1984 Olympic Scientific Congress proceedings* (vol. 8, pp. 31-41). Champaign, IL: Human Kinetics.

Harrington, T., Cracr, M., Crichton, K., Racog, D., and Anderson, I. (1993). Overuse ballet injury of the base of the second metatarsal: A diagnostic problem. *American Journal of Sports Medicine,* 21(4): 591-598.

Henderson, J., Brown, S., Price, S., and Darr, N. (1993). Foot pressures during a common ballet jump in standing and supine positions. *Medical Problems of Performing Artists,* 8(4): 126-131.

Hershman, E., and Mailly, T. (1990). Stress fractures. *Clinics in Sports Medicine,* 9(1): 183-214.

Hertel, J., Denegar, C., Monroe, M., and Stokes, W. (1999). Talocrural and subtalar joint instability after lateral ankle sprain. *Medicine and Science in Sports and Exercise,* 31(11): 1501-1508.

Hintermann, B. (1999). Biomechanics of the unstable ankle joint and clinical implications. *Medicine and Science in Sports and Exercise,* 31(7 Suppl.): S459-S469.

Hockenbury, R. (1999). Forefoot problems in athletes. *Medicine and Science in Sports and Exercise* 31(7 Suppl.): S448-S449.

Hockney, R. (1999). Forefoot problems in athletes. *Medicine and Science in Sports and Exercise,* 31(7 Suppl.): S448-S458.

Howse, J. (1983). Disorders of the great toe in dancers. *Clinics in Sports Medicine,* 2(3): 499-505.

Howse, J., and Hancock, S. (1988). *Dance technique and injury prevention.* New York: Theatre Arts Books/Routledge.

Hughes, L. (1985). Biomechanical analysis of the foot and ankle for predisposition to developing stress fractures. *Journal of Orthopaedic and Sports Physical Therapy,* 7(3): 96-101.

Hutchinson, M., Cahoon, S., and Atkins, T. (1998). Chronic leg pain: Putting the diagnostic pieces together. *The Physician and Sportsmedicine,* 26(7): 37-46.

Jorgensen, U. (1985). Achillodynia and loss of heel pad shock absorbency. *American Journal of Sports Medicine,* 13(2): 128-132.

Kadel, N., Micheli, L., and Solomon, R. (2000). Os trigonum impingement syndrome in dancers. *Journal of Dance Medicine and Science,* 4(3): 99-102.

Kadel, N., Teitz, C., and Kronmal, R. (1992). Stress fractures in ballet dancers. *American Journal of Sports Medicine,* 20(4): 446-449.

Karpovich, P.V., and Manfredi, T.G. (1973). Mechanism at rising on the toes. *Research Quarterly,* 42: 395-404.

Khan, K., Brown, J., Way, S., Vass, N., Crichton, K., Alexander, R., Baxter, A., Butler, M., and Wark, J. (1995). Overuse injuries in classical ballet. *Sports Medicine,* 19(5): 341-357.

Khan, K., Gelber, N., Slater, K., and Wark, J. (1997). Dislocated tibialis posterior tendon in a classical ballet dancer. *Journal of Dance Medicine and Science,* 1(4): 160-162.

Khan, K., Roberts, P., Nattrass, C., Bennell, K., Mayes, W., Way, S., Brown, J., McMeeken, J., and Wark, J. (1997). Hip and ankle range of motion in elite classical ballet dancers and controls. *Clinical Journal of Sports Medicine,* 7: 174-179.

Kleiger, B. (1987). Foot and ankle injuries in dancers. In A. Ryan and R. Stephens (eds.), *Dance medicine: A comprehensive guide* (pp. 116-134). Chicago: Pluribus Press.

Konradsen, L., and Ravin, M. (1990). Ankle instability caused by prolonged peroneal reaction time. *Acta Orthopaedica Scandinavica,* 61: 388-390.

Korkola, M., and Amendola, A. (2001). Exercise-induced leg pain. *The Physician and Sportsmedicine,* 29(6): 35-50.

Kortebein, P., Kaufman, K., Basford, J., and Stuart, M. (2000). Medial tibial stress syndrome. *Medicine and Science in Sports and Exercise,* 32(3 Suppl.): S27-S33.

Kravitz, S., Murgia, C., Huber, S., Fink, K., Shaffer, M., and Varela, L. (1986). Bunion deformity and the forces generated around the great toe: A biomechanical approach to analysis of pointe dance, classical ballet. In C. Shell (ed.), *The dancer as athlete: The 1984 Olympic Scientific Congress proceedings* (vol. 8, pp. 213-225). Champaign, IL: Human Kinetics.

Kreighbaum, E., and Barthels, K. (1996). *Biomechanics: A qualitative approach for studying human movement.* 4th ed. Needham Heights, MA: Allyn & Bacon.

Lane, S. (1990). Severe ankle sprains: Treatment with an ankle-foot orthosis. *The Physician and Sportsmedicine,* 16(11): 43-51.

Leach, R., and Corbett, M. (1979). Anterior tibial compartment syndrome in soccer players. *American Journal of Sports Medicine,* 7(4): 258-259.

Leanderson, J., Eriksson, E., Nilsson, C., and Wykman, A. (1996). Proprioception in classical ballet dancers: A prospective study of the influence of an ankle sprain on proprioception in the ankle joint. *American Journal of Sports Medicine,* 24(3): 370-374.

Levangie, P., and Norkin, C. (2001). *Joint structure and function.* Philadelphia: Davis.

Liederbach, M. (2000). General considerations for guiding dance injury rehabilitation. *Journal of Dance Medicine and Science,* 4(2): 54-65.

Liederbach, M., and Hiebert, R. (1997). The relationship between eccentric and concentric measures of ankle strength and functional equinus in classical dancers. *Journal of Dance Medicine and Science,* 1(2): 56-61.

Lokiec, F., Siev-Ner, I., and Pritsch, M. (1991). Chronic compartment syndrome of both feet. *Journal of Bone and Joint Surgery,* 73B(1): 178-179.

Lundon, K., Melcher, L., and Bray, K. (1999). Stress fractures in ballet: A twenty-five year review. *Journal of Dance Medicine and Science,* 3(3): 101-107.

Magee, D. (1997). *Orthopedic physical assessment.* Philadelphia: Saunders.

Malone, T., and Hardaker, W. (1990). Rehabilitation of foot and ankle injuries in ballet dancers. *Journal of Orthopaedic and Sports Physical Therapy,* 11(8): 355-361.

Marotta, J., and Micheli, L. (1992). Os trigonum impingement in dancers. *American Journal of Sports Medicine,* 20(5): 533-536.

Marshall, P. (1988). The rehabilitation of overuse foot injuries in athletes and dancers. *Clinics in Sports Medicine,* 7(1): 176-191.

Marshall, P., and Hamilton, W. (1992). Cuboid subluxation in ballet dancers. *American Journal of Sports Medicine,* 20(2): 169-175.

Martens, M., Backaert, M., Vermaut, G., and Mulier, J. (1984). Chronic leg pain in athletes due to a recurrent compartment syndrome. *American Journal of Sports Medicine,* 12(2): 148-151.

Martire, J. (1994). Differentiating stress fracture from periostitis: The finer points of bone scans. *The Physician and Sportsmedicine,* 22(10): 71-81.

Matheson, G., Clement, D., McKenzie, D., Taunton, J., Lloyd-Smith, D., and Macintyre, J. (1987). Stress fractures in athletes, a study of 320 cases. *American Journal of Sports Medicine,* 15(1): 46-58.

Mayers, L., Judelson, D., and Bronner, S. (2003). The prevalence of injury among tap dancers. *Journal of Dance Medicine and Science,* 7(4): 121-125.

McCarthy, P. (1989). Managing bursitis in the athlete: An overview. *The Physician and Sportsmedicine,* 17(11): 116-125.

McCrory, J., Martin, D., Lowery, R., Cannon, D., Curl, W., Read, H., Hunter, D., Craven, T., and Messier, S. (1999). Etiologic factors associated with Achilles tendinitis in runners. *Medicine and Science in Sports and Exercise,* 31(10): 1374-1381.

Mercier, L.R. (1995). *Practical orthopedics.* 4th ed. St. Louis: Mosby.

Michael, R., and Holder, L. (1985). The soleus syndrome: A cause of medial tibia stress (shin splints). *American Journal of Sports Medicine,* 13(2): 87-94.

Micheli, L. (1987). The traction apophysitises. *Clinics in Sports Medicine,* 6(2): 389-404.

Micheli, L., and Solomon, R. (1990). Stress fractures in dancers. In R. Solomon, S. Minton, and J. Solomon (eds.), *Preventing dance injuries: An interdisciplinary perspective* (pp. 133-153). Reston, VA: American Alliance for Health, Physical Education, Recreation and Dance.

Molnar, M., and Esterson, J. (1997). Screening students in a pre-professional ballet school. *Journal of Dance Medicine and Science,* 1(3): 118-121.

Moore, K., and Agur, A. (1995). *Essential clinical anatomy.* Baltimore: Williams & Wilkins.

Moore, K., and Dalley, A. (1999). *Clinically oriented anatomy.* Philadelphia: Lippincott Williams & Wilkins.

Nawoczenski, D., Owen, M., Ecker, M., Altman, B., and Epler, M. (1985). Objective evaluation of peroneal response to sudden inversion stress. *Journal of Orthopaedic and Sports Physical Therapy,* 7(3): 107-109.

Nigg, B., Nursae, M., and Stefanyshyn, D. (1999). Shoe inserts and orthotics for sport and physical activities. *Medicine and Science in Sports and Exercise,* 31(7 Suppl.): S421-S428.

Norris, R. (1990). Some common foot and ankle injuries in dancers. In R. Solomon, S. Minton, and J. Solomon (eds.), *Preventing dance injuries: An interdisciplinary perspective* (pp. 293-304). Reston, VA: American Alliance for Health, Physical Education, Recreation and Dance.

O'Malley, M., Hamilton, W., Munyak, J., and De Franco, M. (1996). Stress fractures at the base of the second metatarsal in ballet dancers. *Foot and Ankle International,* 17(2): 89-94.

Omey, M., and Micheli, L. (1999). Foot and ankle problems in the young athlete. *Medicine and Science in Sports and Exercise,* 31(7 Suppl.): S470-S486.

Potter, P., Jones, I., and Math, B. (1996). The effect of plantar fasciitis on ground reaction forces in Scottish Highland dancers. *Medical Problems of Performing Artists,* 11: 51-56.

Quirk, R. (1983). Ballet injuries: The Australian experience. *Clinics in Sports Medicine,* 2(3): 507-514.

Rasch, P.J. (1989). *Kinesiology and applied anatomy.* Philadelphia: Lea & Febiger.

Robbins, S., and Hanna, A. (1987). Running-related injury prevention through barefoot adaptations. *Medicine and Science in Sports and Exercise,* 19(2): 148-156.

Roberts, W. (1999). Plantar fascia injection. *The Physician and Sportsmedicine,* 27(9): 101-102.

Rovere, G., Clarke, T., Yates, C., and Burley, K. (1988). Retrospective comparison of taping and ankle stabilizers in preventing ankle injuries. *American Journal of Sports Medicine,* 16: 228-233.

Ryan, A., and Stephens, R. (eds.). (1987). *Dance medicine: A comprehensive guide.* Chicago: Pluribus Press.

Safran, M., Benedetti, R., Bartolozzi III, A., and Mandelbaum, B. (1999). Lateral ankle sprains: A comprehensive review. Part I: Etiology, pathoanatomy, histopathogenesis, and diagnosis. *Medicine and Science in Sports and Exercise,* 31(7 Suppl.): S429-S437.

Safran, M., Zachazewski, J., Benedetti, R., Bartolozzi III, A., and Mandelbaum, B. (1999). Lateral ankle sprains: A comprehensive review. Part 2: Treatment and rehabilitation with an emphasis on the athlete. *Medicine and Science in Sports and Exercise,* 31(7 Suppl.): S438-S447.

Salter-Pedersen, M., and Wilmerding, V. (1998). Injury profiles of student and professional flamenco dancers. *Journal of Dance Medicine and Science,* 2(3): 108-114.

Sammarco, G. (1980). Biomechanics of the foot. In V. Frankel and M. Nordin (eds.), *Basic biomechanics of the skeletal system* (pp. 193-220). Philadelphia: Lea & Febiger.

Sammarco, G. (1982). The dancer's forefoot. *Emergency Medicine,* May 30: 49-57.

Sammarco, G., and Miller, E. (1979). Partial rupture of the flexor hallucis longus tendon in classical ballet dancers. *Journal of Bone and Joint Surgery,* 61A(1): 149-150.

Sammarco, G., and Tablante, E. (1997). Lateral ankle instability in ballet dancers. *Journal of Dance Medicine and Science,* 1(4): 156-159.

Schafle, M., Requa, R., and Garrick, J. (1990). A comparison of patterns of injury in ballet, modern and aerobic dance. In R. Solomon, S.C. Minton, and J. Solomon (eds.), *Preventing dance injuries: An interdisciplinary perspective* (pp. 1-14). Reston, VA: American Alliance for Health, Physical Education, Recreation and Dance.

Scheller, A., Kasser, J., and Quigley, T. (1980). Tendon injuries about the ankle. *Orthopaedic Clinics of North America,* 11(4): 631-641.

Schon, L., and DeStefano, A. (1999). Evaluation and treatment of posterior tibialis tendinitis: A case report and treatment protocol. *Journal of Dance Medicine and Science,* 3(1): 24-27.

Scranton, P., Pedegana, L., and Whitesel, J. (1982). Gait analysis: Alterations in support phase forces using supportive devices. *American Journal of Sports Medicine,* 10(1): 6-11.

Shea, M., and Fields, K. (2002). Plantar fasciitis: Prescribing effective treatments. *The Physician and Sportsmedicine,* 30(7): 21-25.

Siev-Ner, I. (2000). Common overuse injuries of the foot and ankle in dancers. *Journal of Dance Medicine and Science,* 4(2): 49-53.

Smith, L., Weiss, E., and Lehmkuhl, L. (1996). *Brunnstrom's clinical kinesiology.* Philadelphia: Davis.

Smith, W., Winn, F., and Parette, R. (1986). Comparative study using four modalities in shinsplint treatments. *Journal of Orthopaedic and Sports Physical Therapy,* 8(2): 77-80.

Soderberg, G. (1986). *Kinesiology: Application to pathological motion.* Baltimore: Williams & Wilkins.

Solomon, R., and Micheli, L. (1986). Technique as a consideration in modern dance injuries. *The Physician and Sportsmedicine,* 14(8): 83-90.

Solomon, R., Micheli, L., and Ireland, M. (1993). Physiological assessment to determine readiness for pointe work in ballet students. *Impulse,* 1: 21-38.

Sommer, H., and Vallentyne, S. (1995). Effect of foot posture on the incidence of medial tibial stress syndrome. *Medicine and Science in Sports and Exercise,* 27(6): 800-804.

Somogyi, D. (2001). Lower leg injuries in dance. *Journal of Dance Medicine and Science,* 5(1): 21-26.

Spilken, T. (1990). *The dancer's foot book.* Princeton, NJ: Princeton Book.

Taube, R., and Wadsworth, L. (1993). Managing tibial stress fractures. *The Physician and Sportsmedicine,* 21(4): 123-130.

Taunton, J., Clement, D., and Webber, D. (1981). Lower extremity stress fractures in athletes. *The Physician and Sportsmedicine,* 9(1): 77-86.

Teitz, C. (1986). First aid, immediate care, and rehabilitation of knee and ankle injuries in dancers and athletes. In C. Shell (ed.), *The dancer as athlete: The 1984 Olympic Scientific Congress proceedings* (vol. 8, pp. 73-81). Champaign, IL: Human Kinetics.

Teitz, C., Harrington, R., and Wiley, H. (1985). Pressures on the foot in pointe shoes. *Foot and Ankle,* 5(5): 216-221.

Thacker, S., Gilchrist, J., Stroup, D., and Kimsey, C. (2002). The prevention of shin splints in sports: A systematic review of literature. *Medicine and Science in Sports and Exercise,* 34(1): 32-40.

Tropp, H., Askling, C., and Gillquist, J. (1985). Prevention of ankle sprains. *American Journal of Sports Medicine,* 13(4): 259-262.

Tudisco, C., and Puddu, G. (1984). Stenosing tenosynovitis of the flexor hallucis longus tendon in a classical ballet dancer: A case report. *American Journal of Sports Medicine,* 12(5): 403-404.

Van Hal, M., Keene, J., Lange, T., and Clancy, W. (1982). Stress fractures of the great toe sesamoids. *American Journal of Sports Medicine,* 10(2): 122-128.

Warren, J. (1983). Visco-elastic orthotics: Sorbothane II. *The Journal of Orthopaedic and Sports Physical Therapy,* Winter: 174-175.

Weiker, G. (1988). Dance injuries: The knee, ankle, and foot. In P. Clarkson and M. Skrinar (eds.), *Science of dance training* (pp. 147-192). Champaign, IL: Human Kinetics.

Whiting, W., and Zernicke, R. (1998). *Biomechanics of musculoskeletal injury.* Champaign, IL: Human Kinetics.

Wiesler, E., Hunter, D., Martin, D., Curl, W., and Hoen, H. (1996). Ankle flexibility and injury patterns in dancers. *American Journal of Sports Medicine,* 24(6): 754-757.

Wilmerding, V., Pedersen, E., Encinias, J., and Encinias, D. (1998). Plantar flexion and dorsiflexion strength in ballet and flamenco dancers (abstract). *Journal of Dance Medicine and Science,* 2(4): 153.

Yakut, Y., Otman, S., Livanelioglu, A., and Uygur, F. (1997). Evaluation of the foot arches in ballet dancers. *Journal of Dance Medicine and Science,* 1(4): 139-142.

Chapter 7

American Academy of Orthopaedic Surgeons. (1965). *Joint motion: Method of measuring and recording.* Chicago: American Academy of Orthopaedic Surgeons.

Barclay, L. (2002). Surgery better than splinting in carpal tunnel syndrome. *Medscape Medical News.* www.medscape.com/viewarticle/441279.

Barclay, L. (2004). Brace therapy, physical therapy each play a role in tennis elbow treatment. *Medscape Medical News.* www.medscape.com/viewarticle/472590.

Bartlett, L., Storey, M., and Simons, B. (1989). Measurement of upper extremity torque production and its relationship to throwing speed in the competitive athlete. *American Journal of Sports Medicine,* 17(1): 89-91.

Basmajian, J., and DeLuca, C. (1985). *Muscles alive—Their functions revealed by electromyography.* Baltimore: Williams & Wilkins.

Brindle, T., Nyland, J., Shapiro, R., Caborn, D., and Stine, R. (1999). Shoulder proprioception: Latent muscle reaction times. *Medicine and Science in Sports and Exercise,* 31(10): 1394-1398.

Briner, W., and Benjamin, H. (1999). Volleyball injuries: Managing acute and overuse disorders. *The Physician and Sportsmedicine,* 27(3): 48.

Brunnstrom, S. (1972). *Clinical kinesiology.* Philadelphia: Davis.

Caillet, R. (1996). *Soft tissue pain and disability.* Philadelphia: Davis.

Carfango, D., and Ellenbecker, T. (2002). Osteoarthritis of the glenohumeral joint: Nonsurgical treatment options. *The Physician and Sportsmedicine,* 30(4): 19-30.

Carter, A., and Erickson, S. (1999). Proximal biceps tendon rupture: Primarily an injury of middle age. *The Physician and Sportsmedicine,* 27(6): 95.

Cavallo, R., and Speer, K. (1998). Shoulder instability and impingement in throwing athletes. *Medicine and Science in Sports and Exercise,* 30(4 Suppl.): S18-S25.

Ciccotti, M., and Charlton, W. (2001). Epicondylitis in the athlete. *Clinic in Sports Medicine,* 20(1): 77-93.

Clearman, R. (1990). Rehabilitation of a dancer with recurrent upper back and shoulder pain: Success with neuromuscular re-education. *Medical Problems of Performing Artists,* Sept.: 113-117.

Cools, M., Witvrouw, E., Declercq, G., Danneels, L., and Cambier, D. (2003). Scapular muscle recruitment patterns: Trapezius muscle latency with and without impingement symptoms. *American Journal of Sports Medicine,* 31: 542-549.

DePalma, M., and Johnson, E. (2003). Detecting and treating shoulder impingement syndrome: The role of scapulothoracic dyskinesis. *The Physician and Sportsmedicine*, 31(7): 25-32.

Duda, M. (1985). Prevention and treatment of throwing-arm injuries. *The Physician and Sportsmedicine*, 13(6): 181-187.

English, C., Maclaren, W., Court-Brown, C., Hughes, S., Porter, R., Wallace, W., Graves, R., Pethick, A., and Soutar, C. (1995). Relations between upper limb soft tissue disorders and repetitive movements at work. *American Journal of Industrial Medicine*, 27: 75-90.

Esenkaya, I., Tuygun, H., and Turkmen, M. (2000). Bilateral anterior shoulder dislocation in a weight lifter. *The Physician and Sportsmedicine*, 28(3): 93-100.

Frankel, V., and Nordin, M. (1980). *Basic biomechanics of the skeletal system*. Philadelphia: Lea & Febiger.

Gerhardt, J., and Rippstein, J. (1990). *Measuring and recording of joint motion: Instrumentation and techniques*. Toronto: Hogrefe & Huber.

Goldman, R., and McCann, P. (1997). The elbow and forearm. In G. Scuderi, P. McCann, and P. Bruno (eds.), *Sports medicine: Principles of primary care* (pp. 242-264). St. Louis: Mosby.

Greenfield, B., Donatelli, R., Wooden, M., and Wilkes, J. (1990). Isokinetic evaluation of shoulder rotational strength between the plane of scapula and the frontal plane. *American Journal of Sports Medicine*, 18(2): 124-127.

Greipp, J. (1985). Swimmer's shoulder: The influence of flexibility and weight training. *The Physician and Sportsmedicine*, 13(8): 92-105.

Groppel, J., and Nirschl, R. (1986). A mechanical and electromyographic analysis of the effects of various counterforce braces on the tennis player. *American Journal of Sports Medicine*, 14(3): 195-200.

Gruchow, H., and Pelletier, D. (1979). An epidemiological study of tennis elbow. *American Journal of Sports Medicine*, 7(4): 234-238.

Hall, S. (1999). *Basic biomechanics*. Boston: McGraw-Hill.

Hall-Craggs, E.C.B. (1985). *Anatomy as a basis for clinical medicine*. Baltimore: Urban & Schwarzenberg.

Hamill, J., and Knutzen, K. (1995). *Biomechanical basis of human movement*. Philadelphia: Lippincott Williams & Wilkins.

Hamilton, N., and Luttgens, K. (2002). *Kinesiology: Scientific basis of human motion*. Boston: McGraw-Hill.

Henry, J. (1984). How I manage dislocated shoulder. *The Physician and Sportsmedicine*, 12(9): 65-69.

Hintermeister, R., Lange, G., Shulteis, J., Bey, M., and Hawkins, R. (1998). Electromyographic activity and applied load during shoulder rehabilitation exercise using elastic resistance. *American Journal of Sports Medicine*, 26(2): 210-220.

Horrigan, J., Shellock, F., Mink, J., and Deutsch, A. (1999). Magnetic resonance imaging evaluation of muscle usage associated with three exercises for rotator cuff rehabilitation. *Medicine and Science in Sports and Exercise*, 31(10): 1361-1366.

Howell, S., and Galinat, B. (1989). The glenoid-labral socket: A constrained articular surface. *Clinical Orthopaedics*, 243(June): 122-125.

Howse, J., and Hancock, S. (1988). *Dance technique and injury prevention*. New York: Theatre Arts Books/Routledge.

Johnson, J., Gauvin, J., and Fredericson, M. (2003). Swimming biomechanics and injury prevention: New stroke techniques and medical considerations. *The Physician and Sportsmedicine*, 31(1): 41-46.

Kammer, S., Young, C., and Niedfeldt, M. (1999). Swimming injuries and illness. *The Physician and Sportsmedicine*, 27(4): 51.

Kao, S. (2003). Carpal tunnel syndrome as an occupational disease. *Journal of the American Board of Family Practice*, 16(6): 533-542.

Kibler, W.B., McMullen, J., and Uhl, T.L. (2001). Shoulder rehabilitation strategies, guidelines and practice. *Orthopaedic Clinics of North America*, 32(3): 621-636.

Kraemer, W., and Fleck, S. (2005). *Strength training for young athletes*. 2nd ed. Champaign, IL: Human Kinetics.

Kreighbaum, E., and Barthels, K. (1996). *Biomechanics: A qualitative approach for studying human movement*. 4th ed. Boston: Allyn & Bacon.

Kulund, D., McCue, F., Rockwell, D., and Gieck, J. (1979). Tennis injuries: Prevention and treatment. *American Journal of Sports Medicine*, 7(4): 249-253.

Levine, W., Arroyo, J., Pollock, R., Flatow, E., and Bigliani, L. (2000). Open revision stabilization surgery for recurrent anterior glenohumeral instability. *American Journal of Sports Medicine*, 28(2): 156-159.

Levine, W., and Flatow, E. (2000). The pathology of shoulder instability. *The American Journal of Sports Medicine*, 28(6): 910-917.

Lyons, P., and Orwin, J. (1998). Rotator cuff tendinopathy and subacromial impingement syndrome. *Medicine and Science in Sports and Exercise*, 30(4 Suppl.): S12-S17.

Magee, D. (1997). *Orthopedic physical assessment*. Philadelphia: Saunders.

McCarthy, P. (1989). Managing bursitis in the athlete: An overview. *The Physician and Sportsmedicine*, 17(11): 115-125.

McClure, P., Bialker, J., Neff, N., Williams, G., and Karduna, A. (2004). Shoulder function and 3-dimensional kinematics in people with shoulder impingement syndrome before and after a 6 week exercise program. *Journal of Orthopaedic and Sports Physical Therapy*, 32: A-8.

Mercier, L.R. (1995). *Practical orthopedics*. 4th ed. St. Louis: Mosby.

Metz, J. (1999). Managing golf injuries. *The Physician and Sportsmedicine*, 27(7): 41-58.

Millar, A. (1987). Injuries to the neck and upper extremity. In A. Ryan and R. Stephens (eds.), *Dance medicine: A comprehensive guide* (pp. 267-273). Chicago: Pluribus Press.

Moore, K., and Agur, A. (1995). *Essential clinical anatomy*. Baltimore: Williams & Wilkins.

Moseley, J., Jobe, F., Pink, M., Perry, J., and Tibone, J. (1992). EMG analysis of the scapular muscles during a shoulder rehabilitation program. *American Journal of Sports Medicine*, 20(2): 128-134.

Moynes, D., Perry, J., Antonelli, D., and Jobe, F. (1986). Electromyography and motion analysis of the upper extremity in sports. *Physical Therapy*, 66(12): 1905-1911.

Myers, J. (1999). Conservative management of shoulder impingement syndrome in the athletic population. *Journal of Sport Rehabilitation*, 8(3): 230-252.

Neer, C. (1983). Impingement lesions. *Clinics in Orthopaedics and Related Research*, 173: 70-77.

Nelson, B., and Arciero, R. (2000). Arthroscopic management of glenohumeral instability. *American Journal of Sports Medicine*, 28(4): 602-613.

Nieman, D. (1999). *Exercise testing and prescription.* Mountain View, CA: Mayfield.

Nirschl, R., and Kraushaar, B. (1996a). Assessment and treatment guidelines for elbow injuries. *The Physician and Sportsmedicine,* 24(5): 42.

Nirschl, R., and Kraushaar, B. (1996b). Keeping tennis elbow at arm's length: Simple, effective strengthening exercises. *The Physician and Sportsmedicine,* 24(5): 61.

Nuber, G., Jobe, F., Perry, J., Moynes, D., and Antonelli, D. (1986). Fine wire electromyography analysis of muscles of the shoulder during swimming. *American Journal of Sports Medicine,* 14(1): 7-11.

O'Connor, D., Marshall, S., and Massy-Westropp, N. (2004). Nonsurgical treatment (other than steroid injection) for carpal tunnel syndrome. *Medscape Medical News.* www.medscape.com/viewarticle/486490.

Park, M., Blaine, T., and Levine, W. (2002). Shoulder dislocation in young athletes. *The Physician and Sportsmedicine,* 30(12): 41-48.

Pearsall, A., and Speer, K. (1998). Frozen shoulder syndrome: Diagnostic and treatment strategies in the primary care setting. *Medicine and Science in Sports and Exercise,* 30(4 Suppl.): S33-S39.

Peterson, J., Bryant, C., and Peterson, S. (1995). *Strength training for women.* Champaign, IL: Human Kinetics.

Rasch, P. (1989). *Kinesiology and applied anatomy.* Philadelphia: Lea & Febiger.

Rasch, P.J., and Burke, R.K. (1978). *Kinesiology and applied anatomy.* 6th ed. Philadelphia: Lea & Febiger.

Reeves, R., Laskowski, E., and Smith, J. (1998). Weight training injuries: Part 2—Diagnosing and managing chronic conditions. *The Physician and Sportsmedicine,* 26(3): 54.

Richards, D. (1999). Injuries to the glenoid labrum: A diagnostic and treatment challenge. *The Physician and Sportsmedicine,* 27(6): 73.

Roberts, W. (2000). Lateral epicondylitis injection. *The Physician and Sportsmedicine,* 28(7): 93-94.

Rodeo, S., Suzuki, K., Yamauchi, M., Bhargava, M., and Warren, R. (1998). Analysis of collagen and elastic fibers in shoulder capsule in patients with shoulder instability. *American Journal of Sports Medicine,* 26(5): 634-643.

Rosenwasser, M., and Wilson, R. (1997). The wrist. In G. Scuderi, P. McCann, and P. Bruno (eds.), *Sports medicine: Principles of primary care* (pp. 265-287). St. Louis: Mosby.

Roy, S., and Irvin, R. (1983). *Sports medicine: Prevention, evaluation, management, and rehabilitation.* Englewood Cliffs, NJ: Prentice Hall.

Sauers, E., Borsa, P., Herling, D., and Stanley, R. (2001). Instrumental measurement of glenohumeral joint laxity and its relationship to passive range of motion and generalized joint laxity. *American Journal of Sports Medicine,* 29(2): 143-149.

Schmitz, M., and Ciullo, J. (1999). Sports medicine feature: The recognition and treatment of superior labral anterior-posterior (SLAP) lesions in the shoulder. *Medscape General Medicine,* 1(1). www.medscape.com/viewarticle/408488.

Shea, K. (2001). Shoulder instability: Updates from AAOS 2001 (abstract). American Academy of Orthopaedic Surgeons 68th annual meeting. *Sports Medicine/Pediatrics.* www.medscape.com/viewprogram/231.

Smith, L., Weiss, E., and Lehmkuhl, L. (1996). *Brunnstrom's clinical kinesiology.* Philadelphia: Davis.

Soderberg, G. (1986). *Kinesiology: Application to pathological motion.* Baltimore: Williams & Wilkins.

Steinbeck, J., and Jerosch, J. (1998). Arthroscopic transglenoid stabilization versus open anchor suturing in traumatic anterior instability of the shoulder. *American Journal of Sports Medicine,* 26(3): 373-378.

Warner, J., Micheli, L., Arslanian, L., Kennedy, J., and Kennedy, R. (1990). Patterns of flexibility, laxity, and strength in normal shoulders and shoulders with instability and impingement. *American Journal of Sports Medicine,* 18(4): 367-375.

Washington, E. (1987). A medical and sociological consideration of break dancers and pop-lockers. In A. Ryan and R. Stephens (eds.), *Dance medicine: A comprehensive guide* (pp. 281-293). Chicago: Pluribus Press.

Weldon, G. (1988). Treatment and prevention of tennis elbow. *Sports Injuries,* 1(8). Chicago: Gatorade Sports Science Institute.

Wells, K., and Luttgens, K. (1976). *Kinesiology: Scientific basis of human motion.* Philadelphia: Saunders.

Werner, A., Mueller, T., Boehm, D., and Gohlke, F. (2000). The stabilization sling for the long head of the biceps tendon in the rotator cuff interval. *American Journal of Sports Medicine,* 28(1): 28-31.

Wolf III, W. (1999). Calcific tendonitis of the shoulder: Diagnosis and simple, effective treatment. *The Physician and Sportsmedicine,* 27(9): 27.

Wolin, P., and Tarbet, J. (1997). Rotator cuff injury: Addressing overhead overuse. *The Physician and Sportsmedicine,* 25(6): 54.

Yamaguchi, K., Wolfe, I., and Bigliani, L. (1997). The shoulder. In G. Scuderi, P. McCann, and P. Bruno (eds.), *Sports medicine: Principles of primary care* (pp. 386-412). St. Louis: Mosby.

Yani, T., Hay, J., and Miller, G. (2000). Shoulder impingement in front-crawl swimming: 1. A method to identify impingement. *Medicine and Science in Sports and Exercise,* 32(1): 21-29.

Chapter 8

Adrian, M.J., and Cooper, J.M. (1989). *Biomechanics of human movement.* Indianapolis: Benchmark Press.

Asmussen, E., and Bonde-Peterson, F. (1974). Apparent efficiency and storage of elastic energy in human muscles during exercise. *Acta Physiologica Scandinavica,* 92: 537-545.

Biewener, A., and Roberts, T. (2000). Muscle and tendon contributions to force, work, and elastic energy savings: A comparative perspective. *Exercise and Sport Sciences Reviews,* 28(3): 99-107.

Bobbert, M., and Casius, R. (2005). Is the effect of a countermovement on jump height due to active state development? *Medicine and Science in Sports and Exercise,* 37(3): 440-446.

Bressel, E., and Cronin, J. (2005). The landing phase of a jump: Strategies to minimize injuries. *Journal of Physical Education, Recreation and Dance,* 76(2): 31-35.

Clarkson, P., Kennedy, T., and Flanagan, J. (1984). A study of three movements in classical ballet. *Research Quarterly for Exercise and Sport,* 55(2): 175-179.

Clippinger, K., and Novak, M. (1981). Preliminary investigation of landing from a grand jete devant. Unpublished manuscript. Seattle: University of Washington.

Dahlstrom, M., Liljedahl, M., Gierup, J., Kaijser, L., and Jansson, E. (1997). High proportion of type I fibers in thigh muscle of young dancers. *Acta Physiologica Scandinavica,* 160(1): 49-55.

Dainty, D.A., and Norman, R. (eds.). (1987). *Standardizing biomechanical testing in sport.* Champaign, IL: Human Kinetics.

Devita, P., and Skelly, W. (1992). Effect of landing stiffness on joint kinetics and energetics in the lower extremity. *Medicine and Science in Sports and Exercise,* 24(1): 108-115.

Dufek, J., and Bates, B. (1990). The evaluation and prediction of impact forces during landings. *Medicine and Science in Sports and Exercise,* 22(3): 370-377.

Elliott, B.C., and Blanksby, B.A. (1979). The synchronization of muscle activity and body segment movements during a running cycle. *Medicine and Science in Sports,* 11(4): 322-326.

Ferber, R., McClay-Davis, I., Hamill, J., Pollard, C., and McKeown, K. (2002). Kinetic variables in subjects with previous lower extremity stress fractures. *Medicine and Science in Sports and Exercise,* 34: S5.

Fitt, S.S. (1996). *Dance kinesiology.* 2nd ed. New York: Schirmer.

Golomer, E., and Fery, Y. (2001). Unilateral jump behavior in young professional female ballet dancers. *International Journal of Neuroscience,* 110: 1-7.

Grahame, R., and Jenkins, J. (1972). Joint hypermobility—Asset or liability? A study of joint mobility in ballet dancers. *Annals of the Rheumatic Diseases,* 31: 109-111.

Griner, B., Boatwright, D., and Howell, D. (2003). Plyometrics: Jump training for dancers. *The Sport Journal,* 6(3). www.thesportjournal.org.

Hall, S.J. (1999). *Basic biomechanics.* Boston: McGraw-Hill.

Hamill, J., and Knutzen, K. (1995). *Biomechanical basis of human movement.* Philadelphia: Lippincott Williams & Wilkins.

Hamilton, N., and Luttgens, K. (2002). *Kinesiology: Scientific basis of human motion.* New York: McGraw-Hill.

Harley, Y., Gibson, A., Harley, E., Lambert, M., Vaughan, C., and Noakes, T. (2002). Quadriceps strength and jumping efficiency in dancers. *Journal of Dance Medicine and Science,* 6(3): 87-94.

Hay, J. (1993). *The biomechanics of sports techniques.* Englewood Cliffs, NJ: Prentice Hall.

Hewett, T., Stroupe, A., Nance, T., and Noyes, R. (1996). Plyometric training in female athletes: Decreased impact forces and increased hamstring torques. *American Journal of Sports Medicine,* 24(6): 765-773.

Hodgson, J. (2001). *Mastering movement: The life and work of Rudolf Laban.* New York: Routledge.

Hreljac, A. (2004). Impact and overuse injuries in runners. *Medicine and Science in Sports and Exercise,* 36(5): 845-849.

Hreljac, A., Marshall, R., and Hume, P. (2000). Evaluation of lower extremity overuse injury potential in runners. *Medicine and Science in Sports and Exercise,* 32(9): 1635-1641.

Inman, V.T., Ralston, H.J., and Todd, F. (1981). *Human walking.* Baltimore: Williams & Wilkins.

Ito, A., Komi, P., Sjodin, B., Bosco, C., and Karlsson, J. (1983). Mechanical efficiency of positive work in running at different speeds. *Medicine and Science in Sports and Exercise,* 15(4): 299-306.

Jensen, C., Schultz, G., and Bangerter, B. (1983). *Applied kinesiology and biomechanics.* New York: McGraw-Hill.

Koceja, D., Burke, J., and Kamen, G. (1991). Organization of segmental reflexes in trained dancers. *International Journal of Sports Medicine,* 12(3): 285-289.

Komi, P., and Bosco, C. (1978). Utilization of stored elastic energy in leg extensor muscles by men and women. *Medicine and Science in Sports and Exercise,* 10: 261-265.

Kovacs, I., Tihanyi, J., Devita, P., Racz, L., Barrier, J., and Hortobagyi, T. (1999). Foot placement modifies kinematics and kinetics during drop jumping. *Medicine and Science in Sports and Exercise,* 31(5): 708-716.

Kram, R. (2000). Muscular force or work: What determines the metabolic energy cost of running? *Exercise and Sport Sciences Reviews,* 28(3): 138-143.

Kreighbaum, E., and Barthels, K. (1996). *Biomechanics: A qualitative approach for studying human movement.* 4th ed. Needham Heights, MA: Allyn & Bacon.

Kyrolainen, H., Belli, A., and Komi, P. (2001). Biomechanical factors affecting running economy. *Medicine and Science in Sports and Exercise,* 33(8): 1330-1337.

Laffaye, G., Bardy, B., and Durey, A. (2005). Leg stiffness and expertise in men jumping. *Medicine and Science in Sports and Exercise,* 37(4): 536-543.

Laws, K. (1995). The physics and aesthetics of vertical movements in dance. *Medical Problems of Performing Artists,* 10(June): 41-47.

Laws, K. (2002). *Physics and the art of dance: Understanding movement.* New York: Oxford Press.

Levangie, P.K., and Norkin, C.C. (2001). *Joint structure and function.* Philadelphia: Davis.

Mann, R., Kotmel, J., Herman, J., Johnson, B., and Schultz, C. (1984). Kinematic trends in elite sprinters. In J. Terauds, K. Barthels, E. Kreighbaum, R. Mann, and J. Crake (eds.), *Sports biomechanics: Proceedings of ISBS* (pp. 17-33). Del Mar, CA: Research Center for Sports.

Mann, R., Moran, G., and Dougherty, S. (1986). Comparative electromyography of the lower extremity in jogging, running, and sprinting. *American Journal of Sports Medicine,* 14(6): 501-510.

McGinnis, P.M. (2005). *Biomechanics of sport and exercise.* 2nd ed. Champaign, IL: Human Kinetics.

McLain, S., Carter, C.L., and Abel, J. (1997). The effect of a conditioning and alignment program on the measurement of supine jump height and pelvic alignment when using the Current Concepts reformer. *Journal of Dance Medicine and Science,* 1: 149-154.

McNair, P., Prapavessis, H., and Callender, K. (2000). Decreasing landing forces: Effect of instruction. *British Journal of Sports Medicine,* 34: 293-296.

McNitt-Gray, J., Koff, S., and Hall, B. (1992). The influence of dance training and foot position on landing mechanics. *Medical Problems of Performing Artists,* 7(3): 87-91.

Mostardi, R., Porterfield, J., Greenberg, B., Goldberg, D., and Lea, M. (1983). Musculoskeletal and cardiopulmonary characteristics of the professional ballet dancer. *The Physician and Sportsmedicine,* 11(12): 53-61.

Onate, J., Guskiewicz, K., and Sullivan, R. (2001). Augmented feedback reduces jump landing forces. *Journal of Orthopaedic Sports Physical Therapy,* 31(9): 511-517.

Poggini, L., Losasso, S., Cerreto, M., and Cesari, L. (1997). Jump ability in novice ballet dancers before and after training. *Journal of Dance Medicine and Science,* 1(2): 46-50.

Prapavessis, H., and McNair, P. (1999). Effects of sensory and augmented feedback on ground reaction forces when landing from a jump. *Journal of Orthopaedic Sports Physical Therapy,* 29: 352-356.

Roniger, R. (2002). Training improves ACL outcomes in female athletes. *Biomechanics,* January. www.biomech.com/db_area/archives/2002/0201.preventive.bio.shtml.

Ryman, R. (1978). A kinematic analysis of selected grand allegro jumps. In D. Woodruff (ed.), *Dance research annual IX: Essays in dance research: From the fifth CORD Conference Philadelphia, Nov. 11-14, 1976* (pp. 231-242). New York: Congress on Research in Dance.

Ryman, R., and Ranney, D. (1979). A preliminary investigation of two variations of the grand battement devant. *Dance Research Journal,* 11: 2-11.

Self, B., and Paine, D. (2001). Ankle biomechanics during four landing techniques. *Medicine and Science in Sports and Exercise,* 33(8): 1338-1344.

Simpson, K., and Kanter, L. (1997). Jump distance of dance landings influencing internal joint forces: I. Axial forces. *Medicine and Science in Sports and Exercise,* 29(7): 916-927.

Simpson, K., and Pettit, M. (1997). Jump distance of dance landings influencing internal joint forces: II. Shear forces. *Medicine and Science in Sports and Exercise,* 29(7): 928-936.

Slocum, D., and James, S. (1968). Biomechanics of running. *Journal of the American Medical Association,* 205(11): 97-104.

Tillman, M., Hass, C., and Brunt, D. (2002). Volleyball landings may explain ACL gender gap. *BioMechanics,* March. www.biomech.com/db_area/archives/2002/0203.sportsmed.bio.shtml.

Vanrenterghem, J., Lees, A., Lenoir, M., Aerts, P., and Clereq, D. (2004). Performing the vertical jump: Movement adaptations for submaximal jumping. *Human Movement Science,* 22(6): 713-727.

Westblad, P., Tsai-Fellander, L., and Johansson, C. (1995). Eccentric and concentric knee extensor muscle performance in professional ballet dancers. *Clinical Journal of Sports Medicine,* 5(1): 48-52.

Wilson, G., Elliot, B., and Wood, G. (1992). Stretch-shorten cycle performance enhancement through flexibility training. *Medicine and Science in Sports and Exercise,* 24(1): 116-123.

Winter, D. (1980). Overall principle of lower limb support during stance phase of gait. *Biomechanics,* 13: 925-927.

Zhang, S., Bates, B., and Dufek, J. (2000). Contributions of lower extremity joints to energy dissipation during landings. *Medicine and Science in Sports and Exercise,* 32(4): 812-819.

Index

Note: Page numbers followed by an italicized *f* or *t* refer to the figure or table on that page, respectively.

About the Author

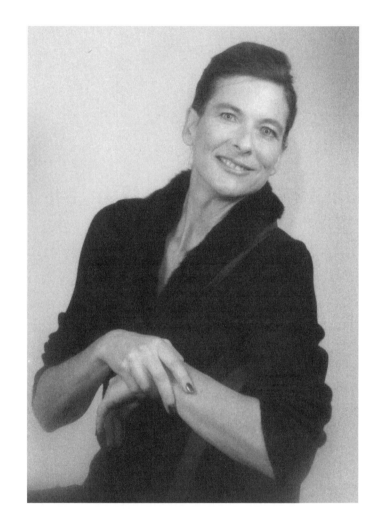

Karen Clippinger received her master's degree in exercise science from the University of Washington in 1984. Her lifelong work has focused on the application of scientific principles to enhance alignment and movement performance while reducing injury risk. She is currently a professor at California State University at Long Beach, where she teaches functional anatomy for dance, Pilates, placement for the dancer, prevention and care of dance injuries, and dance science related to teaching technique. Ms. Clippinger has also taught dance anatomy and kinesiology courses at UCLA, Scripps College, the University of Washington, and the University of Calgary. She serves as a faculty member for Body Arts and Science International.

Prior to her appointment at CSULB, Ms. Clippinger worked as a clinical kinesiologist for 22 years. She has also served as a consulting kinesiologist for the Pacific Northwest Ballet since 1981 and has consulted for the U.S. race walking team, the U.S. Weightlifting Federation, and the California Governor's Council on Physical Fitness and Sports.

Ms. Clippinger has given more than 350 presentations in the United States and abroad. She has taught workshops at many universities and has authored numerous articles and chapters. She wrote an exercise column for *Shape Magazine* for four years and served as one of the founding coeditors in chief of the *Journal of Dance Medicine and Science* from 1996 to 2005.

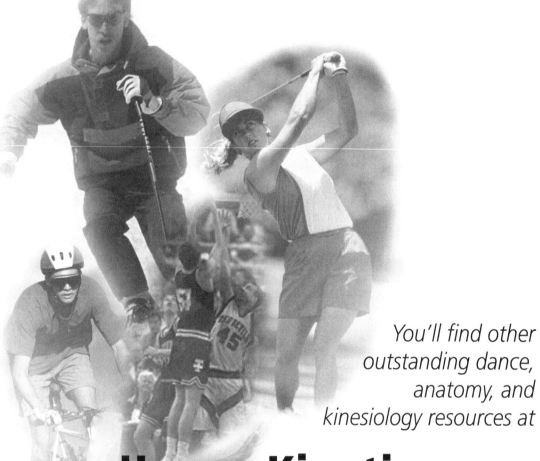

You'll find other outstanding dance, anatomy, and kinesiology resources at

www.HumanKinetics.com

In the U.S. call

1-800-747-4457

Australia...08 8372 0999
Canada 1-800-465-7301
Europe...+44 (0) 113 255 5665
New Zealand......................................0064 9 448 1207

 HUMAN KINETICS
The Information Leader in Physical Activity
P.O. Box 5076 • Champaign, IL 61825-5076 USA